Workbook and Competency Evaluation Review

MOSBY'S TEXTBOOK FOR Long-Term Care NURSING ASSISTANTS

SEVENTH EDITION

D0162912

RELDA T. KELLY, RN, MSN

Professor Emeritus, Kankakee Community College
Kankakee, Illinois
Parish Nurse, Wesley United Methodist Church
Bradley, Illinois

Procedure Checklists by

HELEN CHIGAROS, RN, BS, MSN, CRRN, CNS

Professor Emeritus, Kankakee Community College
Director, Azzarelli Outreach Clinic, St. Teresa Roman
    Catholic Church
Parish Nurse, St. Teresa Roman Catholic Church
Kankakee, Illinois

Competency Evaluation Review by

SYLVIA CREWS, RN, MSN-L

Registered Nurse-Transition of Care Nurse
Matrix Medical Network
Scottsdale, Arizona

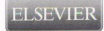
ELSEVIER

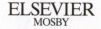

3251 Riverport Lane
St. Louis, Missouri 63043

WORKBOOK AND COMPETENCY EVALUATION REVIEW FOR
MOSBY'S TEXTBOOK FOR LONG-TERM CARE NURSING ASSISTANTS,
SEVENTH EDITION

ISBN: 978-0-323-32080-1

International Standard Book Number: 978-0-323-32080-1

Senior Content Strategist: *Nancy O'Brien*
Content Development Manager: *Ellen Wurm-Cutter*
Senior Content Development Specialist: *Maria Broeker*
Publishing Services Manager: *Jeff Patterson*
Senior Project Manager: *Tracey Schriefer*

Printed in the United States of America
Last digit is the print number: 9 8 7 6 5

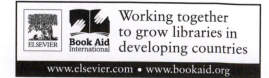

Reviewers

Christi A. Laurent, MSN, RN

Program Director—Patient Care Assisting
Nursing Sciences
Gwinnett Technical College
Lawrenceville, Georgia

Mary Kenneally Smith, RN, MBA

Retired Program Coordinator
Health Care Continuing Education
Health and Human Services
Central Piedmont Community College
Charlotte, North Carolina

Preface

This workbook is written to be used with *Mosby's Textbook for Long-Term Care Nursing Assistants*, Seventh Edition. You will not need other resources to complete the exercises in this workbook.

It is designed to help you apply what you have learned in each chapter of the textbook. You are encouraged to use this book as a study guide. Each chapter is thoroughly covered in the multiple-choice questions, which will help prepare you to take the NATCEP test. In addition, other exercises such as fill-in-the-blank, matching, and crossword puzzles are used in many chapters. Independent Learning Activities at the end of each chapter may be used to apply the information you will learn in a practical setting. The section titled Optional Learning Activities may be used as an alternative exercise to give you more practice in studying the materials.

In addition, Procedure Checklists that correspond with the procedures in the textbook are provided.

These checklists are designed to help you become skilled at performing procedures that affect quality of care. In addition to NNAAP® skills being identified for you, icons indicate skills that are on the textbook companion CD, in Mosby's Nursing Assistant Video Skills 4.0, and on the Evolve student learning resources website (video clips).

The Competency Evaluation Review includes a general review section and two practice exams to help you prepare for the written certification exam. It also features a skills review guide to help you practice procedures required for certification. Answers to the two practice exams can be found on the Evolve student learning resources website.

Assistive personnel are important members of the health team. Completing the exercises in this workbook will increase your knowledge and skills. The goal is to prepare you to provide the best possible care and to encourage pride in a job well done.

1 THE NURSING ASSISTANT WORKING IN LONG-TERM CARE

FILL IN THE BLANKS: KEY TERMS

Accountable
Acute illness
Alzheimer's disease (AD)
Assisted living residence (ALR)
Board and care home
Case management
Chronic illness
Delegate
Group home

Hospice
Independence
Interdisciplinary team
Job description
Licensed practical nurse (LPN)
Licensed vocational nurse (LVN)
Medicaid
Medicare
Nursing assistant

Nursing center
Nursing facility (NF)
Nursing home
Nursing task
Nursing team
Registered nurse (RN)
Responsibility
Skilled nursing facility (SNF)

1. A person who has completed a 1-year nursing program and passed a licensing test is a

   _____.

2. A _____ provides health care to persons who need regular or continuous care.

3. Another name for a nursing center or a nursing facility is a

   _____.

4. _____ means a person is not relying on or requiring care from others.

5. A sudden illness from which the person should recover is an

   _____.

6. A facility that provides nursing care for residents who have many or severe health problems or who need rehabilitation is called a

   _____.

7. A _____ is an ongoing illness, slow or gradual in onset, that has no cure; the illness can be controlled and complications prevented with proper treatment.

8. An _____ provides housing, personal care, supportive services, health care, and social activities in a home-like setting.

9. Being responsible for one's actions and the actions of others who performed tasks is being

   _____.

10. RNs, LPNs/LVNs, and nursing assistants provide nursing care as part of the

    _____.

11. _____ is a disease that affects the brain tissue; there is increasing memory loss and confusion.

12. To _____ is to authorize another person to perform a nursing task in a certain situation.

13. _____ is a federal health insurance plan for persons 65 years of age or older and younger people with certain disabilities.

14. A _____ provides rooms, meals, laundry, and supervision to a few independent residents, often in a home setting.

15. A nursing center or nursing home may be called a

    _____.

16. A _____ is a document that describes what the center expects you to do.

17. A person who has completed a 2-, 3-, or 4-year nursing program and who has passed a licensing test is a

    _____.

18. Nursing care that can be delegated to nursing assistants when it does not require an RN's professional knowledge or judgment is a

    _____.

19. A nursing care pattern where an RN coordinates a person's care is

    _____.

20. A _____ gives basic nursing care under the supervision of a licensed nurse.

21. Another name for a licensed practical nurse is

_____.

22. The many health care workers whose skills and knowledge focus on the person's total care are the

_____.

23. _____ is a health care payment program sponsored by state and federal governments.

24. A health care agency or program for persons who are dying is a

_____.

25. Another name for a board and care home is a

_____.

26. The duty or obligation to perform some act or function is

_____.

CIRCLE THE BEST ANSWER

27. Residents who live in a board and care home
    A. Receive care that meets the person's basic needs
    B. Stay there for a short time while recovering from an illness or surgery
    C. Are in a program for persons who are dying
    D. Are in a closed unit that provides a safer environment

28. Some assisted living facilities are part of
    A. A hospital
    B. A retirement community or nursing center
    C. A hospice
    D. A skilled care facility

29. Skilled nursing facilities provide
    A. Supportive care
    B. More complex care than nursing centers do
    C. A closed unit for residents who have Alzheimer's disease or other dementia
    D. Care for persons who are dying

30. Nursing centers provide health care and nursing care to
    A. Cure an acute illness
    B. Persons who need regular or continuous care
    C. Help the person recover after surgery
    D. Cure a chronic illness

31. Colds and influenza can cause major health problems for older and disabled persons. These are called
    A. Chronic illnesses
    B. Communicable diseases
    C. Emotional illnesses
    D. Disabilities

32. Rehabilitation or restorative care helps
    A. The person to have a complete return of all functions
    B. To provide supportive care that meets basic physical needs
    C. To keep the person safe
    D. Persons return to their highest possible level of physical and mental function

33. Children and pets usually can visit when a dying person is in
    A. An Alzheimer's unit
    B. A hospital
    C. A hospice
    D. A subacute care center

34. An Alzheimer's unit is a closed unit that provides
    A. A safer environment for residents to wander freely
    B. A program for persons who are dying
    C. A place for residents who suffer from deconditioning after an acute illness
    D. A program for residents with a communicable disease

35. Which of these workers or areas in a health care center is under the director of nursing in the organizational chart?
    A. Nursing assistant
    B. Medical director
    C. Case manager
    D. Social worker

36. The director of nursing is responsible for
    A. Coordinating resident care for a certain shift
    B. Planning and presenting educational programs
    C. The entire nursing staff
    D. All resident care and the actions of the nursing staff on a unit

37. Who coordinates care for a certain shift in the nursing center?
    A. Doctor
    B. Staff nurse
    C. Shift manager
    D. Director of nursing

38. Which of the following describes an RN?
    A. Completes a 1-year nursing program and passes a licensing test
    B. Completes studies that qualify the person to become the medical director of the nursing center
    C. Has formal training to give care and passes a competency examination
    D. Completes a 2-, 3-, or 4-year nursing program and has passed a licensing test

39. The nursing assistant gives basic nursing care under the supervision of
    A. The center administrator
    B. The director of nursing
    C. A licensed nurse
    D. Another nursing assistant

40. Medicare is a federal health insurance plan that has benefits for
    A. Persons 65 years of age and older
    B. Families with low incomes
    C. Individuals and families who buy the insurance
    D. Groups of individuals who buy the insurance
41. Part B of Medicare
    A. Pays for hospital costs and some SNF costs
    B. Benefits only persons 65 years of age and older
    C. Is administered by the Social Security Administration
    D. Helps pay for doctor's visits, outpatient hospital care, physical and occupational therapists, and some home care
42. A MS-DRG (Medicare severity-adjusted diagnosis-related group) plan
    A. Covers only persons 65 years of age and older
    B. Is used for hospital costs
    C. Pays for care in an SNF
    D. Limits the choice of where to go for care
43. If a person has managed care, the insured person will have costs covered based on
    A. Health care available in the community
    B. The age of the person
    C. His or her physical needs
    D. The pre-approval process used by the person's insurer
44. Nursing centers require certification to
    A. Signal quality and excellence
    B. Receive Medicare and Medicaid funds
    C. Operate and provide care
    D. Meet state and federal standards
45. A nursing assistant could prevent common nursing center deficiencies by
    A. Protecting residents from abuse, mistreatment, and neglect when giving care
    B. Hiring only people with no legal history of abusing, neglecting, or mistreating residents
    C. Applying physical restraints to keep residents safe
    D. Ignoring other caregivers who may be abusing or neglecting residents
46. Until the 1980s, nursing assistants
    A. Attended nursing assistant classes approved by the state
    B. Were not used in giving basic nursing care
    C. Received on-the-job training from nurses
    D. Worked only in hospitals
47. State laws that regulate nursing assistant roles and functions are determined by
    A. OBRA
    B. The Nurse Practice Act
    C. The state medical society
    D. Insurance companies
48. If you do something beyond the legal limits of your role, you could be
    A. Protected by the Nurse Practice Act
    B. Practicing nursing without a license
    C. Protected by the nurse who supervises your work
    D. Accused of a criminal act
49. OBRA requires that the nursing assistant training and competency evaluation program have at least

    _____ hours of instruction.
    A. 16
    B. 75
    C. 120
    D. 200
50. Which of these areas of study is included in a training program for nursing assistants?
    A. Giving feedings through the naso-gastric tube
    B. Changing sterile dressings independently
    C. Phlebotomy (drawing blood)
    D. Elimination procedures
51. The competency evaluation for nursing assistants has 2 parts. They are
    A. A written test and a skills test
    B. A multiple-choice test and a true-false test
    C. A skills test and a complete bed bath demonstration
    D. A written test and an oral question-and-answer test
52. If you fail the competency evaluation the first time it is taken, you
    A. Can retest one more time
    B. Must repeat your training program
    C. Can retest two more times (for a total of three times)
    D. Can retest as often as necessary free of charge
53. Which of the following information is contained in the nursing assistant registry?
    A. Every place you have worked
    B. Date of birth
    C. Number of dependents
    D. A credit report
54. OBRA requires that retraining and a new competency evaluation test must be taken if you have not worked as a certified nursing assistant for
    A. 24 months
    B. 5 years
    C. 1 consecutive year
    D. 6 months
55. If you wish to work as a CNA in another state, you should
    A. Present your certificate to the nursing center where you wish to work
    B. Apply to that state's nursing board for endorsement, reciprocity, or equivalency
    C. Never tell that state that you lost your certification in another state
    D. Take a nursing assistant course and pass the NATCEP in that state

56. Your work as a nursing assistant is supervised by
    A. A licensed nurse
    B. The doctor
    C. The director of nursing
    D. A nursing assistant with more experience
57. When in-service programs or training is scheduled, the nursing assistant
    A. Must attend those that are required
    B. Needs to attend only if the program is scheduled on a day he or she is scheduled to work
    C. Cannot attend if the program is scheduled during the workday
    D. Does not need to attend if it means he or she must come to work early or stay late
58. You are alone in the nurses' station and you answer the phone. Dr. Smith begins to give you verbal orders. You should
    A. Hang up the phone
    B. Politely give him your name and title and ask him to wait while you get the nurse
    C. Quickly write down the orders and give them to the nurse
    D. Politely give him your name and title and ask him to call back later when the nurse is there
59. As a nursing assistant you may give medications if
    A. The nurse is busy and asks you to give them
    B. The resident is in the shower and the nurse leaves the medications at the bedside
    C. You have completed a state-required medication and training program on giving medications
    D. You are feeding the resident and the nurse asks you to mix the medications with the food
60. The nurse asks you to carry out a task you do not know how to do. You should
    A. Ignore the order since it is something you cannot do
    B. Perform the task as well as you can
    C. Ask another nursing assistant to show you how to carry out the task
    D. Promptly explain to the nurse why you cannot carry out the task
61. The nurse asks you to assist him as he changes sterile dressings. You should
    A. Assist him as needed
    B. Tell him you cannot assist with performing any sterile procedures
    C. Tell him this is something you do cannot do
    D. Report his request to the supervisor
62. Who can tell the person or the family a diagnosis or prescribe treatments?
    A. The director of nursing
    B. The RN
    C. The doctor
    D. An experienced nursing assistant

63. When you read a job description, you should not take a job if it requires you to
    A. Carry out duties you do not like to do
    B. Maintain required certification
    C. Attend in-service training
    D. Function beyond your training limits
64. Which of the following would be wrong?
    A. An RN delegates a task to an LPN/LVN.
    B. An LPN/LVN delegates a task to a nursing assistant.
    C. An RN delegates a task to a nursing assistant.
    D. A nursing assistant delegates a task to another nursing assistant.
65. When a nurse considers delegating tasks, the decision
    A. Should always result in the best care for the person at the time
    B. Depends on whether the nurse likes the nursing assistant
    C. Depends on how busy the nurse is that day
    D. Depends on how well the nurse likes the person.
66. You have been caring for Mr. Watson for several weeks. The nurse tells you she will give his care today. Her delegation decision is based primarily on
    A. How well you performed his care yesterday
    B. Changes in Mr. Watson's condition
    C. Whether the nurse knows you or not
    D. How much supervision you need
67. Which of the following is one of the five rights of delegation?
    A. The right task
    B. The right delegation
    C. The right time
    D. The right team members
68. You may refuse to carry out a task if
    A. The team members you like cannot help you
    B. You do not know how to use the supplies or equipment
    C. You are too busy
    D. You do not like the resident

FILL IN THE BLANKS

Write out the meaning of each abbreviation.

69. CNA _____

70. LNA _____

71. LPN/LVN _____

72. AD _____

73. NF _____

74. SNF _____

75. DON _____

76. MS-DRG _____

77. MS-DRGs are for_____costs.

78. RUG _____

79. RUGs are for _____
payments.

80. CMG _____

81. CMGs are used for _____
centers.

82. HMO _____

83. PPO _____

84. OBRA _____

85. NATCEP _____

86. NCBSN _____

87. RN _____

MATCHING

Match the types of health care service with the correct example.

88. _____ Provides health care and nursing care for residents who have many or severe health problems or who need rehabilitation.

89. _____ Provides rooms, meals, laundry, and supervision to a few independent residents.

90. _____ Provides a unit closed off from the rest of the center. This provides a safe setting for residents to wander freely.

91. _____ Health care agency or program for people who are dying.

92. _____ Provides housing, personal care, supportive services, health care, and social activities in a home-like setting.

A. Skilled care facility
B. Hospice unit
C. Board and care home
D. Alzheimer's unit
E. Assisted living residence

OPTIONAL LEARNING EXERCISES
Comparing Long-Term Care Centers

93. A board and care home provides _____
_____ in a
home-like setting. What is the resident usually
able to do with little help? _____
_____
_____ What happens if the person has
an emergency in the middle of the night? _____
_____

94. An assisted living residence provides
_____
_____
in a home-like setting. Help given includes
_____
_____ . There is access
to _____ .

95. A nursing center provides health care to persons
_____ .
The facility is required to employ _____
nurses on the staff.

96. A skilled nursing facility provides health and
nursing care for residents who have _____
_____ .

97. Long-term care centers help and encourage residents to

A. Focus on _____ .

B. Do as much _____ .

C. Change habits _____
_____ .

D. Understand and accept the limits of
_____ .

98. A hospice is an agency or program for _____ _____. What needs are met by a hospice? _____ _____

99. An Alzheimer's unit is designed for persons with _____ _____. An Alzheimer's unit is closed off from the rest of the center because these residents may _____ _____.

100. Persons on a rehabilitation or subacute care unit often stay there for _____ _____.

Health Team Members (Table 1-1)

Name the health team member who provides the service described.

101. Mr. Williams needs assistance to regain skills to dress, shave, and feed himself (ADL). He is assisted by the _____.

102. The nurse has a concern about a drug action, so calls the _____.

103. Mrs. Young needs the corns on her feet treated. The nurse notifies the _____ _____

104. Ms. Stewart has the responsibility of doing physical examinations, health assessments, and health educations in the center where she works. She is a _____

105. Mr. Gomez keeps turning up the volume on his TV. His hearing is tested by the _____ _____

106. The _____ meets with a new resident and his family to discuss his nutritional needs.

107. Mr. Fox had a stroke and has weakness on his left side. The _____ assists him by developing a plan that focuses on restoring function and preventing disability from his illness.

108. The doctor orders x-rays after Mr. Jackson falls. The x-rays are done by the _____ _____

109. Mr. Ling has chronic lung disease and needs respiratory treatments. These are given by the _____

110. Ms. Walker plans the recreational needs of a nursing center. She is an _____

111. After a stroke, Mr. Stubbs has difficulty swallowing. He is evaluated by the _____

112. When the doctor orders blood tests, the samples are collected by the _____

OBRA Requirements Related to the Nursing Assistant

113. The nursing assistant must meet federal and state training and competency requirements in order to work in _____ _____

114. OBRA requires _____ hours of instruction. _____ hours of supervised practical training are required. Where can the practical training take place? _____ or _____.

115. OBRA requires 15 areas of study. Write the area of study where you learn the skill for each example.

   A. _____ You make a bed.

   B. _____ You close Mr. Smith's door to give him privacy.

   C. _____ You tell Mrs. Forbes the time of day and the day of week frequently during the day.

   D. _____ You apply lotion to a resident's dry skin.

   E. _____ You assist a resident to put on his shirt.

   F. _____ When assigned to a new unit, you find the location of the fire alarm.

   G. _____ You wash your hands before and after giving care.

   H. _____ You get help to move a resident from his bed to the chair.

   I. _____ When speaking to Mr. Jackson, you maintain good eye contact.

   J. _____ The nurse tells you to exercise a resident's extremities (limbs).

K. _____ You shave Mr. Stewart.

L. _____ You position a urinal for a resident in bed.

M. _____ You assist Mrs. Young to walk in the hall.

N. _____
You notice Mrs. Peck has an elevated temperature and her skin is warm.

O. _____ You cut up the meat on Mr. Johnson's plate before helping him to eat.

INDEPENDENT LEARNING ACTIVITIES

Gather the following information about long-term care centers in your area.

- How many board and care homes are located in your area? Choose one home and answer the following questions.
  - Is this home attached to a nursing center or is it a separate center?
  - What services are provided?
  - How many residents are in the home?
  - How many staff members work there? How many staff members are RNs? LPNs? Nursing assistants? What care is provided by nursing assistants?
- How many nursing centers are located in your area? Choose one center and answer the following questions.
  - What types of residents are accepted in the center? (For example, does the center consider level of care needed, the resident's disease, or method of payment?)
  - How many residents live in the center?
  - How many staff members work there? How many staff members are RNs? LPNs? Nursing assistants? What care is provided by nursing assistants?
- How many nursing centers in your area provide skilled nursing care? Choose one center and answer the following questions.
  - How many residents live in the center?
  - How many staff members work there? How many staff members are RNs? LPNs? Nursing assistants? What care is provided by nursing assistants?
- How many assisted living facilities are located in your area? Choose one facility and answer the following questions.
  - Is this facility independent or part of a long-term care center?
  - How many residents live in the facility?
  - What kind of living quarters do the residents have? (For example, does each resident have an apartment or studio? Do residents share kitchen facilities or does each person have a kitchen?)
  - How many staff members work there? How many staff members are RNs? LPNs? Nursing assistants? What care is provided by nursing assistants?
- Find a nursing center that has an Alzheimer's unit and answer the following questions.
  - How is the unit identified? Is it a separate wing? Separate floor? Is the unit closed off?
  - How is the unit different from other units in the center?
  - Do the staff members who work on this unit receive special training? If so, what extra training are they given? What duties are assigned to nursing assistants on this unit?
- Does your area have a hospice program? If so, answer the following questions about the program.
  - Is this program located within a center or does it provide care in the person's facility or home?
  - What type of care is provided?
  - What special training is given to the staff? What duties can be performed by a nursing assistant?
- Obtain a copy of the Nurse Practice Act for your state. How are nursing assistant roles, functions, education, and certification requirements addressed? Are there separate laws for nursing assistants? What rules and regulations apply to nursing assistants?
- Obtain a job description for a nursing assistant. You may be able to ask for this at the facility where you had your clinical experience. What information is contained on the job description about:
  - Who will direct or supervise the nursing assistant?
  - What competencies is the nursing assistant expected to have?
  - What professional requirements are listed?
  - What other skills or requirements are listed?

2 RESIDENT RIGHTS, ETHICS, AND LAWS

FILL IN THE BLANKS: KEY TERMS

Abuse
Assault
Battery
Boundary crossing
Boundary sign
Boundary violation
Civil law
Crime
Criminal law
Defamation
Ethics

False imprisonment
Fraud
Invasion of privacy
Involuntary seclusion
Law
Libel
Malpractice
Neglect
Negligence
Ombudsman
Professional boundary

Professional sexual misconduct
Protected health information
Representative
Self-neglect
Slander
Standard of care
Tort
Treatment
Vulnerable adult
Will

1. Separating a person from others against his or her will, keeping the person in a certain area, or keeping the person from his or her room without consent is

   _____.

2. A _____ is a person 18 years of age or older who has a disability or condition that makes him or her at risk for being wounded, attacked, or damaged.

3. When an act, behavior, or thought warns of a boundary crossing or violation it is a

   _____.

4. _____ is negligence by a professional person.

5. Saying or doing something to trick, fool, or deceive another person is _____.

6. _____ is concerned with offenses against the public and society in general.

7. A _____ is a legal statement about how a person wishes to have property distributed after death.

8. _____ is identifying information and information about the person's health care that is maintained or sent in any form.

9. A brief act or behavior outside of the helpful zone is

   _____.

10. An _____ is someone who supports or promotes the needs and interests of another person.

11. A rule of conduct made by a government body is a

    _____.

12. _____ is the unauthorized touching of a person's body without the person's consent.

13. The willful infliction of injury, unreasonable confinement, intimidation, or punishment that results in physical harm, pain, or mental anguish is

    _____.

14. _____ is making false statements orally.

15. Injuring a person's name and reputation by making false statements to a third person is

    _____.

16. _____ is knowledge of what is right and wrong conduct.

17. Intentionally attempting or threatening to touch a person's body without the person's consent is

    _____.

18. A _____ is a wrong committed against a person or the person's property.

19. _____ are laws concerned with relationships between people.

20. A _____ is any person who has the legal right to act on the resident's behalf when he or she cannot do so for himself or herself.

21. _____ is an act, behavior, or comment that is sexual in nature.

22. An act or behavior that meets your needs, not the person's, is a _____ _____.

23. Violating a person's right not to have his or her name, photograph, or private affairs exposed or made public without giving consent is _____.

24. _____ is the skills, care, and judgment required by the health team member under similar circumstances.

25. _____ separates helpful behaviors from behaviors that are not helpful.

26. An act that violates a criminal law is a _____.

27. _____ is the unlawful restraint or restriction of a person's movement.

28. Defamation through written statements is _____.

29. A _____ is an unintentional wrong in which a person does not act in a reasonable and careful manner and causes harm to a person or to the person's property.

30. The care provided to maintain or restore health, improve function, or relieve symptoms is _____.

31. _____ is the failure to provide the person with goods or services needed to avoid physical harm, mental anguish, or mental illness.

32. A person's behaviors that threaten his or her health or safety is _____.

CIRCLE THE BEST ANSWER

33. A resident in long-term care has the right to
    A. Have a private room in which to live
    B. Have personal choice in what to wear and how to spend his or her time
    C. Have all meals delivered from outside the facility
    D. Have friends live with him or her at the facility

34. Under OBRA, if a resident is incompetent (not able) to exercise his or her rights, who can exercise these rights for the person?
    A. The doctor
    B. A responsible party such as a partner, adult child, or court-appointed guardian
    C. The charge nurse
    D. A neighbor

35. If a resident refuses treatment, what should you do?
    A. Avoid giving any care to the person and move on to other duties
    B. Report the refusal to the nurse
    C. Tell the resident the treatment must be done and continue to carry out the treatment
    D. Tell the resident's family so they can make him accept the treatment

36. A student wants to observe a treatment but the resident does not want her to be present. What is the correct action?
    A. The student cannot watch, as this violates the resident's right to privacy.
    B. The student may observe from the doorway, where the resident cannot see her.
    C. The staff nurse tells the resident he must allow the student to watch.
    D. The nurse calls the resident's wife to get her permission.

37. The resident should be given personal choice whenever it
    A. Is safely possible
    B. Does not interfere with scheduled activities
    C. Is approved by the director of nursing
    D. Is ordered by the doctor

38. If a resident voices concerns about care and the center promptly tries to correct the situation, this action meets the resident's right to
    A. Participate in a resident group
    B. Voice a grievance
    C. Personal choice
    D. Freedom from abuse, mistreatment, and neglect

39. When a resident volunteers to take care of houseplants at the center, this is an acceptable part of
    A. The care plan
    B. A requirement to receive care or care items
    C. Paying the cost of his care
    D. The doctor's orders

40. When a resident and the family plan activities together, this meets the resident's right to
    A. Privacy
    B. Freedom from restraint
    C. Freedom from mistreatment
    D. Take part in resident and family groups

41. The resident you are caring for has many old holiday decorations covering her night-stand. If you throw away these items without her permission you are denying her right to
    A. Privacy
    B. Work
    C. Keep and use personal items
    D. Freedom from abuse

42. A staff member tells a resident he cannot leave his room because he talks too much. This action denies the resident
    A. The right to be free from involuntary seclusion
    B. Freedom from restraint
    C. Care and security of personal possessions
    D. Personal choice

43. When a resident is given certain drugs that affect his mood, behavior, or mental function, it may deny his right to
    A. Freedom from abuse, mistreatment, and neglect
    B. Personal choice
    C. Privacy
    D. Freedom from restraint

44. Which of these actions will promote courteous and dignified care?
    A. Calling the resident by a nickname he does not choose
    B. Assisting with dressing the resident in clothing appropriate for the time of day
    C. Changing the resident's hairstyle without her permission
    D. Leaving the bathroom door open so you can see the person

45. You ask a resident if you may touch him. This is an example of
    A. Courteous and dignified interactions
    B. Courteous and dignified care
    C. Providing privacy and self-determination
    D. Maintaining personal choice and independence

46. Assisting a resident to ambulate without interfering with his independence is an example of
    A. Courteous and dignified interaction
    B. Courteous and dignified care
    C. Providing privacy and self-determination
    D. Maintaining personal choice and independence

47. You provide privacy and self-determination for a resident when you
    A. Knock on the door before entering and wait to be asked in
    B. Allow the resident to smoke in designated areas
    C. Listen with interest to what the person is saying
    D. Groom his beard as he wishes

48. You allow the resident to maintain personal choice and independence when you
    A. Obtain her attention before interacting with her
    B. Provide extra clothing for warmth, such as a sweater or lap robe
    C. Assist him to take part in activities according to his interests
    D. Use curtains or screens during personal care and procedures

49. Which of these activities would be carried out by an ombudsman?
    A. Organize activities for a group of residents
    B. Accompany residents to a religious service at a house of worship
    C. Investigate and resolve complaints made by a resident
    D. Assist the resident to choose friends

50. Which of the following is part of the code of conduct for a nursing assistant?
    A. Carry out any task assigned to you
    B. Take a co-worker's medication for a headache
    C. Recognize the limits of your role and your knowledge
    D. Plan your work so you can go to lunch with your friend

51. Which of the following is an example of boundary crossing?
    A. You avoid caring for a friend or family member.
    B. You hug a person every time you see him or her.
    C. You share information about your personal relationships or problems.
    D. You protect the person's privacy.

52. A boundary violation would be
    A. Keeping secrets with the person
    B. Giving a person a brief hug when he or she is upset
    C. Trading assignments with other staff so you can care for a person
    D. Changing how you dress when you work with a person

53. If a person or family member offers you a gift, you maintain professional boundaries by
    A. Accepting the gift and thanking the person
    B. Refusing the gift by saying: "I don't need this"
    C. Thanking the person but explaining that you cannot accept gifts from those you care for
    D. Giving the gift to someone else

54. A nurse failed to do what a reasonable and careful nurse would have done. Legally, this is called
    A. Fraud
    B. A tort
    C. Negligence
    D. Malpractice

55. You may be accused of negligence if you
    A. Fail to test the temperature of a hot soak and the person is burned
    B. Imply or suggest that a person is stealing from the staff
    C. Threaten to restrain a person
    D. Tell the person or the family that you are a nurse

56. If you fail to identify a person properly and perform a treatment on him intended for another, you are
    A. Committing a crime
    B. Legally responsible (liable) for your actions
    C. Not responsible legally but are unethical
    D. Guilty of an intentional tort

57. A nursing assistant writes a note to a friend that injures the name and reputation of a person by making false statements. This is called
    A. Libel
    B. Slander
    C. Malpractice
    D. Negligence
58. The nursing assistant would violate the Health Insurance Portability and Accountability Act of 1996 (HIPAA) if he or she
    A. Says or does something that tricks or deceives a person
    B. Gives out information about the person's health care
    C. Signs a legal document for a resident
    D. Makes false statements about a resident to a third person
59. A nursing assistant tells a resident she is a nurse. She has committed
    A. Fraud
    B. Libel
    C. Slander
    D. Negligence
60. When a caregiver threatens to "tie down" a person, the caregiver is guilty of
    A. Physical abuse
    B. Assault
    C. Invasion of privacy
    D. Battery
61. If a resident says he does not want you to dress him and you go ahead and touch him, you can be accused of
    A. Fraud
    B. Battery
    C. Assault
    D. False imprisonment
62. If you are asked to obtain a resident's signature on an informed consent, you should
    A. Make sure the resident is mentally competent
    B. Refuse. You are never responsible for obtaining a written consent
    C. Make sure the resident understands what he is signing
    D. Ask a family member to witness the signed consent
63. If a person is confused or unconscious, informed consent
    A. Is not necessary
    B. Cannot be obtained and so no treatments can be given
    C. Can be given by a husband, wife, son, daughter, or legal representative
    D. Can be given by the director of nursing
64. You can refuse to sign a will if
    A. You are named in the will
    B. You do not believe the person is of sound mind
    C. Your nursing center has policies that do not allow employees to witness wills
    D. All of the above
65. Which of the following is a form of abuse?
    A. Assisting the person to take a shower
    B. Telling the person he or she will never see family members again
    C. Expecting a person to feed and dress himself within his abilities
    D. Feeding the person in a dining room

66. When a person refuses medical treatment for a serious illness or is not taking needed drugs, this may be a warning sign of
    A. Elder abuse
    B. Physical abuse
    C. Self-neglect
    D. Involuntary seclusion
67. What kind of abuse occurs when an elderly person is left to sit in urine or feces?
    A. Neglect
    B. Involuntary seclusion
    C. Mental abuse
    D. Sexual abuse
68. An example of verbal abuse can be
    A. Failing to answer a call light
    B. Locking a person in a room
    C. Oral or written statements that speak badly of a person
    D. Making threats of harm to a person
69. Depriving a person of a basic need is
    A. Physical abuse
    B. Involuntary seclusion
    C. Emotional or mental abuse
    D. Sexual abuse
70. Which of the following may be a sign of elder abuse?
    A. The person answers questions openly.
    B. The family makes sure the hearing aids have new batteries.
    C. A caregiver is present during all conversations.
    D. All medications are taken as scheduled.
71. If you suspect an elderly person is being abused, you should
    A. Call the police
    B. Discuss the situation and your observations with the nurse
    C. Discuss the situation with the family
    D. Notify community agencies that investigate elder abuse
72. A husband does not allow his wife to use the car, to leave the home, or to visit with family and friends. This is a form of domestic violence called
    A. Verbal abuse
    B. Social abuse
    C. Physical abuse
    D. Economic abuse

FILL IN THE BLANKS: ABBREVIATIONS

73. CMS _____

74. HIPAA _____

75. OBRA _____

MATCHING

Match the examples with the correct tort.

    A. Negligence
    B. Malpractice
    C. Libel
    D. Slander
    E. False imprisonment
    F. Assault
    G. Battery
    H. Fraud
    I. Invasion of privacy

76. _____ While cleaning a resident's dentures, the nursing assistant drops and breaks them.
77. _____ A nursing assistant opens a resident's mail and reads it without permission.
78. _____ Instead of allowing the resident a choice, the nursing assistant tells him he will have a shower whether he wants one or not.
79. _____ An individual touches a person's body without the person's consent.
80. _____ An individual tricks or fools another person.
81. _____ An individual restrains or restricts a resident's freedom of movement without a physician's order.
82. _____ A nurse gives a treatment to the wrong person.
83. _____ A nursing assistant injures the name and reputation of a resident by making false statements to a third person.
84. _____ A nursing assistant writes notes falsely accusing another nursing assistant of stealing her purse.

OPTIONAL LEARNING EXERCISES

OBRA-Required Actions That Promote Dignity and Privacy (Box 2-2)

Match the action to promote dignity and privacy with the examples.

    A. Courteous and dignified interaction
    B. Courteous and dignified care
    C. Privacy and self-determination
    D. Maintain personal choice and independence

85. _____ File fingernails and apply polish as resident requests
86. _____ Cover the resident with a blanket during a bath
87. _____ Gain the person's attention before giving care
88. _____ Show interest when a person tells stories about the past
89. _____ Open containers and arrange food at meal times
90. _____ Close the door when the person asks for privacy

91. _____ Allow a resident to smoke in a designated area
92. _____ Take the resident to his weekly card game

Code of Conduct for Nursing Assistants (Box 2-3)

Fill in the blank with the correct code of conduct.

93. You cover the person and close the door when giving care. _____

94. You delay going on break when you find a person has soiled, wet linens that need to be changed.

_____

95. A classmate offers to share her antibiotic prescription with you, but you refuse.

_____

96. You report to the nurse that you gave a treatment to the wrong person.

_____

97. You refuse to share information about a person you are caring for with your mother. _____

_____

98. You return the person's shampoo to his room after a shower. _____

INDEPENDENT LEARNING ACTIVITIES

- Visit a nursing center and ask for a copy of the Resident Rights. Compare it to the information in this chapter. What is the same? What is different?
- When you visit a nursing center, ask if they have an ombudsman. If so, ask for an appointment to meet with this person. Ask the ombudsman the following questions.
  - What are the primary responsibilities he or she has in the center?
  - How often does he or she meet with residents?
  - What kind of problems has he or she helped to resolve?
- Make a list of tasks that would conflict with your moral or religious beliefs.
  - How would you feel about performing these tasks in your job?
  - What would you say about these tasks to your employer or co-workers?
- Role-play a situation in which you are asked to perform one of the tasks you identified in the previous activity. Have one student play the person asking you to perform the task. Have a second student observe and answer these questions.
  - What was your reaction when asked?
  - In what way did you communicate your discomfort?
  - What suggestions did you offer to make sure the task was done?

3 WORK ETHICS

FILL IN THE BLANKS: KEY TERMS

Confidentiality
Courtesy
Gossip
Harassment

Preceptor
Priority
Professionalism

Stress
Stressor
Work ethics

1. A staff member who guides another staff member

   is a _____.

2. A _____ is the event or factor
   that causes stress.

3. Trusting others with personal and private

   information is _____.

4. _____ are behaviors in the
   workplace.

5. _____ is to spread rumors or
   talk about the private matters of others.

6. The response or change in the body caused by any
   emotional, physical, social, or economic factor is

   _____.

7. _____ is a polite,
   considerate, or helpful comment or act.

8. _____ means to trouble,
   torment, offend, or worry a person by one's
   behavior or comments.

9. A _____ is the most
   important thing at the time.

10. _____ is following laws,
    being ethical, having good work ethics, and having
    the skills to do your work.

CIRCLE THE BEST ANSWER

11. Work ethics involves
    A. How well you do your skills
    B. What religion you practice
    C. How you treat and work with others
    D. Cultural beliefs and attitudes

12. Your diet will maintain your weight if
    A. You avoid salty and sweet foods
    B. You take in fewer calories than your energy
       needs require
    C. It includes foods with fats and oils
    D. The number of calories taken in equals your
       energy needs

13. Most adults need about _____ hours of sleep
    daily.
    A. 7
    B. 10
    C. 4
    D. 12

14. Exercise is needed for
    A. Rest and sleep
    B. Muscle tone and circulation
    C. Good body mechanics
    D. Good nutrition

15. Smoking odors
    A. Disappear quickly when the person finishes
       smoking
    B. Can be covered up by chewing gum
    C. Are noticed only by the smoker
    D. Stay on the person's breath, hands, clothing,
       and hair

16. The most important reason why a person must
    not work under the influence of alcohol or drugs
    is that it
    A. Affects the person's safety
    B. Causes the person to be disorganized
    C. Makes co-workers angry
    D. Is not allowed by your nursing center

17. Which of these is part of good personal hygiene
    for work?
    A. Bathe every other day to prevent dry skin
    B. Brush your teeth once a day
    C. Cut toenails straight across
    D. Keep fingernails long and polished

18. Tattoos should be covered when working
    because they
    A. May offend others
    B. Can become infected
    C. May spread infection
    D. Increase the risk of skin injuries

19. When working, the nursing assistant usually
    may wear
    A. Jewelry in a pierced eyebrow, nose, lip, or
       tongue
    B. Wedding and engagement rings
    C. Multiple earrings in each ear
    D. Nail polish

20. When working, the nursing assistant may wear
    A. Sandals or open-toed shoes
    B. Hair that is off the collar and away from the face
    C. Perfume, cologne, or after-shave
    D. Colored or patterned underwear
21. Displaying good work ethics at your clinical experience site may help you find a job because
    A. You will pass the course
    B. It will show you care
    C. You will get better grades
    D. The staff always looks at students as future employees
22. You should be well-groomed when looking for a job because it
    A. Shows you are cooperative
    B. Makes a good first impression
    C. Shows you are respectful
    D. Shows you have values and attitudes that fit with the center
23. How does an employer know you can perform required job skills?
    A. They will request proof of training and will check your record in the state nursing assistant registry.
    B. They will have you give a demonstration of your skills.
    C. You will be asked many questions about performing certain skills.
    D. You will be required to take a written test.
24. You usually get a job application from
    A. The personnel office or the human resources office
    B. A friend who works at the center
    C. The director of nursing
    D. The receptionist in the lobby of the center
25. A résumé includes
    A. Contact information
    B. A summary of your hobbies and interests
    C. Information about your personal life
    D. A letter of reference from your friend
26. You should take a dry run to a job interview to
    A. Show you follow directions well
    B. Show you listen well
    C. Make sure you will be on time for the interview
    D. Look over the center to see if you want to work there
27. When you are interviewing, it is correct to
    A. Have a glass of wine before going
    B. Use good eye contact when speaking to the interviewer
    C. Wear a sweatsuit and athletic shoes
    D. Shake hands very gently

28. What is a good way to share your list of skills with the interviewer?
    A. Tell the person verbally what you can do
    B. Ask for a list of skills and check off the ones you know
    C. Bring a list of your skills and give it to the interviewer
    D. Tell the interviewer you will send a list of your skills as soon as possible
29. It is important to ask questions at the end of the interview because it
    A. Will show the interviewer you are interested in the job
    B. Will help you decide if the job is right for you
    C. Shows you have good communication skills
    D. Shows you are dependable
30. If you are assigned a preceptor, the person may be
    A. An RN
    B. Another nursing assistant
    C. An LPN/LVN
    D. Any of the above
31. What is a common reason for losing a job?
    A. Not knowing how to perform a task
    B. Frequent absences or tardiness
    C. Being disorganized
    D. Lacking self-confidence
32. If you are scheduled to begin work at 3 PM, you should arrive
    A. At 3 PM
    B. At 2:30 PM
    C. Early enough to be ready to work at 3 PM
    D. As close to 3 PM as you can
33. You can avoid being part of gossip by
    A. Remaining quiet when you are in a group where gossip is occurring
    B. Talking about residents and family members only to co-workers
    C. Repeating comments only in writing
    D. Removing yourself from a group or situation where gossip is occurring
34. Privacy and confidentiality for residents are rights protected by
    A. Your job description
    B. Resident rights under OBRA
    C. An agreement between the resident and the nurse
    D. Doctor's orders
35. When you are working, you should not wear
    A. Clothing that is wrinkled or needs to be mended
    B. A loose-fitting shirt
    C. A shirt with the top button open
    D. White socks

36. Slang or swearing should not be used at work because
    A. Words used with family and friends may offend residents and family members
    B. The resident may not understand you
    C. The resident may have difficulty hearing
    D. Co-workers may overhear it
37. You should say "please" and "thank you" to others because
    A. Courtesies mean so much to people; they can brighten someone's day
    B. It shows respect to the person
    C. It is required by your job
    D. It shows you like the person
38. When you are working, it is acceptable to
    A. Take a pen to use at home
    B. Sell cookies for your child's school project
    C. Use a pay phone or a cell phone on your break to make a call
    D. Make a copy of a letter on the copier in the nurses' station
39. When you leave and return to the unit for breaks or lunch, you should
    A. Tell each resident
    B. Tell any family members present
    C. Tell the nurse
    D. All of the above
40. Safety practices are important to follow because
    A. They help you to be more organized
    B. Negligent behavior affects the safety of others
    C. They save the center money
    D. You will get promoted more quickly
41. When setting priorities, which of these is not important?
    A. Planning care so you can have breaks and lunch with your friends
    B. Giving care to the person who has the greatest or most life-threatening needs
    C. Finding out what tasks need to be done at a set time
    D. Finding out what tasks need to be done at the end of your shift
42. Stress occurs
    A. Only when you have unpleasant situations in your life
    B. Because you do not handle your problems well
    C. Because you are in the wrong job
    D. Every minute of every day and in everything you do
43. What physical effects of stress can be life-threatening?
    A. High blood pressure, heart attack, strokes, ulcers
    B. Increased heart rate, faster and deeper breathing
    C. Anxiety, fear, anger, depression
    D. Headaches, insomnia, muscle tension

44. Which of these actions is harassment?
    A. Offending others with gestures or remarks
    B. Offending others with jokes or pictures
    C. Making a sexual advance or requesting sexual favors
    D. All of the above
45. If you resign from a job, it is good practice to give
    A. One-week's notice
    B. Two-weeks' notice
    C. Four-weeks' notice
    D. No notice
46. Good work ethics helps residents to
    A. Feel safe, secure, loved, and cared for
    B. Receive adequate care
    C. Recover from their illnesses
    D. Have more freedom to go to activities

OPTIONAL LEARNING EXERCISES

47. List places you can find out about job openings.

    A. _____

    B. _____

    C. _____

    D. _____

    E. _____

    F. _____

    G. _____

    H. _____

Guidelines for Completing a Job Application (Box 3-3)

48. If a job application asks you to print in black ink, why is it a poor idea to use blue ink?

    _____

    _____

49. How can writing illegibly on a job application affect getting a job? _____

    _____

50. Why is it important to give information about employment gaps or leaving a job? _____

    _____

51. If you lie on a job application, it is _____.

    If you do this, what can happen? _____

    _____

Qualities and Traits for Good Work Ethics (Box 3-2)

Match the qualities and traits for good work ethics with the examples.

A. Caring
B. Dependable
C. Considerate
D. Cheerful
E. Empathetic
F. Trustworthy
G. Respectful
H. Courteous
I. Conscientious
J. Honest
K. Cooperative
L. Enthusiastic
M. Self-aware

52. _____ While working with Mr. Smith, you try to understand and feel what it must be like to be paralyzed on one side.

53. _____ You realize you are very good at giving basic care. You know you need to improve your communication skills.

54. _____ When caring for elderly residents, you try to do small things to make them happy or to find ways to ease their pain.

55. _____ You thank co-workers when they help you and remember to wish residents happy birthday as appropriate.

56. _____ When Mrs. Gibson is upset and angry, you remember to respect her feelings and to be kind.

57. _____ You report blood pressure and temperature readings accurately to the nurse.

58. _____ You realize that giving care to residents is important and you are excited about your work.

59. _____ Your supervisor tells you she knows she can count on you because you are always on time and perform delegated tasks as assigned.

60. _____ Even though Mr. Acevado has different cultural and religious views than yours, you value his feelings and beliefs.

61. _____ Before you left home today, you had an argument with your child. When you get to work, you make every effort to put that aside and be pleasant and happy.

62. _____ The nurse discusses a resident problem with you and says she knows you will keep the information confidential.

63. _____ When you are assigned to give care to resident, you make sure his care is done thoroughly and exactly as instructed.

64. _____ Your co-worker says she needs help to turn her resident and you cheerfully offer to help.

INDEPENDENT LEARNING ACTIVITIES

- How well do you take care of your own health? What can you do to improve your health practices?
  - Do you maintain a healthy weight by eating calories adequate for your energy needs? What can you do to improve your diet?
  - How much sleep do you get each night?
  - How do you practice good body mechanics at all times, not just at work?
  - How many hours do you exercise each week? What type of exercise do you do?
  - When did you last have your eyes checked? Do you wear glasses if they were prescribed?
  - Do you smoke? How much? Have you considered any smoking cessation programs?
  - Are you taking any drugs that affect your thinking, feeling, behavior, and function? Did a doctor prescribe them or are you self-medicating? Have you talked with your doctor about the effects of any drugs you are taking?
  - Do you drink alcohol? How much? Have you been told it affects your behavior? Have you considered finding a program to help you quit drinking alcohol?
- Have you ever applied for a job? How did you feel when you were being interviewed? After reading this chapter, how would you handle a future interview?
- Role-play a job interview with a classmate. Take turns playing the interviewer and the job applicant. Use the lists in this chapter to ask questions. Practice answers that you can use in a real interview.
- Think of three people you could use as references when applying for a job. Ask their permission to use them as references. If they agree, make a list of the people and their titles, addresses, and telephone numbers to use when you apply for a job. Why would each of these people be a good reference?

CROSSWORD

Use the terms in Box 3-2 to complete the crossword.

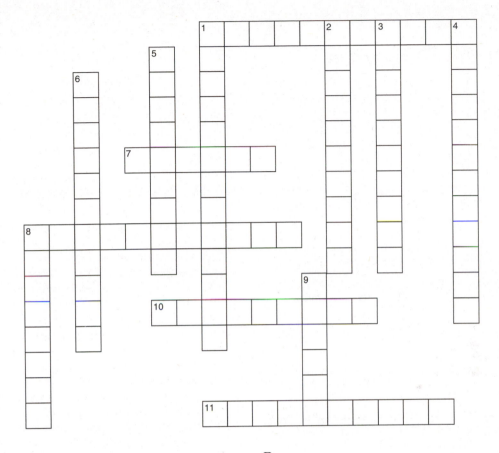

Across

1. Respect the person's physical and emotional feelings
7. Have concern for the person
8. Willing to help and work with others
10. Be polite and courteous to residents, families, and visitors
11. See things from the person's point of view

Down

1. Be careful, alert, and exact in following directions
2. Report to work on time and when scheduled
3. Do not judge or condemn residents and treat them with dignity and respect
4. Be eager, interested, and excited about your work
5. Know your feelings, strengths, and weaknesses
6. Residents and staff have confidence in you. They trust you to keep information confidential.
8. Greet and talk to people in a pleasant manner
9. Accurately report the care given, your observations, and any errors

4 COMMUNICATING WITH THE HEALTH TEAM

FILL IN THE BLANKS: KEY TERMS

Abbreviation
Chart
Communication
Conflict
Kardex

Medical record
Word element
Prefix
Progress note
Recording

Reporting
Root
Suffix

1. A _____ is a word element placed before the root; it changes the meaning of the word.

2. An _____ is a shortened form of a word or phrase.

3. _____ is the exchange of information—a message sent is received and interpreted by the intended person.

4. A _____ is a clash between opposing interests and ideas.

5. A type of card file that summarizes information found in the medical record is a

   _____.

6. A part of a word is a _____.

7. The _____ is another name for the medical record.

8. _____ is a verbal account of care and observations.

9. A written description of the care given and the person's response and progress is the

   _____.

10. A word element placed after a root that changes the meaning of the word is a

    _____.

11. A word element containing the basic meaning of

    the word is the _____.

12. A _____ is a written account of a person's condition and response to the treatment and care.

13. The written account of care and observations is

    _____.

CIRCLE THE BEST ANSWER

14. For communication to be effective
    A. Use words that have the same meaning for the sender and the receiver
    B. Use terms that are unfamiliar to residents and families
    C. Add unrelated information to the message
    D. Answers should not be specific

15. The medical record will include
    A. Physical examination results
    B. The Kardex
    C. Change-of-shift reports
    D. Hospital records

16. To prevent errors and improper placement of records, the medical record is
    A. Kept in the resident's room
    B. Placed in a locked cabinet
    C. Stamped with the person's name, room number, and other identifying information on each page
    D. Printed on colored paper

17. Before a nursing assistant reads a person's chart, he should
    A. Know the center's policy
    B. Ask the nurse for permission
    C. Ask the doctor's permission
    D. Sign a sheet to get permission

18. If a resident asks to see the chart, you should
    A. Give it to him or her because the person always has a right to see the chart
    B. Read the chart and tell the person what it says
    C. Report the request to the nurse
    D. Tell the person that residents are not allowed to see their charts

19. The admission sheet is used to
    A. Find out the person's physical condition
    B. Help the person become familiar with the center
    C. Learn identifying information about a person
    D. Carry out a physical examination

20. Progress notes are usually written
    A. Every shift
    B. When there is a change in the person's condition
    C. Each day
    D. Once a year
21. OBRA requires that summaries of care be written
    A. Once a day
    B. Once every month
    C. At least every 3 months
    D. Once a year
22. What information is included on the activities of daily living flow sheet?
    A. Doctor's orders
    B. Vital signs
    C. Care plan
    D. Old records
23. Information in an electronic flow sheet
    A. Cannot be entered by the nursing assistant
    B. Is not confidential
    C. Is often faster and easier than paper charting
    D. Is entered only at the end of the shift
24. If you make an error when recording in a paper chart, you should follow center policy. Many centers require you to
    A. Erase it
    B. Use correction fluid to cover it
    C. Throw away the page and start over
    D. Draw a line through the incorrect part and date and initial the line
25. The resident and family can
    A. Attend any resident care conference held on the unit
    B. Accompany the staff on walking rounds
    C. Refuse actions suggested by the health team at a conference
    D. Add written notes to the chart

Choose the word that is spelled correctly for each of the definitions in questions 26 to 35.
26. Slow heart rate
    A. Bradecardia
    B. Bradycardia
    C. Bradacordia
    D. Bradicardia
27. Difficulty urinating
    A. Dysuria
    B. Dysurya
    C. Dysuira
    D. Disuria
28. Paralysis on one side of the body
    A. Hemyplegia
    B. Hemaplegia
    C. Hemoplega
    D. Hemiplegia
29. Opening into the ileum
    A. Ileostomie
    B. Ileostomy
    C. Ileastoma
    D. Illiostomy

30. Blue color or condition
    A. Cyonosis
    B. Cyinosis
    C. Cyanosis
    D. Cianosys
31. Opening into the trachea
    A. Tracheastomy
    B. Trachiostomy
    C. Tracheostome
    D. Tracheostomy
32. Pain in a nerve
    A. Neuralgia
    B. Neurolgia
    C. Nourealgia
    D. Neurilegia
33. Examination of a joint with a scope
    A. Arthoscopie
    B. Arthroscopy
    C. Arethroscopy
    D. Artheroscope
34. Rapid breathing
    A. Tachepnea
    B. Tachypinea
    C. Tachypnea
    D. Tachypnia
35. Removal of the gallbladder
    A. Cholecystectomy
    B. Cholcystectomy
    C. Cholicystetomy
    D. Cholecistectomy
36. When you are given a computer password, you
    A. Must never change it
    B. Can share it with a co-worker
    C. Should never tell anyone your password
    D. Can use another person's password when entering the computer
37. Computers should not be used to
    A. Send messages and reports to the nursing unit
    B. Store resident records and care plans
    C. Send e-mails that require immediate reporting
    D. Monitor blood pressures, temperatures, and heart rates
38. When you answer the telephone, do not put callers on hold if
    A. The person has an emergency
    B. It is a doctor
    C. The call needs to be transferred to another unit
    D. You are too busy to find the nurse
39. If you have a conflict with a co-worker, you should
    A. Ask the nurse in charge to schedule you at different times
    B. Ignore the person
    C. Identify the cause of the conflict and try to resolve it
    D. Talk to other co-workers to explain your side of the story

40. When a conflict occurs, what is the first step you should take?
    A. Talk with other co-workers to see if they also have a conflict with the person.
    B. Confront the person and demand that he or she meet with you.
    C. Identify or define the real problem.
    D. Assume that the conflict will resolve itself if you ignore it.
41. Why is it important to resolve a conflict at work?
    A. Unkind words or actions may occur.
    B. The work environment becomes unpleasant.
    C. Care is affected.
    D. All of the above.

FILL IN THE BLANKS: ABBREVIATIONS

42. ADL _____

43. EHR _____

44. EMR _____

45. EPHI _____

46. HIPAA _____

47. MDS _____

48. OBRA _____

49. PHI _____

50. POC _____

MATCHING

Match each common health care term with the correct definition.

   A. Activities of daily living
   B. Assist device
   C. Atrophy
   D. Call light
   E. Care plan
   F. Cognitive function
   G. Contracture
   H. Dementia
   I. Dysphagia
   J. Dyspnea
   K. Feces
   L. Fever
   M. Fowler's position
   N. Incontinence
   O. Pressure ulcer
   P. Prone
   Q. Semi-Fowler's position
   R. Supine
   S. Vital signs
   T. Voiding

51. _____ Urinating
52. _____ Part of a call system that allows persons to signal the nurses' station for help
53. _____ A semi-sitting position; the head of the bed is raised between 45 and 60 degrees
54. _____ Difficult, labored, or painful breathing
55. _____ Lack of joint mobility caused by abnormal shortening of a muscle
56. _____ Not being able to control urination or defecation
57. _____ Involves memory, thinking, reasoning, ability to understand, judgment, and behavior
58. _____ Decrease in size or wasting away of tissue
59. _____ Temperature, pulse, respirations, and blood pressure
60. _____ Activities usually done during a normal day in a person's life
61. _____ Head of bed is raised 30 degrees, or head of bed is raised 30 degrees and knee portion is raised 15 degrees
62. _____ Written guide about the person's care; provides staff with approaches to reach the resident's goals
63. _____ Semi-solid mass of waste products in the colon that is expelled through the anus
64. _____ Loss of cognitive and social function caused by changes in the brain
65. _____ Localized injury to skin and/or underlying tissue, usually over a bony prominence
66. _____ Difficulty swallowing
67. _____ Back-lying or dorsal recumbent position
68. _____ Any item used by the person or staff to promote the person's function or safety
69. _____ Lying on the abdomen with the head turned to one side
70. _____ Elevated body temperature

FILL IN THE BLANKS

71. Next to each time, write the time using the 24-hour clock.

    A. _____ 11:00 AM   G. _____ 3:00 AM
    B. _____ 8:00 AM   H. _____ 4:50 AM
    C. _____ 4:00 PM   I. _____ 5:30 PM
    D. _____ 7:30 AM   J. _____ 10:45 PM
    E. _____ 6:45 PM   K. _____ 11:55 PM
    F. _____ 12 NOON   L. _____ 9:15 PM

Write the definition of each prefix.

72. auto- _____

73. brady- _____

74. dys- _____

75. ecto- _____

76. leuk- _____

77. macro- _____

78. neo- _____

79. supra- _____

80. uni- _____

Write the definition of each root word.

81. adeno _____

82. angio _____

83. broncho _____

84. cranio _____

85. duodeno _____

86. entero _____

87. gyneco _____

88. masto _____

89. pyo _____

Write the definition of each suffix.

90. -asis _____

91. -genic _____

92. -megaly _____

93. -oma _____

94. -phasia _____

95. -plegia _____

96. -ptosis _____

97. -scopy _____

98. -stasis _____

Using the abbreviations listed on the inside back cover of the textbook, write the correct abbreviations.

99. Before meals _____

100. After meals _____

101. With _____

102. Cancer _____

103. Discontinued _____

104. Lower left quadrant _____

105. Every day _____

106. Range-of-motion _____

LABELING

Convert the times from standard to military time and from military time to standard time. Use Figure 4-9 as a guide.

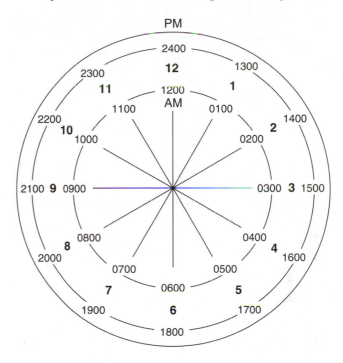

107. 2:00 AM = _____

108. 10:30 AM = _____

109. 5:00 AM = _____

110. 9:30 AM = _____

111. 5:45 PM = _____

112. 10:45 PM = _____

113. 0600 = _____ AM/PM

114. 1145 = _____ AM/PM

115. 1800 = _____ AM/PM

116. 2200 = _____ AM/PM

Identify the 4 abdominal regions. Use RUQ, LUQ, RLQ, LLQ as labels.

117.

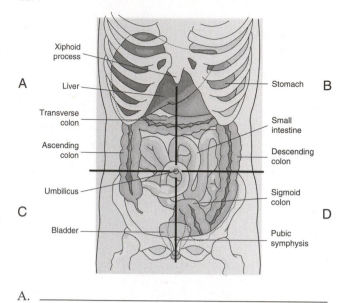

A. _____

B. _____

C. _____

D. _____

OPTIONAL LEARNING EXERCISES

- Class Experiment: It is often difficult to describe fluids in a clear and precise manner. Set up the following examples that imitate situations where you need to describe intake, output, or drainage.
  - Bloody drainage: Mix a teaspoon of ketchup and a teaspoon of water. Pour on the center of a paper napkin.
  - Urine: Pour a tablespoon of tea on the center of a paper towel.
  - Bleeding: Smear a teaspoon of red jelly on the center of a paper towel.
  - Broth: Pour 4 ounces of tea into a bowl.
    - Describe as accurately as possible what you see in terms of amounts, colors, and textures.
    - Compare your notes with classmates to see if you are using words that all have the same meaning.
    - What words were used that were clear to understand? What words were used that had more than one meaning?
- Case Study: *Mr. Larsen was admitted to a subacute care center after his abdominal surgery 1 week ago. This morning the nursing assistant gave Mr. Larsen a shower and assisted him to sit in a comfortable chair. The nursing assistant noticed that he sat very still and held his arms across his abdomen. He asked for a pillow and held it tightly against his abdomen.*

- Imagine you are the patient and answer the following questions.
  - What would you like the nursing assistant to ask you?
  - How would you communicate your feelings to the nursing assistant?
  - How could you let the nursing assistant know that you have pain without telling him or her?
- Imagine you are the nursing assistant and answer the following questions.
  - As the nursing assistant, what observations would be important to make about Mr. Larsen?
  - What questions could you ask Mr. Larsen?
  - What nonverbal communication would give you information about Mr. Larsen?
- Case Study: *Mrs. Miller was admitted to the health care center since you last worked 3 days ago. You have just started your shift and have been assigned to Mrs. Miller.*
  - What information would you need to know before giving care? Why?
  - What information would be important to provide to the on-coming shift?
  - What methods would you use to communicate this information?

Class Experiment	
Substance	**Observations**
Bloody drainage	
Urine	
Bleeding	
Broth	

INDEPENDENT LEARNING ACTIVITIES

Answer These Questions About Situations in Which You May Need to Communicate With Others.

- When have you had a problem with communicating?
  - Why was it difficult? How did you handle this?
- Think about a situation in which you feel you communicated your point well.
  - What made the communication successful? How could you use a similar technique in caring for residents?
- How would you communicate with a person who speaks a language that you do not speak or understand?
  - What methods could you use to explain what you are going to do?
  - How would you communicate with a person from a different culture?

- Make flash cards of the prefixes, suffixes, and root words listed in Chapter 4.
  - Put the meaning of each one on the back of the appropriate card.
  - Work alone or with a partner. By looking at the cards, practice identifying the correct meaning of each term.

- The next time you or a member of your family visit the doctor and are instructed to fill a prescription, look at what the doctor has written.
  - Do you see any abbreviations that you learned in this chapter? What do they mean? How did this chapter help you understand what was written?

5 ASSISTING WITH THE NURSING PROCESS

FILL IN THE BLANKS: KEY TERMS

Assessment
Comprehensive care plan
Evaluation
Goal
Implementation
Interdisciplinary team (IDT)

Medical diagnosis
Nursing diagnosis
Nursing intervention
Nursing process
Objective data
Observation

Planning
Signs
Skilled care
Subjective data
Symptoms
Triggers

1. Daily services provided by the RN and/or therapist for rehabilitation or other complex services is

   _____.

2. _____ are things a person tells you about that you cannot observe through your senses.

3. _____ is to perform or carry out measures in the care plan; a step in the nursing process.

4. The method that RNs use to plan and deliver nursing care is the _____

   _____.

5. Another name for subjective data is

   _____

6. A written guide about the care a person should receive is the _____

   _____.

7. _____ is collecting information about the person; a step in the nursing process.

8. Another name for objective data is

   _____

9. The _____ describes a health problem that can be treated by a nursing measure; a step in the nursing process.

10. Information that is seen, heard, felt, or smelled is

    _____ or signs.

11. A step in the nursing process that is used to measure whether goals in the planning step were met is called _____.

12. _____ is setting priorities and goals; a step in the nursing process.

13. A _____ is an action or measure taken by the nursing team to help the person reach a goal.

14. A _____ is that which is desired in or by the person as a result of nursing care.

15. Using the senses of sight, hearing, touch, and smell to collect information is _____.

16. The identification of a disease or condition by a doctor is a _____.

17. _____ is information that is collected from the MDS for the Care Area Assessments (CAAs).

18. The _____ are the members of departments found in a nursing home.

CIRCLE THE BEST ANSWER

19. Which of these is one of the steps in the nursing process?
    A. Subjective data
    B. Objective data
    C. Observation
    D. Evaluation

20. The nursing process focuses on
    A. The doctor's orders
    B. The person's nursing needs
    C. Tasks and procedures that are needed
    D. Reducing the cost of health care

21. The nursing process
    A. Helps all nursing team members to do the same things for the person
    B. Stays the same from admission to discharge
    C. Cannot be used in home care
    D. Can be used only for adults
22. When you observe by using your senses, you assist the nurse to
    A. Assess the person
    B. Plan for care
    C. Implement care for the person
    D. Evaluate the person
23. Which of these is an example of objective data?
    A. Mrs. Hewitt complains of pain and nausea.
    B. Mr. Stewart tells you he has a dull ache in his stomach.
    C. You are taking Mrs. Jensen's blood pressure and notice her skin is hot and moist.
    D. Mrs. Murano tells you she is tired because she could not sleep last night.
24. A Minimum Data Set (MDS) is used
    A. For nursing center residents
    B. In all health care settings
    C. In acute care settings
    D. In home care
25. The MDS is completed and updated
    A. Shortly after admission
    B. Each quarter
    C. Annually
    D. All of the above
26. Information is recorded in a point of care (POC) module to
    A. Record care given and observations made
    B. Assess the resident
    C. Document the doctor's orders
    D. List medications ordered and given to the person
27. A nursing diagnosis
    A. Identifies a disease or condition
    B. Helps to identify drugs or therapies used by the doctor
    C. Describes a health problem that can be treated by nursing measures
    D. Identifies only physical problems
28. When a nurse uses the nursing process, the person is given
    A. Only 1 nursing diagnosis
    B. No more than 5 nursing diagnoses
    C. As many nursing diagnoses as are needed
    D. Nursing diagnoses that involve only physical needs
29. Planning involves
    A. Setting priorities and goals
    B. Choosing nursing interventions to help the person reach a goal
    C. Revising the care plan as a person's needs change
    D. All of the above

30. OBRA requires an interdisciplinary care planning conference
    A. For each person
    B. To meet agency guidelines
    C. To assess the person
    D. To implement the care plan
31. What part of the nursing process is being carried out when you give personal care to a person?
    A. Assessment
    B. Planning
    C. Implementation
    D. Evaluation
32. An assignment sheet usually includes information about
    A. Each person's care
    B. Evaluation of the goals for care
    C. An assessment of the person
    D. The nursing diagnoses for the person
33. Nurses measure which goals have been met in the

    _____ part of the nursing process.
    A. Assessing
    B. Planning
    C. Implementation
    D. Evaluation

FILL IN THE BLANKS: ABBREVIATIONS

34. ADL _____

35. CAA _____

36. IDT _____

37. MDS _____

38. NANDA-I _____

39. OBRA _____

40. POC _____

41. RN _____

FILL IN THE BLANKS

42. When you make observations while you give care, what senses are used?

    A. _____

    B. _____

    C. _____

    D. _____

43. Each of the following is either subjective or objective data. In the blank next to each statement, place an "S" for subjective or an "O" for objective.

    A. _____ Sleepy

    B. _____ Chest pain

    C. _____ Skin cool

    D. _____ Cyanosis of nails

    E. _____ Labored breathing

    F. _____ Gas pain

    G. _____ Pain when urinating

    H. _____ Productive cough

    I. _____ Breath has fruity odor

    J. _____ Pulse rapid

44. Name the body system or other area you are observing in each of these examples. (Box 5-1)
    A. Is the abdomen firm or soft?

    _____

    B. Is the person sensitive to bright lights?

    _____

    C. Are sores or reddened areas present?

    _____

    D. What is the frequency of the person's cough?

    _____

    E. Can the person bathe without help?

    _____

    F. Can the person swallow food and fluids?

    _____

    G. What is the position of comfort?

    _____

    H. Does the person answer questions correctly?

    _____

    I. Does the person complain of stiff or painful

    joints? _____

45. When planning care, needs that are required for life

    and survival must be met before _____

    _____.

46. A comprehensive care plan is

    A. Developed for _____.
    B. Suggestions are welcomed from all

    _____

    C. It tells the health team members what care

    _____

47. The assignment sheet tells you about

    A. _____

    B. _____

    C. _____

OPTIONAL LEARNING EXERCISES

List at least three nursing interventions for each of these nursing diagnoses and goals.

48. Nursing Diagnosis: Feeding Self-Care Deficit related to weakness in right arm
    Goal: Patient will eat 75% of each meal by 2/1.
    Nursing Interventions:

    A. _____

    B. _____

    C. _____

49. Nursing Diagnosis: Hygiene Self-Care Deficit related to forgetfulness
    Goal: Patient will be assisted to maintain good hygiene throughout hospital stay.
    Nursing Interventions:

    A. _____

    B. _____

    C. _____

INDEPENDENT LEARNING ACTIVITIES

- Ask permission to look at the nursing care plans used at the agency where you had your clinical experience. Answer the following questions about the nursing care plans.
  - How do the nurses develop the plans? What resources do they use?
  - How often are the plans reviewed and revised?
  - How are the plans used by the nursing assistants?
  - How do nursing assistants help to develop and revise the nursing interventions?
  - How do the nurses communicate the information on the nursing care plan?

6 · UNDERSTANDING THE RESIDENT

FILL IN THE BLANKS: KEY TERMS

Agnostic
Atheist
Body language
Comatose
Culture
Disability

Esteem
Holism
Need
Nonverbal communication
Optimal level of function
Paraphrasing

Religion
Self-actualization
Self-esteem
Verbal communication

1. Experiencing one's potential is called
   _____.

2. _____ is thinking well of
   oneself, seeing oneself as useful, and being well
   thought of by others.

3. A person's highest potential for mental and
   physical performance is the _____
   _____.

4. A _____ is that which is
   necessary or desirable for maintaining life and
   mental well-being.

5. Communication that uses the written or spoken
   word is called _____.

6. _____ is lost, absent, or
   impaired physical or mental function.

7. _____ is communication that
   does not involve words.

8. An _____ is a person who
   believes it is impossible to know if a god exists

9. The characteristics of a group of people—language,
   values, beliefs, habits, likes, dislikes, customs—
   passed from one generation to the next is called
   _____.

10. The worth, value, or opinion one has of a person is
    _____.

11. _____ is spiritual beliefs,
    needs, and practices.

12. A person who is _____ has
    an inability to respond to stimuli.

13. Restating the person's message in your own words
    is called _____.

14. _____ sends messages
    through facial expressions, gestures, posture, and
    body movements.

15. _____ is a concept that
    considers the whole person.

16. A person who denies the existence of a god or deity
    is an _____.

CIRCLE THE BEST ANSWER

17. Who is the most important person in the nursing
    center?
    A. The director of nursing
    B. The resident
    C. The doctor
    D. The nurse

18. Which of these losses may have happened to an
    older resident?
    A. Loss of home and family members
    B. Loss of the person's role in the family or
       community
    C. Loss of body functions
    D. All of the above

19. When speaking about the resident, which of these
    statements is best?
    A. "Mrs. Jones in 135 needs a pain pill."
    B. "Granny Jones needs something for pain."
    C. "135 needs a pain pill."
    D. "Janie is complaining of pain."

20. What is the main reason you call a resident by
    a title such as Mr., Mrs., or Miss?
    A. It best identifies the person.
    B. It gives the person dignity and respect.
    C. It is polite.
    D. It shows the person you are in charge.

21. When is it acceptable to call a person by his or her first name or another name?
    A. You have cared for the person for several months.
    B. The person is confused.
    C. The person asks you to use the name.
    D. The person has difficulty hearing.

22. Which of these needs is affected when the person has a disability or illness?
    A. Physical
    B. Social
    C. Psychological
    D. All of the above

23. What needs are most important for survival?
    A. Physical
    B. Safety and security
    C. Love and belonging
    D. Self-esteem

24. It is important for the person to know what to expect when care is given because the person will
    A. Be combative
    B. Feel safer and more secure
    C. Have a more meaningful relationship
    D. Experience his or her potential

25. What need is rarely, if ever, totally met?
    A. Physiological
    B. Safety and security
    C. Self-esteem
    D. Self-actualization

26. Mrs. Young is a new resident. She will feel more secure when you
    A. Give her explanations of routines and procedures only one time
    B. Spend as little time as possible in her room
    C. Use new equipment without telling her what it is
    D. Listen to her concerns and explain all routines and procedures as often as needed

27. Mrs. Peck never has visitors and is becoming weaker and unable to care for herself. What need is not being met?
    A. Physiological
    B. Safety and security
    C. Love and belonging
    D. Self-esteem

28. When a resident asks to see a spiritual leader or adviser, what should you do?
    A. Tell the resident no one is available to see him or her until the Sabbath.
    B. Ignore the request because a visit is not on the schedule.
    C. Tell the resident to have his or her family get in touch with the spiritual leader.
    D. Report this to the nurse at once.

29. When you are caring for a person of a different culture or religion, you should
    A. Expect all people to follow the same practices
    B. Judge the person by your standards
    C. Remember that each person is unique
    D. Ignore the cultural or religious practices

30. A person who is ill and disabled is often very angry because
    A. The care he or she is receiving is poor
    B. He or she is angry at the situation
    C. He or she does not like you
    D. He or she has a bad temper

31. How can you help Mr. Clay maintain his optimal level of functioning?
    A. Give him complete care.
    B. Encourage him to be as independent as possible.
    C. Avoid staying with him to visit.
    D. Do not respond promptly when he asks for help.

32. Mrs. Nelson is alert and oriented. Why would she require care in a nursing center?
    A. She has trouble remembering where she is.
    B. She cannot tell you what she needs or wants.
    C. She has physical problems, so she requires help.
    D. She does not know who she is.

33. Which of these is a reason why confusion and disorientation may be temporary?
    A. The person has a disabling disease.
    B. The person has recently been admitted to the nursing center.
    C. The person needs complete help with all activities of daily living (ADL).
    D. The person is terminally ill.

34. Mrs. Smithers is admitted to the nursing center. The nurse tells you she will only be here short-term. You know the reason for most short-term admissions is to
    A. Provide quality care to dying residents
    B. Give complete care to the resident
    C. Help the resident recover from fractures, acute illness, or surgery
    D. Prevent injury of the resident

35. Respite care provides
    A. Time to recover from surgery or acute illness
    B. Recovery from temporary confusion
    C. Care for a dying person
    D. The caregiver a chance to take a vacation, tend to business, or rest

36. A person who needs life-long care has a disability that occurs
    A. Due to birth defects or childhood illnesses or injuries
    B. Because of mental illness
    C. Because of the aging process
    D. Because the person is dying

37. If a resident is comatose, how would you know the person is in pain?
    A. The person cries and lies very still.
    B. The person asks for pain medications.
    C. Pain is shown by grimacing and groaning.
    D. You cannot tell if the person is in pain.

38. Which of these ways to deal with a person with behavior issues would be helpful?
    A. Argue with the person to show him he is wrong.
    B. Avoid going into the room unless you must give care.
    C. Carry out care and tasks without talking to the person.
    D. Stay calm and professional if the anger and hostility is directed at you.
39. Which of these would help effective communication?
    A. Use words that have the same meaning to both you and the person.
    B. Give long, detailed explanations to questions.
    C. Change the subject when the person seems confused.
    D. Use medical terminology when talking to the person.
40. Mrs. Stevens cannot speak. Which of these would be an example of her verbal communication?
    A. She may use touch.
    B. Her body language sends messages.
    C. She uses gestures to communicate.
    D. She writes messages on a note pad.
41. When you go to Mrs. Hart's room, you can tell she is not happy or not feeling well because
    A. Her hair is well-groomed
    B. She has a slumped posture
    C. She smiles when you enter the room
    D. She is watching TV and does not carry on a conversation
42. You show that you listen effectively when you
    A. Look across the room to avoid eye contact
    B. Lean away from the person with your arms folded
    C. Change the subject if the person seems upset
    D. Respond to the person by nodding your head
43. Which of these is an example of paraphrasing?
    A. "You don't know how long you will be here."
    B. "Do you want to take a tub bath or a shower?"
    C. "Tell me about living on a farm."
    D. "Can you explain what you mean?"
44. When you say: "Mr. Davis, have you taken a shower this morning?" you are
    A. Paraphrasing his thoughts
    B. Asking a direct question
    C. Focusing his thoughts
    D. Asking an open-ended question
45. Responses to open-ended questions generally are
    A. Longer and give more information than responses to direct questions
    B. "Yes" or "no" answers
    C. Able to make sure you understand the message
    D. Focused on dealing with a certain topic

46. Mr. Parker often rambles and tells long stories in which his thoughts wander. You need to know if he had a bowel movement today, so you will
    A. Make a clarifying statement
    B. Ask an open-ended question
    C. Make a focusing statement
    D. Paraphrase his thoughts
47. What is best if the person takes long pauses between statements?
    A. You do not need to talk. Just being there helps.
    B. Try to cheer the person up by talking.
    C. Leave the room.
    D. Find another resident to talk with the person.
48. Mrs. Duke has visitors and you need to give care. What would you do?
    A. Give the care while visitors are present.
    B. Politely ask the visitors to leave the room.
    C. Tell the visitors to give the care.
    D. Tell the visitors they must leave the nursing center.

FILL IN THE BLANKS: BASIC NEEDS

49. List the basic needs for life as described by Maslow from the lowest level to the highest level.

    A. _____

    B. _____

    C. _____

    D. _____

    E. _____

OPTIONAL LEARNING EXERCISES
Basic Needs
Physical needs

50. What are the 6 physical needs required for survival?

    _____

51. The lower-level needs must be met before the

    _____ needs.

Safety and security

52. Safety and security needs relate to feeling safe from

    _____, _____, and

    _____.

53. Why do many people feel a loss of safety and security when admitted to a nursing center?

    A. _____

    B. _____

    C. _____

    D. _____

Love and belonging

54. The need for love and belonging relates to

_____, _____, and

_____

55. These needs also involve _____

_____

56. How can you help a resident feel loved and

accepted? _____

_____

Self-esteem

57. What does self-esteem relate to?

A. _____

B. _____

C. _____

58. Why is it important to encourage residents to do as

much as possible for themselves? _____

_____

Self-actualization

59. What does self-actualization involve?

_____, _____, and

_____

60. What happens if self-actualization is postponed?

_____

Cultural and Religious Practices

61. How can you help a resident to observe religious practices if services are held in the nursing center?

_____

62. If the resident wants to have a visit from a spiritual

leader, you should tell _____.

63. If the resident wants a spiritual leader or adviser

to visit in the room, you should _____,

_____ _____, and

_____

64. If a person has religious objects in the room, you

should treat the items with _____

and should not _____

without permission.

65. If a person refuses a particular food due to a religious custom, you should offer

_____

66. A person tells you he has no belief in a god. This

person is an _____.

67. An _____ does not deny that a
god exists but does not believe it can be

_____.

Cultural Health Care Beliefs

Mexican americans

68. If hot causes the illness, _____
is used for the cure.

69. Hot and cold are found in _____,

_____, and _____.

Vietnamese americans

70. Hot is given to balance _____
illnesses.

71. Cold is given to balance _____
illnesses.

Cultural Sick Practices

72. How do Vietnamese American folk practices treat these illnesses?

A. Common cold _____

B. Headache and sore throat _____

73. What illnesses do these Russian American folk practices treat?

A. _____ An ointment is
placed behind the ears and temples and also at the back of the neck.

B. _____ A dough made of
dark rye flour and honey is placed on the spinal column.

Cultural Touch Practices

74. What may touch mean to persons from these countries?

A. Philippines _____

B. Mexico _____

C. United Kingdom _____

75. Men who are from India may not wish to shake

hands with a _____.

76. The head is not touched by persons from

_____ because it is considered

the center of the _____.

77. People from _____ do not like
touching strangers. They prefer health care workers

of the same _____

78. A person from Ireland would embrace only

_____ and _____.

Cultural Facial Expressions

79. These cultures may have persons who smile readily.

    A. _____

    B. _____

    C. _____

    D. _____

80. _____ may conceal negative emotions with a smile.

Cultural Eye Contact Practices

81. Why would you avoid making direct eye contact with a person from an American Indian, African, or Latin American culture? _____

    _____

82. In certain Indian cultures, eye contact is avoided with persons of _____ or

    _____ socio-economic classes.

83. In Iraq, _____ and

    _____ avoid direct eye contact.

Case Study

You have completed your duties for the morning and have some free time. Mr. Donal is a resident in the nursing center. He rarely has visitors and you try to spend time with him when you can. Fill in the blanks in the following statements about communication techniques you use when you visit with Mr. Donal.

84. You sit in a chair next to Mr. Donal so you can see each other. This position will help you to be at

    his _____ and can maintain good

    _____.

85. You should lean _____ Mr. Donal to show interest.

86. Mr. Donal says: "I know this is the best place for me but I miss my flower garden at home." You respond: "You miss your home." This is an

    example of _____.

87. You ask Mr. Donal: "You told me you did not sleep well last night. Can you tell me why?" He replies: "There was a lot of noise in the hall." This is an

    example of a _____.

88. You say to Mr. Donal: "Tell me about your flower

    garden at home." This is an _____
    question.

89. When you ask: "Can you explain what that means?" you are asking a person to

    _____

90. Mr. Donal says that he "hurts all over" and then begins to talk about the weather. You say: "Tell me

more about where you hurt. You said you hurt all over." This statement helps in _____

_____ the topic.

91. Mr. Donal begins to cry when he talks about his flower garden. How can you show caring and

    respect for his situation and feelings? _____

    _____.

92. When Mr. Donal begins to cry, you quickly begin to talk about the activities planned this morning.

    Changing the subject is a _____

    _____.

INDEPENDENT LEARNING ACTIVITIES

- Refer to the discussion about basic needs in Chapter 6 on p. 79. Think about how well you are meeting your own needs.
  - Do you smoke? What need may be affected by smoking?
  - What kinds of foods and fluids do you eat? Is your diet meeting your basic needs for food and water?
  - How much rest and sleep do you get each day? How much do you need to feel well rested?
  - How safe do you feel at home? At school? In your community? How do your feelings affect your ability to hold a job or attend school?
  - Who are the people who make you feel loved? Who helps you when you have problems?
  - What are you doing that helps you meet the need for self-actualization?
- Answer the following questions about your personal health care practices.
  - What health care practices are followed in your family? How are these practices related to your cultural or religious beliefs?
  - How often do you go to the doctor? For regular check-ups? Only when ill?
  - When do you go to the dentist? Once or twice a year for cleaning and check-ups? Only when you have a toothache?
  - When a family member is in a health care center, how does your family respond? Does someone stay with the person and do all of the care? Or do family members visit for brief periods and let health care workers provide all of the care? Is the family response related to any cultural or religious practices?
- Look at your answers to both sets of questions above.
  - How well are you meeting your basic needs? How could you improve in meeting your needs? What changes would be the most beneficial?
  - How much influence on your practices comes from cultural or religious traditions in your family? Are these influences helping you or hindering you to meet your needs?

7 BODY STRUCTURE AND FUNCTION

FILL IN THE BLANKS: KEY TERMS

Artery
Capillary
Cell
Digestion
Hemoglobin

Hormone
Immunity
Menstruation
Metabolism
Organ

Peristalsis
Respiration
System
Tissue
Vein

1. The substance in red blood cells that carries oxygen and gives blood its color is

   _____.

2. _____ is protection against a disease or condition.

3. The process of supplying the cells with oxygen and removing carbon dioxide from them is

   _____.

4. The process of physically and chemically breaking down food so it can be absorbed for use by the

   cells is _____.

5. _____ is the burning of food for heat and energy by the cells.

6. A blood vessel that carries blood away from the

   heart is the _____.

7. _____ is the involuntary muscle contractions in the digestive system that move food through the alimentary canal.

8. Organs that work together to perform special

   functions form a _____.

9. The basic unit of body structure is a _____.

10. Groups of tissues with the same function form an

    _____.

11. A _____ is a tiny blood vessel.

12. A group of cells with similar function is

    _____.

13. _____ is the process in which the lining of the uterus breaks up and is discharged from the body through the vagina.

14. A chemical substance secreted by the glands into

    the bloodstream is a _____.

15. A _____ is a blood vessel that carries blood back to the heart.

CIRCLE THE BEST ANSWER

16. A cell is
    A. Found only in muscles
    B. The basic unit of body structure
    C. Able to live without oxygen
    D. A group of tissues

17. The control center of a cell is the
    A. Membrane
    B. Protoplasm
    C. Cytoplasm
    D. Nucleus

18. Genes control
    A. Cell division
    B. Tissues
    C. Traits inherited by children
    D. Organs

19. Connective tissue
    A. Covers internal and external body surfaces
    B. Receives and carries impulses to the brain and back to body parts
    C. Anchors, connects, and supports other body tissues
    D. Allows the body to move by stretching and contracting

20. Living cells of the epidermis contain
    A. Blood vessels and many nerves
    B. Sweat and oil glands
    C. Pigment that gives skin its color
    D. Hair roots

21. Sweat glands help
    A. The body to regulate temperature
    B. To keep the hair and skin soft and shiny
    C. To protect the nose from dust, insects, and other foreign objects
    D. The skin to sense pleasant and unpleasant sensations
22. Long bones
    A. Allow skill and ease in movement
    B. Bear the weight of the body
    C. Protect organs
    D. Allow various degrees of movement and flexion
23. Blood cells are manufactured in
    A. The heart
    B. The liver
    C. Blood vessels
    D. Bone marrow
24. Joints move smoothly because of the
    A. Cartilage
    B. Synovial fluid
    C. Muscle
    D. Ligaments
25. A joint that moves in all directions is a
    A. Ball and socket
    B. Hinge
    C. Pivot
    D. All of the above
26. Voluntary muscles are
    A. Found in the stomach and intestines
    B. Attached to bones
    C. Cardiac muscle
    D. Tendons
27. Muscles produce heat by
    A. Contracting
    B. Relaxing
    C. Maintaining posture
    D. Working automatically
28. The central nervous system (CNS) consists of
    A. A myelin sheath
    B. Nerves throughout the body
    C. The brain and spinal cord
    D. Cranial nerves
29. The medulla controls
    A. Muscle contraction and relaxation
    B. Heart rate, breathing, blood vessel size, and swallowing
    C. Reasoning, memory, and consciousness
    D. Hearing and vision
30. Cerebrospinal fluid
    A. Cushions shocks that could injure the structure of the brain and spinal cord
    B. Controls voluntary muscles
    C. Lubricates movement
    D. Controls involuntary muscles
31. The cranial nerves conduct impulses between the
    A. Brain and the head, neck, chest, and abdomen
    B. Brain and the skin and extremities
    C. Brain and internal body structures
    D. Spinal cord and lower extremities
32. When you are frightened, the _____ nervous system is stimulated.
    A. Sympathetic
    B. Parasympathetic
    C. Central
    D. Cranial
33. Receptors for vision and nerve fibers of the optic nerve are found in the
    A. Sclera
    B. Choroids
    C. Retina
    D. Cornea
34. What structure of the ear is involved in balance?
    A. Malleus
    B. Auditory canal
    C. Tympanic membranes
    D. Semicircular canals
35. Hemoglobin in red blood cells gives blood its red color and carries
    A. Oxygen
    B. Food to cells
    C. Waste products
    D. Water
36. Red blood cells live for
    A. About 9 days
    B. 3 or 4 months
    C. 4 days
    D. A year
37. White blood cells or leukocytes
    A. Protect the body against infection
    B. Are necessary for blood clotting
    C. Carry food, hormones, chemicals, and waste products
    D. Pick up carbon dioxide
38. The left atrium of the heart
    A. Receives blood from the lungs
    B. Receives blood from the body tissues
    C. Pumps blood to the lungs
    D. Pumps blood to all parts of the body
39. Arteries
    A. Return blood to the heart
    B. Pass food, oxygen, and other substances into the cells
    C. Pick up waste products, including carbon dioxide, from the cells
    D. Carry blood away from the heart
40. In the lungs, oxygen and carbon dioxide are exchanged
    A. In the epiglottis
    B. Between the right bronchus and the left bronchus
    C. By the bronchioles
    D. Between the alveoli and capillaries

41. The lungs are protected by
    A. The diaphragm
    B. The pleura
    C. A bony framework of the ribs, sternum, and vertebrae
    D. The lobes
42. Food is moved through the alimentary canal (gastro-intestinal tract) by
    A. Chyme
    B. Peristalsis
    C. Swallowing
    D. Bile
43. Water is absorbed from chyme in the
    A. Small intestine
    B. Stomach
    C. Esophagus
    D. Large intestine
44. Digested food is absorbed through tiny projections called
    A. Jejunum
    B. Ileum
    C. Villi
    D. Colon
45. A function of the urinary system is to
    A. Remove waste products from the blood
    B. Rid the body of solid waste
    C. Rid the body of carbon dioxide
    D. Burn food for energy
46. A person usually feels the need to urinate when the bladder contains about
    A. 1000 mL of urine
    B. 500 mL of urine
    C. 250 mL of urine
    D. 125 mL of urine
47. Testosterone is needed for
    A. Male secondary sex characteristics
    B. Female secondary sex characteristics
    C. Sperm to be produced
    D. Ova to be produced
48. The prostate gland lies
    A. In the scrotum
    B. In the testes
    C. Just below the bladder
    D. In the penis
49. The ovaries secrete progesterone and
    A. Estrogen
    B. Testosterone
    C. Ova
    D. Semen
50. When an ovum is released from an ovary, it travels first through the
    A. Uterus
    B. Fallopian tube
    C. Endometrium
    D. Vagina
51. Menstruation occurs when
    A. The hymen is ruptured
    B. An ovum is released by the ovary
    C. The endometrium breaks up
    D. Fertilization occurs
52. A fertilized cell implants in the
    A. Ovary
    B. Fallopian tubes
    C. Endometrium
    D. Vagina
53. The master gland is the
    A. Thyroid gland
    B. Parathyroid gland
    C. Adrenal gland
    D. Pituitary gland
54. Thyroid hormone regulates
    A. Growth
    B. Metabolism
    C. Proper functioning of nerves and muscles
    D. Energy produced during activity
55. If too little insulin is produced by the pancreas, the person has
    A. Tetany
    B. Slow growth
    C. Diabetes
    D. Slowed metabolism
56. When antigens (an unwanted substance) enter the body, white blood cells called lymphocytes increase the production of
    A. Antibodies
    B. Phagocytes
    C. B cells
    D. T cells

FILL IN THE BLANKS: ABBREVIATIONS

57. CNS _____

58. GI _____

59. mL _____

60. RBC _____

61. WBC _____

MATCHING

Match the musculo-skeletal term with the correct description.

    A. Periosteum
    B. Joint
    C. Cartilage
    D. Synovial fluid
    E. Striated muscle
    F. Smooth muscle
    G. Cardiac muscle
    H. Tendons

62. _____ Connective tissue at the end of long bones
63. _____ Skeletal muscle
64. _____ Membrane that covers bone

65. _____ Connects muscle to bone
66. _____ The point at which two or more bones meet
67. _____ Muscle found only in heart
68. _____ Involuntary muscle
69. _____ Acts as a lubricant so the joint can move smoothly

Match the nervous system term with the correct description.
   A. Sclera
   B. Cornea
   C. Retina
   D. Cerumen
   E. Middle ear
   F. Inner ear
   G. Brainstem
   H. Cerebral cortex
   I. Autonomic nervous system
   J. Peripheral nervous system

70. _____ Contains eustachian tubes and ossicles
71. _____ Has 12 pairs of cranial nerves and 31 pairs of spinal nerves
72. _____ White of the eye
73. _____ Outside of the cerebrum; controls highest function of brain
74. _____ Inner layer of eye; receptors for vision are contained here
75. _____ Controls involuntary muscles, heartbeat, blood pressure and other functions
76. _____ Light enters the eye through this structure
77. _____ Contains the midbrain, pons, and medulla
78. _____ Waxy substance secreted in the auditory canal
79. _____ Contains the semicircular canal and cochlea

Match the circulatory system term with the correct description.
   A. Plasma
   B. Erythrocytes
   C. Hemoglobin
   D. Leukocytes
   E. Thrombocytes
   F. Pericardium
   G. Myocardium
   H. Endocardium
   I. Arteries
   J. Veins
   K. Capillaries

80. _____ The part of blood that is mostly water
81. _____ The thin sac covering the heart
82. _____ Very tiny blood vessels

83. _____ The substance in blood that picks up oxygen
84. _____ Carry blood away from the heart
85. _____ White blood cells
86. _____ Carry blood toward the heart
87. _____ Red blood cells
88. _____ The thick muscular portion of the heart
89. _____ Platelets; necessary for clotting
90. _____ The membrane lining the inner surface of the heart

Match the respiratory system term with the correct description.
   A. Epiglottis
   B. Larynx
   C. Bronchiole
   D. Trachea
   E. Alveoli
   F. Diaphragm
   G. Pleura

91. _____ Air passes from the larynx into this structure
92. _____ A two-layered sac that covers the lungs
93. _____ Piece of cartilage that acts like a lid over the larynx
94. _____ Separates the lungs from the abdominal cavity
95. _____ The voice box
96. _____ Several small branches that divide from the bronchus
97. _____ Tiny one-celled air sacs

Match the digestive system term with the correct description.
   A. Liver
   B. Chyme
   C. Colon
   D. Duodenum
   E. Jejunum
   F. Saliva
   G. Pancreas
   H. Gallbladder

98. _____ Structure in which more digestive juices are added to chyme
99. _____ Semi-liquid food mixture formed in the stomach
100. _____ Portion of the GI tract that absorbs food
101. _____ Stores bile
102. _____ Portion of the GI tract that absorbs water
103. _____ Produces bile
104. _____ Moistens food particles in the mouth
105. _____ Produces digestive juices

Match the urinary system term with the correct description.

    A. Bladder
    B. Glomerulus
    C. Kidney
    D. Meatus
    E. Nephrons
    F. Tubules
    G. Ureter
    H. Urethra

106. _____ Basic working unit of the kidney
107. _____ Bean-shaped structure that produces urine
108. _____ A cluster of capillaries in the tubule
109. _____ Structure that allows urine to pass from the bladder
110. _____ A tube attached to the renal pelvis of the kidney
111. _____ Hollow muscular sac that stores urine
112. _____ Opening at the end of the urethra
113. _____ Fluid and waste products form urine in this structure

Match the reproductive system term with the correct description.

    A. Scrotum
    B. Testes
    C. Seminal vesicle
    D. Gonads
    E. Fallopian tube
    F. Endometrium
    G. Labia
    H. Vulva

114. _____ Male sex glands
115. _____ Two folds of tissue on each side of the vagina
116. _____ Sac between the thighs that contains the testes
117. _____ External genitalia of female
118. _____ Testicles; sperm are produced here
119. _____ Attached to uterus; ova travel through this structure
120. _____ Stores sperm and produces semen
121. _____ Tissue lining the uterus

Match the endocrine system term with the correct description.

    A. Epinephrine
    B. Estrogen
    C. Insulin
    D. Parathormone
    E. Testosterone
    F. Thyroxine

122. _____ Released by the pancreas; regulates sugar in blood
123. _____ Sex hormone secreted by the testes
124. _____ Sex hormone secreted by the ovaries
125. _____ Regulates metabolism
126. _____ Regulates calcium levels in the body
127. _____ Stimulates the body to produce energy during emergencies

Match the immune system term with the correct description.

    A. Antibodies
    B. Antigens
    C. Phagocytes
    D. Lymphocytes
    E. B cells
    F. T cells

128. _____ Normal body substances that recognize abnormal or unwanted substances
129. _____ Type of cell that destroys invading cells
130. _____ Type of white blood cell that digests and destroys microorganisms
131. _____ Type of cell that causes production of antibodies
132. _____ An abnormal or unwanted substance
133. _____ Type of white blood cell that produces antibodies

LABELING

134. Name the parts of the cell.

    A. _____

    B. _____

    C. _____

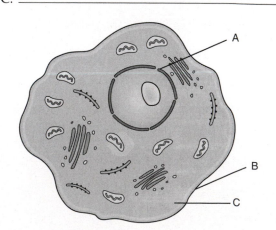

135. Name each type of joint.

A. _____

B. _____

C. _____

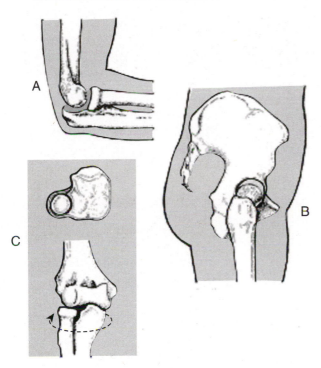

136. Name the parts of the brain.

A. _____

B. _____

C. _____

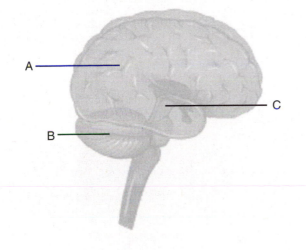

137. Name the 4 chambers of the heart.

A. _____

B. _____

C. _____

D. _____

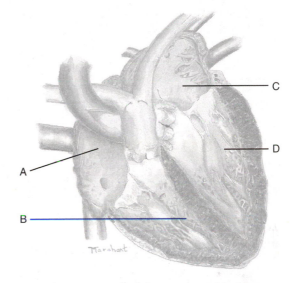

138. Name the structures of the respiratory system.

A. _____

B. _____

C. _____

D. _____

E. _____

F. _____

G. _____

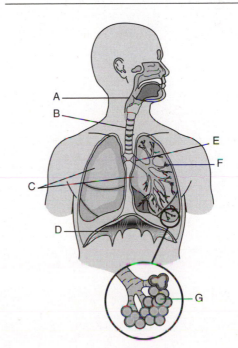

139. Name the structures of the digestive system.

A. _____

B. _____

C. _____

D. _____

E. _____

F. _____

G. _____

H. _____

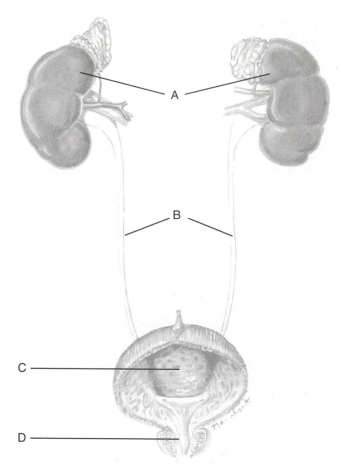

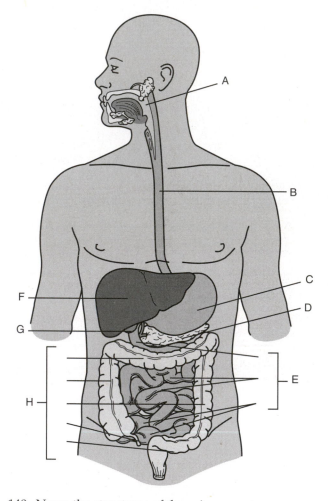

140. Name the structures of the urinary system.

A. _____

B. _____

C. _____

D. _____

(See illustration on column 2)

141. Name the structures of the male reproductive system.

A. _____

B. _____

C. _____

D. _____

E. _____

F. _____

G. _____

H. _____

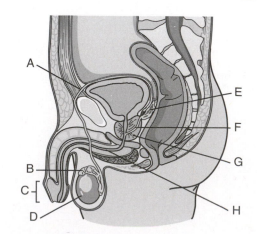

142. Name the external female genitalia.

A. _____

B. _____

C. _____

D. _____

E. _____

F. _____

Marchant

OPTIONAL LEARNING EXERCISES

143. Explain the function of each part of the cell.

A. Cell membrane _____

B. Nucleus _____

C. Cytoplasm _____

_____

D. Protoplasm _____

_____

E. Chromosomes _____

_____

F. Genes _____

_____

144. List the structures contained in the 2 skin layers.

A. Epidermis _____

_____

B. Dermis _____

_____

145. Explain the function of the types of bone.

A. Long bones _____

B. Short bones _____

C. Flat bones _____

D. Irregular bones _____

146. Describe how each type of joint moves and give an example of each type.

A. Ball and socket _____

Example: _____

B. Hinge _____

Example: _____

C. Pivot _____

Example: _____

147. Explain what happens when muscles contract.

_____

_____

_____

148. Explain the function of the three main parts of the brain. Include the function of the cerebral cortex and the midbrain, pons, and medulla.

A. Cerebrum _____

_____

Cerebral cortex _____

_____

B. Cerebellum _____

_____

C. Brainstem _____

Midbrain and pons _____

_____

Medulla _____

_____

149. Explain how the sympathetic and parasympathetic nervous systems balance each other.

_____

_____

_____

_____

150. Explain what happens to each of these structures when light enters the eye.

    A. Choroid _____

    B. Cornea _____

    C. Lens _____

    D. Retina _____

    _____

151. Explain how each of these structures helps to carry sound in the ear.

    A. Ossicles _____

    B. Cochlea _____

    C. Auditory nerve _____

152. Where are red blood cells destroyed as they wear out? _____

153. When an infection occurs, what do white blood cells do? _____

    _____

154. Explain the function of the 4 atria (chambers) of the heart.

    A. Right atrium _____

    B. Left atrium _____

    C. Right ventricle _____

    D. Left ventricle _____

155. Explain where each of these veins carries blood.

    A. Inferior vena cava _____

    _____

    B. Superior vena cava _____

    _____

156. Explain what happens in the alveoli.

    _____

    _____

    _____

    _____

157. After food is swallowed, explain what happens in each of these parts of the digestive tract.

    A. Stomach _____

    _____

    B. Duodenum _____

    C. Jejunum and ileum _____

    D. Colon _____

    E. Rectum _____

    F. Anus _____

158. Explain what happens in these structures of the kidney.

    A. Glomerulus _____

    B. Collecting tubules _____

    C. Ureters _____

    D. Urethra _____

    E. Meatus _____

159. Sperm is produced in the testicles. What happens to the sperm in each of these structures?

    A. Testes _____

    B. Vas deferens _____

    C. Seminal vesicle _____

    D. Ejaculatory duct _____

    E. Prostate gland _____

    F. Urethra _____

160. What is the function of the endometrium?

    _____

    _____

161. Menstruation occurs about every _____ days. Ovulation usually occurs on or about day

    _____ of the cycle.

162. What is the function of each of these pituitary hormones?

    A. Growth hormone _____

    B. Thyroid-stimulating hormone _____

    C. Adrenocorticotropic hormone _____

    D. Antidiuretic hormone _____

    E. Oxytocin _____

163. What is the function of insulin? _____

    _____

    _____

    What happens if too little insulin is produced?

    _____

164. What happens when the body senses an antigen?

    _____

INDEPENDENT LEARNING ACTIVITIES

- Listen to a friend's chest with a stethoscope.
  - What sounds do you hear?
  - What body systems are making the sounds?
  - Are you able to count any of the sounds you hear? What are you counting?
- Listen to your lower abdomen with a stethoscope.
  - What sounds can you hear?
  - What causes sound in the abdomen? What body system is involved in this activity?
- What is occurring when you hear your "stomach growl"? What is the term for this activity that you learned in Chapter 7?
- Look at a friend's eyes in a dimly lit area and observe the size of the pupils.
  - What size are the pupils? Are they both the same size?
  - Shine a flashlight in one eye. What happens to the pupil?
  - What happens when you move the light away? If you see a change, how quickly does it occur?

FILL IN THE BLANKS: KEY TERMS

Development	Dyspnea	Growth
Developmental task	Geriatrics	Menopause
Dysphagia	Gerontology	Presbyopia

1. When menstruation stops it is called

   _____.

2. _____ is a skill that must be completed during a stage of development.

3. Difficult, labored, or painful breathing is

   _____.

4. _____ is difficulty swallowing.

5. The care of aging people is

   _____.

6. The study of the aging process is

   _____.

7. _____ is age-related farsightedness.

8. Changes in mental, emotional, and social function

   are _____.

9. Physical changes that are measured and that occur

   in a steady, orderly manner are _____

   _____.

CIRCLE THE BEST ANSWER

10. In 2010, how many people were 65 years of age and older?
    A. 4,200,000
    B. 15,400,000
    C. 40,300,000
    D. 100,000

11. Most older people live
    A. In a nursing center
    B. Alone
    C. In a family setting
    D. With non-relatives

12. A stage of growth and development in late adulthood is
    A. Adjusting to aging parents
    B. Developing new friends and relationships
    C. Developing a satisfactory sex life
    D. Developing leisure time activities

13. A person is in the oldest-old age range when he or she is
    A. 65 to 74 years of age
    B. 75 to 84 years of age
    C. 60 to 65 years of age
    D. 85 years of age or older

14. As aging occurs
    A. Illness and disability always result
    B. Physical changes are slow
    C. The person is lonely and isolated
    D. Most persons live in nursing centers

15. Social changes include
    A. A decline in mental function
    B. Physical disabilities
    C. A need to find activities to replace the work role
    D. Decreased physical strength

16. It may be difficult to meet all self-esteem needs when retired because
    A. The person can do whatever he or she wants
    B. Work helps meet love, belonging, and self-esteem needs
    C. A retired person develops new relationships
    D. Physical strength decreases

17. Retired people may feel fulfilled and useful when they
    A. Travel
    B. Work part-time or do volunteer work
    C. Live alone
    D. Live with adult children

18. Money problems can result with retirement because
    A. Income is reduced
    B. The person lives alone
    C. The person is unable to work
    D. The person plans for retirement with savings and investments

19. Loneliness may be a bigger problem for foreign-born persons because
    A. Families from other cultures do not care about older persons
    B. The person is not accepted by native-born persons
    C. They may not have anyone to talk to in their native language
    D. They have more chronic illnesses

20. An older person can adjust to social relationship changes by
    A. Avoiding visits with family members
    B. Developing hobbies and church and community activities
    C. Asking for a private room and having meals in his or her room
    D. Staying at home alone to save money

21. When children care for older parents
    A. The older person may feel unwanted and useless
    B. The older person may feel more secure
    C. Tension may develop among the children and the family
    D. All of the above

22. What causes wrinkles to appear on an older person?
    A. Decreases in oil and sweat gland secretions
    B. Fewer nerve endings
    C. Loss of elasticity, strength, and fatty tissue layer
    D. Poor circulation

23. Skin breakdown may heal slowly in older people because
    A. Older people eat a poor diet
    B. Blood vessels are fragile
    C. The skin has more nerve endings
    D. Secretions from oil and sweat glands decrease

24. Bones may break easily because
    A. Joints become stiff and painful
    B. Joints become slightly flexed
    C. Bones lose strength and become brittle
    D. Vertebrae shorten

25. Older persons can prevent bone loss and loss of muscle strength by
    A. Staying active, exercising, and eating a healthy diet
    B. Taking hormones
    C. Resting with their feet elevated
    D. Taking vitamins

26. Dizziness may increase in older people because
    A. They have difficulty sleeping
    B. Blood flow to the brain is decreased
    C. Nerve cells are lost
    D. Brain cells are lost

27. Painful injuries and disease may go unnoticed because
    A. The person is confused
    B. Touch and sensitivity to pain are reduced
    C. Memory is shorter
    D. Blood flow is reduced

28. Eyes are irritated easily because
    A. The lens yellows
    B. The eye takes longer to adjust to changes in light
    C. Tear secretion is less
    D. The person becomes farsighted

29. If severe circulatory changes occur, the person
    A. May be encouraged to walk long distances
    B. May need to rest during the day
    C. May not do any kind of exercise
    D. Should exercise only once a week

30. A person with dyspnea can breathe easier when
    A. Lying flat in bed
    B. Covered with heavy bed linens
    C. Allowed to stay in one position on bedrest
    D. Resting in the semi-Fowler's position

31. Dulled taste and smell decreases
    A. Peristalsis
    B. Appetite
    C. Saliva
    D. Swallowing

32. Older persons need
    A. Fewer calories
    B. Less fluids
    C. More calories
    D. A low-protein diet

33. Many older persons have to urinate several times during the night because
    A. Bladder infections are common
    B. Urine is more concentrated
    C. Bladder muscles weaken and bladder size decreases
    D. Urinary incontinence may occur

34. Sexual activity in older persons changes because
    A. Orgasms for men and women are less intense or forceful
    B. The vaginal secretions increase
    C. An erection lasts longer
    D. Sex hormones increase

35. An advantage of an older person living with family is
    A. The person and family are together all of the time
    B. The family can provide care during illness or disability
    C. The person is with others the same age
    D. The person will have a private bedroom

36. Most adult day-care centers
    A. Require that the person perform some self-care
    B. Accept only persons capable of self-care
    C. Provide complete care
    D. Provide respite care

37. A common dining room and meals usually are not provided when the person lives in
    A. An apartment building
    B. Congregate housing
    C. A board and care home
    D. A residential hotel

38. Assisted living facilities provide
    A. Nursing care
    B. A place for family members to live with the person
    C. Shared household chores and expenses
    D. Social contact with other residents
39. Continuing care retirement communities (CCRCs) may have
    A. Independent living units
    B. Food service and help nearby
    C. Additional services as the person's needs change
    D. All of the above
40. Nursing centers are housing options for older persons who
    A. Need only companionship
    B. Cannot care for themselves
    C. Need care during the daytime while the family works
    D. Are developmentally disabled
41. Moving to a nursing center
    A. Is an exciting change for the older person
    B. Can cause a loss of identity
    C. Is always a permanent move
    D. Allows the person to have more personal freedom
42. A quality nursing center is
    A. Approved by the medical society
    B. Medicare-certified and Medicaid-certified
    C. Licensed by the state board of nursing
    D. Operated by the local health department
43. A quality nursing center is required to have
    A. An area with hot tubs and saunas
    B. All common areas, residents' rooms, and doorways designed for wheelchair use
    C. Toilet facilities that are shared by all residents
    D. A private room for each resident
44. OBRA's environment requirements include
    A. Hand rails, assist devices, and other surfaces in good repair
    B. A private bathroom for each resident
    C. Requiring residents to provide furniture for their rooms
    D. Using tablecloths and cloth napkins in the dining room

FILL IN THE BLANKS: ABBREVIATIONS

45. CCRC _____

46. CMS _____

47. OBRA _____

MATCHING

Match the physical change during the aging process with the body system affected.

48. _____ Reduced blood flow to kidneys
49. _____ Arteries narrow and are less elastic
50. _____ Forgetfulness
51. _____ Gradual loss of height
52. _____ Decreased strength for coughing
53. _____ Decreased secretion of oil and sweat glands
54. _____ Difficulty digesting fried and fatty foods
55. _____ Heart pumps with less force
56. _____ Bladder muscles weaken
57. _____ Difficulty seeing green and blue colors
58. _____ Difficulty swallowing
59. _____ Lung tissue less elastic
60. _____ Bone mass decreases
61. _____ Testosterone level decreases
62. _____ Facial hair in some women

A. Integumentary
B. Musculo-skeletal
C. Nervous
D. Circulatory
E. Respiratory
F. Digestive
G. Urinary
H. Reproductive

OPTIONAL LEARNING EXERCISES

Nursing Concerns Related to Physical Changes

63. When bathing an older person, what kind of soap should be used? _____

    Often no soap is used on the _____

64. If a nick or cut occurs on the feet, it can lead to a

    _____. This can

    happen because the feet usually have

    _____.

65. Skin disorders rarely cause death if they are

    _____.

66. When bone mass decreases, why is it important to

    turn an older person carefully? _____

    _____

67. Why does an older person often have a gradual

    loss of height? _____

    _____

68. What types of exercise help prevent bone loss and

    loss of muscle strength?

    _____

    _____

69. Older persons have changes in the nervous system. When the changes listed below happen, what physical problems occur?
    A. Nerve conduction and reflexes are slower

    _____

    _____

    B. Blood flow to the brain is reduced

    _____

    _____

C. Changes in brain cells

_____

_____

_____

70. When you are eating with an older person, you notice she puts salt on vegetables that taste fine to you. What may be a reason she does this?

    _____

    _____

71. A female nurse has a high-pitched voice and several residents seem to have difficulty hearing her. They do not complain about hearing the male charge nurse. What may be a reason for the difference? _____

    _____

72. How can you help the circulation of persons

    confined to bed? _____
    What other body system will be helped by this

    activity? _____

73. What can the nursing assistant do to prevent respiratory complications from bedrest?

    _____

74. The stomach and colon empty slower and flatulence and constipation are common in the older person. What causes these problems?

    _____

75. How does good oral hygiene and denture care

    improve food intake?

    _____

76. Why should you plan to give most fluids to the

    older person before 1700 (5:00 PM)? _____

    _____

INDEPENDENT LEARNING ACTIVITIES

- Interview an older person who lives independently. Use the following questions to find out what concerns the person has about remaining independent.
  - What physical problems does the person have, if any?
  - What activities are more difficult than they were when the person was younger?
  - What does the person use to provide safety? (Walkers, canes, alarms, daily phone calls, etc.)
  - What comfort measures are needed to decrease pain or help the person sleep?
  - What are transportation needs? Does the person drive? How does the person grocery shop? Visit with family and friends? Attend social functions?

- How are social needs met? How often does the person go out to socialize? How often does the person have visitors?
- Interview an older person and talk about life when the person was young.
  - Observe facial expression and tone of voice when the person talks about events remembered. What changes do you see?
  - Compare how well the person remembers events of long ago with those that happened recently.
  - How do you feel differently about the person after hearing about his or her youth?

9 SEXUALITY

FILL IN THE BLANKS: KEY TERMS

Bisexual
Erectile dysfunction (ED)
Heterosexual
Homosexual

Impotence
Sex
Sexuality

Transgender
Transsexual
Transvestite

1. _____ is a broad term used to describe people who express their sexuality or gender in other than the expected way.

2. Another name for impotence is _____

   or _____.

3. _____ is the physical, psychological, social, cultural, and spiritual factors that affect a person's feelings and attitudes about his or her sex.

4. _____ is a person who dresses like the other sex for emotional and sexual relief; cross-dresser.

5. A person attracted to both sexes is

   _____.

6. A _____ is a person who believes that he or she is a member of the other sex.

7. A _____ is a person who is attracted to members of the same sex.

8. The physical activities involving the reproductive organs that are done for pleasure or to have

   children is _____.

9. A person who is attracted to members of the other

   sex is _____.

10. The inability of the male to have an erection is

    erectile dysfunction or _____.

CIRCLE THE BEST ANSWER

11. Sexuality
    A. Involves the personality and the body
    B. Is the physical activities involving reproductive organs
    C. Is unimportant in old age
    D. Is done for pleasure or to have children

12. A women who is attracted to men is
    A. Homosexual
    B. Heterosexual
    C. Lesbian
    D. Bisexual

13. Transvestites are often
    A. Homosexual
    B. Transsexual
    C. Married and heterosexual
    D. Bisexual

14. Diabetes, spinal cord injuries, and multiple sclerosis may cause
    A. Impotence
    B. Menopause
    C. Sexual aggression
    D. Heterosexuality

15. Which of these is true about sexuality and older persons?
    A. An orgasm is more forceful in older persons than in younger persons.
    B. Older persons are unable to have intercourse.
    C. Older persons do not lose sexual needs and desires.
    D. Love and affection become less important as the person ages.

16. When older adult couples live in a nursing center, OBRA requires that they
    A. Are allowed to share the same room
    B. Are placed in separate rooms
    C. Are not encouraged to be intimate
    D. Cannot share a bed

17. If a person in a nursing center becomes sexually aroused, you should
    A. Report this to the nurse immediately
    B. Tell the person that the behavior is not allowed
    C. Stay with the person
    D. Allow for privacy

46

18. If a person touches you in the wrong way, you should
    A. Ignore it and realize that the person is not responsible
    B. Tell the person you do not like him or her
    C. Tell the person that those behaviors make you uncomfortable
    D. Refuse to give care to the person
19. If you do not share a person's sexual attitudes, values, practices, or standards, you should
    A. Not judge or gossip about the person
    B. Avoid the person
    C. Tell him or her your feelings
    D. Discuss the person's relationships with other staff members

FILL IN THE BLANKS

20. Sexuality develops when the baby's

    _____.

21. Children know their own sex at age _____.

22. Bisexuals often _____ and have

    _____.

23. Sexual function may be affected chronic illnesses such as
    A. _____
    B. _____
    C. _____
    D. _____
24. What reproductive surgeries may affect sexuality?
    A. Men _____
    B. Women _____
25. Some older people do not have intercourse. They may express their sexual needs or desires by

    _____

    _____
26. When you are assisting persons, what grooming practices will promote sexuality for residents?
    A. Men _____
    B. Women _____

27. What can you do to allow privacy for a person and a partner?
    A. Close _____.
    B. Remind the person about _____
    C. Tell other _____
    D. Knock _____
28. Masturbation is a normal _____.
29. What health-related problems may cause a person to touch his or her genitals?
    A. _____ or _____
       system disorders
    B. Poor _____
    C. Being _____ or _____ from
       urine and feces

OPTIONAL LEARNING EXERCISES

Mr. and Mrs. Davis are 78-year-old residents in a nursing center, where they share a room. They need assistance with ADL, but are mentally alert. They are an affectionate couple and care deeply for each other. Answer these questions about meeting their sexual needs.

30. Mr. Davis has diabetes and high blood pressure. What effect can these disorders have on sexuality?

    _____

    _____
31. What is an important thing you could do when Mr. and Mrs. Davis ask for privacy?

    _____

INDEPENDENT LEARNING ACTIVITIES

- Consider this situation about a sexually aggressive person. Answer the questions about how you would respond.
  SITUATION: John James is 72 years old and has paraplegia because of an accident several years ago. His caregivers report that recently he has begun to make sexually suggestive remarks. While you are giving his morning care, he touches you several times in private areas and makes frequent sexually suggestive remarks. The other nursing assistants tell you they just ignore him or joke with him about the actions.
- What would you say to Mr. James when he touches you in private areas?
- How would you respond to his suggestive remarks?

- What would you say to your colleagues who suggest you ignore or joke with Mr. James?
- Has this type of situation ever happened to you? How did you handle it then? What would you do differently after studying this chapter?
- Consider this situation about caring for a person who is gay. Answer the questions about how you would respond.

  SITUATION: *Bobbie Freeman is 45 years old and has had gallbladder surgery. While assisting her to ambulate, she begins to talk about her friend Judy. She tells you that they have been lovers for 15 years.*

- What would you say to a person who tells you she is gay?
- What effect would this information have on the care you provide for the person?
- Has this type of situation ever happened when you were caring for a person? How did you respond? How would you respond differently after studying this chapter?

10 SAFETY

FILL IN THE BLANKS: KEY TERMS

Coma
Dementia
Disaster
Electrical shock
Ground
Hazard

Hazardous substance
Hemiplegia
Incident
Paralysis
Paraplegia

Quadraplegia
Suffocation
Tetraplegia
Workplace violence

1. The loss of cognitive and social function caused by changes in the brain is _____.

2. Anything in the person's setting that may cause injury or illness is a _____.

3. Paralysis from the neck down is _____.

4. _____ is any chemical in the workplace that can cause harm.

5. A _____ is a sudden catastrophic event in which many people are injured and killed and property is destroyed.

6. _____ occurs when breathing stops from the lack of oxygen.

7. Paralysis on one side of the body is _____.

8. A _____ is a state of being unaware of one's surroundings and being unable to react or respond to people, places, or things.

9. That which carries leaking electricity to the earth and away from an electrical appliance is a _____.

10. _____ is paralysis from the waist down.

11. _____ occurs when electrical current passes through the body.

12. Violent acts directed toward persons at work or while on duty is _____.

13. An _____ is any event that has harmed or could harm a resident, staff member, or visitor.

14. _____ means loss of muscle function, loss of sensation, or loss of both muscle function and sensation.

15. Another name for quadriplegia is _____.

CIRCLE THE BEST ANSWER

16. To protect the person from harm you need to
    A. Use restraints
    B. Follow the person's care plan
    C. Limit mobility
    D. Lock all doors

17. A person's risk of accidents increases because of
    A. Obesity
    B. Poor diet
    C. Age
    D. Carelessness

18. People with dementia are at risk of injury because they
    A. No longer know what is safe and what is dangerous
    B. Are in a coma
    C. Have problems sensing heat and cold
    D. Have poor vision

19. Medications can be a risk factor for accidents because side effects can
    A. Affect hearing
    B. Reduce ability to sense heat and cold
    C. Cause loss of balance or lack of coordination
    D. Cause hemiplegia

20. Identifying the person is most important because
    A. You must give the right care to the right person
    B. Visitors may ask for your help to find someone
    C. You need to call the person by the right name
    D. You will have to give care to 2 people if you give it to the wrong person first

21. Which of these is a reliable way to identify the person?
    A. Look at the name above the bed.
    B. Use the person's ID bracelet given by the center.
    C. Ask the person's roommate to identify him or her.
    D. Just call the person by name.

22. Burns from smoking can be prevented if
    A. Smoking is allowed when the person is in bed
    B. Residents are allowed to smoke only in smoking areas
    C. No smoking is allowed
    D. Smoking materials are kept at each person's bedside

23. It is most important to store personal care items according to center policy because
    A. This keeps the person's unit tidy
    B. Everyone will be able to find the items
    C. These items can cause harm when swallowed
    D. It maintains privacy for the resident

24. Suffocation can be caused by
    A. Cutting food into small, bite-sized pieces
    B. Making sure dentures fit properly and are in place
    C. Giving oral food and fluids to a person with a feeding tube
    D. Checking the care plan for swallowing problems

25. If a person clutches the throat and is unable to speak, he or she has a
    A. Sore throat
    B. Dangerous level of carbon monoxide
    C. Severe airway obstruction
    D. Mild airway obstruction

26. When a severe foreign body airway obstruction occurs and the person is conscious, you should first
    A. Place the person in bed and go for help
    B. Perform abdominal thrusts until the object is expelled
    C. Do a finger sweep to remove the object
    D. Ask the person to cough to expel the object

27. An electrical appliance owned by the resident cannot be used if it
    A. Has a three-pronged plug
    B. Is connected directly to a wall outlet
    C. Has not been checked by the maintenance staff
    D. The cord is in good repair

28. An electrical shock is especially dangerous because it can
    A. Start a fire
    B. Damage equipment
    C. Affect the heart and cause death
    D. Violate OBRA regulations

29. If you are shocked by electric equipment, you should
    A. Take the item to the nurse
    B. Try to see what is wrong with the equipment
    C. Make sure it has a ground prong
    D. Test the equipment in a different outlet

30. Wheelchair brakes are locked when
    A. Transporting the person
    B. Taking a wheelchair up or down stairs
    C. A person is transferring to or from the wheelchair
    D. Storing the wheelchair

31. When moving a person on a stretcher, it is correct to
    A. Use safety straps or side rails only when the person is confused
    B. Unlock the stretcher before transferring the person
    C. Leave the person alone if he or she is alert
    D. Stand at the head of the stretcher. Your co-worker stands at the foot

32. A example of a health hazard caused by chemicals would be
    A. A burn from an explosion
    B. Damage to the kidneys, nervous system, lungs, skin, eyes, or mucous membranes
    C. Using oxygen in a room
    D. An ungrounded electrical plug

33. What should be done if a label is missing from a hazardous substance?
    A. Take the container to the nurse
    B. Return the container to the cupboard or shelf
    C. Use the substance as usual
    D. Leave the container where you found it and go for help

34. Where will you find information about a hazardous substance?
    A. The nurse
    B. The care plan
    C. SDS (Safety Data Sheet)
    D. The doctor's orders

35. When you are cleaning up a hazardous substance, you should
    A. Work from dirty areas to clean areas using circular motions
    B. Wear personal protective equipment when instructed to do so by the nurse
    C. Dispose of hazardous waste in sealed bags or containers
    D. Use paper towels and discard them in the regular trash

36. _____ requires a hazard communication program so that employees know how to handle hazardous substances.
    A. Omnibus Budget Reconciliation Act of 1987 (OBRA)
    B. Occupational Safety and Health Administration (OSHA)
    C. Joint Commission on Accreditation of Healthcare Organizations (JCAHO)
    D. Safety Data Sheet (SDS)

37. Where would you find the Safety Data Sheets (SDSs) for hazardous materials?
    A. Attached to the substance
    B. In the administrator's office
    C. In a binder at a certain place on each nursing unit
    D. In the patient's chart
38. If a resident is receiving oxygen, he or she is at special risk for
    A. Burns
    B. Suffocation
    C. Poisoning
    D. Electrical shock
39. A person receiving oxygen should wear
    A. Fireproof clothing
    B. Disposable clothing
    C. Cotton gown or pajamas
    D. Clothing made with wool or synthetic fabrics
40. If a fire occurs, what should you do first?
    A. Rescue people in immediate danger.
    B. Sound the nearest fire alarm and call the switchboard operator.
    C. Close doors and windows to confine the fire.
    D. Use a fire extinguisher on a small fire that has not spread to a larger area.
41. When using a fire extinguisher, the "P" in the word *PASS* means
    A. Pull the fire alarm
    B. Pull the safety pin
    C. Rescue person in immediate danger
    D. Push the handle or lever down
42. If evacuating is necessary, residents who are
    A. Closest to the outside door are rescued first
    B. Able to walk are rescued last
    C. Closest to the fire are taken out first
    D. Are helpless are rescued last
43. If there is a disaster, you
    A. Are expected to go to your nursing center immediately
    B. Should follow procedures for the nursing center
    C. Should stay away or leave to get out of the way
    D. May go home to check on your family
44. Why is workplace violence a big concern in health care?
    A. Nurses and nursing assistants have the most contact with residents and families.
    B. Acutely disturbed and violent persons may seek health care.
    C. Agency pharmacies are a source of drugs and therefore a target for robberies.
    D. All of the above.
45. Which of these would be effective in dealing with an agitated or aggressive person?
    A. Stand away from the person at a safe distance so he cannot hit or kick you.
    B. Close the door to keep the person away from others.
    C. Sit quietly with the person in her room. Hold her hand to calm her.
    D. Tell the person that his behavior is unacceptable.
46. Which of these could *not* be used as a weapon by an aggressive person?
    A. Your jewelry or scarf
    B. Long hair that is worn up and off the collar
    C. Keys, scissors, or other items
    D. Tools or items left by maintenance staff
47. Risk management involves
    A. Training the staff to understand SDSs
    B. Identifying and controlling risks and safety hazards
    C. Firing employees who have accidents
    D. Hiring security staff to prevent injuries
48. When you are filling out a valuables list or envelope, which of these would be the best description?
    A. "A diamond in a gold setting"
    B. "A one-carat diamond in a 14K gold setting"
    C. "A white stone in a yellow setting"
    D. "A white diamond-like stone in a gold-like setting"
49. Which of these would *not* be reported as an accident or error?
    A. Forgetting to give care
    B. Giving the wrong care
    C. Assisting a co-worker to give care
    D. Losing a resident's dentures

FILL IN THE BLANKS: ABBREVIATIONS

50. AED _____
51. C _____
52. CPR _____
53. EMS _____
54. F _____
55. FBAO _____
56. ID _____
57. OBRA _____
58. OSHA _____

59. PASS _____

60. RACE _____

61. SDS _____

MATCHING

Match each safety measure with the risk of injury it prevents.
  A. Burns
  B. Suffocation
  C. Poisoning
  D. Fire
  E. Electrical
  F. Wheelchair
  G. Stretcher

62. _____ Do not let the person use an electric blanket

63. _____ Keep soap and shampoo in a safe place

64. _____ Be sure that residents smoke only in smoking areas

65. _____ Keep electrical items away from water

66. _____ Make sure that casters face forward

67. _____ Do not leave the person alone

68. _____ Do not give the resident a shower or tub bath when there is an electrical storm

69. _____ Keep matches away from confused and disoriented persons

70. _____ Report loose teeth or dentures to the nurse

71. _____ Do not let the person stand on the footplates of a wheelchair

72. _____ Do not touch a person who is experiencing an electrical shock

73. _____ Move all residents from the area if you smell gas or smoke

74. _____ Do not allow smoking near oxygen tanks or concentrators

75. _____ Fasten safety straps when the person is positioned properly

FILL IN THE BLANKS

76. Before giving care, use the _____ to identify the person.

77. _____ is a gas produced by the burning of fuel.

78. Forceful _____ can remove the object causing a mild airway obstruction.

79. The abdominal thrust is not used for very _____ persons or _____ women.

80. If a ground (three-pronged) plug is not used, it can cause _____ and possible _____.

81. Before using a hazardous substance, you check the _____ for safety information.

82. If a person is receiving oxygen therapy, _____ signs are placed on the door and near the bed.

83. Color-coded wristbands are used to promote the person's safety and prevent harm. Explain what these colors mean:
  A. Red _____
  B. Yellow _____
  C. Purple _____
  D. Pink _____

84. If an incident that has harmed a person occurs, you should _____ at once.

OPTIONAL LEARNING EXERCISES

85. What factors related to age make older persons more at risk for accidents?
  A. _____ strength
  B. Poor balance makes it hard to avoid _____
  C. Less sensitive to _____ and _____

86. How does impaired smell and touch increase accident risks?
  A. Person may not detect _____ or _____ odors
  B. Person has problems sensing _____ and _____
  C. Decreased _____ sense

87. When identifying a person, why is just calling the name not enough? _____ _____

88. Warning labels on hazardous substances identify
  A. _____
  B. _____
  C. _____
  D. _____
  E. _____

89. If a person is receiving oxygen therapy, why are wool blankets and synthetic fabrics removed from the room? _____

90. What does RACE mean when a fire occurs?

    A. R _____

    _____

    B. A _____

    _____

    C. C _____

    _____

    D. E _____

91. When using a fire extinguisher, what does the word *PASS* stand for?

    A. P _____

    B. A _____

    C. S _____

    D. S _____

92. What kinds of threats are considered workplace violence?

    A. _____

    B. _____

    C. _____

93. What information is required on an incident report?

    A. _____

    B. _____

    C. _____

    D. _____

    E. _____

    F. _____

Indicate the related safety measure from textbook Box 10-4, Safety Measures to Prevent Equipment Accidents, and Box 10-5, Wheelchair and Stretcher Safety.

94. The nursing assistant tells the resident that his shower will be delayed until the storm passes.

    _____

95. The nursing assistant tells the nurse that she has never used the portable foot bath before.

    _____

96. The nursing assistant dries her hands carefully before plugging in a razor. _____

97. An electric fan will not work and the staff member follows the correct procedure to have it repaired.

    _____

98. The nursing assistant moves an electrical cord that is lying across a heat vent. _____

99. The nursing assistant makes sure that the person has both feet on the wheelchair footplates.

    _____

    _____

100. The nursing assistant notices that one wheel is flat on a wheelchair and reports it to the nurse.

    _____

    _____

101. The nursing assistant locks the wheelchair when the person is sitting in it next to her bed.

    _____

    _____

Indicate the safety measures you should follow when handling hazardous materials. (Box 10-6)

102. When cleaning up a hazardous material, how do you know what equipment to wear?

    _____

103. When a spill occurs, what is the correct way to wipe it up? _____

    _____

104. The nurse tells the nursing assistant that the resident is having an x-ray done in her room.

    _____

    _____

105. The staff opens the windows when cleaning up a hazardous material. _____

    _____

What fire prevention measure is being practiced in each of these examples? (Box 10-7)

106. The resident is taken to the smoking area in his wheelchair. _____

_____

107. When cleaning the smoking area, the staff uses a metal can partially filled with sand. _____

_____

108. When heating food for a resident, the nursing assistant remains in the kitchen. _____

_____

Answer how each of these are related to preventing or controlling workplace violence. (Box 10-8)

109. How can jewelry serve as a weapon? _____

_____

110. Why is long hair worn up? _____

_____

111. Why are few pictures, vases, and other items kept in some areas? _____

112. What type of glass protects nurses' stations, reception areas, and admitting areas? _____

_____

113. What clothing items should be worn by staff to assist the ability to run? _____

_____

Answer how each of these practices will help affect personal safety. (Box 10-9)

114. Where should you park your car in a parking garage?

_____

_____

115. What items should you keep in the car for safety?

_____

_____

116. Why is a "dry run" important? _____

_____

117. If you think someone is following you, what should you do? _____

_____

118. If someone wants your wallet or purse, what should you do? _____

_____

119. How can you use your car keys as a weapon?

_____

_____

_____

120. How can you use your thumbs as a weapon?

_____

_____

121. What part of the body can you attack on either a man or a woman? _____

_____

INDEPENDENT LEARNING ACTIVITIES

- Safety is important to everyone and needs to be practiced at all times. Check the following items or areas in your own home to determine whether it is safe.
  - What areas are adequately lighted for safety? What areas need improved lighting?
  - Check electrical cords and plugs on appliances and lamps. How many have frayed cords? Ungrounded plugs? Other problems that make them unsafe to use?
  - How many smoke detectors do you have in your home? When were the batteries last replaced? How can you check the smoke detector to make sure it is working correctly?
  - How many scatter rugs are used on slippery surfaces? How many have some type of backing to prevent slipping?
  - Where are hazardous materials (medications, cleaning solutions, painting supplies, etc.) stored? Which of these could be reached by children? What could be done to store them more safely?
- Make a list of good safety practices in your home. Make a list of safety practices that could be improved.
- Develop a plan for your home and family that helps everyone know how to escape if a fire occurs.
  - Make sure every person knows at least two escape routes from the sleeping area.
  - Practice how to check a door for heat before opening.
  - Arrange a place to meet once you are outside the building.

11 PREVENTING FALLS

FILL IN THE BLANKS: KEY TERMS

Bed rail
Gait belt
Transfer belt

1. A device used to support a person who is unsteady

   or disabled is a _____.

2. A _____ is a device that
   serves as a guard or barrier along the side of the bed.

3. Another name for a transfer belt is a

   _____.

CIRCLE THE BEST ANSWER

4. Most falls occur in
   A. Hallways
   B. Resident rooms and bathrooms
   C. Outside areas
   D. Dining areas
5. Falls are more likely to occur
   A. After midnight
   B. During shift changes
   C. At meal time
   D. In the morning after breakfast
6. Which of these would help to prevent falls?
   A. Answer call light promptly.
   B. Take the person to the bathroom once per shift.
   C. Always keep side rails up.
   D. Have the person wear socks to walk in his or
      her room.
7. What can be done to prevent falls when assisting a
   person in the shower?
   A. Support the person with your hand while he or
      she is standing in the shower.
   B. Make sure that grab bars are secure and the
      person can reach them.
   C. Always use a gait belt when giving a shower.
   D. Only give tub baths to prevent falls in the shower.
8. Bed rails
   A. Are used for all older persons
   B. Are considered restraints by OBRA
   C. Prevent falls
   D. Are never used when giving care
9. When giving care, the bed wheels are
   A. Unlocked
   B. Locked
   C. Unlocked on the side of the bed where you are
      working
   D. Locked when moving the bed

10. A transfer belt is
    A. Always applied over clothing
    B. Applied with the buckle over the spine
    C. Applied very loosely
    D. Always applied next to the skin
11. If a person begins to fall, you should
    A. Try to prevent the fall
    B. Call for help and hold the person up
    C. Ease the person to the floor
    D. Stand back and let the person fall

FILL IN THE BLANKS

12. Most falls occur between _____

    and _____.

13. Meeting basic needs may help to

    _____.

14. Grab bars are in _____ and

    by _____ and _____.

15. Tubs and showers may be made safer if they have

    _____ surfaces.

16. Alarms are used on the bed, chair, door, floor mat,

    and belt to sense _____

    _____.

17. The need for bed rails is noted in the person's

    _____ and _____.

18. You raise the bed to give care. What safety
    measures are taken during care to prevent the
    person from falling?

    A. For the person who uses side rails, _____

       _____

    B. If you need to leave the bedside for any reason,

       raise _____.

    C. For the person who does not use bed rails,

       a co-worker stands _____

    D. Never leave the person _____

       _____

    E. Always lower the bed _____

       _____.

19. Hand rails in hallways and stairways give support to persons who are _____ _____.

20. When a transfer belt is applied, you should be able to slide your _____ under the belt.

21. The transfer belt buckle is never applied over the _____.

22. When a person starts to fall, you should protect the person's _____ as you ease the person to the floor.

OPTIONAL LEARNING EXERCISES

23. Why are falls more likely to happen during shift changes? The staff are _____ _____. Confusion can occur about _____ _____.

24. Why should floor coverings be one color in areas where older persons are living? _____ _____

25. Why are falls prevented when the person's phone, lamp, and personal belongings are at the bedside? _____

26. Before using a transfer/gait belt, check with the nurse and the care plan to determine if the person has any of these conditions:
    A. _____
    B. _____
    C. _____
    D. _____
    E. _____
    F. _____
    G. _____
    H. _____

27. What kind of footwear and clothing will help to prevent falls?
    A. Footwear _____ _____
    B. Clothing _____ _____

28. Why is it important to answer call lights promptly? _____ _____

29. If a person needs bed rails, keep them up at all times except _____

30. For a person who uses bed rails, always raise the far bed rail if you _____.

31. If a person does not use bed rails and you are giving care, how do you protect the person from falling? _____ _____.

32. Wheels are locked at all times except when _____.

33. If a person starts to fall, you _____ _____. This lets you control _____.

INDEPENDENT LEARNING ACTIVITIES

- Look at the nursing center where you are assigned to answer these questions about safety.
    - How quickly are call lights answered? How does the staff know who should answer each light?
    - If you are there during a shift change, how does the staff make sure that residents do not fall?
    - What safety measures do you see being used? (Use Box 11-2 as a guide to check for these measures.)
    - How many residents use bed rails? What are the reasons these residents need bed rails?
- Practice easing a falling person to the floor with a classmate.
    - How did you support the person?
    - How did using the transfer/gait belt help to control the fall?
    - What was easy and what was difficult about this practice?
    - How did this practice help you to feel more confident about helping a falling person?

12 RESTRAINT ALTERNATIVES AND SAFE RESTRAINT USE

FILL IN THE BLANKS: KEY TERMS

Chemical restraint
Freedom of movement
Medical symptom

Physical restraint
Remove easily

1. Any change in place or position of the body or any part of the body that the person is physically able to control is _____.

2. A _____ is any manual method or mechanical device, material, or equipment attached to or near the person's body that he or she cannot remove easily and that restricts freedom of movement or normal access to one's body.

3. Any drug that is used for discipline or convenience and not required to treat medical symptoms is a

   _____.

4. A _____ is an indication or characteristic of a physical or psychological condition.

5. _____ is when the manual method, device, material, or equipment used to restrain the person can be removed intentionally by the person in the same manner it was applied by the staff.

CIRCLE THE BEST ANSWER

6. Restraints may be used
   A. Whenever the nurse feels they are necessary
   B. For the immediate physical safety of the person or others
   C. To make sure the person does not fall
   D. To decrease work for the staff

7. The decision to find ways to meet the person's safety needs is made by
   A. The doctor
   B. The nurse and family
   C. The health team at a resident care conference
   D. The nursing assistants giving care

8. Research shows that restraints
   A. Prevent falls
   B. Cause falls
   C. Are used whenever the nurse decides
   D. Are necessary protective devices

9. A person's harmful behaviors may be caused by
   A. Being afraid of a new setting
   B. Being too hot or too cold
   C. Being hungry or thirsty
   D. All of the above

10. Guidelines about using restraints are part of
    A. FDA regulations
    B. State agencies
    C. OBRA and CMS regulations
    D. All of the above

11. The Centers for Medicare & Medicaid Services (CMS) rules for restraint use say they
    A. May be used to discipline or punish a person
    B. Must be discontinued at the earliest possible time
    C. May be as restrictive as needed as decided by the staff
    D. May be used to keep a person confined to the bed or room

12. Which of these can be a physical restraint?
    A. A soft chair with a footstool to elevate the feet
    B. A bed without rails
    C. A chair with a lap-top tray attached (Geri-chair)
    D. A drug that helps a person function at his or her highest level

13. The most serious risk from restraints is
    A. Cuts, bruises, and fractures
    B. Death from strangulation
    C. Falls
    D. Depression, anger, and agitation

14. After receiving instructions about the correct use of a restraint, you should
    A. Ask for help to apply it to a person
    B. Demonstrate proper application before using it on a person
    C. Watch someone else apply it to a person
    D. Apply it to the person independently

15. Which of these is a chemical restraint?
    A. A vest restraint
    B. A chair with an attached tray
    C. A drug that affects the person's mental function
    D. Sheets tucked in so tightly they restrict movement

16. In order to use a restraint, the nurse must
    A. Get permission from the family
    B. Have a written doctor's order
    C. Get permission from the health care team
    D. Receive OBRA permission
17. Unnecessary restraint is
    A. False imprisonment
    B. Needed to give good care
    C. Acceptable if the person does not resist
    D. Acceptable if used for short periods of time
18. OBRA requires informed consent. This consent is obtained by
    A. The person's legal representative
    B. The doctor or nurse
    C. The person
    D. The nursing assistant
19. When restraining a combative and agitated person, it should be done
    A. Slowly by only one person
    B. By the nurse
    C. With enough help to protect the person and staff from injury
    D. In a public area so the person is distracted
20. The person who is restrained must be observed at least every
    A. 5 minutes
    B. 15 minutes
    C. Hour
    D. 2 hours
21. Wrist restraints are used when a person
    A. Tries to get out of bed
    B. Moves his wheelchair without permission
    C. Pulls at tubes used in medical treatments
    D. Slides out of a chair easily
22. Belt restraints
    A. Are more restrictive than other restraints
    B. May allow the person to turn from side to side
    C. Must be released by the staff
    D. Can be used only in bed
23. A vest restraint
    A. Always crosses in the front
    B. Is applied next to the skin under clothing
    C. Must be secured very tightly to be safe
    D. Crosses in the back

24. When applying wrist restraints
    A. Tie the straps to the bed rail
    B. Tie firm knots in the straps
    C. Place the restraints over clothing
    D. Place the soft part toward the skin
25. When you apply mitt restraints
    A. Make sure the person's hand is clean and dry
    B. Pad the mitt with soft material
    C. Make sure the mitt is securely tied so the hand cannot move
    D. Make sure you can slide 3 or 4 fingers between the wrist and the restraint
26. When using a vest restraint in bed
    A. The straps are secured to the movable part of the bed frame
    B. The straps are secured to the bed rail
    C. The vest crosses in the back
    D. The person can turn over
27. How can you improve the quality of life for a person with restraints?
    A. Provide water or other fluids frequently.
    B. Check often to make sure breathing and circulation are normal.
    C. Treat the person with kindness, caring, respect, and dignity.
    D. All of the above.

FILL IN THE BLANKS: ABBREVIATIONS

Write out the meaning of each abbreviation.

28. CMS _____

29. FDA _____

30. OBRA _____

31. TJC _____

MATCHING

Match each legal aspect of restraint use with the correct statement.

32. _____ The person must understand the reason for the restraints.

33. _____ Restraints are not used to punish or penalize uncooperative persons.

34. _____ The care plan must include measures to protect the person and to prevent the person from harming others.

35. _____ The doctor gives the reason for the restraint, what to use, and how long to use the restraint.

36. _____ The restraint allows the greatest amount of movement or body access possible.

37. _____ If told to apply a restraint, you must clearly understand the need.

A. Restraints must protect the person.
B. A doctor's order is required.
C. The least restrictive method is used.
D. Restraints are used only after other measures fail to protect the person.
E. Unnecessary restraint is false imprisonment.
F. Informed consent is required for restraint use.

Match each safety guideline with the correct example.

38. _____ The nurse gives you the printed instructions about applying and securing the restraint safely.

39. _____ When the restraint is removed, range-of-motion exercises are done or the person is ambulated.

40. _____ Some people become more confused because they do not know what is happening to them.

41. _____ Persons in immediate danger of harming themselves or others are restrained quickly.

42. _____ Restraints are used for as short a time as possible.

43. _____ Injuries and deaths have occurred from improper restraint and poor observation.

A. Observe for increased confusion and agitation
B. Protect the person's quality of life
C. Follow the manufacturer instructions
D. Apply restraints with enough help to protect the person and staff from injury
E. Observe the person at least every 15 minutes or more often as noted in the care plan
F. Remove or release the restraint, re-position the person, and meet basic needs at least every 2 hours

FILL IN THE BLANKS

44. When using restraints, what information is reported and recorded?

    A. _____

    B. _____

    C. _____

    D. _____

    E. _____

    F. _____

    G. _____

    H. _____

    I. _____

    J. _____

    K. _____

    L. _____

    M. _____

45. Persons restrained in a supine position must be monitored constantly because they are a great risk for _____.

46. You should carry scissors with you because in an emergency _____.

LABELING

47. Explain what is being done in the figure.

_____

_____

_____

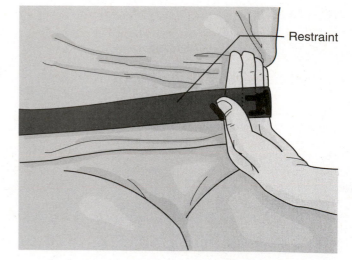

Restraint

OPTIONAL LEARNING EXERCISES

48. Drugs or drug dosages are chemical restraints if they

    A. _____

    B. _____

49. How does a restraint increase incontinence?

    _____

    _____

50. What life-long habits and routines could be included in the nursing care plan as alternatives to restraints? _____

    _____

    _____

51. Why would a person in restraints be at risk for dehydration? _____

    _____

52. Why would videotapes of family and friends or visiting with family be good alternatives to restraints? _____

    _____

INDEPENDENT LEARNING ACTIVITIES

- *Role play:* One person is a nursing assistant and one is a person who is restrained. An active physical restraint is applied as the person sits in a chair or wheelchair. Once the restraint is in place, the nursing assistant leaves and does not return for 15 minutes. Discuss the following questions after the experiment.
  - How did the person feel when the restraints were applied? What did the nursing assistant tell the person about the restraints?
  - Did the nursing assistant ask the person if toileting was needed? If the person was thirsty?
  - Was the chair comfortable? Was there any padding? Did the nursing assistant check for wrinkles? Could the person move around to re-position himself or herself for comfort?

- How was the person able to get help during the 15 minutes of being alone?
- What diversions were offered while the person was restrained? TV or radio? Reading materials? A window with a pleasant view? If any of these were provided, who chose the channel, station, book, or view?
- Was the person told someone would return in 15 minutes? Was a clock or watch available to see the time? How long did it seem?
- What was learned from this experience by both people?

13 PREVENTING INFECTION

FILL IN THE BLANKS: KEY TERMS

Asepsis
Biohazardous waste
Carrier
Clean technique
Communicable disease
Contagious disease
Contamination
Disinfection
Germicide
Healthcare-associated infection (HAI)

Immunity
Infection
Infection control
Medical asepsis
Microbe
Microorganism
Non-pathogen
Normal flora
Pathogen
Reservoir

Spore
Sterile
Sterile field
Sterile technique
Sterilization
Surgical asepsis
Vaccination
Vaccine

1. A human or animal that is a reservoir for microbes but does not have signs and symptoms of infection is a _____.

2. A _____ is a small living plant or animal seen only with a microscope.

3. Protection against a certain disease is

_____

4. A preparation that contains dead or weakened microbes and is given to produce immunity against an infectious disease is a _____.

5. A work area free of all pathogens and

non-pathogens is a _____.

6. _____ is items contaminated with blood, body fluids, secretions, and excretions that may be harmful to others.

7. _____ is the administration of a vaccine to produce immunity against an infectious disease.

8. _____ is the practices used to remove or destroy pathogens and to prevent their spread from one person or place to another person or place.

9. A communicable disease is also called a _____

_____

10. An _____ is a disease state resulting from the invasion and growth of microorganisms in the body.

11. _____ is the practice that keeps equipment and supplies free of all microbes.

12. A _____ is a disease caused by pathogens that spread easily.

13. The process of destroying pathogens is

_____.

14. A _____ is an infection acquired in a health care agency.

15. _____ is being free of disease-producing microbes.

16. Another name for a microorganism is a

_____.

17. The environment in which microbes live and grow

is a _____ or host.

18. Medical asepsis is also called _____

_____

19. The process of becoming unclean is

_____

20. The absence of all microbes is _____

_____

21. Surgical asepsis is also called _____

_____

22. A bacterium protected by a hard shell that forms

around microbes is a _____.

23. _____ are microbes that usually live and grown in a certain location.

24. A disinfectant applied to the skin, tissue, or

non-living objects is a _____

25. A microbe that does not usually cause an infection is a _____.

26. _____ is a process of destroying all microbes.

27. A microbe that is harmful and causes an infection is a _____.

28. Practices and procedures that prevent the spread of infection is _____.

CIRCLE THE BEST ANSWER

29. Germs are a type of microbe called
    A. Protozoa
    B. Fungi
    C. Viruses
    D. Bacteria
30. *Rickettsiae* are transmitted to humans by
    A. Plants
    B. Other humans
    C. Insect bites
    D. One-celled animals
31. In order to live and grow, all microbes need
    A. Oxygen
    B. A reservoir
    C. A hot environment
    D. Plenty of light
32. Normal flora
    A. Are always pathogens
    B. Are always non-pathogens
    C. Become pathogens when transmitted from their natural site to another site
    D. Cause signs and symptoms of an infection
33. Multidrug-resistant organisms
    A. Are killed easily by antibiotics
    B. Are normal flora
    C. Can resist the effects of antibiotics
    D. Are not a serious problem
34. If a person has a MRSA infection, this means the person
    A. Is infected with normal flora and is not infectious
    B. Has a methicillin-resistant staphylococcus infection
    C. Has a vancomycin-resistant enterococcus infection
    D. Can be cured easily with antibiotics
35. When caring for a person with a *C. difficile* infection, it is important to
    A. Wear a face mask and gown
    B. Use only alcohol-based hand sanitizers
    C. Wash hands with soap and warm water
    D. Make sure the person eats all of the meals served
36. Which of these is a sign or symptom of infection?
    A. Normal vital signs (temperature, pulse, and respirations)
    B. Increased activity and energy
    C. Sores on mucous membranes
    D. Increased appetite

37. The source of infection is
    A. A break in the skin
    B. A human or animal
    C. Poor nutritional status
    D. A pathogen
38. In the chain of infection, one portal of exit is
    A. Blood
    B. Humans and animals
    C. A pathogen
    D. A carrier
39. Healthcare-associated infections often occur when
    A. Insects are present
    B. Hand washing is poor
    C. Medical asepsis is used correctly
    D. A person is in isolation
40. The practice that keeps equipment and supplies free of all microbes is
    A. Medical asepsis
    B. Clean technique
    C. Contamination
    D. Surgical asepsis
41. What is the easiest and most important way to prevent the spread of infection?
    A. Sterilize all equipment.
    B. Use only disposable equipment.
    C. Keep all residents in isolation.
    D. Practice good hand washing (hand hygiene).
42. When washing hands you should
    A. Use hot water
    B. Keep hands lower than the elbows
    C. Turn off faucets after lathering
    D. Keep hands higher than elbows
43. Clean under fingernails by rubbing your fingers against your palms
    A. Each time you wash your hands
    B. If you have long nails
    C. Only for the first hand washing of the day
    D. For at least 10 seconds
44. To avoid contaminating your hands, turn off the faucets
    A. After soap is applied
    B. Before drying hands
    C. With clean, dry paper towels
    D. With your elbows
45. When cleaning dirty equipment
    A. Wear personal protective equipment (PPE)
    B. Rinse in hot water first
    C. Use the clean utility room
    D. Remove any organic materials with a paper towel
46. What should be done with non-disposable equipment when a resident leaves a facility?
    A. Send it home with the family.
    B. Discard it.
    C. Clean, disinfect, and then sterilize it.
    D. Give it to another resident.

47. How are re-usable items such as wheelchairs or commodes disinfected?
    A. Sterilized using surgical asepsis
    B. Cleaned with germicides
    C. Boiling water or steam is used
    D. Dusted with a dry cloth
48. Residents with dementia are protected from infection when the staff
    A. Keep the person confined to his or her room
    B. Wear gloves when in contact with the person
    C. Practice isolation precautions when caring for the person
    D. Assist them with hand washing
49. Isolation precautions are used
    A. For all residents
    B. During a sterile procedure
    C. To prevent the spread of communicable or contagious diseases
    D. When cleaning a room after a resident is discharged
50. You can make a person in isolation more comfortable if you
    A. Organize your work so you can stay to visit with the person
    B. Avoid going to the room to allow the person to rest
    C. Keep the room dark and quiet
    D. Make sure no visitors enter the room
51. When you don personal protective equipment (PPE), you
    A. May go in and out of the room to get supplies
    B. Must remove it before leaving the room
    C. May take it off and keep it in the room to don later
    D. Hang it up to dry it if becomes wet while giving care
52. Standard Precautions are used
    A. For a person with a respiratory infection
    B. For a person with a wound infection
    C. For a person with tuberculosis
    D. In the care of all residents
53. A person placed in airborne precautions may have
    A. Meningitis, pneumonia, or influenza
    B. A wound infection
    C. Mumps, rubella, or pertussis
    D. Measles, chicken pox, or tuberculosis
54. Health team members are restricted from the room when the person has an airborne infection if
    A. The person has skin lesions
    B. The team member is susceptible to the infection
    C. The person is sneezing or coughing
    D. The skin lesions are not covered
55. When a person has contact precautions, a gown should be worn
    A. At all times
    B. When making a safety check of the person
    C. When you are delivering a food tray
    D. When clothing may have direct contact with the person

56. Gloves worn in Standard Precautions
    A. Do not need to be changed when performing several tasks for the same person
    B. Do not need to be changed as you care for different persons
    C. Should be changed before giving care to a different person
    D. Are worn only when the person has an infection
57. If you are allergic to latex gloves, you should
    A. Wash hands each time you remove the gloves
    B. Make sure the gloves have powder inside
    C. Report the allergy to the nurse
    D. Never wear any gloves
58. When wearing gloves you know that
    A. The inside of the glove is contaminated
    B. Slightly used gloves can be saved and re-used
    C. You may need more than one pair of gloves for a task
    D. Gloves are easier to put on when hands are damp
59. When removing gloves
    A. Pull the glove down over your hand so it is inside out
    B. Pull off the gloves by the fingers
    C. Reach inside one glove with the other gloved hand to pull it off
    D. Hold the discarded gloves tightly in your hands
60. Hands are washed or decontaminated
    A. After removing gloves
    B. For 5 minutes between residents
    C. Only when moving between residents
    D. Only if gloves were not worn
61. When donning a gown, what is tied first?
    A. Strings at the back of the neck
    B. The waist strings at the back
    C. Mask ties
    D. It does not matter
62. When removing protective apparel, which of these is done first?
    A. Remove the goggles or face shield.
    B. Remove the gloves.
    C. Remove the gown.
    D. Untie the gown.
63. When removing a mask, touch only the ties or elastic bands because
    A. The front of the mask is contaminated
    B. The front of the mask is sterile
    C. Your gloves are contaminated
    D. Your hands are contaminated
64. Re-usable eyewear is contaminated after use and
    A. Should be discarded
    B. Should be autoclaved
    C. Is washed with soap and water and then a disinfectant
    D. Is rinsed in cool running water

65. How are contaminated items identified when sent to the laundry or trash collection?
    A. Bags are transparent so materials are visible.
    B. They are labeled as "contaminated."
    C. They are always double-bagged.
    D. They are labeled with a *BIOHAZARD* symbol.
66. How are specimen containers handled in an isolation room?
    A. All are double-bagged.
    B. They are put in the biohazard bag.
    C. Testing must be done in the room.
    D. Special specimen containers are needed.
67. If a resident in isolation precautions must be transported to another area
    A. The person wears a mask as required by Transmission-Based Precautions
    B. The person wears PPE as required
    C. The elevator is disinfected before anyone else can use it
    D. The wheelchair or stretcher stays with the person and is used only for him or her
68. Which of these will help a person in isolation meet the need for love, belonging, and self-esteem?
    A. Avoid the room so you do not disturb the person.
    B. Let the person see your face before putting on the mask.
    C. Discourage the person from using the telephone to contact friends.
    D. Remind the person often that he or she has a contagious disease.
69. Persons with dementia in isolation may have increased confusion and agitation because
    A. The infection increases confusion
    B. Personal protective equipment may increase these behaviors
    C. They feel dirty and undesirable
    D. They do not receive any visitors
70. What viruses are bloodborne pathogens?
    A. Influenza and pneumococcus
    B. Measles and chicken pox
    C. HIV and HBV
    D. Staphylococcus and streptococcus
71. Which of these items can transmit bloodborne pathogens?
    A. Laundry soiled with blood or other potentially infectious materials
    B. Items caked with dried blood
    C. Contaminated sharps
    D. All of the above
72. How do staff members know what to do if exposed to a bloodborne pathogen?
    A. Training and information must be provided upon employment and yearly by employers.
    B. Information is provided on the Internet.
    C. They may attend classes offered at colleges or hospitals.
    D. The nurse tells them what they need to know.

73. The hepatitis B (HBV) vaccine
    A. Requires only 1 vaccination
    B. Must be given every year
    C. Involves 3 injections
    D. Is required by law
74. Which of these is a work practice control to reduce exposure risks?
    A. Discard contaminated needles and sharp instruments in regular trash containers.
    B. Shear (break) contaminated needles before discarding them.
    C. Do not store food or drinks where blood or potentially infectious materials are kept.
    D. Wash hands only if you have not worn gloves.
75. Personal protective equipment
    A. Is free to employees
    B. Is purchased by staff members
    C. Must be worn by all employees instead of regular uniforms
    D. Must be laundered by the employee
76. If glass is broken
    A. It can be picked up carefully with gloved hands
    B. It is cleaned up with a brush and dustpan
    C. A person specially trained to remove biohazardous materials is required to clean it up
    D. It is wiped up with wet paper towels
77. When discarding regulated waste, the containers are
    A. Colored red and labeled with the *BIOHAZARD* symbol
    B. Labeled as "contaminated" in red letters
    C. Melt-away bags
    D. Cloth re-usable bags
78. If an exposure incident occurs
    A. Report it only if you had a skin break or needle-stick
    B. You can have free medical evaluation and follow-up
    C. Wait at least 90 days before having a blood test
    D. See your own doctor to maintain confidentiality in the workplace
79. If a sterile item touches a clean item
    A. It can still be used
    B. It is no longer sterile
    C. It should be handled with sterile gloves
    D. It can be placed on the sterile field
80. When working with a sterile field, you should
    A. Always wear a mask
    B. Keep items within your vision and above your waist
    C. Keep the door open
    D. Wear clean gloves
81. When arranging the inner package of sterile gloves
    A. Have the right glove on the left and the left glove on the right
    B. Have the fingers pointing toward you
    C. Have the right glove on the right and the left glove on the left
    D. Straighten the gloves to remove the cuff

82. When picking up the first sterile glove
    A. Touch only the cuff and inside of the glove
    B. Reach under the cuff with your fingers
    C. Grasp the edge of the glove with your hand
    D. Slide your hand into the glove without touching it with the other hand

FILL IN THE BLANKS: ABBREVIATIONS

Write out the meaning of each abbreviation.

83. AIIR _____

84. CDC _____

85. C. diff _____

86. cm _____

87. HAI _____

88. HBV _____

89. HIV _____

90. MDRO _____

91. MRSA _____

92. OPIM _____

93. OSHA _____

94. PPE _____

95. TB _____

96. VRE _____

MATCHING

Match the kind of asepsis being used to each example.
    A. Medical asepsis (clean technique)
    B. Surgical asepsis (sterile technique)

97. _____ An item is placed in an autoclave.
98. _____ Each person has his or her own toothbrush, towel, washcloth, and other personal care items.
99. _____ Hands are washed before preparing food.
100. _____ Non-disposable items are cleaned, disinfected, and then sterilized.
101. _____ All pathogens, including spores, are destroyed.
102. _____ Hands are washed every time you use the bathroom.

Match each statement to the link in the chain of infection it would control.
    A. Reservoir (host)
    B. Portal of exit
    C. Method of transmission
    D. Portal of entry
    E. Susceptible host

103. _____ Provide the person with tissues to use when coughing or sneezing.
104. _____ Make sure linens are dry and wrinkle-free to protect the skin.
105. _____ Use leak-proof plastic bags for soiled tissues, linens, and other materials.
106. _____ Wear protective equipment.
107. _____ Hold equipment and linens away from your uniform.
108. _____ Assist with cleaning or clean the genital area after elimination.
109. _____ Clean from cleanest area to the dirtiest.
110. _____ Label bottles.
111. _____ Follow the care plan to meet the person's nutritional and fluid needs.
112. _____ Make sure drainage tubes are properly connected.
113. _____ Do not use items that are on the floor.
114. _____ Assist the person with coughing and deep-breathing exercises as directed.
115. _____ Do not sit on a person's bed. You will pick up microorganisms and transfer them.

Match each practice to the correct principle for surgical asepsis.
    A. A sterile item can touch only another sterile item
    B. A sterile field or sterile items are always kept within your vision and above your waist
    C. Airborne microbes can contaminate sterile items or a sterile field
    D. Fluids flow downward, in the direction of gravity
    E. The sterile field is kept dry, unless the area below it is sterile
    F. The edges of a sterile field are contaminated
    G. Honesty is essential to sterile technique

116. _____ Consider any item as contaminated if unsure of its sterility.
117. _____ Wear a mask if you need to talk during the procedure.
118. _____ Place all sterile items inside the 1-inch margin of the sterile field.
119. _____ Do not turn your back on a sterile field.
120. _____ Prevent drafts by closing the door and avoiding extra movements.
121. _____ Avoid spilling and splashing when pouring sterile fluids into sterile containers.
122. _____ If you cannot see an item, it is contaminated.
123. _____ You know when you contaminated an item or a field. Report it to the nurse.
124. _____ Hold wet items down.

LABELING

125. The illustration shows how to remove gloves. List the steps of the procedure shown in each drawing

A. (1) _____

    (2) _____

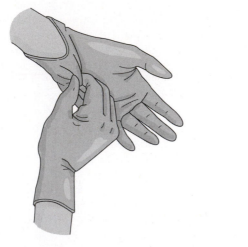

B. (1) _____

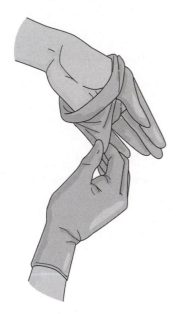

C. (1) _____

    (2) _____

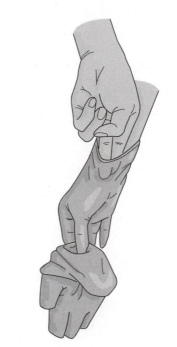

D. (1) _____

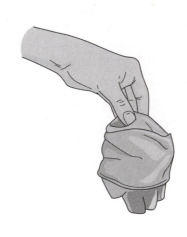

126. In this figure, color the part of the sterile field that would not be sterile.

How wide is this space? _____

133. What information does the nursing assistant need from the nurse or care plan when the person requires isolation precautions?

A. _____

B. _____

C. _____

134. If a person has measles and you are susceptible, what should you do? _____

_____

135. If a person in airborne precautions must leave the room, the person must wear

_____.

136. How is preventing the spread of infection an important part of your job? _____

_____

_____

OPTIONAL LEARNING EXERCISES

127. Compare medical asepsis to surgical asepsis.

Medical asepsis is _____

_____ .

Surgical asepsis is _____

_____

_____ .

128. Why are hands and forearms kept lower than elbows in hand washing? _____

_____

129. What is the least time you should wash hands?

_____

130. Why is lotion applied after hand washing?

_____

_____

131. Gloves are worn in Standard Precautions when contact is likely with

A. _____

B. _____

C. _____

D. _____

E. _____

132. Masks, goggles, and face shields are worn for procedures and tasks that are likely to cause

_____

137. How does wearing gloves protect you and the person? It protects you _____

_____ . It protects the person

_____

_____ .

138. Why is a gown turned inside out as you remove it?

_____

_____

139. If you are wearing gloves, gown, eyewear, and mask, in what order are they donned? _____

_____

140. When you remove gloves, gown, eyewear, and mask, in what order are they taken off? _____

_____

141. Why is a moist mask or gown changed?

_____

142. What basic needs may not be met when a person is in isolation? _____

_____

143. In addition to blood, what are other potentially infectious materials (OPIM)?

A. _____

_____

_____

B. _____

_____

_____

C. _____

_____

_____

144. What information is included in training about bloodborne pathogens?

A. _____

_____

B. _____

_____

C. _____

_____

D. _____

_____

E. _____

_____

F. _____

_____

G. _____

_____

H. _____

_____

I. _____

_____

J. _____

_____

145. How are containers used for contaminated sharps

identified? _____

_____

146. OSHA requires these measures for safely handling and using personal protective equipment.

A. _____

B. _____

C. _____

D. _____

E. _____

F. _____

G. _____

H. _____

147. If you are asked to assist with a sterile procedure, what information do you need before beginning?

A. _____

B. _____

C. _____

D. _____

E. _____

F. _____

INDEPENDENT LEARNING ACTIVITIES

• Hand washing practices are important to use whenever you are to prevent the spread of infection. Use this exercise to make yourself aware of your own habits.
  • Make a list of when you washed your hands for 1 day.
    • How did you wash your hands? Did you use the method taught in this chapter?
    • How many times did you wash your hands at work? At home?
    • How many times did you realize you had forgotten to wash your hands? What were the reasons you forgot?
  • How can you improve your hand washing practices? What will you change after studying this chapter?

CROSSWORD

Fill in the crossword by choosing words from this list.

Asepsis   Germicide   Latex   PPE
Biohazard   HAI   Microbe   Reservoir
Carrier   HBV   MSRA   Virus
Contamination   HIV   OPIM   VRE

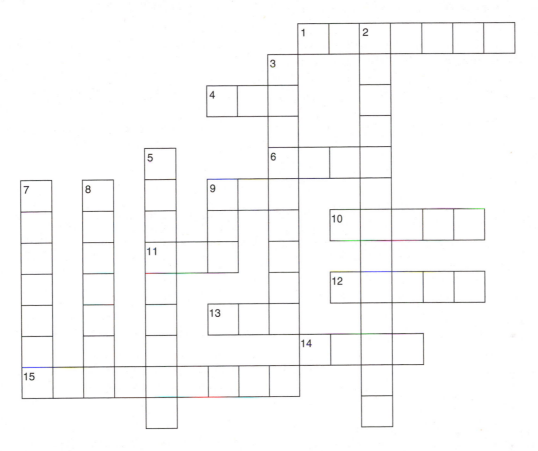

Across

1. Small living plant or animal
4. Abbreviation for personal protective equipment—gloves, mask, gown, and goggles or face shield worn to protect yourself
6. Abbreviation for methicillin-resistant *Staphylococcus aureus*—a bacterium that can cause serious wound infections and pneumonia
9. Abbreviation for infection acquired in a health care agency
10. One type of microbe; it grows in living cells
11. Abbreviation for human immunodeficiency virus
12. A rubber product used to make some gloves; some people are allergic to this
13. Abbreviation for vancomycin-resistant *Enterococcus*—a bacterium that can cause urinary tract, wound, pelvic, and other infections
14. Human body fluids, any tissue or organ, and HIV-containing cells that may cause infections
15. Humans and animals where a pathogen can grow and multiply

Down

2. The process of becoming unclean
3. Disinfectant applied to skin, tissue, and non-living objects
5. Symbol placed on contaminated linens or contaminated items before removing them from a person's room
7. A reservoir that does not have signs or symptoms of infection but can pass the infection to others
8. Being free of disease-producing microbes
9. Hepatitis B virus

14 BODY MECHANICS AND SAFE RESIDENT HANDLING, POSITIONING, AND TRANSFERS

FILL IN THE BLANKS: KEY TERMS

Base of support
Body alignment
Body mechanics
Dorsal recumbent position
Ergonomics
Fowler's position

Friction
Lateral position
Logrolling
Posture
Prone position
Semi-prone side position

Shearing
Side-lying position
Sims' position
Supine position
Transfer

1. _____ is another name for lateral position.

2. _____ or posture is the way the head, trunk, arms, and legs are aligned with one another.

3. When the skin sticks to a surface while muscles slide in the direction the body is moving, it is called _____.

4. The _____ is the same as the back-lying or supine position.

5. The area on which an object rests is the _____.

6. _____ is a left side-lying position in which the upper leg is sharply flexed so that it is not on the lower leg and the lower arm is behind the person.

7. A semi-sitting position with the head of the bed elevated 45 to 90 degrees is _____.

8. Lying on the abdomen with the head turned to one side is _____.

9. _____ is using the body in an efficient and careful way

10. The back-lying or dorsal recumbent position is also called the _____.

11. _____ is another name for body alignment.

12. _____ is turning the person as a unit, in alignment, with one motion.

13. _____ is the science of designing the job to fit the worker.

14. When the person lies on one side or the other it is the side-lying or _____ position.

15. Another name for the Sims' position is _____.

16. Using the body in an efficient and careful way is _____.

17. _____ is the rubbing of one surface against another.

CIRCLE THE BEST ANSWER

18. Using good body mechanics will
    A. Prevent good posture
    B. Cause back injuries
    C. Reduce the risk of injury, especially to the back
    D. Cause muscle injury

19. For a wider base of support
    A. Keep your feet close together
    B. The head, trunk, arms, and legs are aligned with one another
    C. Stand with your feet apart
    D. Make sure you are in good physical condition

20. When you bend your knees and squat to lift a heavy object, you are
    A. Using good body alignment
    B. In danger of injury
    C. Likely to strain your back
    D. Using good body mechanics

21. If you need to move a heavy object
    A. Push, slide, or pull the object
    B. Always work alone
    C. Bend at the waist to lift from the floor
    D. Keep feet close together

22. The risk of work-related musculo-skeletal disorders (MSDs) increases
    A. When the worker does not exercise regularly
    B. When the worker is small and weak
    C. When a task involves repeating an action to move persons
    D. Only when the staff member is using poor body mechanics

23. If you have pain when standing or rising from a seated position, you
    A. May have a back injury
    B. Are using poor body mechanics
    C. Have worked too many hours
    D. Should exercise more

24. Which of these nursing tasks are known to be a high risk for musculo-skeletal disorders (MSDs)?
    A. Using good body mechanics when transferring a person
    B. Getting help when lifting or moving heavy objects
    C. Picking up a person from the floor to the bed
    D. Lifting with forceful movement

25. Which of these activities will help prevent back injury?
    A. Reach across the bed to give care.
    B. Bend at the waist to pick up an object from the floor.
    C. Lift an object above your shoulder.
    D. Get help from a co-worker to move heavy objects.

26. When caring for a person, regular position changes and good alignment
    A. Cause pressure ulcers and contractures
    B. Promote comfort and well-being
    C. Interrupt rest and sleep
    D. Decrease circulation

27. A resident who depends on the nursing team for position changes needs to be positioned
    A. At least every 2 hours
    B. Once an hour
    C. Every 15 minutes
    D. Once a shift

28. Linens need to be clean, dry, and wrinkle-free to help prevent
    A. Pressure ulcers
    B. Contractures
    C. Breathing problems
    D. Frequent repositioning

29. Most older persons have limited range of motion in their necks and so do not tolerate
    A. Lateral position
    B. Sims' position
    C. Fowler's position
    D. Prone position

30. When positioning a person in the supine position, the nurse may ask you to place a pillow under the person's lower legs to
    A. Improve the circulation
    B. Assist the person to breathe easier
    C. Lift the heels off of the bed
    D. Prevent swelling of the legs and feet

31. A small pillow is positioned against the person's back in the
    A. Lateral position
    B. Prone position
    C. Supine position
    D. Semi-Fowler's position

32. In the chair position, a pillow is not used
    A. To position paralyzed arms
    B. To support the feet
    C. Under the upper arm and hand
    D. Behind the back if restraints are used

33. To prevent injuries when moving older persons
    A. Move the person without help
    B. Grab the person under the arms
    C. Allow the person to move himself or herself
    D. Move the person carefully to prevent injury or pain

34. To prevent work-related injuries, OSHA recommends that
    A. Manual lifting be minimized or eliminated when possible
    B. Manual lifting be used at all times
    C. You never lift any person or object alone
    D. You always use mechanical lifts for any lifting

35. When moving residents, it is best if you move the person
    A. By yourself
    B. With at least 2 staff members
    C. Using a mechanical lift
    D. Only with staff members that you like

36. When moving a person up in bed, prevent hitting the head-board with the head by
    A. Keeping the person in good body alignment
    B. Placing the pillow upright against the head-board
    C. Placing your hand on the person's head
    D. Asking the person to bend his or her neck forward

37. Which of these would be correct when you are using manual lifting?
    A. Reach across the bed to grasp the person.
    B. Stand with your feet wide apart and bend your knees.
    C. Keep the bed in the lowest position.
    D. Do not ask co-workers for help.

38. If a person with dementia resists being moved, you should
    A. Move the person by yourself
    B. Proceed slowly and use a calm, pleasant voice
    C. Leave the person alone and do not re-position him or her
    D. Tell the person firmly that he or she must cooperate with being moved

39. When you are delegated to move a person in bed, you need to know
    A. Whether the person has eaten recently
    B. Whether the person is awake
    C. How many workers are needed to move the person safely
    D. Whether the person wishes to be moved at this time

40. When the person can bear some weight, can sit up with help, and may be able to pivot to transfer, you know that the person's level of dependence is
    A. Code 4
    B. Code 3
    C. Code 2
    D. Code 1

41. When turning a person, it is important to
    A. Place the person in the prone position
    B. Make sure the person's face, nose, and mouth are not obstructed by a pillow
    C. Always turn the person toward you
    D. Only use logrolling

42. Why are beds raised to move persons in bed?
    A. It prevents the person from falling out of bed.
    B. It reduces friction and shearing.
    C. It prevents pulling on drainage tubes.
    D. This reduces bending and reaching.

43. How can you reduce friction and shearing?
    A. Raise the head of the bed to a sitting position before moving the person.
    B. Roll the person to re-position him or her.
    C. Pull the person up in bed by grasping under the arms.
    D. Massage the skin.

44. When raising a person's head and shoulders
    A. It is best to have help with an older person to prevent pain and injury
    B. A mechanical lift should be used
    C. You can always do this alone
    D. A transfer belt will be needed

45. In order to correctly raise the head and shoulders
    A. Both of your hands are placed under the person's back
    B. The person puts his near arm under your near arm and behind your shoulder
    C. Use a lift sheet to raise the person up
    D. Your free arm rests on the edge of the bed

46. You may move a person up in bed alone if the
    A. Person can assist and use a trapeze
    B. Rest of the staff is busy and cannot help
    C. Nurse tells you to use a lift sheet or slide sheet
    D. Nurse tells you have to move the person alone

47. What is the position of the bed when you are moving a person up in bed?
    A. Fowler's
    B. Flat
    C. As flat as possible for the person's condition
    D. Semi-Fowler's

48. The person is moved
    A. On the "count of 3"
    B. On the "count of 2"
    C. When the person says he or she is ready
    D. As soon as all workers are in position

49. An assist device such as a lift sheet is used
    A. For most residents
    B. Only for a person with a dependence level of Code 1
    C. Only for a person with a dependence level of Code 4
    D. For a person with dementia

50. Where is the lift sheet positioned?
    A. Under the head and shoulders
    B. Under the buttocks
    C. From the head to above the knees or lower
    D. From the hips to below the knees

51. When using a lift sheet as an assist device, the workers should
    A. Roll the sheet up close to the person
    B. Grasp the sheet at the edges
    C. Move one side of the sheet at a time
    D. Grasp the sheet only at the top edge

52. A person is moved to the side of the bed before turning because
    A. It makes it easier to turn the person
    B. It prevents injury to the person
    C. Otherwise, after turning, the person lies on the side of the bed and not in the middle
    D. It prevents friction and shearing

53. When you move a person in segments, you should
    A. Begin by first moving the hips and legs
    B. First place your arms under the person's neck and shoulders and grasp the far shoulder
    C. Move the center part of the body by placing one arm under the waist and one arm under the legs
    D. First move the legs and feet

54. When using a drawsheet to move a person to the side of the bed, support the
    A. Back
    B. Knees
    C. Head
    D. Hips

55. After the person is turned
    A. Give the person good personal care
    B. Position him or her in good body alignment
    C. Elevate the head of the bed
    D. Elevate the bed to its highest position

56. When delegated to turn a person, you get the information you need
    A. From the doctor's orders
    B. By asking your co-workers
    C. From the nurse and care plan
    D. By asking the person how he or she wants to be turned

57. When a person is turned, musculo-skeletal injuries, skin breakdown, and pressure ulcers could occur if a person is not in
    A. A special bed
    B. Good body alignment
    C. Good body mechanics
    D. The middle of the bed

58. How do you decide whether to turn the person toward you or away from you?
    A. Check the doctor's order.
    B. It depends on the person's condition and the situation.
    C. Use the method you like best.
    D. Ask the person which way is best.

59. Why do you need 2 or 3 staff members to logroll a person?
    A. A person who is being logrolled is usually in pain.
    B. It is important to keep the spine straight and in alignment.
    C. The person probably has a Code 4 level of dependence and needs extra help.
    D. No assist devices are used when you logroll.

60. When preparing to logroll a person, place a pillow
    A. At the head of the bed
    B. Between the knees
    C. Under the head
    D. Under the shoulders

61. What information do you need before dangling a person?
    A. The person's diagnosis
    B. When the person ate last
    C. The person's dependence level
    D. Whether the person likes to dangle

62. What should you do if a person who is dangling becomes faint or dizzy?
    A. Lay the person down.
    B. Go and report this to the nurse.
    C. Tell the person to take deep breaths.
    D. Have the person move his or her legs back and forth in circles.

63. When preparing to dangle a person, the head of the bed should be
    A. Flat
    B. Slightly raised
    C. In a sitting position
    D. At a comfortable height for the person

64. When preparing to transfer a person, you should
    A. Arrange the room so there is enough space for a safe transfer
    B. Keep furniture in the position the resident likes
    C. Remove all furniture from the room
    D. Ask the person how to arrange the furniture

65. The person being transferred should wear non-skid footwear to
    A. Protect the person from falls
    B. Allow the person to bend the feet more easily
    C. Promote comfort for the person
    D. Keep the feet warm

66. Lock the bed, wheelchair, or assist device wheels when transferring to
    A. Help the staff use good body mechanics
    B. Prevent damage to the equipment being used
    C. Prevent the bed and the device from moving during the transfer
    D. Make sure the person is kept in good body alignment

67. When a person is transferring from a chair or wheelchair, help the person out of bed on
    A. The right side of the bed
    B. His or her strong side
    C. His or her weak side
    D. The side of the bed that is most convenient for the staff

68. Which of these is the preferred method for chair or wheelchair transfers?
    A. Use a gait/transfer belt.
    B. Have the person put his or her arms around your neck.
    C. Put your arms around the person and the grasp the shoulder blades.
    D. Always use a mechanical lift.

69. When a person is seated in a wheelchair, you can increase the person's comfort by
    A. Placing pillows around the person
    B. Making sure nothing covers the vinyl seat and back
    C. Covering the back and seat with a folded bath blanket
    D. Removing any cushions or positioning devices

70. When you transfer a person, the nurse may ask you to take and report what before and after the transfer?
    A. Blood pressure
    B. Pulse rate
    C. Respirations
    D. Temperature

71. When using a transfer belt, you can prevent the person from sliding or falling by
    A. Moving the person quickly from the bed to wheelchair
    B. Blocking the person's weak leg with your legs or knees
    C. Straddling your legs around the person's strong leg
    D. Planning the transfer so the person moves his or her weak side first

72. When you are transferring a person back to bed from a chair or wheelchair, the person should be positioned
    A. With the weak side near the bed
    B. With the strong side near the bed
    C. With the chair in the same position as it was when the person got out of bed
    D. Where you have the most space to work

73. A mechanical lift is used
    A. For all persons regardless of the level of dependence
    B. For persons who are too heavy for the staff to transfer
    C. When staff members prefer to use it instead of lifting manually
    D. Only when ordered by the doctor
74. When you are delegated to use a mechanical lift, you need to know
    A. Whether the doctor has ordered using the mechanical lift
    B. What sling the person prefers
    C. How many staff members are needed to perform the task safely
    D. When the mechanical device was used last
75. As a person is lifted in the sling of the mechanical lift, he or she
    A. May hold the swivel bar
    B. May hold the straps or chains
    C. Should keep the arms folded across the chest
    D. Should keep the legs outstretched
76. When transferring a person from a wheelchair to the toilet
    A. The toilet should have a raised seat
    B. The toilet seat should be removed
    C. Always position the wheelchair next to the toilet
    D. Unlock the wheelchair to allow movement during the transfer
77. A slide board may be used to transfer a person from a wheelchair to a toilet if
    A. The person can stand and pivot
    B. There is enough room to position the wheelchair next to the toilet
    C. The staff member does not want to use a transfer belt
    D. The person has lower body strength
78. When moving a person who weighs more than 200 pounds to a stretcher, OSHA recommends
    A. Using a lateral sliding aid and 2 staff members
    B. Using a lateral sliding aid and 3 staff members
    C. Using a lateral sliding aid or a friction-reducing device and 2 staff members
    D. Using a drawsheet, turning pad, or large incontinence underpad
79. During transport on the stretcher, the person is moved feet first so
    A. The staff member at the feet can clear the pathway
    B. The staff member at the head can watch the person's breathing and color
    C. The person can see where he or she is going
    D. The person does not become disoriented

FILL IN THE BLANKS

Write out the meaning of each abbreviation.

80. ID _____

81. OSHA _____

82. MSD _____

83. Where are strong, large muscles that are used to lift and move heavy objects located?
    A. _____
    B. _____
    C. _____
    D. _____

84. Back injuries are a major risk when lifting. For good body mechanics, you should
    A. _____
    B. _____

85. Describe these risk factors for musculo-skeletal disorders (MSDs) in nursing centers.
    A. Force _____
       _____
    B. Repeating action _____
       _____
    C. Awkward postures _____
       _____
    D. Heavy lifting _____
       _____

86. Early signs and symptoms of MSDs are
    A. _____
    B. _____
    C. _____

87. What nursing tasks are known to be high risk for MSDs?
    A. _____
    B. _____
    C. _____
    D. _____
    E. _____
    F. _____
    G. _____
    H. _____

I. _____

J. _____

K. _____

L. _____

M. _____

N. _____

O. _____

P. _____

88. Instructions to re-position a person are received

from the _____ and the

_____.

89. If you are delegated the task to position the person, what information do you need?

A. _____

B. _____

C. _____

D. _____

E. _____

F. _____

G. _____

H. _____

I. _____

J. _____

K. _____

90. What measures are needed for good alignment when the person is in Fowler's position?

A. _____

B. _____

C. _____

91. In supine position?

A. _____

B. _____

C. _____

92. In prone position?

A. _____

B. _____

C. _____

93. In lateral position?

A. _____

B. _____

C. _____

D. _____

E. _____

F. _____

94. In Sims' position?

A. _____

B. _____

C. _____

D. _____

95. In chair position?

A. _____

B. _____

C. _____

96. To prevent injuries in older persons with fragile bones and joints, what safety measures must be used?

A. _____

B. _____

C. _____

D. _____

E. _____

F. _____

G. _____

97. To promote mental comfort when handling, moving, or transferring the person, you should

A. _____

B. _____

98. To promote physical comfort when handling, moving, or transferring the person, you should

A. _____

_____

B. _____

_____

C. _____

_____

D. _____

_____

99. When lifting manually, you use good body mechanics when you

    A. _____

    B. _____

    C. _____

    D. _____

    E. _____

100. Explain how a person is lifted and transferred for each level of dependence.

    A. Code 4: Total Dependence _____

    _____

    B. Code 3: Extensive Assistance _____

    _____

    C. Code 2: Limited Assistance _____

    _____

    D. Code 1: Supervision _____

    _____

    E. Code 0: Independent _____

    _____

101. When you move a person in bed, report and record

    A. _____

    B. _____

    C. _____

    D. _____

    E. _____

102. Friction and shearing can be reduced when moving a person in bed by

    A. _____

    B. _____

103. You can sometimes move a person up in bed alone if the person can use a _____

104. When moving a person up in bed and the person can assist

    A. Flex _____

    B. Ask the person to grasp the _____

    C. Tell the person to move _____

105. An assist device is used to move persons

    A. Who are recovering from _____

    _____

    B. Older _____

106. What assist devices, other than mechanical lifts, are used to move persons to the side of the bed?

    _____

    _____

107. Before turning and repositioning a person, what information do you need from the nurse and the care plan?

    A. _____

    B. _____

    C. _____

    D. _____

    E. _____

    F. _____

    G. _____

    H. _____

108. What observations are reported and recorded after turning a person?

    A. _____

    B. _____

    C. _____

    D. _____

    E. _____

109. After turning and repositioning a person, it is common to place pillows

    A. _____

    B. _____

    C. _____

    D. _____

110. When a person is logrolled, the spine must be

    _____.

111. Logrolling is used to turn these persons:

    A. _____

    B. _____

    C. _____

    D. _____

112. When a person is dangling, the circulation can be stimulated by having the person move

    _____.

113. What observations should be reported and recorded after dangling a person?

    A. _____

    B. _____

    C. _____

    D. _____

    E. _____

    F. _____

    G. _____

114. While a person is dangling, check the person's condition by

    A. Asking _____

    B. Checking _____

    C. Checking _____

    D. Noting _____

115. A person can transfer from the bed to the chair with a stand and pivot transfer if

    A. _____

    _____

    B. _____

    _____

    C. _____

    _____

116. During a chair or wheelchair transfer, the person must not put his or her arms around your neck

    because _____

    _____.

117. Locked wheelchairs may be considered restraints

    if the person _____.

118. When using a transfer belt to transfer a person to a chair or wheelchair, grasp the

    belt at _____ and grasp

    _____ the belt.

119. If you transfer a person to a chair without a

    transfer belt, place your hands _____ and

    around the person's _____.

120. For what reasons would you use the slings listed?

    A. Standard full sling _____

    B. Extended length sling _____

    C. Bathing sling _____

    D. Toileting sling _____

    E. Amputee sling _____

121. What information do you need when you are delegated to use a mechanical lift?

    A. _____

    B. _____

    C. _____

    D. _____

    E. _____

    F. _____

122. To promote mental comfort when using a mechanical lift, you should explain

    _____ and show the person

    _____.

123. A slide board can be used when transferring a person to and from a toilet if

    A. _____

    B. _____

    C. _____

    D. _____

124. If a person weighs more than 200 pounds and is being moved to a stretcher, OSHA recommends the use of one of the following.

    A. _____

    B. _____

    C. _____

LABELING

125. Identify the positions in each of the illustrations.

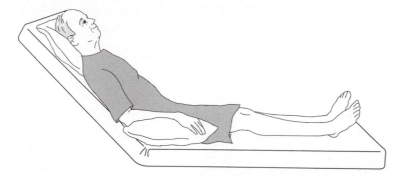

A. _____

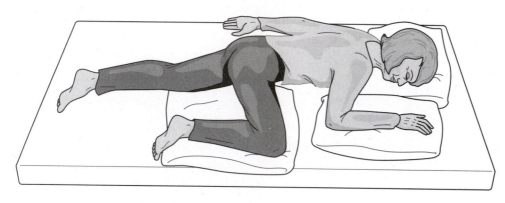

B. _____

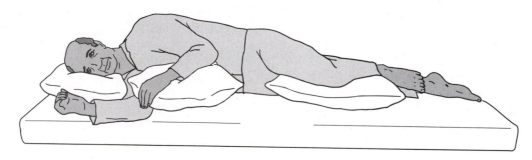

C. _____

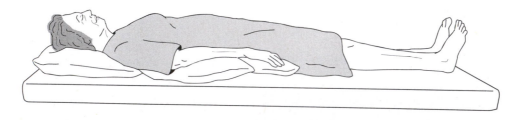

D. _____

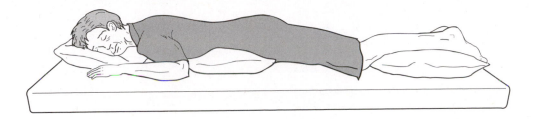

E. _____

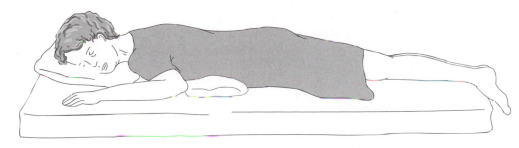

F. _____

OPTIONAL LEARNING EXERCISES

126. According to OSHA, certain activities can lead to back injuries. Read the examples below and state the factor that could cause a back injury in each activity. (Factors listed in textbook)

A. The nursing assistant does not raise the level of the bed when changing linens. _____

_____

B. While you are walking with Mr. Smith, he slips and starts to fall. _____

_____

C. Mrs. Tippett slides down in bed and looks uncomfortable. _____

_____

D. You assist Mrs. Miller to use the toilet in her small bathroom. _____

E. Water is spilled on the hallway floor.

_____

_____

F. You lean across the bed to hold the person in position while the nurse changes a dressing.

_____

_____

127. When caring for a person, regular position changes and good alignment promote

A. _____

B. _____

C. _____

D. _____

Position changes and good alignment prevent

E. _____

F. _____

128. If you need to move a person with dementia, the person may resist because he or she may not

_____. What measures in the care plan will help you give safe care?

A. _____

B. _____

C. _____

129. What type of pad is not strong enough to be used during a lift?

_____

130. For a safe lift, the underpad must

A. _____

_____

B. _____

_____

C. _____

_____

131. When you turn a person and re-position him or her, what must be done to the level of the bed before you leave the room?

    _____

132. When two staff members are logrolling a person without a turning sheet, where does each person stand?
    A. First worker stands near _____

    B. Co-worker stands near _____

133. What should you do if the mechanical lift available is different than ones you have used

    before? _____

INDEPENDENT LEARNING ACTIVITIES

- After learning about using good body mechanics in this chapter, think about how well you practice good body mechanics in your daily life and answer these questions.
    - How much do the books you carry with you each day weigh? How do you carry them? When carrying them, where is your base of support? Is your body in good alignment?
    - Do you have small children whom you pick up? How do you lift them? What methods listed in the chapter do you use?
    - When carrying groceries into the house, do you carry them held close to the body? How well are you using good body mechanics?
    - At the end of the day, how do you feel? How could using good body mechanics help you avoid any discomfort?
- Work with classmates and practice the following activities. Each of you should take a turn as the resident.
    - Practice moving a person up in bed with and without assist devices. Answer the following questions after you have completed this exercise.
        - Which method was easier for the worker? For the person being moved?
        - How did you feel when you were being moved? Did anyone explain what was being done?
    - Practice transferring a person who is weak on one side to a chair from the bed and then return the person to the bed. Answer the following questions after you complete the exercise.
        - As the worker: How did you position the chair? How did the chair position change when you returned the person to bed?

- As the person: How safe did you feel during the transfer? What could the worker have done to help you feel safe? What else could the staff have done to make you more comfortable?
- Practice logrolling a person with and without a turning sheet. Answer the following questions after you have completed the exercise.
    - As the worker: How many workers were used to logroll the person? Which method was easier—with or without the turning sheet? How well do you think the workers did with the turns? Did the spine stay straight?
    - As the person: How did you feel? Did you understand what was being done? Was the turn smooth or did you feel as if your spine twisted?
- Ask your instructor if you can use a mechanical lift to practice with each other. If the instructor approves this exercise, answer the following questions after practicing.
    - As the worker: What did you do before beginning the lift? What questions did you ask? What other information should you have gathered before starting?
    - As the person: How did you feel when you were lifted? Did you feel as if you understood what was happening? What other information would have helped make you more comfortable?
- Overall, how will these practices help you as you move residents? What would you do differently now that you have practiced these exercises?

15 THE RESIDENT'S UNIT

FILL IN THE BLANKS: KEY TERMS

Fowler's position
Full visual privacy
High-Fowler's position

Resident unit
Reverse Trendelenburg's position

Semi-Fowler's position
Trendelenburg's position

1. The personal space, furniture, and equipment provided for the individual by the nursing center is the _____.

2. In _____, the head of the bed is raised 30 degrees; or the head of the bed is raised 30 degrees and the knee portion is raised 15 degrees.

3. _____ is a semi-sitting position; the head of the bed is raised 45 to 60 degrees.

4. The head of the bed is raised and the foot of the bed is lowered in _____.

5. In _____, the head of the bed is lowered and the foot of the bed is raised.

6. The person has the means to be completely free from public view while in bed when they have

_____.

7. The bed is in a semi-sitting position; the head of the bed is raised between 60 and 90 degrees in

_____.

CIRCLE THE BEST ANSWER

8. When residents share a room
   A. You may rearrange items and furniture in the room as needed
   B. Each person has a private area of the room
   C. They may use each other's belongings
   D. They generally share furniture such as a dresser

9. OBRA requires that nursing centers maintain a temperature range of
   A. 68°F to 74°F
   B. 61°F to 71°F
   C. 71°F to 81°F
   D. 78°F to 85°F

10. Persons who are older and those who are ill
    A. May need cooler room temperatures
    B. May need higher temperatures for comfort
    C. Are insensitive to room temperature changes
    D. Will need a warmer room at night

11. Which of these factors that affect comfort cannot be controlled by the nursing staff?
    A. Illness
    B. Temperature
    C. Noise
    D. Odors

12. If an older person complains of a draft
    A. Have the person go to bed
    B. Give the person a hot shower
    C. Offer a lap robe or a warm sweater to wear
    D. Pull the privacy curtain around the person

13. If unpleasant odors occur, these may be controlled when you
    A. Use spray deodorizers around all residents
    B. Provide good hygiene to prevent body and breath odors
    C. Make sure incontinent persons are taken to the toilet once an hour
    D. Empty laundry hampers once a shift

14. A person with dementia may react to loud noises, especially
    A. At night
    B. When the room is well lighted
    C. During meal time
    D. When he or she is in an area with others present

15. Which of these measures will reduce noises in a nursing center?
    A. Have drapes in rooms.
    B. Use only metal equipment.
    C. Wait for the nurse to answer the telephone.
    D. Talk loudly in halls so others can hear you clearly.

16. Soft, non-glare lighting is used with dementia residents because it
    A. Helps residents to relax
    B. Increases agitation in residents
    C. Improves orientation in residents with dementia
    D. Helps residents to see more clearly

17. Cranks on manual beds are kept down when not in use to
    A. Prevent residents from operating the bed
    B. Prevent anyone walking past the crank from bumping into it
    C. Keep the bed in the correct position
    D. Make sure they are ready to use at all times

18. How can the staff prevent a person from adjusting an electric bed into unsafe positions?
    A. Lock the bed into a position.
    B. Unplug the bed.
    C. Put the person in a bed that cannot be repositioned.
    D. Keep reminding the person not to change the position.
19. What bed position may adjust the head of the bed and the knee portion to prevent sliding down in bed?
    A. Fowler's
    B. Semi-Fowler's
    C. Trendelenburg's
    D. Reverse Trendelenburg's
20. If a person becomes trapped in the hospital bed system, you should
    A. Call for the nurse at once
    B. Call 911
    C. Make sure the person is comfortable
    D. Lower the bed rails
21. If a person becomes trapped between the end of the bed rail and the side edge of the head-board, the area is called
    A. Zone 1
    B. Zone 2
    C. Zone 6
    D. Zone 7
22. Which of these items can be placed on the over-bed table?
    A. Urinals
    B. Personal care items
    C. Soiled linens
    D. Bedpans
23. Where are the bedpan and urinal kept in the bedside table?
    A. Wherever the person wants
    B. The top shelf or drawer
    C. The bottom shelf or drawer
    D. The middle shelf or drawer
24. OBRA requires that the resident unit always has
    A. Two chairs
    B. A straight-back chair
    C. A reclining chair
    D. At least one chair for personal and visitor use
25. Privacy curtains
    A. Are sometimes used in rooms with more than one bed
    B. Are always pulled completely around the bed when care is given
    C. Can block sounds and conversations
    D. May be open when giving personal care
26. Personal care items
    A. Are often supplied by the nursing center
    B. Must be provided by the resident
    C. Must be ordered by the doctor
    D. Are required by OBRA

27. When the resident is weak on the left side, the call light
    A. Is placed on the left side
    B. Is removed from the room
    C. Is placed on the right side
    D. Is replaced by an intercom
28. If a confused person cannot use a call light
    A. Explain often how to use the call light
    B. Use an intercom instead
    C. Remove the call light
    D. Check the person often
29. Elevated toilet seats
    A. Help residents with joint problems
    B. Make wheelchair transfers more difficult
    C. Are required by OBRA
    D. Are used on all toilets in a nursing center
30. When a person uses a bathroom call light
    A. It flashes above the room door and at the nurses' station
    B. It makes the same sound as the room call light
    C. It activates the intercom
    D. The signal sounds and flashes only above the bathroom door
31. Closet and drawer space
    A. Is shared by persons in a room with more than one person
    B. Can be opened and searched by a staff member at any time
    C. Cannot be searched without the resident's permission
    D. Is not required in a nursing center
32. What equipment may be in rehabilitation centers but usually is not found in long-term care centers?
    A. Televisions
    B. Commode chairs
    C. Blood pressure equipment or wall outlets for oxygen and suctioning
    D. Electric beds
33. Residents can bring some furniture and personal items to use in the room as long as the items
    A. Do not interfere with the rights of others
    B. Match the color and decoration in the room
    C. Can be cared for by the resident or the family
    D. Do not need to be attached to the wall

FILL IN THE BLANKS

34. What are three factors that affect comfort and that usually cannot be controlled?

    A. _____

    B. _____

    C. _____

35. What factors that affect comfort can be controlled?

    A. _____

    B. _____

    C. _____

    D. _____

    E. _____ .

36. Describe the entrapment zones that can occur in a hospital bed system.

    A. Zone 1 _____

    B. Zone 2 _____

    _____

    C. Zone 3 _____

    D. Zone 4 _____

    _____

    E. Zone 5 _____

    F. Zone 6 _____

    _____

    G. Zone 7 _____

37. The resident is allowed to bring personal items to make his space as home-like as possible. The health team must make sure the resident's choices

    A. _____

    B. _____

    C. _____

LABELING

38. In this figure

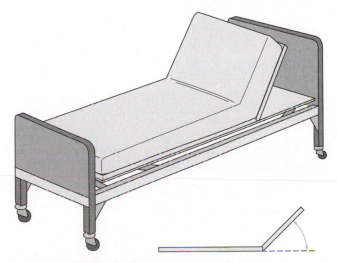

    A. What is the bed position called?

    _____

    B. What is the angle of the head of the bed?

    _____

39. In this figure

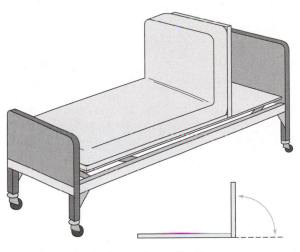

    A. What is the bed position called?

    _____

    B. What is the angle of the head of the bed?

    _____

40. In this figure

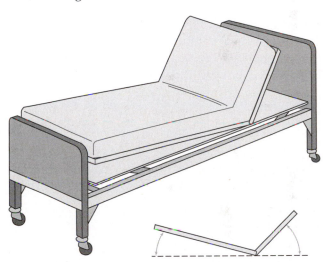

    A. What is the bed position called?

    _____

    B. What is the angle of the head of the bed?

    _____

    C. The angle of the knee portion of the bed?

    _____

    D. Raising the knee portion of the bed can

    _____ .

41. In this figure

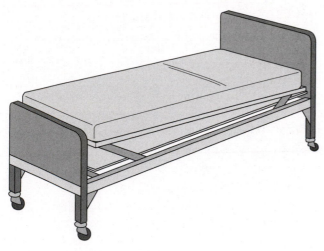

A. What is the bed position called?

_____

B. What is the position of the head of the bed and the foot of the bed?

_____

C. This position requires a _____ .

42. In this figure

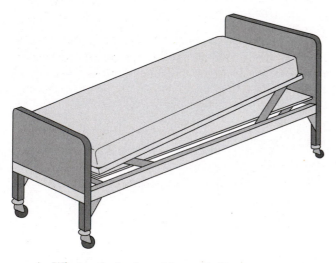

A. What is the bed position called?

_____

B. What is the position of the head of the bed and the foot of the bed? _____

_____

C. This position requires a

_____ .

OPTIONAL LEARNING EXERCISES

43. In these situations, how would you help protect a resident from drafts?
    A. The person is dressing for the day.

    _____

    _____

    B. The person is sitting in a wheelchair.

    _____

    _____

    C. You are assisting a resident who is going to bed for the night. _____

    _____

    D. You are giving personal care to the resident.

    _____

    _____

44. How can you help eliminate odors in these situations?
    A. You are caring for a person who is frequently incontinent. _____

    _____

    B. The person is vomiting and has wound drainage. _____

    _____

    C. The person uses the bathroom by herself.

    _____

    D. The person keeps a urinal at his bedside and uses it himself during the day.

    _____

45. When the staff talk loudly and laugh in the hallways, some persons may think that

    _____ .

46. Why do persons with dementia react more to loud noises at night? _____

    _____

47. How can the staff reduce noises and increase resident comfort?
    A. Control _____
    B. Handle _____
    C. Keep _____
    D. Answer _____

48. What are 2 situations when bright lights are helpful for a resident with poor vision?

_____ and

_____ .

49. In dementia units, how does adjusting lighting help the residents?

A. Soft, non-glare _____ .

B. Brighter _____ .

50. The bed in the flat position is used for

A. _____

B. _____

51. Semi-Fowler's position has 2 definitions. They are

A. _____

B. _____

52. How do you position the bed when semi-Fowler's position is ordered? _____

_____

53. In order to raise the foot of the bed with Trendelenburg's position, you may put _____

_____ .

54. When the nursing team uses the over-bed table as a work area, what are the only items that can be placed on it? _____

55. What are your responsibilities in these situations regarding the call light?

A. The resident is sitting in a chair next to the bed.

_____

B. The person is weak on the right side.

_____

C. The person calls out instead of using the call light. _____

_____

D. The resident is embarrassed because she soiled the bed after signaling for assistance.

_____

E. The bathroom light in a room rings while you are busy in another room. _____

_____

56. List the OBRA requirement that relates to each of these items in the resident unit.

A. Number of residents in a room _____

B. Windows _____

C. Closets _____

D. Call system _____

E. Odors, noise, lighting _____

_____

F. Hand rails _____

INDEPENDENT LEARNING ACTIVITIES

- When you are in the health care center as a student, find an empty resident room and practice using the equipment. Answer the following questions about the equipment.
  - Where are the controls for the bed?
    - How do you operate the head of the bed?
    - How do you operate the knee control of the bed?
    - How do you adjust the height of the bed?
  - Where is the call light located?
  - Where are the controls for the television and radio?
  - Does the center have an intercom system? How is it used?
- Ask the staff the following questions about the call lights.
  - How does the staff know when a resident turns on the call light?
  - When a resident uses a bathroom call light, how does the staff know the difference?
- Think about what temperature is comfortable for you and answer the following questions. This exercise will help you understand the importance of individual preferences for residents in the health care center.
  - What is the usual temperature of your home?
  - Who decides what the temperature will be in your home? Partner, spouse, roommate, children?
  - Would the temperature you prefer be comfortable for an infant? An older person? Why or why not?
- Think about the noises in your home and how they affect you. This exercise will help you understand why noise levels in the nursing center can affect the residents.
  - When you study, do you turn on the TV or radio? Listen to music? Prefer complete silence?
  - What noises do you like when going to sleep? TV? Radio? Soft music?
  - Does everyone in your household agree on how loud or soft to play a radio or TV? How are conflicts about noise levels resolved?
  - If you are in noisy surroundings, how do you react? How does it affect your ability to think? To rest? To study? How does it affect your relationship with others?

16 BEDMAKING

FILL IN THE BLANKS: KEY TERMS

Cotton drawsheet
Drawsheet
Waterproof drawsheet

1. A drawsheet made of plastic, rubber, or absorbent material used to protect the mattress and bottom linens from dampness and soiling is a

   _____.

2. A _____ is a small sheet placed over the middle of the bottom sheet.

3. A drawsheet made of cotton that helps keep the mattress and bottom linens clean and dry is a

   _____.

CIRCLE THE BEST ANSWER

4. In nursing centers, bed linens are changed
   A. Only if the person asks for a change
   B. Every day
   C. On the person's bath or shower day
   D. Once a week on a scheduled day

5. Follow Standard Precautions and the Bloodborne Pathogen Standard when you
   A. Handle any bed linens
   B. Make the bed every morning
   C. May have contact with wet, soiled, or damp linens soiled with the person's blood, body fluids, secretions, or excretions
   D. Place clean linens on the bed

6. When handling linens and making beds, you should
   A. Put the dirty linens on the floor
   B. Hold the linens away from your body and uniform
   C. Shake linens in the air to straighten them
   D. Use any extra linens for another resident

7. A closed bed
   A. Is made with the person in the bed
   B. Has the top linens fan-folded back so the person can get into bed
   C. Is made for residents who are up for most or all of the day
   D. Has the linens fan-folded length-wise to the side of the bed

8. When making a bed, you use good body mechanics when you
   A. Bend from the waist when removing and replacing the linens
   B. Stretch across the bed to smooth the linens
   C. Raise the bed to a comfortable height
   D. Lock the wheels

9. If extra clean linens are brought to a person's room, you should
   A. Return the unused linens to the linen room
   B. Store the extra linens in the person's closet
   C. Put the unused linens in the dirty laundry
   D. Use the linens for a person in the next room

10. An open bed
    A. Is made with the person in it
    B. Lets the person get into the bed with ease
    C. Is not in use until bedtime; the top linens are not folded back
    D. Is made to transfer a person from a stretcher to the bed

11. Which of these linens will be collected first?
    A. Bath towel
    B. Bath blanket
    C. Mattress pad
    D. Top sheet

12. When you remove dirty linens, it is correct to
    A. Gather all the linens in one large roll
    B. Roll each piece of dirty linen away from you
    C. Place disposable pads in the laundry hamper with the dirty linens
    D. Replace all linens with clean linens every day

13. A waterproof drawsheet
    A. Can cause discomfort and skin breakdown
    B. Is used to keep linens tight and wrinkle-free
    C. Is used for all residents
    D. Is disposable and can be placed in the trash when soiled

14. When you are delegated to make a bed, why do you need to know the person's schedule for treatments, therapies, and activities?
    A. You need to make sure the bed is flat.
    B. It is best to change linens after the treatment or when the person is out of the room.
    C. You need to unlock beds that have been locked in a certain position.
    D. You will then know what type of bed to make.

15. When assigned to make a bed, what information do you need from the nurse or care plan?
    A. How the person wants the bed made
    B. Whether the person is confused
    C. When the bed was changed last
    D. How to position the person and the positioning devices needed

16. When a person is discharged from a hospital or nursing center, what is done in addition to changing the bed?
    A. New pillows are placed on the bed.
    B. The bed frame and mattress are cleaned and disinfected.
    C. The bed is sterilized.
    D. The bedspread and blanket may be reused.

17. When making a bed with a flat sheet, position the bottom sheet with
    A. The lower edge even with the top of the mattress
    B. The hem-stitching facing downward, away from the person
    C. The large hem at the bottom and the small hem at the top
    D. The center crease across the bed

18. When the top sheet, blanket, and bedspread are in place on the bed
    A. Each one is tucked under the mattress separately
    B. The sheet and blanket are tucked together and the bedspread is allowed to hang loose over them
    C. All three are tucked together under the foot of the bed and the corners are mitered
    D. All three are allowed to hang loose over the foot of the bed

19. The pillow is placed on the bed
    A. So the open end of the pillowcase is away from the door
    B. So the seam of the pillowcase is toward the foot of the bed
    C. So it is leaning against the head of the bed
    D. So the open end of the pillowcase is toward the door

20. If you are making an occupied bed for a person who is comatose, it is important to
    A. Keep the bed in the low position
    B. Unlock the wheels
    C. Use special linens
    D. Explain each step of the procedure to the person before it is done

21. A bath blanket is used when making an occupied bed to
    A. Protect the person from injury
    B. Provide warmth and privacy for the person
    C. Protect the bed linens
    D. Protect the person from dirty linens

22. To provide safety when making an occupied bed for a person who does not use bed rails, you should
    A. Have a co-worker work on the opposite side of the bed
    B. Push the bed against the wall
    C. Always keep one hand on the person while you are making the bed
    D. Only change linens when the person is out of the bed for tests or therapies

23. When making an occupied bed, privacy is provided when you
    A. Close the door and pull curtains around the bed
    B. Ask the roommate to leave the room
    C. Work alone so there is only one worker in the room
    D. Lock the door so no one can enter the room

24. Which of these steps is done when making a surgical bed?
    A. Fan-fold linens length-wise to the side of the bed farthest from the door.
    B. Remove all linens from the bed if the person is arriving from the hospital.
    C. Remove the mattress pad, as it is never used on a surgical bed.
    D. Cover the person with a bath blanket.

25. You allow the person the right of personal choice when you
    A. Allow the person to use bed linens from home
    B. Decide which linens will look best in the room
    C. Tell the person you will make the bed at 9 AM
    D. Choose the pillows and blanket the person needs for comfort

FILL IN THE BLANKS

26. Number the following list from 1 to 13 in the order you would collect the linens to make a bed.

    _____ Pillowcase(s)

    _____ Top sheet

    _____ Gown or pajamas

    _____ Bottom sheet (flat or fitted)

    _____ Mattress pad

    _____ Bedspread

    _____ Waterproof drawsheet

    _____ Bath blanket

    _____ Hand towel

    _____ Cotton drawsheet

    _____ Bath towel(s)

    _____ Blanket

    _____ Washcloth

OPTIONAL LEARNING EXERCISES

27. When is a complete linen change made in a nursing center? _____

_____

28. Clean, dry, and wrinkle-free linens are important to promote _____ and to prevent _____ and

_____.

29. What should you do to keep beds neat and clean?

   A. _____

   B. _____

   C. _____

   D. _____

   E. _____

   F. _____

30. When handling linens, practice medical asepsis. Explain why each of the following actions would be *poor* medical asepsis.

   A. Holding the linens close to your body and

   uniform _____

   B. Shaking the linens to straighten them

   _____

   C. Placing the dirty linens on the floor

   _____

31. Family and visitors may question the quality

   _____ and the quality

   _____ if the bed is unmade, messy, or dirty.

INDEPENDENT LEARNING ACTIVITIES

- When you make beds at home this week, practice the methods you learned in this chapter.
  - What linens did you collect? In what order did you collect the linens?
  - Did you remember to make as much of one side of the bed as possible before moving to the other side?
  - What step could *not* be carried out at home that would have helped you to use good body mechanics?
  - Think about the methods you used to change your bed before reading this chapter. How will you change your bedmaking practices now that you have studied this chapter?

- Practice with a classmate and take turns as a resident who must have an occupied bed made. Ask the following questions about your feelings.
  - In what ways was your privacy protected?
  - Did the caregiver offer you any choices before making your bed? What were these choices?
  - Did you feel safe at all times? If not, what made you feel unsafe?
  - What was uncomfortable during the bed change?
  - How were you positioned after the bed was made?
- It is sometimes difficult for a new nursing assistant to remember the order in which to collect linens. Make a list in a pocket notebook or on a 3- × 5-inch index card so you can carry it with you when you are working.

17 HYGIENE

FILL IN THE BLANKS: KEY TERMS

AM care
Aspiration
Denture
Early morning care

Evening care
Morning care
Oral hygiene
Pericare

Perineal care
Plaque
PM care
Tartar

1. Another name for PM care is _____.

2. _____ is cleansing the genital and anal areas; it is sometimes called pericare.

3. Sometimes evening care is called _____.

4. Routine care performed before breakfast or early morning care is called _____.

5. _____ is mouth care or measures that keep the mouth and teeth clean.

6. Hardened plaque on teeth is _____.

7. _____ occurs when breathing fluid, food, vomitus, or an object into the lungs.

8. Care given after breakfast when hygiene measures are more thorough is called _____.

9. Another name for perineal care is _____.

10. _____ is a thin film that sticks to the teeth. It contains saliva, microbes, and other substances.

11. Another name for AM care is _____.

12. An artificial tooth or a set of artificial teeth is a

_____.

CIRCLE THE BEST ANSWER

13. If a person needs help with personal hygiene, you can find out what needs they have by
    A. Following the nurse's directions and the care plan
    B. Asking the family
    C. Asking other staff members
    D. Making your own decisions

14. You should assist a person with personal hygiene
    A. Only when the person asks
    B. Only in the morning
    C. Whenever help is needed
    D. Only when it is your assignment

15. When giving personal hygiene, you need to remember to protect the person's right to
    A. Privacy and personal choice
    B. Care and security of personal possessions
    C. Activities
    D. Environment

16. When giving routine care before breakfast, you should
    A. Assist with activity by ambulating the person
    B. Give a complete bath
    C. Change wet or soiled linens and garments
    D. Change all of the bed linens for every person

17. Which of these is done every time you assist with hygiene measures throughout the day?
    A. Assisting with dressing and hair care
    B. Face and hand washing
    C. Assisting with ambulation
    D. Helping the person change into sleepwear

18. If good oral hygiene is not done regularly, the person may develop tartar, which will lead to
    A. A dry mouth
    B. Periodontal disease
    C. A bad taste in the mouth
    D. Plaque

19. The nurse may be assisted in assessing the person's need for mouth care by the
    A. Nursing assistant
    B. Physical therapist
    C. Doctor
    D. Dietitian

20. Teeth are flossed
    A. When brushing the teeth is not possible
    B. When the person is in a coma
    C. When you do not have time to give complete oral hygiene
    D. To remove food from between the teeth

21. Which of these steps is correct when flossing the teeth?
    A. Floss dentures in the same way you floss natural teeth.
    B. Use a new piece of floss for each section of the mouth.
    C. Move the floss gently up and down between the teeth.
    D. Move to a new section of floss when moving from the upper to lower teeth.

22. Sponge swabs are used for
    A. Persons who are unconscious
    B. Cleaning dentures
    C. Oral care on children
    D. Oral care on all residents

23. You follow Standard Precautions and the Bloodborne Pathogen Standard when giving oral hygiene because
    A. You will not spread bacteria to the person
    B. It will help you avoid bad breath odors from the person
    C. Gums may bleed during mouth care
    D. You will avoid any loose teeth or rough dentures

24. When the person is able to perform oral hygiene in bed, you arrange the items on
    A. The over-bed table
    B. The bedside table
    C. The sink counter
    D. The bed

25. When you are brushing the person's teeth, you should
    A. Let the person rinse the mouth with water
    B. Use only a sponge swab to clean the teeth
    C. Have the person floss his or her teeth
    D. Wear gloves only if bleeding occurs

26. When providing mouth care for an unconscious person, position the person on one side with the head turned well to the side to
    A. Make it easier to brush the teeth
    B. Make the person more comfortable
    C. Prevent the risk of aspiration
    D. Make it easier for the person to breathe

27. When giving oral hygiene to an unconscious person who wears dentures, you should
    A. Remove the dentures, clean them, and replace them in the mouth
    B. Know that dentures are not worn when the person is unconscious
    C. Clean the dentures in the mouth without removing them
    D. Insert your fingers to keep the mouth open

28. Mouth care is given to an unconscious person
    A. After each meal
    B. When AM and PM care is given
    C. At least every 2 hours
    D. Once a day

29. A padded tongue blade is used when giving oral hygiene to an unconscious person to:
    A. Keep the mouth open
    B. Clean the teeth
    C. Clean the tongue
    D. Prevent aspiration

30. When cleaning dentures at a sink, line the sink with a towel to
    A. Prevent infections
    B. Prevent the dentures from falling on a hard surface
    C. Dry the dentures
    D. Clean the dentures

31. If dentures are not worn after cleaning, store them in
    A. Cool water or a denture soaking solution
    B. Hot water
    C. A soft towel
    D. Soft tissues or a napkin

32. If the person cannot remove the dentures, you can use which of these to get a good grip on the slippery dentures?
    A. Gloves
    B. Washcloth
    C. Gauze squares
    D. Bare hands

33. Older persons usually need a complete bath or shower twice a week because
    A. They are less active
    B. They are often ill
    C. They have increased perspiration
    D. Dry skin often occurs with aging

34. If a person has dry skin, which of these will help keep it soft?
    A. Soaps
    B. Lotions and oils
    C. Frequent baths or showers
    D. Deodorants and antiperspirants

35. If a person with dementia resists bathing, you should:
    A. Hurry through the bath
    B. Speak firmly in a loud voice
    C. Try giving a partial bath or try giving the bath later
    D. Use restraints so the person will not harm you

36. When choosing skin care products for bathing, you should use
    A. Soap
    B. Products the person prefers or those listed in the care plan
    C. Bath oils
    D. Creams and lotions
37. The water temperature for a complete bed bath is usually between 110°F and 115°F (43.3°C and 46.1°C) for adults. For older persons, the temperature
    A. Should be between 110°F and 115°F (43.3°C and 46.1°C)
    B. May need to be lower
    C. Should be whatever you feel is comfortable
    D. May need to be warmer
38. When applying powder
    A. Shake or sprinkle the powder directly on the person
    B. Sprinkle a small amount of powder on your hands or a cloth
    C. Apply a thick layer of powder
    D. You should never use powder on any older person
39. A complete bed bath is given to
    A. Those who cannot bathe themselves
    B. Persons with dementia or confusion
    C. All residents who need help with hygiene
    D. A person who walks independently
40. When you are giving a complete bed bath, the bed linens are changed
    A. Only if needed
    B. Before the bath begins
    C. After the bath
    D. After the person gets out of bed
41. The person is offered the bedpan, urinal, or commode or is taken to the bathroom
    A. Before the bath begins
    B. After the bath ends
    C. During the bath, before perineal care is done
    D. Only if this step is part of the care plan
42. During the bed bath, the bath blanket is placed
    A. Over the top linens
    B. Under the top linens
    C. Over the person as the top linens are removed
    D. Under the person
43. Do not use soap when washing
    A. The face, ears, and neck
    B. Around the eyes
    C. The abdomen
    D. The perineal area
44. How do you avoid exposing the person when washing the chest?
    A. Keep the bath blanket over the area.
    B. Keep the top linens over the chest.
    C. Place a bath towel over the chest cross-wise.
    D. Make sure the curtains are closed.

45. Bath water is changed during a bed bath
    A. Every 5 minutes
    B. Only if the person asks you to change it
    C. Before giving perineal care
    D. After washing the face, ears, and neck
46. Which of these persons may respond well to a towel bath?
    A. Person with dementia
    B. Person who has been incontinent
    C. Person with breaks in the skin
    D. Person who needs a partial bath
47. A partial bath involves bathing
    A. Areas the person cannot reach
    B. The face, hands, axillae (underarms), back, buttocks, and perineal area
    C. The arms, legs, and feet
    D. The chest, abdomen, and underarms
48. When giving any type of bath, you should
    A. Wash from the dirtiest to cleanest areas
    B. Allow the skin to air-dry to avoid rubbing
    C. Provide for privacy
    D. Decide what is best for the person
49. A tub bath should not last longer than
    A. 10 minutes
    B. 15 minutes
    C. 20 minutes
    D. 30 minutes
50. If a person is weak or unsteady, which of these should be used when the person showers?
    A. Shower chair
    B. Transfer belt
    C. Wheelchair
    D. Stretcher
51. Which of these would be good time management when giving a tub bath or shower?
    A. Take the person to the shower room and then collect your equipment.
    B. Ask a co-worker to give the shower for you.
    C. Ask a co-worker to make the person's bed while you give the bath.
    D. Clean and disinfect the tub or shower before returning the person to his or her room.
52. When assisting with a tub bath or shower, which of these steps is done first?
    A. Help the person undress and remove footwear.
    B. Assist or transport the person to the tub or shower room.
    C. Put the occupied sign on the door.
    D. Place a rubber bath mat in the tub or on the shower floor.
53. The best position for a back massage is
    A. Prone position
    B. Supine position
    C. Side-lying position
    D. Semi-Fowler's position

54. Back massages are dangerous for persons
    A. Who are bedridden
    B. With lung disorders
    C. Who have arthritis
    D. Who have intact skin
55. When giving a back massage, the strokes
    A. Start at the shoulders and go down to the buttocks
    B. Should be light and gentle
    C. Start at the buttocks and go up to the shoulders
    D. Are continued for at least 10 minutes
56. When cleaning the perineal area
    A. You do not need to wear gloves
    B. Work from the anal area to the urethral area
    C. Work from the urethral area to the anal area
    D. Work from the dirtiest area to the cleanest area
57. When gathering equipment for perineal care, you will need
    A. 1 washcloth
    B. 2 washcloths
    C. At least 3 washcloths
    D. At least 4 washcloths
58. When giving perineal care to a male, you
    A. Retract the foreskin if he is uncircumcised
    B. Wash from the scrotum to the tip of the penis
    C. Use one washcloth for the entire procedure
    D. Leave the foreskin retracted after finishing the care
59. If a family member or friend offers to help provide hygiene to a person
    A. You should check the center policy
    B. The person must consent to this
    C. Accept the offer and allow him or her to give the care
    D. Tell the family member or friend that this is not allowed

MATCHING

Match the skin care product with the benefits or the problem that may occur if you use the product.
    A. Soaps
    B. Bath oils
    C. Creams and lotions
    D. Powders
    E. Deodorants and antiperspirants

60. _____ Absorbs moisture and prevents friction
61. _____ Makes showers and tubs slippery
62. _____ Protects skin from the drying effect of air and evaporation
63. _____ Excessive amounts can cause caking and crusts that can irritate the skin
64. _____ Masks and controls body odors
65. _____ Tends to dry and irritate skin

66. _____ Keeps skin soft and prevents drying of skin
67. _____ Removes dirt, dead skin, skin oil, some microbes, and perspiration

FILL IN THE BLANKS

68. C is an abbreviation for _____.
69. F is an abbreviation for _____.
70. HS means _____.
71. ID is an abbreviation for _____.
72. The _____ and _____ must be intact to prevent microbes from entering the body and causing an _____.
73. The religion of East Indian Hindus requires at least _____ a day.
74. Some Hindus believe that bathing after _____ causes injury.
75. When is oral hygiene given to a person?
    _____
    _____
76. When you are delegated to give oral hygiene, what observations should you report?
    A. _____
    B. _____
    C. _____
    D. _____
    E. _____
    F. _____
77. If flossing is done only once a day, the best time to floss is at _____.
78. When giving oral care to an unconscious person, explain what you are doing because you always assume _____.
79. When following the rules for bathing in Box 17-1, you protect the skin by these actions:
    A. Rinse _____
    B. Pat _____
    C. Dry _____

80. What methods can be used to measure the water temperature when giving a bed bath?

    A. _____

    B. _____

81. When you place a person's hands in the basin during the bed bath, you may have the person

_____ the hands and fingers.

82. When assisting a person to take a partial bath, you know that most people need help washing the

_____.

83. When a person has been on bedrest, safety is a concern because the bath can make the person feel

_____, _____, or _____.

84. When the shower room has more than one stall or cabinet, you must protect the person's right

_____. What can you do to protect this right?

    A. _____

    B. _____

85. When giving a tub bath or shower, you use safety measures to protect the person from

_____, _____,

and _____.

86. When giving a back massage and the person does not want the buttocks exposed, you should _____

_____.

87. When you are delegated to give a back massage, what observations should you report and record?

    A. _____

    B. _____

    C. _____

    D. _____

88. When you are assisting a person with perineal care, what terms can you use to help the person

understand what you are going to do? _____

_____

LABELING

89. Look at the figure and answer the following questions.

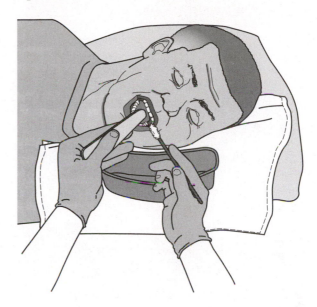

    A. Why is the person positioned on his side?

    _____

    B. What is the purpose of the padded tongue blade?

    _____

90. In this figure, what is the staff member using to

remove the upper denture? _____

Why? _____

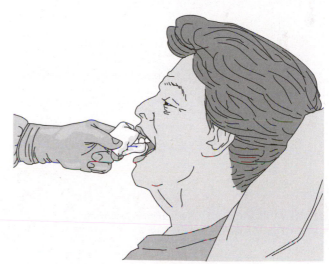

91. In this figure, explain what the staff member is doing. _____ Why is the towel positioned vertically on the person?

_____

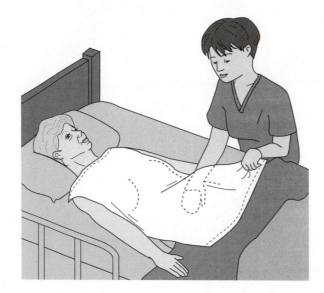

OPTIONAL LEARNING EXERCISES

92. Hygiene promotes comfort, safety, and health. Answer the following questions about hygiene.

    A. Why is intact skin important? _____

    _____.

    B. What other areas must be clean to maintain intact skin? _____

    _____

    C. Besides cleansing, what are the other benefits of good hygiene? _____

    _____

    D. What are 2 other reasons that hygiene is important? _____

    _____

93. What factors cause mouth dryness in an unconscious person?

    A. _____

    B. _____

    C. _____

94. The factors listed above cause crusting on the _____ and _____

    _____.

95. Oral hygiene keeps the mouth and teeth _____. It also prevents _____ and _____.

96. What are the benefits of bathing?

    A. Cleans _____

    B. Also cleans _____

    C. Removes _____

    D. Bath is _____ and

    _____

    E. Stimulates _____

    F. Exercises _____

    G. You can make _____

    H. You have time _____

97. When you are bathing a person with dementia, what measures are important to help the person through the bath?

    A. _____

    B. _____

    C. _____

    D. _____

    E. _____

    F. _____

    G. _____

    H. _____

    I. _____

    J. _____

    K. _____

    L. _____

    M. _____

    N. _____

98. You are delegated to give Mrs. Johnson a bath. Before beginning, what information do you need?

    A. _____

    B. _____

    C. _____

    D. _____

    E. _____

    F. _____

    G. _____

    H. _____

99. As you are bathing Mrs. Johnson, what observations should you make to report and record?

A. _____

B. _____

C. _____

D. _____

E. _____

F. _____

G. _____

H. _____

I. _____

J. _____

100. When you are preparing to give perineal care to Mrs. Johnson, how many washcloths should you gather? _____

Why? _____

_____

_____

INDEPENDENT LEARNING ACTIVITIES

- Ask several classmates the following questions to better understand personal preferences about hygiene.
  - Do you prefer a shower or tub bath?
  - What time of day do you usually bathe?
  - What skin care products do you use to keep your skin healthy?
  - What special measures do you use when brushing your teeth? Special brush? Toothpaste? Do you floss? How often?
- As part of your preparation for caring for residents, you may give a classmate a back massage and receive a back massage. Answer these questions about how you felt when you were the "resident."
  - How did the lotion feel on your back? Was it warm or cold?
  - Which strokes were relaxing? Which were more stimulating?
  - How long do you think the back massage lasted? Did you look at the clock to see the actual time?
  - What would you like to tell the person giving the back massage that would improve the back massage?
  - How will this practice help you when you give a back massage to another person?
- As part of your preparation for caring for residents, you may give a classmate oral hygiene. Answer these questions about how you felt when you were the "resident."
  - What did the "nursing assistant" tell you before beginning the oral hygiene?
  - What choices were offered? Position? Equipment? Products?
  - How did it feel to have someone else give you oral hygiene? Flossing your teeth?
  - How clean did your teeth feel when the oral hygiene was completed?
  - What would you like to tell the person who gave the oral hygiene that would help improve the procedure?
  - How will this experience help you when you give oral hygiene to a resident?

18 GROOMING

FILL IN THE BLANKS: KEY TERMS

Alopecia
Anticoagulant
Bed bugs
Dandruff

Hirsutism
Lice
Mite
Pediculosis

Pediculosis capitis
Pediculosis corporis
Pediculosis pubis

1. A very small spider-like organism is a
_____.

2. The infestation with lice is _____.

3. _____ is an excessive amount of dry, white flakes from the scalp.

4. The infestation of the body with lice is
_____.

5. Hair loss is _____.

6. _____ is the infestation of the pubic hair with lice.

7. Excessive body hair in women and children is
_____.

8. The infestation of the scalp with wingless insects is
_____.

9. A drug that prevents or slows blood-clotting time is an _____.

10. Another name for pediculosis is _____.

11. Small, flat insects that feed on the blood of sleeping people and animals are _____.

CIRCLE THE BEST ANSWER

12. Hair care, shaving, and nail and foot care are important to residents because they also affect the need for
    A. Safety and security
    B. Love and belonging and self-esteem
    C. Basic physical needs
    D. Self-actualization

13. If you see any signs of lice, you should report them to the nurse because
    A. Lice bites can cause severe infections
    B. Lice are easily spread to other persons through clothing, furniture, bed linens, and sexual contact
    C. Lice can cause the person's hair to fall out
    D. Lice will cause the hair to mat and tangle

14. The nurse tells you that a person you are caring for has scabies. When giving care, you observe
    A. Dry, white flakes on the scalp
    B. A rash in the underarm area, on the thighs, and in the genital area
    C. White or yellow oval nits on the hair
    D. Tan to grayish-white objects the size of sesame seeds in the pubic hair

15. Who chooses how you will brush, comb, and style a person's hair?
    A. The person
    B. You
    C. The nurse
    D. The care plan

16. If long hair becomes matted or tangled, you should
    A. Braid the hair
    B. Cut the hair to remove the tangles and matting
    C. Talk to the nurse and ask for directions
    D. Get the family's permission to change the hairstyle

17. When caring for a person with hair that is curly, coarse, and dry, which of these would you do?
    A. Braid or cut the hair.
    B. Use a wide-toothed comb.
    C. Start at the ends and work toward the scalp.
    D. Use a fine-tooth comb

18. When shampooing a person who has small braids
    A. Undo the hair and re-braid it each time it is shampooed
    B. The braids are left intact for shampooing
    C. Undo the braids only at night
    D. Comb out the braids once a week

19. If a woman's hair is done by the beautician
    A. Wash her hair only once a week
    B. Shampoo her hair on the day she goes to the beautician
    C. Make sure she wears a shower cap during the tub bath or shower
    D. Wash her hair each time she gets a shower or tub bath
20. If a person has limited range of motion in the neck, he or she is not shampooed
    A. At the sink or on a stretcher with the head tipped back
    B. In the tub or shower with the head tipped forward
    C. During a tub bath
    D. In bed
21. What observation is made and reported when shampooing?
    A. The hair color
    B. The presence of nits or lice
    C. The texture of the hair
    D. The hairstyle
22. If a person receives anticoagulants and needs shaving
    A. An electric razor is used
    B. Use disposable safety razors
    C. It must be done by the nurse or barber
    D. It should be done only during the shower or bath
23. When using safety razors (blade razors)
    A. The same razor can be used for several persons until it becomes dull
    B. Use the resident's own razor several times
    C. Discard the razor blade or disposable razor in the sharps container
    D. Be careful when shaving a person who takes anticoagulants
24. Why is an electric razor used when shaving a person with dementia?
    A. They usually bleed easily.
    B. The person may resist care and move suddenly.
    C. It is faster than using a safety razor.
    D. The person's skin is tender and sensitive.
25. When shaving a person with a safety razor, wear gloves
    A. To protect the person from infections
    B. To prevent contact with blood
    C. When applying shaving cream
    D. To maintain sterile technique
26. When caring for a mustache and beard, you should
    A. Wash and comb the mustache or beard daily
    B. Allow only the barber to groom the mustache or beard
    C. Wash with shampoo and conditioner
    D. Trim a mustache or beard when needed
27. Nursing assistants can trim nails
    A. Whenever they have time
    B. On all persons
    C. Only if center policy allows them to do so
    D. If the person agrees to the care

28. When caring for the fingernails, you should
    A. Cut the nails with small scissors
    B. Shape the nails with an emery board or nail file
    C. Clip the nails straight across with nail clippers
    D. Soak the hands for 15 to 20 minutes
29. When changing clothing, remove the clothing from
    A. The weak side first
    B. The lower limbs first
    C. The right side last
    D. The strong or "good" side first
30. When you are undressing a person, it is usually done
    A. In the bed in the supine position
    B. With the person sitting in a chair
    C. With the person standing at the bedside
    D. In the bathroom
31. When you are changing the person's clothes, you use good body mechanics by
    A. Having a good base of support
    B. Holding objects close to your body
    C. Raising the bed to a good working level
    D. Lifting with the large muscles
32. To provide warmth and privacy when changing clothes, you
    A. Keep the top sheets in place
    B. Cover the person with a bath blanket
    C. Close the curtains
    D. Close the door
33. When changing the gown of a person with an IV
    A. Turn off the IV
    B. Lay the IV bag on the bed and remove the gown
    C. Slide the gathered sleeve over the tubing, hand, arm, and IV site
    D. Disconnect the IV
34. When you have finished changing the gown of a person with an IV, always
    A. Re-start the pump
    B. Re-connect the IV
    C. Ask the nurse to check the flow rate
    D. Check the flow rate

FILL IN THE BLANKS

35. Write the meaning of the following abbreviations
    A. C _____
    B. F _____
    C. ID _____
    D. IV _____
36. When you are giving care, report these signs and symptoms of lice to the nurse at once
    A. _____
    B. _____
    C. _____
    D. _____
    E. _____

37. When you brush and comb the hair, you should report and record

A. _____

B. _____

C. _____

D. _____

E. _____

F. _____

G. _____

H. _____

38. If you give hair care to a person in bed after a linen change, collect falling hair by _____

_____ .

39. Brush and comb matted hair by starting at the

_____ and working up to the _____ .

40. You can protect the person's eyes during shampooing by asking the person to hold a _____

_____ .

41. What delegation guidelines do you need when shaving a person?

A. _____

B. _____

C. _____

D. _____

E. _____

F. _____

G. _____

H. _____

42. What should be reported at *once* when you are shaving a person?

A. _____

B. _____

C. _____

43. When you are shaving the face and underarms with a safety razor, shave in the direction of the

_____ .

44. When shaving legs with a safety razor, shave

_____ .

45. When using an electric shaver, shave

_____ .

46. When you are delegated to give nail and foot care, report and record

A. _____

B. _____

C. _____

D. _____

E. _____

47. Foot care for persons with diabetes or poor

circulation is provided by _____

or _____ .

48. When undressing the person who cannot raise the head and shoulders

A. _____

B. _____

C. _____

D. _____

E. _____

49. When dressing the person who cannot raise the hips and buttocks

A. _____

B. _____

C. _____

D. _____

E. _____

50. Before changing the hospital gown of a person with an IV, what information do you need from the nurse and the care plan?

A. _____

B. _____

OPTIONAL LEARNING EXERCISES

51. You are caring for a person who is receiving cancer treatments. What effect could this treatment have

on the person's hair? _____

_____ .

52. Dandruff not only occurs on the scalp, but it may

involve the _____ .

53. How are each of these problems treated?

    A. Lice _____

    _____

    B. Scabies _____

    _____

    C. Bed bugs _____

    _____

54. Brushing the hair increases _____

    to the scalp. It also brings _____
    along the hair shaft.

55. Why do older persons usually have dry hair?

    _____

56. What water temperature is usually used when

    shampooing the hair? _____

57. How can the beard be softened before shaving?

    _____

    _____

58. After shaving, why do some people apply after-shave or lotion?

    A. Lotion _____

    B. After-shave _____

59. Injuries to the feet of a person with poor circulation are serious because poor circulation

    _____.

60. When changing clothing or hospital gowns, what rules should be followed?

    A. _____

    B. _____

    C. _____

    D. _____

    E. _____

    F. _____

61. How does grooming improve quality of life?

    A. Promotes _____

    B. Helps the person's _____

    and _____

    C. Whenever possible, it allows for

    _____

    D. Treats personal _____ and

    _____.

INDEPENDENT LEARNING ACTIVITIES

- Role-play this situation with a classmate. Take turns being the resident and the nursing assistant. Remember to keep your left arm and leg limp when you are the resident.
  - **Situation:** *Mr. Olsen is a 58-year-old resident who has weakness on the left side. You are assigned to take off his sleepwear and dress him for the day. You need to remove his pajamas and dress him in a shirt, a pullover sweater, slacks, socks, and shoes.*
    - How did you provide privacy?
    - How was Mr. Olsen positioned for the clothing change?
    - What difficulties did you have when you removed his pajamas?
  - Which arm did you re-dress first? What difficulty did you have getting his arms into the shirt?
  - How did you put on the sweater? What was most difficult about this?
  - What was the most difficult part of putting on the slacks?
  - How did you put on the socks and shoes?
  - What did you learn from this role-play situation? Did you follow the procedure in the chapter to assist you?
  - Discuss with each other how it felt to have someone dress you when you were "Mr. Olsen."

19 NUTRITION AND FLUIDS

FILL IN THE BLANKS: KEY TERMS

Anorexia
Aspiration
Calorie
Daily Value (DV)

Dehydration
Dysphagia
Edema
Graduate

Intake
Nutrient
Nutrition
Output

1. _____ is the amount of fluid taken in.

2. The _____ is how a serving fits into the daily diet. It is expressed in a percentage based on a daily diet of 2000 calories.

3. The loss of appetite is _____.

4. The amount of fluid lost is _____.

5. A substance that is ingested, digested, absorbed, and used by the body is a _____.

6. _____ is difficulty swallowing.

7. The breathing of fluid, food, vomitus, or an object into the lungs is _____.

8. The many processes involved in the ingestion, digestion, absorption, and use of food and fluids by the body is _____.

9. The fuel or energy value of food is a _____.

10. A decrease in the amount of water in body tissues is _____.

11. A _____ is a measuring container for fluid.

12. _____ is the swelling of body tissues with water.

CIRCLE THE BEST ANSWER

13. When a person has a poor diet and poor eating habits, he or she is likely to have
    A. Decreased risk for infection
    B. Improved wound healing
    C. Increased risk for accidents and injuries
    D. Decreased risk of acute and chronic diseases

14. Body fuel for energy is found in
    A. Vitamins
    B. Minerals
    C. Fats, proteins, and carbohydrates
    D. Water

15. The *Dietary Guidelines for Americans, 2010* help people
    A. Recover from chronic illnesses
    B. Promote over-all health
    C. Develop a vegetarian diet
    D. Aim to include 2500 mg of sodium in their diet each day

16. *Dietary Guidelines for Americans, 2010* recommends
    A. Eating a diet with more than 300 mg of cholesterol
    B. Including raw fish or shellfish in the diet
    C. Reducing daily sodium intake to less than 2300 mg for healthy people
    D. Eating plenty of refined grain foods, especially those that contain solid fats

17. What type of fat should be kept as low as possible in the diet, according to the *Dietary Guidelines for Americans, 2010*?
    A. Trans fatty acids
    B. Saturated fatty acids
    C. Monosaturated fatty acids
    D. Polyunsaturated fatty acids

18. According to the *Dietary Guidelines for Americans, 2010*, persons over 51 years of age and those with certain chronic diseases should reduce sodium intake to
    A. Less than 1000 mg a day
    B. No more than 3500 mg a day
    C. No more than 1500 mg a day
    D. No more than 5000 mg a day

19. In *Dietary Guidelines for Americans, 2010*, building healthy eating patterns includes
    A. Eating the same foods every day
    B. Eating only fruits and vegetables
    C. Selecting an eating pattern that meets nutrient needs over time
    D. Taking a multi-vitamin to supplement the diet

20. The MyPlate plan recommends increasing
    A. The size of portions eaten
    B. Fruits and vegetables to half of your plate
    C. Sodium intake
    D. Intake of sugary drinks
21. Which of these is an example of moderate physical activity?
    A. Playing singles tennis
    B. Walking at about 2 miles per hour
    C. Participating in water aerobics
    D. Swimming freestyle laps
22. Dairy products in the My Plate plan should
    A. Supply more than half of the calories in the diet
    B. Be a very small amount of the calories in the diet
    C. Be mostly fat-free or low-fat (1%) products
    D. Be mostly high-fat products
23. Vegetables in the MyPlate plan should be
    A. High in cholesterol
    B. Served only uncooked
    C. Always dark green in color
    D. Fresh, frozen, or canned
24. Oils are
    A. One of the food groups in the MyPlate plan
    B. Low in calories
    C. Liquid at room temperatures
    D. Solid at room temperature
25. Which nutrient is needed for tissue growth and repair?
    A. Carbohydrates
    B. Fats
    C. Vitamins
    D. Protein
26. Which vitamin is needed for the formation of substances that hold tissue together?
    A. Vitamin K
    B. Vitamin C
    C. Vitamin A
    D. Vitamin B_{12}
27. Food labels are important because they help people
    A. Determine the cost of the food
    B. Know all of the vitamins and minerals in the food
    C. Know the total amount of fat and the amount of saturated and trans fats
    D. Determine the flavor of the food
28. A cultural group that eats a diet of rice with meat, fish, and vegetables that is high in sodium is found in
    A. The Philippines
    B. China
    C. Poland
    D. Mexico
29. Which of these religious groups forbids eating all pork and pork products?
    A. Seventh-Day Adventists
    B. Islam or Muslims
    C. Church of Jesus Christ of Latter-Day Saints
    D. Roman Catholics

30. People with limited incomes often buy
    A. More protein foods
    B. Foods high in carbohydrates
    C. Foods high in vitamins and minerals
    D. Fatty foods
31. When people buy cheaper foods, the diet may lack
    A. Fats
    B. Starchy foods
    C. Protein and certain vitamins and minerals
    D. Sugars
32. Appetite can be stimulated by
    A. Illness and medications
    B. Decreased senses of taste and smell
    C. Aromas and thoughts of food
    D. Anxiety, pain, and depression
33. When a person has swallowing difficulties, he or she will be given foods that
    A. Are thickened
    B. Are easy to chew
    C. Have been pureed and are very liquid
    D. Can be given through a feeding tube
34. During illness
    A. Appetite increases
    B. Fewer nutrients are needed
    C. Nutritional needs increase to fight infection and heal tissue
    D. The person will prefer protein foods
35. As a person ages, changes in the GI system can cause
    A. Increases in taste and smell
    B. Increases in secretion of digestive juices
    C. Difficulty swallowing
    D. A decrease in the appetite
36. Requirements for food served in long-term care centers are made by
    A. MyPlate
    B. OBRA and CMS
    C. The nursing center
    D. The public health department
37. A requirement for food served in long-term care centers is
    A. All food served must be cut up or ground
    B. The person's diet is well-balanced, nourishing, and tastes good
    C. All food is served at room temperature
    D. No salt or sugar is added to the food
38. A general diet
    A. Is ordered for person with difficulty swallowing
    B. Has no dietary limits or restrictions
    C. May have restricted amounts of sodium
    D. Increases the amount of sugar in the diet
39. The body needs no more than _____ of sodium each day.
    A. 2400 mg
    B. 3000 mg
    C. 5000 mg
    D. 1000 mg

40. When the body tissues swell with water, what organ has to work harder?
    A. Kidneys
    B. Liver
    C. Heart
    D. Lungs
41. When you are caring for a person with diabetes, you should
    A. Serve the person's meals and snacks when the person requests food
    B. Give the person extra salt or sugar as requested
    C. Give the person extra food and snacks whenever requested
    D. Serve meals and snacks at regular times
42. A person may be given a mechanical soft diet because
    A. Nausea and vomiting have occurred
    B. The person has chewing difficulties
    C. The person has been advanced from a clear-liquid diet
    D. The person has constipation
43. If you are serving a meal to a person on a fiber- and residue-restricted diet, the meal would *not* include
    A. Raw fruits and vegetables
    B. Strained fruit juices
    C. Canned or cooked fruit without skin or seeds
    D. Plain pasta
44. A person who has serious burns would receive a
    A. Sodium-controlled diet
    B. Fat-controlled diet
    C. High-calorie diet
    D. High-protein diet
45. When a person has dysphagia, the thickness of the food served is chosen by the
    A. Person
    B. Nursing assistant
    C. Family
    D. Speech-language pathologist, dietitian, and doctor or nurse
46. A thickened liquid on a dysphagia diet is served
    A. From a cup
    B. In a bowl
    C. By stirring immediately before serving
    D. According to the care plan
47. When assisting a person with dysphagia, you can help prevent aspiration while the person is eating by placing him or her in
    A. Semi-Fowler's position
    B. Fowler's position or upright in a chair
    C. The side-lying position
    D. The supine position
48. If fluid intake exceeds fluid output, the person may
    A. Have edema in the tissues
    B. Be dehydrated
    C. Have vomiting and diarrhea
    D. Have increased urinary output

49. How much fluid is needed every day for normal fluid balance?
    A. 1500 mL
    B. 1000–1500 mL
    C. 2000–2500 mL
    D. 3000–4000 mL
50. If the person you are caring for has an order for restricted fluids, which of these should you do?
    A. Offer a variety of liquids.
    B. Thicken all fluids.
    C. Remove the water pitcher from the room.
    D. Do not allow the person to swallow any liquids during oral hygiene.
51. When you are keeping I&O records, you should measure all of these except
    A. Milk, water, coffee, and tea
    B. Mashed potatoes and creamed vegetables
    C. Gelatin and popsicles
    D. Ice cream, custard, and pudding
52. When you are measuring I&O, you need to know that 1 ounce equals
    A. 10 mL
    B. 500 mL
    C. 100 mL
    D. 30 mL
53. When you are using the graduate to measure output, you read the amount by
    A. Holding the graduate at waist level and reading the amount
    B. Looking at the graduate while it is held above eye level
    C. Keeping the container at eye level
    D. Setting the graduate on the floor and reading it
54. When I&O is ordered, which of the following is measured as output?
    A. Perspiration
    B. Solid stool
    C. Drainage from suction
    D. Solid foods
55. A quietly confused person may sometimes be served meals in a _____ dining program.
    A. Social
    B. Family
    C. Low-stimulation
    D. Restaurant-style
56. Which of the following needs to be done before the person is served a meal?
    A. Give complete personal care.
    B. Change all linens.
    C. Make sure the person is clean and dry.
    D. Make sure the person has been shaved or has make-up applied.
57. What should you do if a food tray has not been served within 15 minutes?
    A. Re-check the food temperatures.
    B. Serve the tray immediately.
    C. Throw the food away.
    D. Serve only the cold items on the tray.

58. How can you make sure the food tray is complete?
    A. Ask the person being served.
    B. Ask the nurse.
    C. Call the dietary department.
    D. Check items on the tray with the dietary card.
59. If you become impatient while feeding a resident with dementia, you should
    A. Refuse to continue caring for the person
    B. Return the person to his or her room
    C. Talk to the nurse
    D. Make the person eat his or her food
60. When you are feeding a person, you should
    A. Not allow the person to assist
    B. Give the person a fork and knife to assist with cutting the food
    C. Feed the person in a private area to maintain confidentiality
    D. Use a spoon because it is less likely to cause injury
61. When feeding a person, liquids are given
    A. Only at the start of feeding
    B. During the meal, alternating with solid foods
    C. At the end of the meal when all solids have been eaten
    D. Only if the person has difficulty swallowing
62. When providing fresh water to residents, you would
    A. Give fresh water once each shift
    B. Put ice in all pitchers
    C. Practice the rules of medical asepsis to prevent the spread of microbes
    D. Give each person one glass of water at a time
63. When you keep track of calorie intake, you include
    A. What time the person ate
    B. Only the liquids that the person drinks
    C. All of the food that was served to the person
    D. What the person ate and how much
64. When residents are included in deciding what foods they eat, the person's right to _____ is being met.
    A. Personal choice
    B. Privacy
    C. Confidentiality
    D. Good nutrition

FILL IN THE BLANKS

65. Write out the meaning of each abbreviation.
    A. CMS _____
    B. DV _____
    C. GI _____
    D. I&O _____
    E. mg _____
    F. mL _____
    G. NPO _____
    H. OBRA _____
    I. oz _____
    J. USDA _____
66. How many calories are in each of these?
    A. 1 gram of fat _____
    B. 1 gram of protein _____
    C. 1 gram of carbohydrate _____

Questions 67 to 71 relate to the Dietary Guidelines for Americans, 2010.

67. The Dietary Guidelines help people
    A. _____
    B. _____
    C. _____
68. Which foods or food components should be reduced in the diet?
    A. _____ to less than 2300 mg
    B. Consume less than 10% of diet from _____
    C. Consume less than 300 mg of _____
    D. Keep _____ consumption as low as possible
69. What foods and nutrients should be increased?
    A. A variety of _____, especially _____
    B. Half of all grains should be _____
    C. Fat-free or low-fat _____
    D. _____ should be chosen in place of meat and poultry
70. What recommendations are made to manage weight?
    A. _____
    B. _____
    C. _____
    D. _____

71. What guidelines are given to build healthy eating patterns?

    A. _____

    B. _____

    C. _____

Questions 72 to 77 relate to MyPlate.

72. What are the 5 food groups included in MyPlate?

    A. _____

    B. _____

    C. _____

    D. _____

    E. _____

73. _____ are also included in food patterns but are not a food group.

74. What foods contain the entire grain kernel?

    A. _____

    B. _____

    C. _____

    D. _____

    E. _____

75. What are 5 vegetable sub-groups?

    A. _____

    B. _____

    C. _____

    D. _____

    E. _____

76. What are the health benefits of milk and milk products?

    A. _____

    B. _____

    C. _____

77. What nutrients are provided in protein foods?

    A. _____

    B. _____

    C. _____

78. If dietary fat is not needed by the body, it is stored as _____.

79. What is the function of each of these nutrients?

    A. Protein _____

    B. Carbohydrates _____

    C. Fats _____

    D. Vitamins _____

    E. Minerals _____

    F. Water _____

80. Which vitamins can be stored by the body?

    _____

81. Which vitamins must be ingested daily?

    _____

82. What vitamin is important for these functions? *Formation of substances that hold tissues together; healthy blood vessels, skin, gums, bones, and teeth; wound healing; prevention of bleeding; resistance to infection* _____

83. Milk and milk products, liver, green leafy vegetables, eggs, breads, and cereals are good sources of which vitamin? _____

84. What mineral allows red blood cells to carry oxygen? _____

85. When the diet does not have enough _____, it may affect nerve function, muscle contraction, and heart function.

86. Calcium is needed for _____

    _____.

87. What information is found on food labels?

    A. _____

    B. _____

    C. _____

88. Those who practice _____ as part of their religion eat only fish with scales and fins.

89. Alcohol and coffee are avoided or discouraged by these religious groups.

    A. _____

    B. _____

    C. _____

90. What religious group may have members who fast from meats on certain Fridays during the year?

    _____

91. Nutritional needs increase during illness when the body must _____ _____ .

92. Why do the diets of people with limited income sometimes lack protein? _____ _____

93. What OBRA requirement relates to the temperature of foods served in long-term care centers? _____ _____

94. What foods are included in a clear-liquid diet? _____ _____ _____

95. When the person receives a full-liquid diet, it will include all of the foods on the clear-liquid diet as well as these foods: _____ _____ _____ .

96. If a person has poorly fitted dentures and has chewing difficulties, the doctor may order a _____ diet.

97. A person who is constipated and has other GI disorders may receive a _____ diet. The foods in this diet increase the amount of _____ to stimulate _____

98. If a person is receiving a high-calorie diet, the calorie intake is increased to _____ _____

99. What vegetable juices are high in sodium? _____

100. When a person is receiving a diabetic diet, the same amount of _____ _____ are eaten each day.

101. If you are feeding a person a dysphagia diet, what observations should be reported to the nurse immediately?

    A. _____ , _____ , or _____ during or after meal

    B. _____ or _____

102. Why is it important to offer water often to older persons? _____ _____

103. When you give oral hygiene to a person who is receiving nothing by mouth, the person must not _____ .

104. List the amount of millimeters in the following

    A. 1 ounce equals _____ mL.

    B. 1 pint equals about _____ mL.

    C. 1 quart equals about _____ mL.

105. What information do you need when you are delegated to measure intake and output?

    A. _____

    B. _____

    C. _____

    D. _____

    E. _____

106. What type of dining programs may be used with persons who are oriented or are quietly confused? _____

107. What can be done to promote comfort when preparing residents for meals?

    A. _____

    B. _____

    C. _____

    D. _____

    E. _____

    F. _____

108. If a food tray is not served within 15 minutes, what should be checked? _____

109. When you are delegated to serve meal trays, what information do you need from the nurse or the care plan?

    A. _____

    B. _____

    C. _____

    D. _____

    E. _____

    F. _____

110. When you are serving meal trays, you make sure the right person gets the right tray by checking

    _____

    _____ .

111. When you are feeding a person, the spoon should

    be filled _____ .

112. Why is it important to sit facing the person when you feed him or her?

    A. _____

    B. _____

    C. _____

113. What should be reported after you have fed a person?

    A. _____

    B. _____

    C. _____

    D. _____

114. What are safety tips from the USDA to keep food safe to eat?

    A. Clean _____

    B. Separate _____

    C. Cook _____

    D. Chill _____

LABELING

115. Enter this information on the intake and output record. Total amounts are for the 8-hour and 24-hour periods. Amounts in ( ) indicate how much a person ate or drank. Use 2400–0800, 0800–1600, and 1600–2400 as 8-hour periods.

0200	*Voided 300 mL*
0600	*Voided 500 mL*
0730	***Breakfast***
	Orange juice (whole glass)
	Milk (½ carton)
	Coffee (1 cup)
0700	*Voided 300 mL*
1000	*Water pitcher filled*
1130	***Lunch***
	Soup (whole bowl)
	Milk (½ carton)
	Tea (1 cup)
	Jell-O (1 serving)
1330	*Voided 450 mL*
1430	*Water pitcher 500 mL (refilled)*

1530	*Vomited 50 mL*
1545	*1 can of soda (whole can)*
1730	***Dinner***
	Soup (whole bowl)
	Tea (1 cup)
	Juice (whole glass)
	Ice cream (all)
1730	*Voided 250 mL*
1830	*Vomited 100 mL*
1915	*Voided 500 mL*
2000	*Milk (1 carton)*
2015	*Voided 300 mL*
2330	*Voided 200 mL*

OSF
ST. JOSEPH MEDICAL CENTER

Bloomington, Illinois

FLUID BALANCE CHART

Water Glass	250cc	Ice Cream	120cc
Styrofoam Cup	180cc	Ice Chips	1/2 amt. of
Cup (coffee)	250cc		cc's in cup
Milk Carton	240cc	Pitcher	
Pop (1 can)	360cc	(Yellow)	1000cc
Broth-Soup	175cc		
Juice Carton	120cc		
Juice Glass	120cc		
Jello	120cc		

DATE _____

	INTAKE			OUTPUT					
				URINE		OTHER		CONT. IRRIGATION	
TIME	ORAL	Parenteral	Amt. cc Absbd.	Method Collected	Amt. (cc)	Method Collected	Amt. (cc)	In	Out
2400-0100		cc from previous shift							
0100-0200									
0200-0300									
0300-0400									
0400-0500									
0500-0600									
0600-0700									
0700-0800									
		8 - hour Sub-total		8-hr T		8-hr T			
0800-0900		cc from previous shift							
0900-1000									
1000-1100									
1100-1200									
1200-1300									
1300-1400									
1400-1500									
1500-1600									
		8 - hour Sub-total		8-hr T		8-hr T			
1600-1700		cc from previous shift							
1700-1800									
1800-1900									
1900-2000									
2000-2100									
2100-2200									
2200-2300									
2300-2400									
		8 - hour Sub-total		8-hr T		8-hr T			
		24 - hour Sub-total		24-hr T		24-hr T			

Source Key:

URINE

V - Voided
C - Catheter
INC - Incontinent
U.C. - Ureteral Catheter

Source Key:

OTHER

G.I.T. - Gastric Intestinal Tube
T.T. - T. Tube
Vom. - Vomitus
Liq S. - Liquid Stool
H.V. - Hemovac

310' Marie Mills

Form No. MF36722 (Rev. 5/97)   **MFI**

116. Label the plate with numbers so that you can describe the location of food to a blind person. How would you tell a visually impaired person who asks you where to find the food items on the plate?

   A. Bread _____

   B. Baked potato _____

   C. Vegetables _____

   D. Meat _____

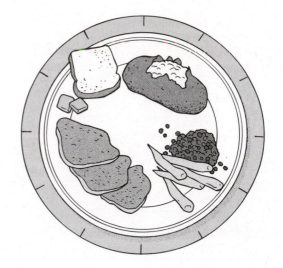

OPTIONAL LEARNING EXERCISES

117. John is 40 years old. The following is his food intake for one day. List the foods in the correct food group from MyPlate and list the number of servings in each group.

BREAKFAST
6 oz orange juice
1 cup oatmeal
½ cup milk
2 slices toast with 1 tablespoon butter
1 cup black coffee

LUNCH
1 cup tomato soup
Grilled cheese sandwich (with 1 oz natural
   cheese and 2 slices bread)
12 oz diet soda

DINNER
2 pork chops (4 oz each)
4 oz baked potato with 2 tablespoons butter
¼ cup green beans
4 oz pudding
1 cup black coffee

SNACKS
1 apple
2 oz peanuts
1 can regular soda
½ cup ice cream

A. Grains _____

   Servings _____

B. Vegetables _____

   Servings _____

C. Fruits _____

   Servings _____

D. Dairy _____

   Servings _____

E. Protein _____

   Servings _____

F. Other, including oils _____

   Servings _____

118. How many servings of each food group should John have? How many did he actually consume?

	Daily Servings	Servings Consumed
A. Grains	_____	_____
B. Vegetables	_____	_____
C. Fruits	_____	_____
D. Dairy	_____	_____
E. Protein	_____	_____

INDEPENDENT LEARNING ACTIVITIES

- Now that you have learned about good nutrition, use this exercise to find out whether you eat a nutritious diet. List your intake for 1 day. Be sure to include the amount of each item—remember, the portion size is important.

  Group the foods and liquids you eat according to the parts of MyPlate. If you wish, you may go to www.ChooseMyPlate.gov and follow the directions there to group the foods. Answer the following questions.
  - How many servings of grains did you eat? How many of these servings were whole grain?
  - How many servings of fruit did you eat? How many were fresh fruit? Canned fruit? Fruit juice? Had added sugars?
  - How many servings of vegetable did you eat? How many were raw? Cooked? How much sodium was contained in prepared vegetables?
  - How many servings of dairy products did you eat? How many were low-fat or fat-free?
  - How many servings of protein foods did you eat? How many were high in fat? Low in fat? High in sodium?
  - How many foods did you eat that count as oils?
  - In which food groups are you meeting your daily needs?
  - In which groups do you need to increase your intake? Decrease your intake?
  - How much physical activity did you include in your daily plan?

- After completing this exercise, what changes in your diet and activity level will you consider?
- Role-play with a classmate and take turns feeding each other as you would a resident. You may choose any spoon-fed foods you wish. (Pudding, gelatin, and soup are suggestions.) You should also give a beverage to the person.

  After you have fed each other, answer the following questions.
  - How were your physical needs met before you were fed? (toileting, handwashing, oral hygiene)
  - Where were you fed? (bed, chair, at a table) Who made the decision about your location?
  - Which food was offered first? Who made the choice of how food was offered? Where you offered a variety of foods?
  - When was a beverage offered? Between food items? Only at the end of feeding? How did the person feeding you decide the order of foods and beverages? The temperature of these items?
  - When you were being fed, how was the nursing assistant positioned? Sitting? Standing? How did the person's position make you feel?
  - What kind of conversation was carried on while you were eating? What chances were offered to rest while you were eating? Did you feel relaxed or rushed?
  - After this exercise, what will you do differently when you feed a resident?

20 NUTRITIONAL SUPPORT AND IV THERAPY

FILL IN THE BLANKS: KEY TERMS

Aspiration
Enteral nutrition
Flow rate
Gastrostomy tube
Gavage

Intravenous (IV) therapy
Jejunostomy tube
Naso-enteral tube
Naso-gastric (NG) tube

Parenteral nutrition
Percutaneous endoscopic
  gastrostomy (PEG) tube
Regurgitation

1. Giving nutrients into the gastrointestinal (GI) tract through a feeding tube is _____ _____.

2. A _____ is a tube inserted through a surgically created opening in the stomach.

3. A feeding tube inserted through the nose into small bowel is a _____ _____.

4. _____ is the backward flow of stomach contents into the mouth.

5. A _____ is a feeding tube inserted into a surgically created opening in the jejunum of the small intestine.

6. The process of giving a tube feeding is called _____.

7. The _____ is the number of drops per minute.

8. _____ is breathing fluid or an object into the lungs.

9. Giving nutrients through a catheter inserted into a vein is _____.

10. _____ is giving fluids through a needle or catheter inserted into a vein.

11. A feeding tube inserted through the nose into the stomach is a _____ _____.

12. A _____ is a feeding tube inserted into the stomach through a small incision made through the skin.

CIRCLE THE BEST ANSWER

13. The doctor may order nutritional support for a person who
    A. Cannot eat enough to meet his or her nutritional needs
    B. Is underweight
    C. Does not like the food served
    D. Is over-weight

14. Which of these tubes are used for short-term nutritional support?
    A. Naso-gastric (NG) tubes
    B. Gastrostomy tubes
    C. Jejunostomy tubes
    D. PEG tubes

15. Opened formula for a gavage feeding can remain at room temperature for
    A. 1 hour
    B. About 8 hours
    C. About 2 hours
    D. Overnight

16. If a person is receiving intermittent (scheduled) feedings, the nurse will
    A. Attach the feeding to a pump
    B. Give feeding four or more times each day
    C. Give the feedings over a 24-hour period
    D. Give the feeding directly from the refrigerator

17. A major risk with tube feedings is
    A. Nausea
    B. Complaints of flatulence
    C. Aspiration
    D. Elevated temperature

18. If a person is receiving a gavage feeding, you should report at once if
    A. The blood pressure is elevated
    B. The person has signs and symptoms of respiratory distress
    C. The pulse rate is within normal range
    D. The person is sleeping

19. You can help prevent regurgitation when a person is receiving gavage by
    A. Positioning the person in a left side-lying position
    B. Maintaining Fowler's or semi-Fowler's position after the feeding
    C. Positioning the person in a supine position
    D. Positioning the person in prone position
20. When a person is receiving nutrition through a tube, frequent mouth care is needed because
    A. It stimulates peristalsis to aid digestion
    B. It prevents discomfort from dry mouth, dry lips, and sore throat
    C. It provides additional fluid intake
    D. It provides additional nutrition
21. Which of these are *never* done by nursing assistants?
    A. Inserting a feeding tube
    B. Removing a feeding tube
    C. Giving tube feedings
    D. Cleaning area around a feeding tube
22. When a person is receiving TPN, the nursing assistant would assist by
    A. Removing the tube
    B. Inserting the tube
    C. Providing frequent oral hygiene and other basic needs
    D. Giving the feedings
23. When caring for a person receiving IV therapy, the nursing assistant should
    A. Adjust the flow rate if it is too fast or too slow
    B. Report to the nurse if no fluid is dripping
    C. Disconnect the IV to give basic care
    D. Change the IV bag when it is empty
24. You may change a dressing on a peripheral IV if
    A. The nurse asks you to do this
    B. You observe that it is loose and soiled
    C. Your state allows nursing assistants to perform the procedure
    D. You think you know how to do this procedure

FILL IN THE BLANKS

25. Write out the meaning of each abbreviation.
    A. GI _____
    B. gtt _____
    C. gtt/min _____
    D. IV _____
    E. mL _____
    F. NG _____

G. NPO _____
H. oz _____
I. PEG _____
J. PICC _____
K. TPN _____

26. Naso-gastric and naso-intestinal tubes are in place for short-term nutritional support, usually for less than _____.
27. Gastrostomy, jejunostomy, and PEG tubes are used for long-term support, usually longer than

_____.

28. Formula is given through a feeding tube at room temperature because cold fluids cause _____.
29. Coughing, sneezing, vomiting, suctioning, and poor positioning can move a tube out of place and are common causes of _____.
30. What can the nursing assistant do to assist the nurse in preventing regurgitation and aspiration?
    A. _____
    B. _____
    C. _____
31. What comfort measures will help a person with a feeding tube who has a dry mouth?
    A. _____
    B. _____
    C. _____
32. The nose and nostrils are cleaned every 4 to 8 hours because a feeding tube can _____

and _____.

33. If your state and job description allow you to be delegated the task of giving a tube feeding, what should the nurse identify and check first?
    A. _____
    B. _____
34. How much flushing solution is used before giving a tube feeding to an adult? _____

_____

35. When a person is receiving TPN, what signs and symptoms should be reported to the nurse at once?

    A. _____

    B. _____

    C. _____

    D. _____

    E. _____

    F. _____

    G. _____

    H. _____

    I. _____

    J. _____

    K. _____

    L. _____

    M. _____

    N. _____

36. When caring for a person receiving IV therapy, what complications at the IV site would you observe and report?

    A. _____

    B. _____

    C. _____

    D. _____

    E. _____

OPTIONAL LEARNING EXERCISES

37. What type of feeding tube would each of these persons probably have in place?

    A. The nurse tells you Mr. S. is expected to have a feeding tube to his stomach for 2 to 3 weeks.

    _____

    B. Mrs. G. has had a feeding tube to her stomach for 9 months. _____,

    _____, or _____

    C. The nurse tells you to observe Mr. H. for irritation of his nose and nostril when you give care. _____ or

    _____

D. The nurse tells you that Mrs. K. is at great risk for regurgitation from her feeding tube. _____

    or _____

38. Why is formula warmed to room temperature when is has been refrigerated?

    _____

39. Why are older persons more at risk for regurgitation and aspiration?

    A. _____

    B. _____

40. What would you do if a person with a feeding tube asks you for something to eat or drink? _____

    _____ He or she may be allowed to

    have _____.

41. Mrs. H. has a feeding tube in her nose. Answer these questions about caring for her nose and nostrils.

    A. How often should the nose and nostrils be cleaned? _____

    B. How is the tube secured to the nose?

    _____

    C. Why is the tube secured to the person's garment at the shoulder? _____

    _____

    D. What are 2 ways the tube can be secured at the shoulder?

    1. _____

    2. _____

42. When giving tube feedings, what answers would you likely get if you asked the nurse these questions?

    A. What feeding method is used? _____

    _____

    B. What size syringe is used? _____

    _____

    C. How is the person positioned for the feeding?

    _____

    D. How is the person positioned after the feeding?

    _____

E. How high is the syringe raised or the feeding bag hung? _____

F. How much fluid is used to flush the tubing?

_____

G. How fast is the feeding given if using a syringe?

_____

43. If a person is receiving TPN, how will you assist the nurse?

A. _____

B. _____

C. _____

44. How can you check the flow rate of an IV?

_____

45. What would you tell the RN at once when you check the flow rate?

A. _____

B. _____

C. _____

46. When you assist the person with an IV in turning and re-positioning, how should the IV bag be handled?

A. _____

B. _____

INDEPENDENT LEARNING ACTIVITIES

- Have you or anyone you know ever needed enteral nutrition? Either answer these questions yourself or ask the person you know to answer them.
  - How long was the tube in place? What type of tube was used?
  - What discomfort or pain was felt?
  - How did having a feeding tube affect your activity? Your personal care and grooming?
- Have you ever had an IV? Answer these questions about the experience.
  - What type of IV did you have? Where was it inserted?
  - How long was the IV in place?
  - How did the IV interfere with your care, grooming, or activity?
- You may care for a person who is not receiving any nutritional support or IV therapy. Answer these questions about how you handle this situation.
  - How would you feel about caring for a person who is not receiving any nutritional support?
  - How would your religious or cultural values affect you in this situation?
  - If the situation made you uncomfortable, what would you do?

CROSSWORD

Fill in the crossword by choosing words from this list.

Aspiration   gtt   naso-enteral   oz
Gastrostomy   IV   naso-gastric   regurgitation
Gavage   Jejunostomy NPO   TPN
GI   mL   PEG

Across
7. Feeding tube inserted through the nose into the small intestine
9. Tube inserted through surgically created opening in the stomach
10. Abbreviation for giving fluids through a needle or catheter inserted into a vein
11. Backward flow of stomach contents into the mouth
13. Abbreviation for total parenteral nutrition
14. Abbreviation for drop
15. Abbreviation for gastro-intestinal

Down
1. Process of giving a tube feeding
2. Feeding tube inserted through the nose into the stomach
3. Abbreviation for feeding tube inserted into the stomach through a small incision made through the skin
4. Feeding tube inserted in a surgically created opening in the jejunum or the small intestine
5. Abbreviation for milliliter
6. Abbreviation for nothing by mouth
8. Breathing fluid, food, vomitus, or an object into the lungs
12. Abbreviation for ounce

21 URINARY ELIMINATION

FILL IN THE BLANKS: KEY TERMS

Catheter
Catheterization
Dysuria
Foley catheter
Functional incontinence
Hematuria
Indwelling catheter
Micturition

Mixed incontinence
Nocturia
Oliguria
Overflow incontinence
Polyuria
Reflex incontinence
Retention catheter
Straight catheter

Stress incontinence
Transient incontinence
Urge incontinence
Urinary frequency
Urinary incontinence
Urinary urgency
Urination
Voiding

1. Abnormally large amounts of urine are called

   _____.

2. _____ is the combination of
   stress incontinence and urge incontinence.

3. A Foley or indwelling catheter is also called a

   _____.

4. The process of inserting a catheter is

   _____.

5. _____ is the involuntary loss
   or leakage of urine.

6. Frequent urination at night is _____.

7. A catheter left in the bladder so urine drains
   constantly into a drainage bag is called a retention,

   Foley, or _____.

8. _____ is temporary or
   occasional incontinence that is reversed when the
   cause is treated.

9. The loss of small amounts of urine from a full

   bladder is _____

   _____.

10. Another word for urination is _____.

11. _____ occurs when the
    person has bladder control but cannot use the toilet
    in time.

12. Another name for micturition or voiding; the
    process of emptying urine from the bladder is

    _____.

13. A _____ is a tube used to
    drain or inject fluid through a body opening.

14. Blood in the urine is _____.

15. A catheter that drains the bladder and then is

    removed is a _____

    _____.

16. Voiding at frequent intervals is _____.

17. An indwelling or retention catheter is also called a

    _____.

18. When urine leaks during exercise and certain
    movements that cause pressure on the bladder,

    it is called _____.

19. Another word for urination or micturition is

    _____.

20. _____ is the need to void at
    once.

21. The loss of urine in response to a sudden, urgent

    need to void is _____

    _____.

22. Painful or difficult urination is _____.

23. The loss of urine at predictable intervals when the

    bladder is full is _____

    _____.

24. A scant amount of urine, usually less than 500 mL

    in 24 hours, is _____.

CIRCLE THE BEST ANSWER

25. Solid wastes are removed from the body by the
    A. Digestive system
    B. Urinary system
    C. Blood
    D. Integumentary system

26. A healthy adult excretes about

    _____ of urine a day.
    A. 500 mL
    B. 1000 mL
    C. 1500 mL
    D. 2000 mL

27. You can provide privacy when the person is voiding by
    A. Warming the bedpan
    B. Staying in the room
    C. Pulling the curtain around the bed
    D. Asking the roommate to leave the room

28. If the person has difficulty starting the urine stream, you can
    A. Play music on the TV
    B. Provide perineal care
    C. Use a stainless steel bedpan
    D. Run water in a nearby sink

29. The urine may be bright yellow if the person eats
    A. Asparagus
    B. Carrots and sweet potatoes
    C. Beets and blackberries
    D. Rhubarb

30. When using a steel bedpan you should
    A. Keep the pan in the utility room
    B. Warm the pan with water and dry it before use
    C. Sterilize the pan after each use
    D. Cool the pan with water and dry it before use

31. When you are getting ready to give a person the bedpan, you should
    A. Raise the head of the bed slightly
    B. Position the person in the Fowler's position
    C. Wash the person's hands
    D. Place the bed in a flat position

32. Urinals are usually placed at the bedside on
    A. Bed rails
    B. Over-bed tables
    C. Bedside stands
    D. The floor

33. If a man is unable to place a urinal to void, you should
    A. Tell the nurse
    B. Ask a male co-worker to help the man
    C. Place the penis in the urinal
    D. Pad the bed with incontinence pads

34. A commode chair is used when
    A. The person is unable to walk to the bathroom
    B. You need to obtain a urine specimen
    C. The person does not want to use the toilet
    D. The bathroom is occupied by another person

35. When you place a commode over the toilet
    A. Restrain the person
    B. Stay in the room with the person
    C. Lock the wheels
    D. Make sure the container is in place

36. Dribbling of urine that occurs with laughing, sneezing, coughing, lifting, or other activities means the person has
    A. Urge incontinence
    B. Stress incontinence
    C. Overflow incontinence
    D. Functional incontinence

37. When you do not answer lights quickly or do not position the call light within the person's reach, it can cause
    A. Overflow incontinence
    B. Mixed incontinence
    C. Reflex incontinence
    D. Functional incontinence

38. When a person with dementia is incontinent, you can provide safe care by
    A. Telling the person it is wrong to be incontinent
    B. Changing the person's wet clothing once every 2 hours to establish a schedule
    C. Reassuring the person if he or she becomes upset when incontinent
    D. Wait for the person to tell you when he or she needs to void

39. It will help prevent urinary tract infections if you
    A. Avoid having the person wear underwear
    B. Decrease fluid intake
    C. Encourage the person to wear cotton underpants
    D. Keep side rails of the bed up

40. When providing perineal care for an incontinent person, you should
    A. Provide perineal care once a day
    B. Dry the perineal area and buttocks after cleaning the area
    C. Remove wet incontinence products, garments, and linens once every 2 hours
    D. Wipe the area with tissue paper or dry washcloths

41. A catheter that is inserted and is then removed is
    A. An indwelling catheter
    B. A straight catheter
    C. A condom catheter
    D. A Foley catheter

42. A person may have an indwelling catheter when
    A. He or she is incontinent
    B. A urine specimen is needed
    C. He or she has a bladder infection
    D. He or she has wounds and pressure ulcers from contact with urine

43. A last resort for incontinence is
    A. Bladder training
    B. Answering call lights promptly
    C. An indwelling catheter
    D. Adequate fluid intake

44. When cleaning a catheter, you should
    A. Wipe 4 inches up the catheter to the meatus
    B. Disconnect the tubing from the drainage bag
    C. Clean the catheter from the meatus down the catheter about 4 inches
    D. Wash and rinse the catheter by washing up and down the tubing

45. The drainage bag from a catheter should not hang from the
    A. Bed frame
    B. Chair
    C. Wheelchair
    D. Bed rail

46. If a catheter is accidentally disconnected from the drainage bag, you should tell the nurse at once and then
    A. Quickly reconnect the drainage system
    B. Clamp the catheter to prevent leakage
    C. Wipe the end of the tube and end of the catheter with antiseptic wipes and reconnect
    D. Discard the drainage bag and get a new bag

47. If a person uses a leg drainage bag, it
    A. Is changed to a drainage bag when the person is in bed
    B. Is attached to the clothing with tape or safety pins
    C. Is attached to the bed rail when the person is in bed
    D. Can be worn 24 hours a day

48. A leg bag needs to be emptied more often than a drainage bag because
    A. It holds less than 1000 mL and the drainage bag holds about 2000 mL
    B. It is more likely to leak than the drainage bag
    C. It holds about 250 mL and the drainage bag holds 1000 mL
    D. It interferes with walking if it is full

49. When you empty a drainage bag, you
    A. Disconnect the bag from the tubing
    B. Clamp the catheter to prevent leakage
    C. Open the clamp on the drain and drain into a graduate
    D. Take the bag into the bathroom to empty it

50. When applying a condom catheter
    A. Apply elastic tape in a spiral around the penis
    B. Make sure the catheter tip is touching the head of the penis
    C. Apply adhesive tape securely in a circle entirely around the penis
    D. Remove and reapply every shift

51. The goal of bladder training is
    A. To keep the person dry and clean
    B. Control of urination
    C. Prevention of skin breakdown
    D. Prevention of infection

52. When you are assisting the person with habit training for bladder rehabilitation
    A. Help the person to the bathroom every 15 or 20 minutes
    B. The voiding is scheduled at regular times to match the person's voiding habits
    C. Clamp the catheter for 1 hour
    D. Tell the person he or she can void only once a shift

53. When you assist with bladder training for a person with an indwelling catheter
    A. Empty the drainage bag every hour
    B. At first, clamp the catheter for 1 hour
    C. At first, clamp the catheter for 3 to 4 hours
    D. Give the person 15 to 20 minutes to start voiding

54. What do the following abbreviations mean?

    A. CMS _____

    B. IV _____

    C. mL _____

    D. UTI _____

FILL IN THE BLANKS

55. What substances increase urine production?

    A. _____

    B. _____

    C. _____

    D. _____

56. A normal position for voiding for women is

    _____. For men, a normal

    position is _____.

57. What can you do to mask urination sounds?

    A. _____

    B. _____

    C. _____

58. Fracture pans are used for persons

    A. _____

    B. _____

    C. _____

    D. _____

    E. _____

    F. _____

59. When a person voids in a bedpan or urinal, what observations about the urine are important?

    A. _____

    B. _____

    C. _____

    D. _____

    E. _____

    F. _____

60. When you are handling bedpans, urinals, and commodes and their contents, you should follow

    _____ and

    _____.

61. When you are delegated to provide a urinal, what guidelines should you follow?

    A. _____

    B. _____

    C. _____

    D. _____

    E. _____

    F. _____

    G. _____

    H. _____

62. When you transfer a person to a commode from bed, you must practice safe transfer practices and

    use a _____ and _____.

63. Name 5 causes of urge incontinence.

    A. _____

    B. _____

    C. _____

    D. _____

    E. _____

64. Stress incontinence is common in women because

    the pelvic muscles weaken from _____

    and with _____.

65. Overflow incontinence may occur in men because

    of a _____.

66. _____ incontinence occurs with nervous system disorders and injuries.

67. When a catheter is inserted after a person voids, it

    is measuring how _____.

68. When you provide perineal care after a person is incontinent, remember to

    A. _____

    B. _____

    C. _____

    D. _____

    E. _____

    F. _____

69. A catheter is secured to the inner thigh or the man's

    abdomen to prevent _____

    _____.

70. When a person has a catheter, what observations should you report and record?

    A. _____

    B. _____

    C. _____

    D. _____

    E. _____

    F. _____

    G. _____

    H. _____

71. When you give catheter care, clean the catheter

    about _____ inches. Clean

    _____ from the meatus with

    _____ stroke.

72. Is the urinary system sterile or non-sterile?

    _____

73. What happens if a drainage bag is higher than the

    bladder? _____ This can

    cause _____.

74. If a drainage system is disconnected accidentally, what should you do?

    A. Tell _____

    B. Do not _____

    C. Practice _____

D. Wipe _____

E. Wipe _____

F. Do not _____

G. Connect _____

H. Discard _____

I. Remove _____

75. Before applying a condom catheter, you should

   A. Provide _____

   B. Observe the penis for _____

76. The catheter is clamped for 1 hour at first and eventually for 3 to 4 hours when

_____ is being done.

LABELING

77. Mark the places you would secure the catheter. Explain why the catheter is secured this way.

_____

_____

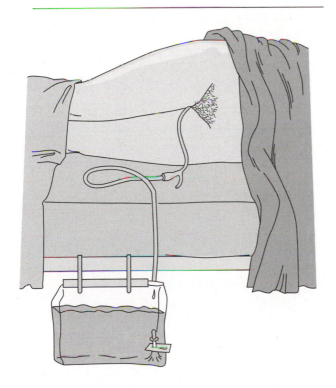

78. Mark the places you would secure the catheter. Explain why the catheter is secured this way.

_____

_____

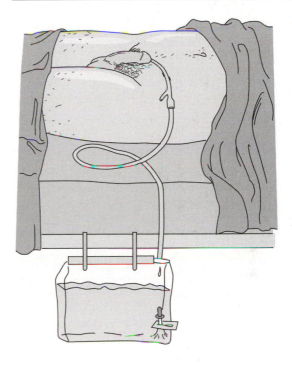

CROSSWORD

Fill in the crossword by answering the clues with words from this list.

Dysuria

Frequency

Hematuria

Incontinence

Nocturia

Oliguria

Polyuria

Urgency

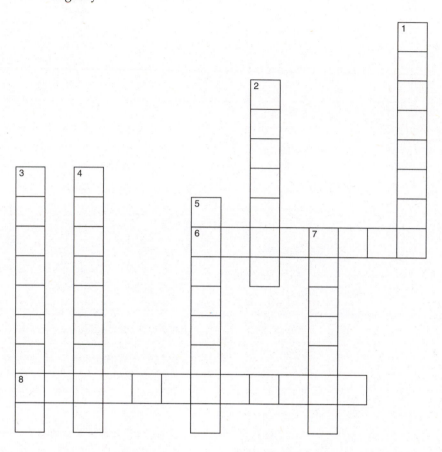

Across

6. Scant amount of urine, usually less than 500 mL in 24 hours
8. Inability to control loss of urine from bladder

Down

1. Production of abnormally large amounts of urine
2. Painful or difficult urination
3. Blood in the urine
4. Voiding at frequent intervals
5. Frequent urination at night
7. Need to void immediately

OPTIONAL LEARNING EXERCISES

79. When a person eats a diet high in salt, it causes the body to _____. When this happens, how does it affect urine output?

_____

80. You would ask the nurse to observe urine that looks or _____. You would also report complaints of _____

_____.

81. A fracture pan can be used with older persons who have _____ or _____

_____.

82. Covering the lap and legs of a person using a commode provides _____ and promotes _____.

83. If you are caring for an incontinent person and you become short-tempered and impatient, you should

_____

What right are you protecting when you do this?

_____

84. Even though catheters are a last resort for incontinent persons, they may be used with weak, disabled, or dying persons to

A. Promote _____

B. Prevent _____

C. Protect _____ and

_____

D. Allow _____

85. Catheters may have diagnostic reasons for use, such as

A. _____

B. _____

86. What can happen if microbes enter a closed drainage system? _____

_____.

87. What type of tape is used to apply a condom catheter? _____ Why?

_____ What can happen if you use the wrong tape? _____

_____

INDEPENDENT LEARNING ACTIVITIES

- Role-play the following situation with a classmate. Take turns playing the person using the bedpan and the nursing assistant. Answer the questions about the activity.

   Situation: *Mrs. Donnelly is a 70-year-old who must use the bedpan. She finds it difficult to move easily and usually does not have enough strength to raise her hips to get on the bedpan. She tells you she will try to help as much as she can.*

   As Mrs. Donnelly:

- When you tried to assist, how easy was it to raise your hips? How did the nursing assistant help you get on the pan?
- When you were rolled onto the bedpan, how did it feel? How well was the pan positioned under you?

- How did you feel about sitting on the pan in bed? Did you feel as if this would be an easy or difficult way to void? Explain your feelings.
- How could the nursing assistant have made this procedure better?

   As the nursing assistant:

- How did you position the bedpan to get ready to slide it under Mrs. Donnelly? Did this method work? How could you improve this?
- When you rolled Mrs. Donnelly onto the pan, how well positioned was she? What adjustments were necessary?
- When you rolled her off the pan, what happened? If urine had been in the pan, what would have occurred?
- How could you change some of your steps to make this procedure better?

22 BOWEL ELIMINATION

FILL IN THE BLANKS: KEY TERMS

Colostomy
Constipation
Defecation
Dehydration
Diarrhea
Enema

Fecal impaction
Fecal incontinence
Feces
Flatulence
Flatus
Ileostomy

Ostomy
Peristalsis
Stoma
Stool
Suppository

1. A surgically created opening for the elimination of body wastes is a _____.

2. The process of excreting feces from the rectum through the anus is a bowel movement or _____

3. The excessive formation of gas in the stomach and intestines is _____

4. A _____ is a cone-shaped solid drug that is inserted into a body opening.

5. The frequent passage of liquid stools is _____

6. _____ is the prolonged retention and buildup of feces in the rectum.

7. _____ is the excessive loss of water from tissues.

8. Gas or air passed through the anus is _____

9. The introduction of fluid into the rectum and lower colon is an _____

10. Excreted feces is _____.

11. An artificial opening between the colon and abdominal wall is a _____

12. _____ is the alternating contraction and relaxation of intestinal muscles.

13. The passage of a hard, dry stool is _____

14. _____ is the inability to control the passage of feces and gas through the anus.

15. An opening that can be seen on the abdominal wall is a _____

16. The semi-solid mass of waste products in the colon is _____

17. A surgically created opening between the ileum and the abdominal wall is an _____.

CIRCLE THE BEST ANSWER

18. People usually have a bowel movement
    A. After every meal
    B. When they have consumed large amounts of fluids
    C. At a regular time and pattern that is normal for the person
    D. Once a week

19. Bleeding in the stomach and small intestines causes stool to be
    A. Brown
    B. Black
    C. Red
    D. Clay-colored

20. The characteristic odor of stool is caused by
    A. Poor personal hygiene
    B. Poor nutrition
    C. Bacterial action in the intestines
    D. Adequate fluid intake

21. When you observe stool that is abnormal
    A. Ask the nurse to observe the stool
    B. Report your observations and discard the stool
    C. Ask the person if the stool is normal for him or her
    D. Record your observations when you finish giving care

22. Which of these could interfere with defecation?
    A. Being able to relax by reading a book or newspaper
    B. Eating a diet with high-fiber foods
    C. Using a bedpan, commode, or bathroom when others are present
    D. Drinking 6 to 8 glasses of water daily

23. A person who must stay in bed most of the time may have irregular elimination and constipation because of
    A. Poor diet
    B. Poor fluid intake
    C. Lack of activity
    D. Lack of privacy

24. Which of these would provide safety for the person during bowel elimination?
    A. Make sure the bedpan is warm
    B. Place the call light and toilet tissue within the person's reach
    C. Provide perineal care
    D. Allow enough time for defecation

25. Constipation can be relieved by
    A. Giving the person a low-fiber diet
    B. Increasing activity
    C. Decreasing fluids
    D. Ignoring the urge to defecate

26. A person tries several times to have a bowel movement and cannot. Liquid feces seep from the anus. This probably means the person has
    A. Diarrhea
    B. Constipation
    C. A fecal impaction
    D. Fecal incontinence

27. When the nurse finds a fecal impaction is present, he or she sometimes tries to relieve it by
    A. Changing the person's diet
    B. Telling the nursing assistant to give more fluids
    C. Removing the fecal mass with a gloved finger
    D. Increasing the activity of the person

28. Good skin care is important when a person has diarrhea because
    A. This prevents odors
    B. Skin breakdown and pressure ulcers are risks
    C. It prevents the spread of microbes
    D. It prevents fluid loss

29. Diarrhea can be very serious in older persons, especially because it
    A. Causes skin breakdown
    B. Causes odors
    C. Can cause dehydration
    D. Increases activity

30. When caring for a person with *Clostridium difficile* (*C. difficile*), you practice good hand hygiene by
    A. Washing your hands in alcohol
    B. Washing your hands with soap and water
    C. Using alcohol-based hand rubs
    D. Wearing sterile gloves

31. When a person has fecal incontinence, it is important to
    A. Increase fluid intake
    B. Help the person with elimination once a shift
    C. Help the person with elimination after meals and every 2 to 3 hours
    D. Tell the person to turn on the call light in time for help to arrive

32. If flatus is not expelled, the person may complain of
    A. Abdominal cramping or pain
    B. Diarrhea
    C. Fecal incontinence
    D. Nausea

33. What is a goal of bowel training?
    A. To give laxatives daily to maintain regular bowel movements
    B. To gain control of bowel movements
    C. To make sure the person has at least one bowel movement each day
    D. To prevent abdominal cramping

34. When bowel training is planned, which of these is included in the care plan?
    A. The amount of stool the person expels
    B. How many bowel movements the person has each day
    C. The usual time of day the person has a bowel movement
    D. The foods that cause flatus

35. When the nurse delegates preparing a soapsuds enema for an adult to you, mix
    A. 2 teaspoons of salt in 1000 mL of tap water
    B. 3 to 5 mL of castile soap in 500 to 1000 mL of tap water
    C. 2 mL of castile soap in 500 mL of tap water
    D. Mineral oil with sterile water

36. When you give an enema of 750 to 1000 mL, it should be given to the person
    A. Within 5 minutes
    B. Over about 30 minutes
    C. Over about 10 to 15 minutes
    D. Over about 20 minutes

37. The person receiving an enema is usually placed in a
    A. Supine position
    B. Prone position
    C. Semi-Fowler's position
    D. Sims' or left side-lying position

38. When you prepare and give an enema, you will
    A. Prepare the solution at 110°F
    B. Insert the tubing 2 to 4 inches into the rectum
    C. Hold the solution container about 18 inches above the bed
    D. Give the enema solution as quickly as possible

39. When the doctor orders enemas until clear
    A. Give one enema
    B. Give as many enemas as necessary to return a clear fluid
    C. Ask the nurse how many times to repeat the enema
    D. Give only tap water enemas

40. If you are giving an enema and the person complains of cramping
    A. Tell the person it is normal and continue to give the enema
    B. Clamp the tube until the cramping subsides
    C. Discontinue the enema immediately and tell the nurse
    D. Lower the bag below the level of the bed

41. When giving a small-volume enema, do not release pressure on the bottle because
    A. It will cause cramping if pressure is released
    B. The fluid will leak from the rectum
    C. Solution will be drawn back into the bottle
    D. It will cause flatulence

42. When giving a small-volume enema
    A. Place the person in the prone position
    B. Insert the enema tip 2 inches into the rectum
    C. Heat the solution to 105ºF
    D. Clamp the tubing if cramping occurs

43. An oil-retention enema is given to
    A. Cleanse the bowel to prepare for surgery
    B. Regulate the person who is receiving bowel training
    C. Relieve flatulence
    D. Soften the feces and lubricate the rectum

44. If you feel resistance when you are giving a cleansing enema
    A. Lubricate the tube more thoroughly
    B. Push more firmly to insert the tube
    C. Stop and report this to the nurse
    D. Ask the person to take a deep breath and relax

45. When you are caring for a person with any type of ostomy, you know
    A. All of the stools are solid and formed
    B. A stoma does not have sensation and is not painful
    C. An ostomy is always temporary and is reconnected after healing
    D. A pouch is worn to protect the stoma

46. Which of these statements is true about an ileostomy?
    A. The stool is solid and formed.
    B. The stoma is an opening into the colon.
    C. The pouch is changed daily.
    D. The skin around the ileostomy can be irritated by the digestive juices in the stool.

47. When caring for a person with a stoma, the pouch is
    A. Changed daily
    B. Changed every 3 to 7 days and when it leaks
    C. Worn only when the person thinks he or she will have a bowel movement
    D. Changed every time the person has a bowel movement

48. The best time to change the ostomy bag is after sleep because
    A. The stoma is less likely to expel stool at this time
    B. The person has more time in the morning
    C. It should be changed before morning care
    D. The person tolerates the procedure better before eating

49. When cleaning the skin around the stoma, you use
    A. Sterile water and sterile gauze squares
    B. Alcohol and sterile cotton
    C. Gauze squares or washcloths and water or soap and other cleansing agents as directed by the nurse
    D. Adhesive remover and sterile cotton balls

50. You give the person with an ostomy the right of personal choice when you
    A. Allow the person to manage the care when able
    B. Choose the time when care is done
    C. Choose the care measures and equipment used
    D. Ask the nurse to determine the care to be done

FILL IN THE BLANKS

51. What do these abbreviations mean?

    A. BM _____

    B. GI _____

    C. oz _____

    D. SSE _____

52. When observing stool, what should be reported to the nurse?

    A. _____

    B. _____

    C. _____

    D. _____

    E. _____

    F. _____

    G. _____

    H. _____

53. What 3 food groups are high in fiber?

    A. _____

    B. _____

    C. _____

54. Name 6 gas-forming foods.

    A. _____

    B. _____

    C. _____

    D. _____

    E. _____

    F. _____

55. Drinking warm fluids such as coffee, tea, hot cider, and warm water will increase _____.

56. How will dehydration affect these?

    A. Skin is _____

    B. Urine is _____

    C. Blood pressure _____

    D. Pulse and respirations _____

57. Persons at risk for developing a *Clostridium difficile* infection are those who are

    A. _____

    B. _____

    C. _____

58. The *Clostridium difficile* microbe is found in the

    _____

59. Flatulence may be caused when the person

    _____ while eating and drinking.

60. When a nurse inserts a suppository for bowel training, how soon would you expect the person to defecate? _____

61. Before giving an enema, make sure that

    A. _____

    B. _____

    C. _____

    D. _____

    E. _____

62. After giving an enema, what should be reported and recorded?

    A. _____

    B. _____

    C. _____

    D. _____

    E. _____

    F. _____

    G. _____

63. Because it is likely you will come in contact with stool while giving an enema, you should follow

    _____ and _____.

64. How can cramping be prevented during an enema?

    A. _____

    B. _____

65. How long does it usually take for a tap water, saline, or soapsuds enema to take effect?

    _____

66. A small-volume enema contains _____ of solution.

67. A person should retain a small-volume enema for

    _____

68. When you start to insert the tube to give an enema, ask the person to _____.

69. What can you place in the ostomy pouch to prevent odors? _____

70. Showers and baths are delayed 1 or 2 hours after applying a new pouch to allow _____

LABELING

Answer Questions 71 through 74 using the illustrations of colostomies.

71. Name the 4 types of colostomies shown

    A. _____

    B. _____

    C. _____

    D. _____

72. Which colostomy will have the most solid and formed stool? _____

73. Which colostomy will have the most liquid stool? _____

74. Which colostomy is a temporary colostomy? _____

Answer Questions 75 through 77 using the following illustration.

Stoma

75. What type of ostomy is shown? _____

76. What part of the bowel has been removed? _____

77. Will the stool from the ostomy be liquid or formed? _____

OPTIONAL LEARNING EXERCISES

78. You are caring for Mr. Evans, who is in a semi-private room. His roommate has a large family and many visitors. Mr. Evans has not had a bowel movement in 3 days, even though he is eating well and taking medications to assist elimination. What could be a reason he has not had a bowel movement? _____

_____

79. Mrs. Weller usually has a bowel movement after breakfast. What are some activities that may assist her to defecate more easily? _____

_____

80. Mrs. Shaffer tells you she cannot digest fruits and vegetables and she refuses to eat them. What may be added to her cereal and prune juice to provide fiber? _____

81. You offer Mr. Murphy _____ of water each day to promote normal bowel elimination.

82. Mr. Hernandez has been taking an antibiotic, which is a drug to treat his pneumonia, and he has developed diarrhea. You think he may have diarrhea because _____

_____.

83. Mr. Hernandez has continued to have diarrhea and the nurse tells you he has *Clostidrium difficile*. His signs and symptoms are

A. _____

B. _____

C. _____

D. _____

E. _____

84. When you care for Mr. Hernandez, you can spread the microbes if your contaminated hands or gloves

A. _____

B. _____

85. You are caring for 83-year-old Mrs. Chen. You helped her to the bathroom 30 minutes ago, where she had a bowel movement. When you enter her room to make her bed, she tells you she needs to use the bathroom for a bowel movement. You know that older people _____

_____

86. The two goals of bowel training are

_____ and _____

_____.

87. Why can tap water enemas be dangerous?

_____

_____ How many tap water enemas can be given? _____

Why? _____

_____

88. Compare small-volume enemas and oil-retention enemas.

    A. Small-volume enemas are given to

    _____. Oil-retention

    enemas are given to _____.

    B. Small-volume enemas take effect in about

    _____ minutes. Oil-
    retention enemas should be retained for at least

    _____ minutes.

    C. An oil-retention enema may be retained for

    _____ hours.

INDEPENDENT LEARNING ACTIVITIES

- Think about times when you have had a problem with bowel irregularity. Answer these questions about how you handled the problems.
    - What causes you to have irregularity? Foods? Illness? Stress? Inactivity?
    - What methods have you used to treat irregularity? Diet? Medication?
    - How does irregularity affect you physically? Your appetite? Energy level? Sleep and rest?
    - How does irregularity affect your mood? Your daily activities?
- Interview a person who has a colostomy or an ileostomy. You may know someone who has an ostomy. Or you may care for someone who has one. Your community may have an ostomy support group that you can contact. Talk to the person and ask the following questions.
    - How long has the person had the ostomy? Is it permanent or temporary?
    - What was the hardest part of learning to live with an ostomy? What was the easiest part?
    - How has living with an ostomy affected the person's life? Has the person's work been affected? Were leisure activities affected?
    - How has the ostomy affected the person's family? What changes have occurred?
    - What equipment works best for the person? How expensive is the equipment? How much time is required each day to care for the ostomy?

23 EXERCISE AND ACTIVITY

FILL IN THE BLANKS: KEY TERMS

Abduction
Adduction
Ambulation
Atrophy
Contracture
Deconditioning
Dorsiflexion

Extension
External rotation
Flexion
Footdrop
Hyperextension
Internal rotation
Orthostatic hypotension

Plantar flexion
Postural hypotension
Pronation
Range of motion (ROM)
Rotation
Supination
Syncope

1. If _____ is present, the foot is bent down at the ankle.

2. A brief loss of consciousness or fainting is _____.

3. Bending a body part is _____.

4. Moving a body part away from the mid-line of the body is _____.

5. _____ is the movement of a joint to the extent possible without causing pain.

6. Turning the joint outward is _____.

7. A drop in blood pressure when the person stands is postural hypotension or _____.

8. _____ occurs when moving a body part toward the mid-line of the body.

9. Turning the joint upward is called _____.

10. Bending the toes and foot up at the ankle is _____.

11. Excessive straightening of a body part is _____.

12. A decrease in size or a wasting away of tissue is _____.

13. Turning the joint is _____.

14. _____ is the straightening of a body part.

15. _____ is another name for orthostatic hypotension.

16. _____ is permanent plantar flexion; the foot falls down at the ankle.

17. The act of walking is _____.

18. _____ is turning the joint downward.

19. The loss of muscle strength from inactivity is _____.

20. _____ is turning the joint inward.

21. The lack of joint mobility caused by abnormal shortening of a muscle is a _____.

CIRCLE THE BEST ANSWER

22. If a person is on bedrest, he or she
    A. May be allowed some activities of daily living (ADL)
    B. Can use the bedside commode for elimination needs
    C. May not perform any activities of daily living
    D. Can use the bathroom for elimination needs

23. Complications of bedrest include
    A. Contractures in fingers, wrists, knees, and hips
    B. Increased muscle strength
    C. Increased appetite and improved muscle strength
    D. Normal blood pressure when getting out of bed

24. If a contracture develops
    A. It will require extra range-of-motion exercises to correct it
    B. You need to position the person in good body alignment
    C. The person is permanently deformed and disabled
    D. It will be relieved as soon as the person is able to walk and exercise
25. When you are caring for a person who has orthostatic hypotension, you should
    A. Raise the head of the bed slowly to Fowler's position
    B. Have the person get out of bed quickly to prevent weakness
    C. Keep the bed flat when getting the person out of bed
    D. Have the person walk around to decrease weakness and dizziness
26. Nursing care that helps prevent complications from bedrest will include
    A. Positioning in good body alignment
    B. Doing all ADL for the person
    C. Changing position once a shift
    D. Allowing the person to sleep as much as possible
27. If a person sitting on the edge of the bed complains of weakness, dizziness, or spots before the eyes, you should
    A. Assist the person to stand
    B. Help the person to sit in a chair or walk around
    C. Help the person to return to Fowler's position
    D. Tell the person it is a normal response and continue to get the person up
28. Bed-boards are used to
    A. Keep the person in alignment by preventing the mattress from sagging
    B. Prevent plantar flexion that can lead to footdrop
    C. Keep the hips abducted
    D. Keep the weight of top linens off the feet
29. Plantar flexion must be prevented to
    A. Keep the feet from bending down at the ankle (footdrop)
    B. Keep the hips from rotating outward
    C. Keep the wrist, thumb, and fingers in normal position
    D. Maintain good body alignment
30. To prevent the hips and legs from turning outward, you can use
    A. Bed cradles
    B. Hip abduction wedges
    C. Trochanter rolls
    D. Splints
31. When a trapeze bar is used for exercise, it will strengthen the
    A. Trunk and hips
    B. Shoulders
    C. Legs and hips
    D. Arms
32. When you move a person's joints through range-of-motion exercises, it is called
    A. Active range-of-motion
    B. Activities of daily living
    C. Active-assistive range-of-motion
    D. Passive range-of-motion
33. A nursing assistant can perform range-of-motion exercises on the _____ only if allowed by center policy.
    A. Shoulder
    B. Neck
    C. Hip
    D. Knee
34. When exercising the wrist, which of these exercises turns the hand toward the thumb?
    A. Abduction
    B. Hyperextension
    C. Radial flexion
    D. Extension
35. Which of these joints is adducted and abducted?
    A. Neck
    B. Hip
    C. Elbow
    D. Knee
36. When you help a person to walk, you should
    A. Apply a gait (transfer) belt
    B. Help the person lean on furniture to walk around the room
    C. Put soft socks on the feet without shoes
    D. Let the person walk without any help
37. When the person is walking with crutches, the person should wear
    A. Soft slippers on the feet
    B. Clothes that fit well
    C. Clothes that are loose
    D. A gait belt
38. When walking with a cane, it is held
    A. On the strong side of the body
    B. On the weak side of the body
    C. In the right hand
    D. On the left side of the body
39. When a person is using a walker, it is
    A. Picked up and moved 3 to 4 inches in front of the person
    B. Moved forward with a rocking motion
    C. Moved first on the left side and then on the right
    D. Picked up and moved about 10 inches in front of the person
40. When you are caring for a person who wears a brace, it is important to report at once
    A. How far the person walks
    B. What care the person can do alone
    C. The amount of mobility in joints when doing range-of-motion exercises
    D. Any redness or signs of skin breakdown when you remove a brace

41. Recreational activity is important because
    A. It forces the person to find new interests
    B. It prevents boredom
    C. Circulation is stimulated and joints and muscles are exercised
    D. It forces the person to do things that do not interest him or her

FILL IN THE BLANKS

42. Write out the meaning of each abbreviation
    A. ADL _____
    B. PT _____
    C. ROM _____

43. To prevent deconditioning, is it important to promote _____ and _____ in all persons to the extent possible.

44. Bedrest is ordered to
    A. _____
    B. _____
    C. _____
    D. _____
    E. _____

45. The nurse tells you the resident is on bedrest but can use the bathroom for elimination. This means the resident is ordered _____.

46. When a person has a contracture, the person is _____ deformed and disabled.

47. When a person is suddenly moved from lying or sitting to a standing position, the blood pressure may _____. This is called _____.

48. Supportive devices such as bed-boards, foot-boards, and trochanter rolls are used to _____ and _____ the person in a certain position.

49. When you use a foot-board, the soles of the feet are _____ against it to prevent _____.

50. A trochanter roll is placed along the body to prevent the hips and legs from _____ _____.

51. Hand rolls or grips prevent _____ of the thumb, fingers, and wrists.

52. A device used to keep the wrist, thumb, and fingers in normal position is a _____.

53. Bed cradles are used because the weight of top linens can cause _____ and _____.

54. A trapeze bar allows the person to lift the _____ off the bed. It also allows the person to _____ and _____ in bed.

55. When a person does exercises with some help, he or she is doing _____ range-of-motion exercises.

56. When range-of-motion exercises are done, what should be reported and recorded?
    A. _____
    B. _____
    C. _____
    D. _____
    E. _____

57. When performing range-of-motion exercises, each movement should be repeated _____ times or the _____.

58. When performing range-of-motion exercises, you should
    A. _____
    B. _____
    C. _____
    D. _____
    E. _____
    F. _____
    G. _____
    H. _____
    I. _____

59. When you help a person to walk, you should walk to the _____ and _____ the person. Provide support with the _____ or have one _____ and the other _____.

60. Many people prefer a walker because it gives more support than a _____.

61. When many recreational activities are offered, it protects the person's right to _____ _____.

LABELING

62. ROM exercises for the _____ joint are shown in these drawings. Name the movements shown in each drawing.

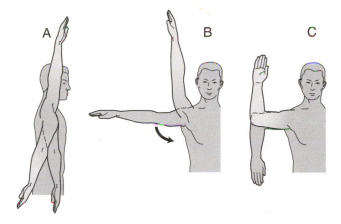

   A. _____

   B. _____

   C. _____

63. ROM exercises for the _____ are shown in these drawings. Name the movements shown in each drawing.

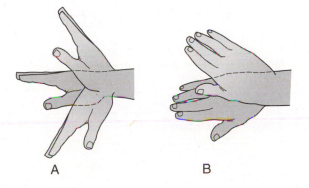

   A. _____

   B. _____

64. ROM exercises for the _____ are shown in these drawings. Name the movements shown in each drawing.

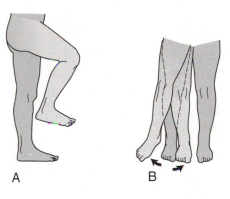

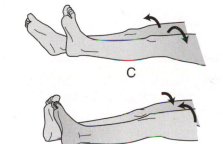

   A. _____

   B. _____

   C. _____

   D. _____

CROSSWORD

Fill in the crossword by choosing words from the following list.

Abduction   Contracture   Footdrop   Rotation
Adduction   Deconditioning   Hyperextension   Supination
ADL   Dorsiflexion   Pronation   Syncope
Ambulation   Extension   PT
Atrophy   Flexion   ROM

Across

4. Loss of muscle strength from inactivity
8. Abbreviation for range of motion
10. Bending a body part
12. Decrease in size or wasting away of tissue
13. Abbreviation for physical therapy
14. Moving a body part away from the mid-line of the body
15. Straightening a body part
16. Brief loss of consciousness; fainting
17. Bending the toes and foot up at the ankle
18. Moving a body part toward the mid-line of the body

Down

1. Foot falls down at the ankle; permanent plantar flexion
2. Abbreviation for activities of daily living
3. Turning a joint
5. Lack of joint mobility caused by abnormal shortening of a muscle
6. Act of walking
7. Excessive straightening of body part
9. Turning the joint downward
11. Turning the joint upward

OPTIONAL LEARNING EXERCISES

65. What kind of range of motion would be used with each of these residents?

    A. The resident needs complete care for bathing, grooming, and feeding. _____

    _____

    B. The resident takes part in many activities in the center. She walks to most activities independently. _____

    C. The resident has weakness on his left side. He is able to feed himself but needs help with bathing and dressing. _____

    _____

66. As you plan to help a person out of bed, you are concerned about orthostatic hypotension. In order to make sure the person is able to stand and get up safely, you plan to take the blood pressure, pulse, and respirations several times. When would you take the blood pressure?

    A. _____

    B. _____

    C. _____

D. _____

E. _____

67. When doing range-of-motion exercises, you should ask the person if he or she has _____ or _____.

68. When performing range-of-motion exercises, you do not

    A. _____

    B. _____

69. When you ambulate a person, what observations are reported and recorded?

    A. _____

    B. _____

    C. _____

    D. _____

    E. _____

70. Why does the nurse assess the skin under braces every shift? _____

    _____

INDEPENDENT LEARNING ACTIVITIES

- Role-play with a classmate and take turns acting as the nursing assistant and a person with left-sided weakness. Perform range-of-motion exercises on the person. Answer the following questions about how you felt after this activity.
  - What did the nursing assistant explain to you before performing the exercises?
  - How were you positioned for exercising? What did the nursing assistant ask about your comfort and personal wishes in the position used?
  - How was your privacy maintained? Was there anything that made you feel exposed or embarrassed?
  - How were your joints supported during the exercises? Did you feel any discomfort or pain during the exercises?
  - What exercises were you encouraged to carry out independently? With some assistance?
  - Which exercises were done first? Were the exercises carried out in an organized pattern? How did you know what exercise would be done next?

- After this activity, what will you do differently when giving range-of-motion exercises to a person?
- With a classmate, role-play assisting a weak, older person to ambulate. Take turns acting as the person and the nursing assistant. Answer the following questions about how you felt and what you learned.
  - What did the nursing assistant tell you before preparing to walk with you? What choices were offered about the time you were to ambulate, what clothing to wear, and where you were going to walk?
  - What safety devices were used? What did the nursing assistant tell you about the devices or equipment used?
  - What assessments were made before you sat up? When you dangled? After walking?
  - How did the nursing assistant make you feel secure during ambulation? How did the nursing assistant hold you?
  - What did you learn from this activity that will help you when you ambulate a person?

24 COMFORT, REST, AND SLEEP

FILL IN THE BLANKS: KEY TERMS

Acute pain
Chronic pain
Circadian rhythm
Comfort
Discomfort
Distraction

Enuresis
Guided imagery
Insomnia
NREM sleep
Pain
Persistent pain

Phantom pain
Radiating pain
Relaxation
REM sleep
Rest
Sleep

1. Another name for discomfort is _____.

2. _____ is pain that is felt suddenly from injury, disease, trauma, or surgery; it generally lasts less than 6 months.

3. _____ is a way to change a person's center of attention.

4. A state of unconsciousness, reduced voluntary muscle activity, and lowered metabolism is

   _____.

5. Pain lasting longer than 6 months is

   _____. It may be constant or occur off and on.

6. _____ is to be free from mental or physical stress.

7. _____ is a state of well-being. The person has no physical or emotional pain and is calm and at peace.

8. To be calm, at ease, and relaxed is to

   _____. The person is free of anxiety and stress.

9. Creating and focusing on an image is

   _____.

10. The stage of sleep when there is rapid eye

    movement is _____.

11. _____ is a chronic condition in which the person cannot sleep or stay asleep throughout the night.

12. The day-night cycle or body rhythm is also called

    _____. This daily rhythm is based on a 24-hour cycle.

13. _____ is pain felt at the site of tissue damage and in nearby areas.

14. To ache, hurt, or be sore is _____.

    It is also called pain.

15. _____ is the phase of deep sleep when there is no rapid eye movement.

16. Pain felt in a body part that is no longer there is

    _____.

17. Urinary incontinence in bed at night is

    _____.

18. Another name for chronic pain is

    _____.

CIRCLE THE BEST ANSWER

19. Rest and sleep are needed to
    A. Restore energy and well-being
    B. Decrease energy needed for daily functions
    C. Increase muscle strength
    D. Increase the appetite

20. OBRA requirements related to comfort, rest, and sleep include
    A. Only 2 people in a room
    B. Bright lighting in all areas
    C. Room temperature between 65°F and 71°F
    D. Adequate ventilation and room humidity

21. When a person complains of pain or discomfort
    A. The person has pain or discomfort
    B. It must be measured carefully to see if the person really has pain or discomfort
    C. You can easily measure to find out how much pain is present
    D. You can tell if the person really has pain or discomfort by the way he or she acts

134

22. When a person complains of pain that is at the site of tissue damage and in nearby areas, this is

_____ pain.
    A. Acute
    B. Chronic
    C. Radiating
    D. Phantom

23. If pain is ignored or denied, it may be because the person thinks pain is a sign of weakness. Which factor that affects pain would this be?
    A. Attention
    B. Past experience
    C. Value or meaning of pain
    D. Support from others

24. A person from Mexico may react to pain by
    A. Showing a strong emotional response
    B. Appearing very stoic
    C. Accepting pain quietly
    D. Viewing it as the will of God

25. When a person has anxiety, the person
    A. May feel increased pain
    B. Will usually feel less pain
    C. May deny having pain
    D. May be stoic and show no reaction to pain

26. When you ask a person "Where is the pain?" you are asking the person to
    A. Describe the pain
    B. Explain the intensity of the pain
    C. Tell you the onset and duration of the pain
    D. Tell you the location of the pain

27. When a person tells you he has pain when coughing or deep breathing, this is
    A. A factor causing pain
    B. A measurement of the onset of pain
    C. Words used to describe the pain
    D. The location of the pain

28. A distraction measure to promote comfort and relieve pain may be
    A. Asking the person to focus on an image
    B. Learning to breathe deeply and slowly
    C. Listening to music or playing games
    D. Contracting and relaxing muscle groups

29. If the nurse has given a person pain medication, it is best if you
    A. Give the person a bath
    B. Walk the person according to the care plan
    C. Wait 30 minutes before giving care
    D. Give care before the medication makes the person sleepy

30. You may help to promote comfort and relieve pain when you
    A. Tell family members and friends to leave the person alone
    B. Keep the room brightly lit and play loud music
    C. Provide blankets for warmth and to prevent chilling
    D. Avoid touching the person to give care or back massages

31. You can help to promote rest when you
    A. Meet physical needs such as thirst, hunger, and elimination needs
    B. Check the person every 10 minutes to ask if he or she is resting
    C. Provide snacks that include caffeine drinks
    D. Give care at a time most convenient to you

32. When caring for an ill or injured person, you know the person may need more rest. You can help the person to get rest by making sure you
    A. Provide plenty of exercise to prevent weakness
    B. Provide rest periods during or after a procedure
    C. Give complete hygiene and grooming measures quickly
    D. Spend time talking with the person to distract him or her

33. During sleep
    A. The person is aware of the environment
    B. Metabolism is increased
    C. Vital signs (blood pressure, temperature, pulse, respirations) increase
    D. There are no voluntary arm or leg movements

34. Some people function better in the morning because of
    A. The circadian rhythm
    B. Getting enough sleep
    C. Interference with the body rhythm
    D. Changes in the work schedule

35. During REM sleep, the person
    A. Is hard to arouse
    B. Has a gradual fall in vital signs
    C. Is easily aroused
    D. Has tension in voluntary muscles

36. Which stage of sleep is usually not repeated during the cycles of sleep?
    A. REM
    B. Stage 1: NREM
    C. Stage 2: NREM
    D. Stage 3: NREM

37. Which age-group requires less sleep than middle-age adults?
    A. Toddlers
    B. Young adults
    C. Adolescents
    D. Older adults

38. Which of these factors increases the need for sleep?
    A. Illness
    B. Weight loss
    C. Emotional problems
    D. Medications and other substances

39. When a person takes sleeping pills, sleep may not restore the person mentally because
    A. Caffeine prevents sleep
    B. Some have difficulty falling asleep
    C. The length of REM sleep is reduced
    D. It upsets the usual sleep routines

40. Exercise should be avoided for 2 hours before sleep because
    A. It requires energy
    B. People usually feel good after exercise
    C. It causes the release of substances in the bloodstream that stimulate the body
    D. The person tires after exercise

41. Persons who are ill, in pain, or hospitalized may experience
    A. Sleep deprivation
    B. Sleepwalking
    C. Insomnia
    D. Increased sleep times

42. If a person has decreased reasoning, red, puffy eyes, and coordination problems, report this to the nurse because the person
    A. Is having a reaction to sleeping medications
    B. Has signs and symptoms of sleep disorders
    C. Needs more exercise before bedtime
    D. May need an increase in sleeping pills

43. Which of these measures would help to promote sleep?
    A. Turn on several lights in the room
    B. Have the person void or make sure that incontinent persons are clean and dry
    C. Encourage the person to take part in an exercise class shortly before bedtime
    D. Offer the person a cup of coffee or tea at bedtime

FILL IN THE BLANKS

44. Write out the meaning of each abbreviation
    A. CPAP _____
    B. NREM _____
    C. REM _____
    D. TENS _____

45. OBRA has requirements about the person's room. List the requirements that relate to each of these.
    A. Suspended curtain _____
    B. Linens _____
    C. Bed _____
    D. Room temperature _____
    E. Persons in room _____

46. Name the type of pain described.
    A. A person with an amputated leg may still sense leg pain. _____
    B. There is tissue damage. The pain decreases with healing. _____

    C. Pain from a heart attack is often felt in the left chest, left jaw, left shoulder, and left arm.
    _____
    D. The pain remains long after healing. Common causes are arthritis and cancer.
    _____

47. What is the reason why persons from the Philippines may appear stoic in reaction to pain?
    _____

48. Older persons may ignore or deny new pain because
    A. _____
    B. _____

49. Persons with dementia may signal pain by changes
    _____.

50. When gathering information about a person in pain, you can use a scale of 1 to 10. Which end of the scale is the most severe pain? _____

51. What happens to vital signs when the person has acute pain? _____

52. When the person uses words such as aching, knife-like, or sore to describe pain, what do you report to the nurse? _____
    _____

53. What body responses may be objective signs or symptoms (signs you can measure or see) that the person has acute pain?
    A. _____
    B. _____
    C. _____
    D. _____

54. What changes in these behaviors may be symptoms of pain?
    A. Speech _____
    B. Affected body part _____
    C. Positioning _____

55. List nursing measures to promote comfort and relieve pain related to these clues.
    A. Position of the person _____
    B. Linens _____
    C. Blankets _____
    D. Pain medications _____
    E. Family members _____

56. If a person is receiving strong pain medication or sedatives, what safety measures are important?

    A. _____

    B. _____

    C. _____

    D. _____

57. When you explain the procedure before performing it, you may help a person to rest better because you met the need for _____.

58. A clean, neat, and uncluttered room can promote rest by meeting _____ needs.

59. The mind and body rest, the body saves energy, and body functions slow during _____.

60. Mental restoration occurs during a phase of sleep called _____.

61. The deepest stage of sleep occurs during _____.

62. If work hours change, it can affect the normal _____ cycle or _____ rhythm.

63. Alcohol tends to cause drowsiness and sleep but it interferes with _____.

64. Insomnia may be caused by

    A. Fear of _____

    B. Fear of not _____

    C. Fear of not being able _____

    D. Physical and emotional _____

65. When a person has dementia and wanders at night, the best approach for some persons is to allow _____.

OPTIONAL LEARNING EXERCISES

66. You are caring for 2 residents who both have arthritis. Mr. Forman tells you this is the first time he has had any health problems. Mrs. Wegman tells you she has had several surgeries and has had 3 children. Which of these 2 persons is likely to be more anxious about the pain and to be unable to handle the pain well? _____ Why?

    _____

67. Mr. Forman tells you his pain seems much worse at night. What could be the reason for this reaction?

    _____

    _____

68. You are caring for Mrs. Reynolds. She tells you she misses her children, who have moved to another state. Today, Mrs. Reynolds is complaining of pain in her abdomen. In spite of providing nursing comfort measures, she still rates her pain at a 7. What is a possible reason Mrs. Reynolds is not getting relief from her pain? _____

    _____

69. When a person is ill, how do these affect sleep?

    A. Treatments and therapies _____

    B. Care devices such as traction or a cast _____

    C. Emotions _____

70. Certain foods affect sleep. Tell how these foods affect sleep and list foods that contain the substances.

    A. Caffeine _____ sleep. It is found in _____

    B. Tryptophan _____ sleep. It is found in _____

INDEPENDENT LEARNING ACTIVITIES

- Form a group with several classmates and share your personal experiences with pain. Discuss the following questions to understand the different ways you respond to pain and treat the pain.
  - What experiences have you had with pain? Accidents? Illnesses? Childbirth? Surgery?
  - What type of pain have you had? Acute? Chronic? Other types?
  - How would you rate your pain on a scale of 1 to 10? How long did it last?
  - How did your family and friends respond to your pain? How much support did you receive from them? How did the support (or lack of it) affect the pain?
  - What measures were used to treat the pain? What was the most effective? The least effective?
  - What did you learn from this discussion with others about their pain? How will this help you as you care for others with pain?
- Form a group with several classmates to talk about differences in sleep habits. Answer these questions to understand differences in personal practices concerning rest and sleep.
  - How many hours do you sleep each day? How many hours of sleep do you think you *should* get each day?
  - If you did not have to follow a schedule (work, school, etc.), when would you go to bed and wake up?
  - What rituals do you perform before going to bed? How is your sleep affected if you cannot perform these rituals?
  - What factors interfere with your sleep? What do you do to avoid these factors?
  - When do you feel most alert? Morning? Afternoon? Night?
  - How do you feel when you wake up? Alert? Pleasant? Grouchy? Tired?
  - How often do you take naps? What time of day do you like to nap? How do you feel when you wake from a nap?
  - How will this discussion help you understand differences in sleep patterns when you are caring for others? How will it affect how you help the persons you care for to get the rest and sleep they need?

25 OXYGEN NEEDS AND RESPIRATORY THERAPIES

FILL IN THE BLANKS: KEY TERMS

Allergy
Apnea
Biot's respirations
Bradypnea
Cheyne-Stokes respirations
Cyanosis
Dyspnea
Hemoptysis
Hemothorax
Hyperventilation

Hypoventilation
Hypoxemia
Hypoxia
Intubation
Kussmaul respirations
Mechanical ventilation
Orthopnea
Orthopneic position
Oxygen concentration
Patent

Pleural effusion
Pnuemothorax
Pollutant
Respiratory arrest
Respiratory depression
Sputum
Suction
Tachypnea
Tracheostomy

1. _____ are respirations that are rapid and deep followed by 10 to 30 seconds of apnea.

2. Bloody sputum is called _____.

3. Bluish color to the skin, lips, mucous membranes, and nail beds is _____.

4. _____ is mucus from the respiratory system that is expectorated through the mouth.

5. Air in the pleural space is a _____.

6. Rapid breathing where respirations are usually greater than 24 per minute is called

   _____.

7. An _____ is a sensitivity to a substance that causes the body to react with signs and symptoms.

8. A _____ is blood in the pleural space.

9. Difficult, labored, or painful breathing is

   _____.

10. Being able to breathe deeply and comfortably only while sitting is _____.

11. The process of withdrawing or sucking up fluid is

    _____.

12. Respirations that are less than 12 per minute are slow breathing or _____.

13. Open or unblocked is called _____.

14. A reduced amount of oxygen in the blood is

    _____.

15. _____ describes slow, weak respirations that occur at a rate of fewer than 12 per minute.

16. Inserting an artificial airway is _____.

17. The lack or absence of breathing is

    _____.

18. _____ is a pattern of respirations that is rapid and deeper than normal.

19. A harmful chemical or substance in the air or water is a _____.

20. _____ is the escape and collection of fluid.

21. _____ are respirations that gradually increase in rate and depth and then become shallow and slow. Breathing may stop for 10 to 20 seconds.

22. The _____ is sitting up and leaning over a table to breathe.

23. When breathing stops, it is _____.

24. Using a machine to move air into and out of the lungs is _____.

25. Very deep and rapid respirations are

    _____.

26. _____ is the amount of hemoglobin containing oxygen.

27. When cells do not have enough oxygen, it is

    called _____.

28. Respirations that are slow, shallow, and sometimes irregular are _____.

29. A _____ is a surgically created opening into the trachea.

CIRCLE THE BEST ANSWER

30. Oxygen (O_2) is carried to cells by the
    - A. Alveoli
    - B. Red blood cells
    - C. Bone marrow
    - D. White blood cells
31. Oxygen needs increase when
    - A. The person is aging
    - B. Medications are taken
    - C. The person has fever or pain
    - D. The person is well-nourished
32. Respiratory depression can occur when
    - A. The person exercises
    - B. Allergies are present
    - C. Narcotics are taken in large doses
    - D. The person smokes
33. Restlessness is an early sign of
    - A. Hypoxia
    - B. Apnea
    - C. Hyperventilation
    - D. Bradypnea
34. Signs of hypoxia may be
    - A. Disorientation and confusion
    - B. Decrease in pulse rate and respirations
    - C. Being relaxed and calm
    - D. The skin, mucous membranes, and nail beds are pink
35. When you prepare a person for a bronchoscopy, you
    - A. Make sure the person does not eat for 6 to 8 hours before the test
    - B. Help the person remove all clothing and jewelry from the waist to the neck
    - C. Place the person in a sitting position
    - D. Keep the person on bedrest for at least 1 hour before the x-ray
36. If you are caring for a person who just had a pulmonary function test, you would expect the person to
    - A. Tell you he or she has chest pain
    - B. Be very tired
    - C. Have hemoptysis
    - D. Complain of nausea and vomiting
37. If a pulse oximeter is being used on a person with tremors or poor circulation, which of these sites would be best to use?
    - A. A toe on a foot that is swollen
    - B. A finger that has nail polish on the nail
    - C. A toe with an open wound
    - D. An earlobe

38. When you are delegated to place a pulse oximeter on a person, report to the nurse if
    - A. The person is sleeping
    - B. The person's pulse rate goes above or below the alarm limit
    - C. You remove nail polish on the nail before attaching the pulse oximeter
    - D. You tape the oximeter in place
39. When a person has breathing difficulties, it is usually easier for the person to breath
    - A. In the supine position
    - B. Lying on one side for long periods
    - C. In the semi-Fowler's or Fowler's position
    - D. In the prone position
40. Deep-breathing and coughing exercises
    - A. Help prevent pneumonia and atelectasis
    - B. Decrease pain after surgery or injury
    - C. Are done once a day
    - D. Cause mucus to form in the lungs
41. When assisting with coughing and deep breathing, you tell the person to
    - A. Inhale through the mouth
    - B. Hold the breath for 30 seconds
    - C. Exhale slowly through pursed lips
    - D. Repeat the exercise 1 or 2 times
42. When a person uses an incentive spirometer, it allows the person to
    - A. Take shallow breaths
    - B. See air movement when inhaling
    - C. See air movement with exhaling
    - D. Exhale quickly
43. If a person is receiving oxygen, you may
    - A. Set the flowmeter rate
    - B. Apply the oxygen device to the person
    - C. Set up the system
    - D. Turn on the oxygen
44. If a person receives oxygen through a nasal cannula, it is important to look for irritation
    - A. On the nose, ears, and cheekbones
    - B. Under the mask
    - C. In the throat
    - D. In the oral cavity
45. If you are near a person receiving oxygen, which of these should you report?
    - A. The humidifier is bubbling.
    - B. The humidifier has enough water.
    - C. The humidifier is not bubbling.
    - D. The person is in a semi-Fowler's position.
46. If a person uses an inhaler, it is important to
    - A. Make sure they use the inhaler frequently
    - B. Notify the nurse quickly if the person cannot catch his or her breath
    - C. Make sure the inhaler is bubbling
    - D. Make sure the person always has the inhaler with him or her

47. When caring for a person with an artificial airway, you should tell the nurse at once if
    A. The vital signs remain stable
    B. Frequent oral hygiene is done
    C. The airway comes out or is dislodged
    D. The person feels as if he or she is gagging

48. Because a person with an endotracheal tube (ET) cannot speak, it is important to
    A. Never ask questions
    B. Avoid talking to the person
    C. Always keep the call light within reach
    D. Avoid explaining what you are going to do

49. The person with an ET can communicate by
    A. Whispering or speaking softly
    B. Using paper and pencil, Magic Slates, or communication boards
    C. Having a family member ask and answer questions
    D. Covering the tube opening

50. If you are caring for a person with an artificial airway, your care should always include
    A. Removing the device to clean it
    B. Comforting and reassuring the person that the airway helps breathing
    C. Suctioning to maintain the airway
    D. Making sure the person never takes a tub bath

51. The stoma or tube must be
    A. Covered when the person is shaving
    B. Covered with plastic when the person is outdoors
    C. Covered with a loose gauze dressing when the person bathing
    D. Uncovered when the person is outdoors

52. When suctioning is done, the nurse
    A. Follows Standard Precautions and the Bloodborne Pathogen Standard
    B. Makes sure a suction cycle is not more than 20 to 30 seconds
    C. Waits about 5 seconds between each suction cycle
    D. Suctions as many times as needed to clear the airway

53. If you are caring for a person who needs suctioning, you know that suctioning is done
    A. On a regular schedule
    B. As needed when signs and symptoms of respiratory distress are observed
    C. When the nurse directs you to do the suctioning
    D. When the person asks for suctioning

54. When the alarm sounds on a machine used for mechanical ventilation, you should first
    A. Report it to the nurse at once
    B. Reset the alarms
    C. Reassure the person that the alarm is normal
    D. Check to see if the person's tube is attached to the ventilator

55. Petrolatum gauze is kept at the bedside of a person with chest tubes to
    A. Cover the insertion site if the chest tube comes out
    B. Lubricate the site of the chest tube
    C. Cleanse the skin around the chest tube
    D. Cover the site of the chest tube insertion to prevent drainage

FILL IN THE BLANKS

56. Write out the meaning of each abbreviation.
    A. CO_2 _____
    B. ET _____
    C. L/min _____
    D. O_2 _____
    E. RBC _____
    F. SpO_2 _____

57. As a person ages, several factors affect the person's oxygen needs. List what happens in each of the areas listed below.
    A. Respiratory muscles _____
    B. Lung tissue _____
    C. Strength for coughing _____
    D. Risk for respiratory _____

58. Three diseases are caused by or are risk factors related to smoking. They are
    A. _____
    B. _____
    C. _____

59. How does alcohol increase the risk of aspiration?
    It depresses the _____ and
    reduces the _____ and increases
    _____.

60. How many respirations per minute occur with
    A. Normal respirations _____
    B. Tachypnea _____
    C. Bradypnea _____

61. What signs and symptoms can be used to describe sputum when reporting and recording these areas of observation?
    A. Color _____
    B. Odor _____
    C. Consistency _____
    D. Hemoptysis _____

62. If a person has difficulty breathing, he or she may prefer a position in which the person is sitting

_____.

This position is called _____

_____.

63. If a person has a productive cough, what respiratory hygiene and cough etiquette should be taught?

A. _____

B. _____

C. _____

D. _____

64. If a person is using an incentive spirometer, how long is the breath held to keep the balls floating?

_____

65. What observations should be reported after a person uses an incentive spirometer?

A. _____

B. _____

C. _____

D. _____

66. When a person wears a mask to receive oxygen, what should you do when the person needs to eat?

_____ How will the person receive oxygen during the meal?

_____

67. Oxygen is humidified because it will _____

_____.

68. When caring for a person with an artificial airway, you may be delegated to

A. Check _____ often

B. Observe for _____

C. Give frequent _____

D. Report to the nurse at once if _____

_____

69. What are the 3 parts of a tracheostomy tube?

A. _____

B. _____

C. _____

Questions 70 to 77 relate to caring for a tracheostomy and assisting the nurse during suctioning. You must know whether your state laws or job description allows you to assist with these procedures.

70. Which part of the tracheostomy tube is removed for cleaning and mucus removal?

_____

71. Which part of the tracheostomy tube is not

removed? _____

72. If a person with a tracheostomy is outdoors, what is used to cover the tracheostomy?

_____

73. A suction cycle takes no more than

_____ seconds. The cycle involves

A. _____

B. _____

C. _____

74. Before, during, and after suctioning, what is checked and observed?

A. _____

B. _____

C. _____

D. _____

75. When you are observing a person with a tracheostomy, what should be reported to the nurse at once?

A. _____

B. _____

C. _____

D. _____

E. _____

76. When a person has mechanical ventilation, what should you say when you enter the room?

_____

When you leave the room? _____

77. If chest tubes are in place, what should be reported to the nurse?

A. Signs and symptoms of _____

and _____

B. Complaints of _____ or

_____

CROSSWORD

Fill in the crossword by choosing words from the following list.

Apnea
Biot's
Bradypnea
Cheyne-Stokes
Dyspnea

Hyperventilation
Hypoventilation
Kussmaul
Orthopnea
Tachypnea

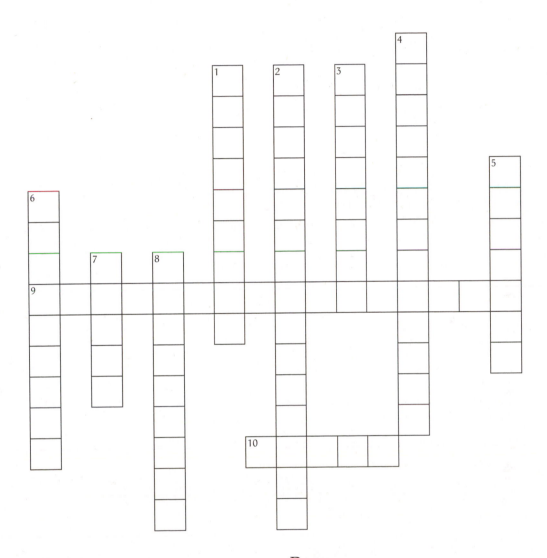

Across

9. Respirations are rapid and deep
10. Rapid and deep respirations followed by 10 or 20 seconds of apnea; occur with nervous disorders

Down

1. Respirations are 24 or more per minute
2. Respirations are slow, shallow, and sometimes irregular
3. Very deep and rapid respirations; signal diabetic coma
4. Respirations gradually increase in rate and depth; common when death is near
5. Difficult, labored, or painful breathing
6. Breathing deeply and comfortably only when sitting
7. Lack or absence of breathing
8. Respirations are fewer than 12 per minute

OPTIONAL LEARNING EXERCISES

Situation: You are caring for Mr. R., age 84, who has *chronic obstructive pulmonary disease.*

78. What position would make it easier for Mr. R. to breathe when he is in bed? _____

_____

79. How can you increase his comfort when he sitting up? _____ What is this position called? _____

_____

Situation: Mrs. F. is receiving oxygen through a nasal cannula at 2 L/min. Her respirations are unlabored at 16 per minute unless she is walking about or doing personal care. Then her respirations are 28 per minute and dyspneic.

80. Where should you check for signs of irritation from the cannula? _____

_____

81. You should make sure there are _____ in the tubing and that Mrs. F. does not _____ of the tubing.

82. What are the abnormal respirations that Mrs. F. has with activity called? _____

_____

83. If you are caring for a person with a tracheostomy, why is the tracheostomy covered when the person is outdoors? _____

_____

84. What is done to protect the stoma in the following situations?

    A. Tub baths or showers _____

    _____

    B. Shaving _____

    C. Shampooing _____

    _____

85. The stoma is never covered with _____ Why? _____

_____

86. What do you need to check before you use an Ambu bag attached to oxygen? _____ Why? _____

_____

87. If a person has mechanical ventilation, where do you find a plan for communication? _____ Why is it important for everyone to use the same signals for communication? _____

_____

88. If a person has chest tubes, why is it important to prevent kinks in the tubing? _____

_____

INDEPENDENT LEARNING ACTIVITIES

- Work with a classmate and carry out these exercises. They will help you understand how it feels to be a person with breathing problems.
    - Have your partner count your respirations while you are at rest. Then exercise by running or jogging in place for at least 2 minutes. Now have your partner check your respirations again. How have they changed? Rate? Rhythm or pattern? Easy or labored?
    - While you exercise, try first to breathe only through your nose. Then try breathing through your mouth. Which way makes you feel you are getting enough air?
    - Place a drinking straw in your mouth and close your lips tightly around it. Now breathe only through the straw while at rest and during exercise. When you are at rest, how comfortable does this feel? Are you getting enough air? How is your air supply during exercise?
- Take a drinking straw and place small pieces of paper in one end so that it is fairly tight. Now try breathing through the straw at rest and during exercise. What is the difference between the open and blocked straw? Imagine that every breath you take feels like it does with the blocked straw. This is how many people with breathing problems feel all the time.
- Try to find a person who has had a type of artificial ventilation discussed in this chapter. Ask the person the following questions.
    - What was the worst part of the experience?
    - How did the person communicate his or her needs with others?
    - What did the staff do that helped make the person comfortable?
    - What would have helped to make the experience better?

26 MEASURING VITAL SIGNS

FILL IN THE BLANKS: KEY TERMS

Apical-radial pulse
Blood pressure (BP)
Body temperature
Bradycardia
Diastole
Diastolic pressure
Fever

Hypertension
Hypotension
Pulse
Pulse deficit
Pulse rate
Respiration
Sphygmomanometer

Stethoscope
Systole
Systolic pressure
Tachycardia
Vital signs

1. A rapid heart rate is _____. The heart rate is over 100 beats per minute.

2. The _____ is taking the apical and radial pulse at the same time.

3. An instrument used to listen to the sounds produced by the heart, lungs, and other body organs is a _____.

4. A condition in which the systolic blood pressure is below 90 mm Hg and the diastolic pressure is below 60 mm Hg is _____.

5. The _____ is the number of heartbeats or pulses felt in 1 minute.

6. The amount of heat in the body that is a balance between the amount of heat produced and amount lost by the body is the _____.

7. _____ is the period of heart muscle contraction.

8. _____ is persistent blood pressure measurements above the normal systolic (140 mm Hg) or diastolic (90 mm Hg) pressures.

9. The instrument used to measure blood pressure is a _____.

10. The beat of the heart felt at an artery as a wave of blood passes through the artery is the _____.

11. Temperature, pulse, respirations, and blood pressure are _____.

12. _____ is a slow heart rate; the rate is less than 60 beats per minute.

13. The amount of force it takes to pump blood out of the heart into the arterial circulation is the _____.

14. The period of heart muscle relaxation is _____.

15. The difference between the apical and radial pulse rates is the _____.

16. _____ is the amount of force exerted against the walls of an artery by the blood.

17. The act of breathing air into and out of the lungs is _____.

18. _____ is the pressure in the arteries when the heart is at rest.

19. Elevated body temperature is _____.

CIRCLE THE BEST ANSWER

20. Vital signs are
    A. Temperature, pulse, respirations, and blood pressure
    B. Temperature, pulse, and respirations
    C. Blood pressure and pulse oximeter reading of oxygen level
    D. Tachycardia, bradypnea, and bradycardia

21. Unless otherwise ordered, take vital signs when the person
    A. Is lying or sitting
    B. Has been walking or exercising
    C. Has just finished eating
    D. Is getting ready to take a shower or tub bath

22. Body temperature is lower in the
    A. Afternoon
    B. Morning
    C. Evening
    D. Night
23. If you are taking vital signs on a person with dementia, it may be better if
    A. You have 2 or 3 co-workers restrain the person
    B. The vital signs are taken when the person is asleep
    C. You take the pulse and respirations at one time and the temperature and blood pressure at another time
    D. You ask the nurse to take the vital signs
24. What should you do if a resident asks his or her vital sign measurements?
    A. You can tell the person the measurements if center policy allows.
    B. Tell the nurse that the person wants to know the measurements.
    C. Tell the person you cannot tell him or her this information.
    D. This information is private and cannot be shared.
25. If you take a rectal temperature, the normal range of the temperature would be
    A. 96.6°F to 98.6°F (35.9°C to 37.0°C)
    B. 97.6°F to 99.6°F (36.5°C to 37.5°C)
    C. 98.6°F to 100.6°F (37.0°C to 38.1°C)
    D. 98.6°F (37°C)
26. If you are taking the temperature of an older person, you would expect the temperature to be
    A. Lower than the normal range
    B. Higher than the normal range
    C. About in the middle of the normal range
    D. The same as a younger adult
27. When recording an axillary temperature of 97.6°F, it is written
    A. 97.6°
    B. 97.6° R
    C. 97.6° Ax
    D. 97.6° axillary
28. When using an electronic thermometer, you can prevent the spread of infection by
    A. Discarding the thermometer after each use
    B. Discarding the probe cover after each use
    C. Keeping a thermometer for each person at the bedside
    D. Sterilizing the thermometer after each use
29. When taking a temperature on a resident with dementia, the best choice is to
    A. Take a rectal temperature
    B. Take an oral temperature
    C. Take an axillary temperature
    D. Use a tympanic membrane or temporal artery thermometer

30. Which pulse is most commonly used?
    A. Carotid
    B. Brachial
    C. Radial
    D. Popliteal
31. A _____ pulse is taken during cardiopulmonary resuscitation (CPR).
    A. Carotid
    B. Temporal
    C. Femoral
    D. Radial
32. When using a stethoscope, you can help to prevent infection by
    A. Warming the diaphragm in your hand
    B. Wiping the ear-pieces and diaphragm with antiseptic wipes before and after use
    C. Placing the diaphragm over the artery
    D. Placing the ear-pieces in your ears so the bend of the tips point forward
33. When a pulse rate is 120 beats per minute, you
    A. Report that the person has bradycardia
    B. Know that this is a normal pulse rate
    C. Report that the person has tachycardia
    D. Report that the pulse is irregular
34. The pulse rate is the number of heartbeats or pulses felt in
    A. 30 seconds
    B. 15 seconds
    C. 1 minute
    D. 5 minutes
35. You cannot get information about pulse _____ with electronic blood pressure equipment.
    A. Force
    B. Rate
    C. Tachycardia
    D. Bradycardia
36. When taking the radial pulse, place
    A. The thumb over the pulse site
    B. 2 or 3 fingers on the middle of the wrist
    C. 2 or 3 fingers on the thumb side of the wrist
    D. The stethoscope on the chest wall
37. The apical pulse is counted for
    A. 30 seconds
    B. 15 seconds
    C. 1 full minute
    D. The amount of time directed by the nurse
38. An apical pulse of 72 is recorded as
    A. Pulse 72
    B. 72 – Apical pulse
    C. 72Ap
    D. P 72

39. An apical-radial pulse is taken by
    A. Taking the radial pulse for 1 minute and then taking the apical pulse for 1 minute
    B. Subtracting the apical pulse from the radial pulse
    C. Having one staff member take the radial pulse at the same time that another staff member takes the apical pulse
    D. Having 2 persons take the apical pulse at the same time

40. When counting respirations, the best way is to
    A. Stand quietly next to the person and watch the chest rise and fall
    B. Keep your fingers or stethoscope over the pulse site so the person thinks you are still counting the pulse
    C. Tell the person to breathe normally so you can count the respirations
    D. Use the stethoscope to hear the respirations clearly and count for 1 full minute

41. Each respiration involves
    A. One inhalation
    B. One exhalation
    C. One inhalation (chest rises) and one exhalation (chest falls)
    D. Counting for 15 seconds and multiplying by four

42. The blood pressure should not be taken on an arm
    A. If the person has had breast surgery on that side
    B. If the arm was used for a blood draw earlier in the day
    C. If it is the dominant arm used for eating and writing
    D. If the person has arthritis in the hand

43. You will find out the size of blood pressure cuff needed
    A. By asking the nurse
    B. By measuring the person's arm
    C. By reading the doctor's orders
    D. By asking the person

44. When taking the blood pressure, you place the stethoscope diaphragm
    A. Over the radial artery on the thumb side of the wrist
    B. Over the brachial artery at the inner aspect of the elbow
    C. Lightly against the skin
    D. Over the apical pulse site

45. When getting ready to take the blood pressure, position the person's arm
    A. Above the level of the heart
    B. Level with the heart
    C. Below the level of the heart
    D. Abducted from the body

46. The blood pressure cuff is inflated between
    A. 100 mm Hg and 120 mm Hg
    B. 2 to 4 mm per second
    C. 160 mm Hg and 180 mm Hg
    D. 180 mm Hg and 200 mm Hg

FILL IN THE BLANKS

47. Write out the meaning of each abbreviation.
    A. BP _____
    B. C _____
    C. F _____
    D. Hg _____
    E. mm _____
    F. mm Hg _____
    G. TPR _____

48. Vital signs are taken when medications are taken that affect _____.

49. When taking vital signs, report to the nurse at once if
    A. _____
    B. _____
    C. _____

50. Sites for measuring temperature are the
    A. _____
    B. _____
    C. _____
    D. _____
    E. _____

51. Which site has the highest baseline temperature?

    _____

52. Which site has the lowest baseline temperature?

    _____

53. When taking an axillary temperature, the axilla must be _____.

54. Tympanic membrane and temporal artery thermometers are used for confused persons because they are _____.

55. When using an electronic thermometer, what does the color of the probe mean?

    A. Blue _____

    B. Red _____

56. When you take a rectal temperature,

    _____ the tip of the thermometer or the end of the covered probe.

57. When taking a tympanic membrane temperature,

    pull up and back on the adult's ear to _____

    _____.

58. The pulse rate for a person 12 years or older is

    between _____ and

    _____ per minute.

59. List words used to describe the following.

    A. Forceful pulse _____

    B. Hard-to-feel pulse _____

60. If a pulse is irregular, count the pulse for

    _____.

61. When you take a pulse, what observations should be reported and recorded?

    A. _____

    B. _____

    C. _____

    D. _____

    E. _____

    F. _____

    G. _____

62. Do not use your thumb to take a pulse because

    _____.

63. When taking an apical pulse, each *lub-dub* sound is

    counted as _____.

64. The radial pulse rate is never greater than the

    _____.

65. A healthy adult has _____ respirations per minute.

66. What observations should be reported and recorded when counting respirations?

    A. _____

    B. _____

    C. _____

    D. _____

    E. _____

    F. _____

    G. _____

    H. _____

67. Each respiration involves _____

    and _____.

68. Respirations are counted for _____ if they are abnormal or irregular.

69. Blood pressure is controlled by

    A. _____

    B. _____

    C. _____

70. Normal ranges for blood pressures are

    A. Systolic _____

    B. Diastolic _____

71. If a person has been exercising, let the person

    rest for _____ before taking the blood pressure.

72. How should the person be positioned to take the

    blood pressure? _____
    Sometimes the doctor orders blood pressure in the

    _____ position.

73. When listening to the blood pressure, the first

    sound you hear is the _____ pressure and the point where the sound disappears

    is the _____ pressure.

LABELING

74. Name the pulse sites shown.

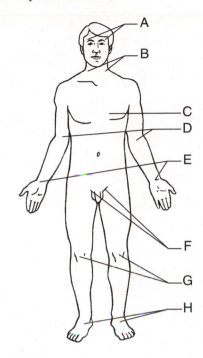

A. _____

B. _____

C. _____

D. _____

E. _____

F. _____

G. _____

H. _____

I. Which pulse is used during cardiopulmonary resuscitation (CPR)?

_____

J. Which pulse is most commonly taken?

_____

K. Which pulse is used when taking the blood pressure? _____

L. Which pulse is found with a stethoscope?

_____

75. Fill in the drawings so the dials show the correct blood pressures.

A. 168/102

B. 104/68

A

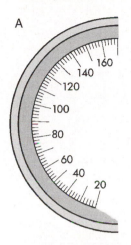
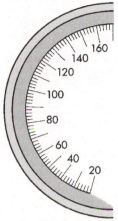

B

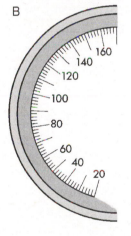
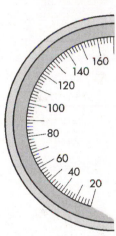

76. Fill in the drawings so the mercury columns show the correct blood pressures.

   A. 152/86

   B. 198/110

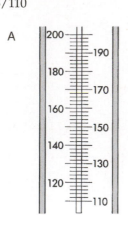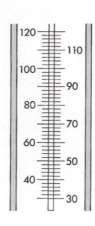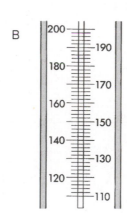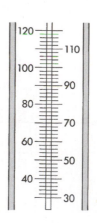

OPTIONAL LEARNING EXERCISES

Taking Temperatures

77. How would you record these temperature readings?

   A. An oral temperature of 97.4°F _____

      36.5°C _____.

   B. A rectal temperature of 99.8°F _____

      38.1°C _____.

   C. An axillary temperature of 96.2°F _____

      36.1°C _____.

Taking Pulses and Respirations

78. You are assigned to take Mrs. Sanchez's pulse and respirations. You note that the pulse rate and respirations are regular, so you take each one for

   _____. When you complete

   counting the pulse, you keep your _____

   and count _____. This is

   done so that Mrs. Sanchez will _____.

79. When you finish counting Mrs. Sanchez's pulse and respirations, your numbers are pulse 36 and respirations 9. What numbers should be

   recorded? Pulse _____

   Respirations _____ Why?

   _____

80. The nurse tells you to take an apical-radial pulse on Mrs. Hellman. Why do you ask a co-worker to help

   you? _____

81. For how long is an apical-radial pulse counted?

   _____ After you have taken

   the apical-radial pulse, how do you find the pulse

   deficit? _____

Taking Blood Pressures

82. You are assigned to take Mr. Hardaway's blood pressure. You know that he goes for dialysis 3 times a week. What do you need to know before you take

   his blood pressure? _____ Why?

   _____

83. When you inflate the cuff, you cannot feel the pulse after you pump the cuff to 130 mm Hg. How high will you inflate the cuff to take Mr. Hardaway's

   blood pressure? _____

84. You should deflate the cuff at an even rate of

   _____ per second.

INDEPENDENT LEARNING ACTIVITIES

- Take turns measuring vital signs on 3 or 4 classmates. If possible, use electronic, tympanic, and temporal thermometers for each person to see if they give similar results. Use the following table to record the results.

Person	Temperature	Pulse	Respiration	Blood Pressure
#1	Electronic Tympanic Temporal	Radial Apical	Rate Rhythm Depth	
#2	Electronic Tympanic Temporal	Radial Apical	Rate Rhythm Depth	
#3	Electronic Tympanic Temporal	Radial Apical	Rate Rhythm Depth	
#4	Electronic Tympanic Temporal	Radial Apical	Rate Rhythm Depth	

Answer the following questions about this exercise.
  - If you used different thermometers, how did the results compare?
  - What differences were there in finding the radial pulses among your classmates?
  - What differences did you find in the rates and rhythms?
  - How were you able to measure respirations so the person did not know you were watching?
  - What differences in rhythm and depth of respirations did you find among your classmates?
  - What differences did you find in locating the brachial artery in different people?
  - How did the sounds of the blood pressure differ among your classmates?
  - What difficulties did you have with any of the measurements taken?

- What will you change about measuring vital signs on a resident after this practice?
- Practice taking an apical-radial pulse with classmates. Take turns acting as the staff members and the person having the pulse taken. Answer the following questions after the exercise is completed.
  - How was privacy maintained for the person having the pulse measured?
  - How did the "staff members" decide who would begin and end the count?
  - What problems did you have in counting for 1 minute?
  - How did the apical and radial counts compare?
  - What will you change about measuring the apical-radial pulses on a resident after this experience?

27 ASSISTING WITH THE PHYSICAL EXAMINATION

FILL IN THE BLANKS: KEY TERMS

Dorsal recumbent position
Genupectoral position
Horizontal recumbent position
Knee-chest position

Laryngeal mirror
Lithotomy position
Nasal speculum
Ophthalmoscope

Otoscope
Percussion hammer
Tuning fork
Vaginal speculum

1. An instrument vibrated to test hearing is a

_____.

2. In the _____ the person lies on the back with the hips at the edge of the exam table; the knees are flexed, the hips are externally rotated, and the feet are in stirrups.

3. The supine position with the legs together is called

the _____.

4. An _____ is a lighted instrument used to examine the external ear and the eardrum (tympanic membrane).

5. A _____ is an instrument used to open the vagina so it and the cervix can be examined.

6. When a person kneels and rests the body on the knees and chest, so that the head is turned to one side, the arms are above the head or flexed at the elbows, the back is straight, and the body is flexed about 90 degrees at the hip, the person is in the

_____.

7. A _____ is an instrument used to tap body parts to test reflexes.

8. An instrument used to examine the mouth, teeth,

and throat is called a _____.

9. An instrument used to examine the inside of the

nose is a _____.

10. The dorsal recumbent position is also called the

_____.

11. An _____ is a lighted instrument used to examine the internal structures of the eye.

12. Another name for the knee-chest position is

_____.

CIRCLE THE BEST ANSWER

13. When weighing a person, have him or her
    A. Wear only socks and shoes and a bathrobe
    B. Remove regular clothes and wear a gown or pajamas
    C. Wear regular street clothes
    D. Remove any clothing worn after being weighed and then weigh the clothes

14. Chair, bed, and lift scales are used when
    A. A person can transfer from a wheelchair to the scale
    B. A person cannot stand
    C. A person can stand and walk independently
    D. A person is in the supine position

15. When a person cannot stand on the scale to have the height measured
    A. Ask the person or the family the person's height
    B. Have the person sit in a chair and use a measuring tape to measure the person from head to toe
    C. Position the person in a supine position in bed and measure with a measuring tape
    D. Estimate the height of the person by observing him or her

16. In nursing centers, residents have a physical examination
    A. Only when the person is admitted
    B. Once a month
    C. At least once a year
    D. Only when the person is ill

17. If a resident is having a physical examination, you may be asked to assist by
    A. Measuring vital signs, height, and weight
    B. Having the person remove all clothing
    C. Explaining why the examination is being done and what to expect
    D. Leaving the person alone after you have taken the vital signs and positioned the person

18. When the doctor is examining the person's mouth, teeth, and throat, you may be asked to hand him or her the
    A. Ophthalmoscope
    B. Percussion hammer
    C. Tuning fork
    D. Laryngeal mirror
19. The right to personal choice for a person having a physical examination is protected during a physical exam when you
    A. Have the person urinate before the examination begins
    B. Tell the person who will do the exam and when it will be done
    C. Keep the person screened and the room door closed
    D. Allow a family member to be present if the person requests it
20. The right to privacy is protected by
    A. Removing all clothes for a complete examination
    B. Explaining the reasons for the examination
    C. Exposing only the body part being examined
    D. Explaining the exam results with a family member present
21. Before the exam begins, you should
    A. Make sure the person has a bowel movement
    B. Have the person void so the bladder is empty
    C. Give the person an enema to empty the colon
    D. Have the person drink a large glass of water
22. After you have taken the person to the exam room and placed the person in position, you should
    A. Put the call light on for the nurse or examiner
    B. Leave the room
    C. Go to the nurse or examiner to report that the person is ready
    D. Open the door so the nurse or examiner knows you are ready
23. When the abdomen, chest, and breasts are to be examined, you will place the person in the
    A. Lithotomy position
    B. Sims' position
    C. Dorsal recumbent (horizontal recumbent) position
    D. Knee-chest position
24. If a person is asked to stand on the floor during an exam, you should
    A. Assist the person to put on shoes or slippers
    B. Place paper or paper towels on the floor
    C. Place a sheet on the floor
    D. Wipe the floor carefully with an antiseptic cleaner before the person stands on it

FILL IN THE BLANKS

25. List the equipment you need to collect when the ears are being examined.
    A. _____
    B. _____
26. List the items needed to examine the eyes.
    A. _____
    B. _____
27. When the nose, mouth, and throat are being examined, you should collect
    A. _____
    B. _____
    C. _____
    D. _____
28. What is done to the balance scale before having the person step on it?
    A. _____
    B. _____
    C. _____
29. When measuring a person in the supine position, the ruler is placed _____.
    _____
30. What are common fears the person may have when a physical examination is done?
    A. _____
    B. _____
    C. _____
    D. _____
    E. _____
    F. _____
    G. _____
    H. _____
31. To maintain the person's right to privacy, who are the only persons who have a right to see the person's body during the exam?
    _____
32. Who are the staff members who need to know the reason for the exam and its results?
    _____

LABELING

Look at the instruments and answer Questions 33 to 37.

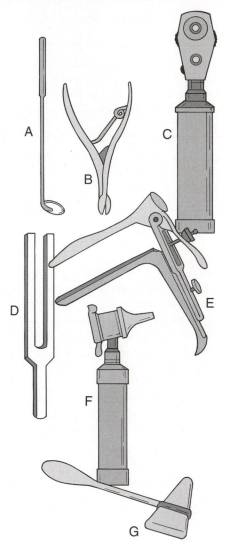

37. The reflexes are examined by using the

    _____.

Look at the positions and answer Questions 38 to 41.

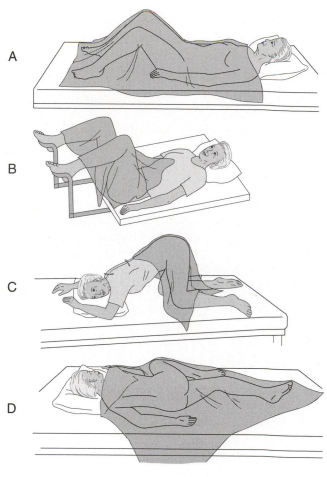

33. Name the instruments.

    A. _____

    B. _____

    C. _____

    D. _____

    E. _____

    F. _____

    G. _____

34. Which instrument is used to examine the nose?

    _____

35. When the eye is examined, the examiner uses the

    _____.

36. If a person has a sore throat, the examiner will look

    at the throat with the _____.

38. Name the positions.

    A. _____

    B. _____

    C. _____

    D. _____

39. Which positions may be used when a rectal examination is done?

    A. _____

    B. _____

40. When the abdomen, chest, and breasts are

    examined, the person is placed in _____

    _____.

41. The _____ is used for a vaginal exam.

OPTIONAL LEARNING EXERCISES

42. When you are delegated the job of preparing a person for an exam, why do you need the following information?

    A. What time is the examination?

    _____

    B. What are 2 reasons it would be helpful to know which examinations will be done?

    _____

    _____

    C. What equipment will you need if you are assigned to take vital signs? _____

    _____

43. You are a female nursing assistant assisting a male examiner with an examination of a female resident. The nurse tells you to stay in the exam room during the entire procedure. Why is this important to the examiner and to the woman? _____

    _____

    _____

INDEPENDENT LEARNING ACTIVITIES

- You probably have had a physical examination at some time. Perhaps you needed one to be a student in this class. Answer the following questions about your experience when you had the physical done to you.
  - Who explained what to expect during the exam? What were you told about any discomfort?
  - What steps were taken to give you privacy? While you changed clothes? During the exam?
  - Who was present during the exam? Were you given a choice of having another person in the room with you and the examiner? How did you feel about having (or not having) another person in the room?
  - How did you know what was being done? How much information were you given about procedures? Positions? Tests?

- What positions were used during the exam? Which positions shown in this chapter were used? How comfortable did you feel? How did the examiner and assistant help make you more comfortable with the positions?
- What questions did you have during the exam? Who was able to answer these? How well were they answered to make you understand what was being done?
- How comfortable did you feel about the exam? What could have been done to make you more comfortable physically and psychologically?
- How did this experience help you understand the feelings of persons you may assist during an exam?

28 COLLECTING AND TESTING SPECIMENS

FILL IN THE BLANKS: KEY TERMS

Acetone
Glucosuria
Glycosuria
Hematoma

Hematuria
Hemoptysis
Ketone
Ketone body

Melena
Sputum

1. Bloody sputum is _____.

2. A ketone is also called _____.

3. A black, tarry stool is _____.

4. _____ is glucosuria, or sugar in the urine

5. _____ is mucus from the respiratory system that is expectorated through the mouth.

6. Acetone is called _____ or ketone body.

7. A substance that appears in urine from the rapid breakdown of fat for energy is _____

_____.

8. Sugar in the urine is called glycosuria or

_____

9. _____ is blood in the urine.

10. A swelling that contains blood is a

_____

CIRCLE THE BEST ANSWER

11. Specimens are collected and tested to
    A. Measure the specimen
    B. Measure output
    C. Detect diseases
    D. Assist the person with personal care
12. When you are collecting a specimen, you should
    A. Use a sterile container for each specimen
    B. Follow the rules of medical asepsis
    C. Label the specimen after taking it to the clean utility room
    D. Carry the specimen to the lab wrapped in a clean paper towel
13. A urine specimen may be placed in a paper bag to
    A. Prevent embarrassing the person
    B. Protect the specimen from light
    C. Follow Standard Precautions
    D. Keep the specimen sterile

14. A random urine specimen is collected
    A. First thing in the morning
    B. After meals
    C. At any time
    D. At bedtime
15. When a person is collecting a random urine specimen, ask the person to put the toilet tissue in
    A. The wastebasket or toilet
    B. The specimen container
    C. The specimen pan
    D. A BIOHAZARD bag
16. When obtaining a midstream specimen, the perineal area is cleaned to
    A. Remove all microbes from the area
    B. Reduce the number of microbes in the urethral area
    C. Follow Standard Precautions and the Bloodborne Pathogen Standard
    D. Reduce infection during the specimen collection
17. When collecting a midstream specimen, which of these is correct?
    A. Collect the entire amount of urine voided.
    B. Collect about 4 oz (120 mL) of urine.
    C. Have the person void and then pass the receptacle into the stream of urine.
    D. Collect several specimens and mix them together.
18. When collecting a 24-hour urine specimen, the urine is kept
    A. Chilled on ice or refrigerated during the 24-hour period
    B. At room temperature
    C. In a sterile container at the nurses' station
    D. In a drainage collection bag at the bedside
19. A 24-hour urine specimen collection is started
    A. At the beginning of a shift
    B. After a meal
    C. At night
    D. After the person voids and that urine is discarded
20. At the end of 24-hour specimen collection
    A. The person voids and that urine is saved
    B. Write down any missed or spilled urine
    C. Record the amount of urine collected
    D. The person voids and that urine is discarded

21. When you test urine with reagent strips (dipsticks), it is important that you
    A. Follow the manufacturer instructions
    B. Use a sterile urine specimen
    C. Wear sterile gloves
    D. Make sure the urine is cold
22. When you are assigned to strain a person's urine, you
    A. Have the person void directly into the strainer
    B. Send all urine to the lab
    C. Have the person void into the receptacle and then pour the urine through the strainer
    D. Discard the strainer if it contains any stones
23. If a warm stool specimen is required, it is
    A. Placed it in an insulated container
    B. Taken to the laboratory at once
    C. Tested at once on the nursing unit
    D. Taken at once to the storage area for transport to the laboratory
24. When collecting a stool specimen, ask the person to
    A. Void and have a bowel movement in a bedpan
    B. Use only a bedpan or commode to collect the specimen
    C. Urinate into the toilet and collect the stool in the specimen pan
    D. Place the toilet tissue in the bedpan, commode, or specimen pan with the stool
25. When collecting the stool specimen
    A. Pour it into the specimen container
    B. Use your gloved hand to obtain a specimen to place in the container
    C. Use a tongue blade to take about 2 tablespoons of stool from the middle of the formed stool
    D. Use a tongue blade to place the entire stool specimen in the container
26. When you test a stool specimen for blood
    A. It must be sent to the laboratory
    B. The specimen must be sterile
    C. You will need to test the entire stool specimen
    D. Use a tongue blade to obtain a small of amount of stool from two different areas
27. A sputum specimen is more easily collected
    A. Upon awakening
    B. After eating
    C. At bedtime
    D. After activity
28. Before obtaining a sputum specimen, ask the person to
    A. Rinse the mouth with clear water
    B. Brush the teeth and use mouthwash
    C. Cough and discard the first sputum expectorated
    D. Sit in an upright position to loosen secretions
29. Postural drainage is used when collecting a sputum specimen to
    A. Collect sterile specimens
    B. Make the sputum specimen more liquid
    C. Stimulate coughing
    D. Help secretions drain by gravity
30. When choosing a site for blood glucose testing, the best choice is
    A. The thumb
    B. The fleshy part of the middle finger
    C. The side toward the tip of the middle or ring finger
    D. The index finger
31. To increase the blood flow in the fingers before a blood glucose test
    A. Apply a warm washcloth or wash the hands in warm water
    B. Massage the fingers vigorously
    C. Apply cool compresses to the fingers and hands
    D. Have the person hang the hand over the edge of the bed for several minutes

FILL IN THE BLANKS

32. Write out the meaning of each abbreviation

    A. BM _____

    B. ID _____

    C. I&O _____

    D. mL _____

    E. oz _____

33. When collecting urine specimens, what observations are reported and recorded?

    A. _____

    B. _____

    C. _____

    D. _____

    E. _____

34. How much urine is collected for a random urine specimen? _____

35. When collecting a midstream urine specimen, the person starts to void and then stops _____. After the specimen container is positioned, the person _____ _____.

36. When you are obtaining a midstream specimen from a female, spread the labia with the thumb and index finger of your _____ hand.

37. When cleaning the female perineum for a midstream specimen, clean from _____.

38. When cleaning the male perineum for a midstream specimen, clean the penis starting _____

39. When you make labels for a 24-hour urine collection to place in the room and bathroom, what information is marked?

    _____

    _____

40. Urine pH measures if the urine is _____ or _____.

41. When you use reagent strips, you read the strip by comparing it to the _____.

42. When you strain urine, you are looking for stones that can develop in the _____.

43. The strainer or gauze is placed in the specimen container if any _____ _____ appear.

44. Stool specimens are studied and checked for

    A. _____

    B. _____

    C. _____

    D. _____

    E. _____

45. After collecting a stool specimen, place the container in a _____.

46. When you are delegated to collect a stool specimen, what observations are reported and recorded?

    A. _____

    B. _____

    C. _____

    D. _____

    E. _____

47. When stools are black and tarry, there is bleeding in the _____.

48. Blood in the stool that is hidden is called

    _____

49. Mouthwash is not used before a sputum specimen is collected because it _____.

50. When you are delegated to collect a sputum specimen, report and record

    A. _____

    B. _____

C. _____

D. _____

E. _____

F. _____

G. _____

H. _____

I. _____

51. When you are assisting a person to collect a sputum specimen, ask the person to take 2 or 3 _____ and _____ the sputum.

52. When preparing to carry out a blood glucose test, how will you make sure

    A. The glucose meter was tested for accuracy?

        _____

    B. You have the correct reagent strips for the meter you are using? _____

        _____

    C. The strips are not too old to use?

        _____

OPTIONAL LEARNING EXERCISES

53. If you are collecting a midstream specimen, what should you do if it is hard for the person to stop the stream of urine? _____

    _____

54. You are caring for a person who is having a 24-hour urine specimen test. He tells you he forgot to save a specimen 1 hour ago. What should you do and why? _____

55. What is normal pH for urine? _____

    What can cause changes in the normal pH?

    _____

56. When the body cannot use sugar for energy, it uses fat. When this happens, _____ appear in the urine.

57. Why is privacy important when collecting a sputum specimen? _____

    _____

INDEPENDENT LEARNING ACTIVITIES

- Answer the following questions about collecting specimens.
  - What specimens may be collected by nursing assistants in your state?
  - What special training is given to make sure that nursing assistants understand how to collect specimens?

- Ask permission to look at specimen containers used at your clinical site. Are any directions included with the containers?
- Where is information about collecting specimens kept at the clinical site?

CROSSWORD

Fill in the crossword by choosing words from this list.

Calculi

Dysuria

Expectorated

Labia

Midstream

Occult

Postural

Random

Specimens

Suctioning

Across

1. Samples
3. Urine specimen that can be collected at any time
6. Hidden, as in blood in the stool
8. Position with head lower than body used to cause fluid to flow down
10. Pain when urinating

Down

2. Expelled, as in sputum, through the mouth
4. Urine specimen that is collected after the person starts to void
5. Stones that develop in the kidneys, ureters, or bladder
7. Removal of sputum from the trachea with a machine

29 ADMISSIONS, TRANSFERS, AND DISCHARGES

FILL IN THE BLANKS: KEY TERMS

Admission   Discharge   Transfer

1. _____ is moving a person from one room or nursing unit to another.

2. The official entry of a person into a nursing center is _____.

3. _____ occurs with the official departure of a person from a nursing center.

CIRCLE THE BEST ANSWER

4. Usually, _____ to a home setting is a happy time.
   A. Admission
   B. Discharge
   C. Transfer
   D. Home care

5. What staff member starts the admissions process?
   A. The doctor
   B. The nurse
   C. The admission coordinator
   D. The activities director

6. When a person with dementia is admitted to a nursing center, the person
   A. Is usually depressed
   B. May have an increase in confusion
   C. May have a decrease in confusion
   D. Usually feels safer in the new setting

7. Persons admitted to a rehabilitation unit from the hospital
   A. Are always admitted by the RN
   B. Are always admitted by the nursing assistant
   C. May be admitted by the nursing assistant after the nurse determines that the person's condition is stable and the person has no discomfort or distress
   D. Are never admitted by the nursing assistant

8. If a person being admitted is arriving by stretcher, you should
   A. Raise the bed to its highest level
   B. Leave the bed closed
   C. Raise the head of the bed to Fowler's position
   D. Lower the bed to its lowest level

9. During admission you can help the person feel more comfortable by
   A. Taking the person to his or her room and leaving the person alone
   B. Telling family members they must leave
   C. Talking quickly and answering questions with short answers
   D. Assisting the person to hang up pictures or display photos

10. When a person is being moved to a new room, who is notified?
    A. The doctor
    B. The social worker
    C. The family and business office
    D. The person's roommate

11. When you are transferring a person, you should
    A. Identify the person by checking the ID bracelet against the transfer slip
    B. Explain the reasons for the transfer
    C. Call the person's family to let them know about the transfer
    D. Wear gloves when gathering the person's belongings

12. If a person wishes to leave the center without the doctor's permission, you should
    A. Tell the person this is not allowed
    B. Prevent the person from leaving
    C. Tell the nurse at once
    D. Try to convince the person to stay

13. When you are assisting a person who is being discharged, you should
    A. Strip the bed and disinfect the equipment in the room while the person is packing
    B. Check off items on the clothing list and personal belongings list
    C. Call the family to ask them to assist the person in getting ready to go home
    D. Give the person prescriptions written by the doctor

FILL IN THE BLANKS

14. OBRA has standards for transfers and discharges. List the ways these standards affect the person's rights.

    A. Reasons for _____ and _____ are part of the person's _____.

    B. The _____ and _____ are told of transfer or discharge plans.

    C. A procedure is followed if the person _____.

    D. An _____ often works with the person and family to ensure that _____.

15. When you are delegated to assist with admissions, transfers, or discharges, what information do you need from the nurse?

    A. _____

    B. _____

    C. _____

    D. _____

    E. _____

    F. _____

    G. _____

    H. _____

    I. _____

    J. _____

16. When a person is being admitted, what identifying information is obtained?

    A. _____

    B. _____

    C. _____

    D. _____

    E. _____

17. During admission, why does the person have a photo taken or receive an ID bracelet? _____

    _____

18. When you are asked to admit a person, what can you do to make a good first impression?

    A. _____

    B. _____

    C. _____

    D. _____

    E. _____

19. What are reasons a person is moved to a new room?

    A. _____

    B. _____

    C. _____

    D. _____

    E. _____

20. According to OBRA and the CMS, reasons for a transfer or discharge are

    A. _____

    B. _____

    C. _____

    D. _____

    E. _____

21. When you transfer a person to a new unit, use good communication skills by

    A. _____

    B. _____

    C. _____

    D. _____

22. When a person is transferred or discharged, the nurse will tell you when to start _____

    and when the person is _____.

23. When you assist with a transfer or discharge, you should report and record

    A. _____

    B. _____

    C. _____

    D. _____

    E. _____

    F. _____

24. To help the person and family cope with admission, transfer, and discharge, you should

    A. Be _____

    B. Be _____

    C. Handle _____

    _____

    D. Treat _____

OPTIONAL LEARNING EXERCISES

Situation: Rosa Romirez, age 65, had a stroke (CVA) last week and is being admitted to a rehabilitation unit in the nursing care center where you work.
Answer the following questions about Mrs. Romirez.

25. Because you know Mrs. Romirez is arriving by wheelchair, you leave the bed

    A. _____

    B. _____

26. The nurse instructs you to collect the equipment needed to admit a new person. You collect

    A. _____

    B. _____

    C. _____

    D. _____

    E. _____

    F. _____

    G. _____

    H. _____

    I. _____

    J. _____

27. When Mrs. Romirez arrives with her husband, it may help them feel more comfortable if you offer

    them _____.

28. You greet Mrs. Romirez by name and ask if she

    prefers a certain _____

When you arrive at work one day, you are told Mrs. Romirez is being transferred to another room and you are asked to assist. Answer the following questions about transferring her.

29. When you transport Mrs. Romirez in a wheelchair,

    she is covered with a _____.

30. What items are taken with Mrs. Romirez to the new

    unit? _____

31. What information is recorded and reported about the transfer?

    A. _____

    B. _____

    C. _____

    D. _____

    E. _____

    F. _____

    G. _____

Several weeks later, you are assigned to care for Mrs. Romirez and find she is going home. Answer the following questions about her discharge.

32. What information and teaching should Mrs. Romirez receive from the health team before discharge?

    A. _____, _____, and

    _____

    B. Teaching about _____ and

    _____

    C. Arrangements for

    (1) _____

    (2) _____

    (3) _____

    D. Appointment with _____

33. Good communication skills should be used when assisting with the discharge. When Mrs. Romirez

    and her family leave, you should _____

    _____.

INDEPENDENT LEARNING ACTIVITIES

- Have a discussion with 3 or 4 classmates to share experiences you have had with admissions to care facilities. You may have had personal experience or you may have observed a friend or family member being admitted. If you have not had this experience, perhaps you can relate the feelings you have had when visiting a doctor's office. Answer the following questions during the discussion.
  - Who was the first person you met when you arrived to be admitted? How were you greeted? Did you feel welcome?
  - How did you arrive at your room? Were you escorted or did you have to find your way?
  - How long did you wait in the room before a staff member came to admit you? How did this affect your feelings about the place?
  - How were you addressed? First name? Last name? Did anyone ask you what you preferred?
  - What information were you given to make you feel more comfortable? What printed information was provided?
  - Overall, how did the admission procedure affect your feelings about the facility? Negative? Positive?
  - How will your personal experience and the experiences of others in this group affect your approach to new persons in a care facility?

30 WOUND CARE

FILL IN THE BLANKS: KEY TERMS

Abrasion
Arterial ulcer
Chronic wound
Clean wound
Clean-contaminated wound
Closed wound
Compress
Constrict
Contaminated wound
Contusion
Dehiscence
Diabetic foot ulcer
Dilate
Dirty wound
Edema

Embolus
Evisceration
Full-thickness wound
Gangrene
Hyperthermia
Hypothermia
Incision
Infected wound
Intentional wound
Laceration
Open wound
Pack
Partial-thickness wound
Penetrating wound
Phlebitis

Puncture wound
Purulent drainage
Sanguineous drainage
Serosanguineous drainage
Serous drainage
Skin tear
Stasis ulcer
Thrombus
Trauma
Ulcer
Unintentional wound
Vascular ulcer
Venous ulcer
Wound

1. A _____ is a break or rip in the skin that separates the epidermis from underlying skin.

2. A cut produced surgically by a sharp instrument is a(n) _____.

3. A shallow or deep crater-like sore of the skin or mucous membrane is an _____.

4. When tissues are injured but the skin is not broken, it is a _____.

5. _____ is thick green, yellow, or brown drainage.

6. When the dermis and epidermis of the skin are broken, it is called a _____.

7. A _____ is a break in the skin or mucous membrane.

8. A wound that is not infected is a _____.

9. A(n) _____ is a partial-thickness wound caused by the scraping away or rubbing of the skin.

10. A _____ is an open wound on the foot caused by complications from diabetes.

11. Thin, watery drainage that is blood-tinged is called _____.

12. A(n) _____ is a wound containing large amounts of microbes that shows signs of infection.

13. Another name for a blood clot is a _____.

14. _____ is an inflammation of a vein.

15. A wound with a high risk of infection is a _____.

16. A condition in which there is death of tissue is _____.

17. A body temperature that is much higher then the person's normal range is _____.

18. A _____ is an open wound with torn tissues and jagged edges.

19. A wound resulting from trauma is an _____.

20. A(n) _____ is an open wound on the lower legs or feet caused by poor arterial blood flow.

21. Clear, watery fluid is _____.

22. A blood clot that travels through the vascular system until it lodges in a distant vessel is called an _____.

23. Another name for an infected wound is

_____.

24. A _____ is a wound that does not heal easily.

25. An open sore on the lower legs or feet cause by poor blood flow through the veins is a

_____.

26. An open wound made by a sharp object is a

_____.

27. A wound created for therapy is a(n)

_____.

28. A _____ is an open wound that breaks the skin and enters a body area, organ, or cavity.

29. _____ is the separation of wound layers.

30. Swelling that is caused by fluid collecting in tissues is _____.

31. A _____ occurs when the dermis, epidermis, and subcutaneous tissue are penetrated. Muscle and bone may be involved.

32. An accident or violent act that injures the skin, mucous membranes, bones, and internal organs is called _____.

33. The separation of the wound along with the protrusion of abdominal organs is

_____.

34. A _____ is another name for a venous ulcer.

35. Bloody drainage is called _____.

36. A closed wound caused by a blow to the body is a

_____.

37. A(n) _____ occurs when the skin or mucous membrane is broken.

38. A soft pad applied over a body part is a

_____.

39. A _____ is a wet or dry application wrapping a body part.

40. To expand or open wider is to _____.

41. A very low body temperature is

_____.

42. _____ means to narrow.

43. A wound that occurs from the surgical entry of the reproductive, urinary, respiratory, or gastrointestinal system is a _____

_____.

44. A _____ is an open sore on the lower legs or feet caused by decreased blood flow through the arteries or veins.

CIRCLE THE BEST ANSWER

45. When you inspect a resident's elbow, you find some of the skin is rubbed away. You would report this to the nurse as a(n)
    A. Laceration
    B. Abrasion
    C. Contusion
    D. Incision

46. When you look at a resident's arm that caught on the wheelchair, the tissue is torn with jagged edges. You know this is a
    A. Puncture wound
    B. Abrasion
    C. Penetrating wound
    D. Laceration

47. Which of these would place a person at risk for skin tears?
    A. The person is obese.
    B. The person is able to walk to the dining room.
    C. The person is very thin.
    D. The person is alert and oriented.

48. Applying lotion will help prevent skin breakdown or skin tears because it may
    A. Prevent loss of fatty layer under the skin
    B. Increase general thinning of the skin
    C. Keep the skin moisturized
    D. Prevent moisture in areas of the body where perspiration occurs

49. Venous ulcers of the feet and legs are caused by
    A. Poorly fitted shoes
    B. Decreased venous blood flow
    C. Increased activity
    D. Increased fluid intake

50. A measure to promote circulation to prevent venous (stasis) ulcers is
    A. Use elastic or rubber band–type garters to hold the person's socks in place
    B. Keep the person's feet flat on the floor while sitting in a chair
    C. Apply elastic stockings or elastic wraps to legs
    D. Massage the legs and feet

51. Elastic stockings
    A. Are usually removed every 8 hours for 30 minutes
    B. Are applied after the person has been out of bed for 30 minutes or more
    C. Normally cause the person to complain of tingling or numbness in the feet
    D. Are removed only at bedtime or for a bath or shower

52. When applying elastic stockings, it is correct to
    A. Position the person in the chair
    B. Turn the stocking inside out down to the heel
    C. Make sure the stocking is large enough to fit loosely
    D. Fold over the top of the stocking if it is too long

53. Elastic stockings and elastic bandages are
    A. Applied loosely to prevent discomfort
    B. Applied starting at the knee
    C. Used with persons at risk for developing a thrombus
    D. Used with all older persons

54. When applying elastic bandages, you should
    A. Apply the bandage so it completely covers the fingers or toes
    B. First apply the bandage to the lowest (distal) part of the wrist, foot, ankle, or knee
    C. Secure the bandage at the back of the leg with a safety pin
    D. Remove the bandage only when it becomes loose or falls off the extremity

55. Common causes of arterial ulcers are
    A. Poor blood flow through the veins
    B. Leg or foot surgery
    C. Smoking, high blood pressure, and diabetes
    D. Surgery on bones and joints

56. When caring for a person at risk for vascular ulcers, you should
    A. Remind the person not to sit with the legs crossed
    B. Assist the person to apply garters to hold up socks or hose
    C. Massage pressure points
    D. Encourage the person to use elastic garters to hold stockings in place

57. When caring for a person with diabetes, it is important to
    A. Massage the feet and ankles frequently
    B. Ask the person if the feet are too cold or too hot
    C. Check the person's feet every day
    D. Tell the person not to wear any shoes

58. During wound healing, what phase is happening when the wound is about 1 year old?
    A. Initial phase
    B. Inflammatory phase
    C. Maturation phase
    D. Proliferative phase

59. The nurse tells you to make sure Mrs. Reynolds supports her abdominal wound when she coughs. The nurse wants this done to protect against
    A. Secondary intention healing
    B. Infection
    C. Scarring
    D. Dehiscence

60. When you are caring for Mrs. Reynolds, you notice thin, watery drainage that is blood-tinged. When you report your observations, you tell the nurse that the wound has _____ drainage.
    A. Purulent
    B. Serosanguineous
    C. Serous
    D. Sanguineous

61. Which of these methods used in wound care will prevent microbes from entering a wound when large amounts of drainage are expected?
    A. Wet-to-dry dressings
    B. Closed drainage system attached to suction
    C. Penrose drain
    D. Nonadherent gauze

62. Transparent adhesive film applied to a wound
    A. Absorbs dead tissue, which is removed when dressings are dry
    B. Allows drainage to be absorbed
    C. Allows air to reach the wound but does not allow fluids and bacteria to reach it
    D. Can be lifted to observe the wound

63. Plastic and paper tape may be used to secure a dressing
    A. Because they allow movement of the body part
    B. When the dressing must be changed frequently
    C. If the person is allergic to adhesive tape
    D. Because they stick well to the skin

64. A wet-to-wet dressing
    A. Is allowed to dry before being removed
    B. Is kept wet at all times
    C. Provides pressure to support the wound
    D. Prevents microbes from entering the wound

65. If you are assigned to change a dressing, which of these is important information to have?
    A. What kind of medication the person receives
    B. The person's diagnosis
    C. When pain medication was given and when it will take effect
    D. The person's age

66. You can make the person more comfortable when changing a dressing by
    A. Changing the dressing immediately after pain medication is given
    B. Avoiding body language that indicates the wound is unpleasant
    C. Encouraging the person to look at the wound
    D. Removing the dressing quickly by pulling the tape and dressing off all at once

67. When you are assigned to change dressings, you should
   A. Follow Standard Precautions and the Bloodborne Pathogen Standard
   B. Use sterile technique
   C. Wear gloves only to remove old dressings
   D. Use one pair of gloves throughout the dressing change

68. Binders promote healing because they
   A. Prevent infection
   B. Prevent drainage
   C. Support wounds and hold dressings in place
   D. Prevent bleeding

69. A binder should be applied
   A. With firm, even pressure over the area
   B. So safety pins are positioned where they are easy to reach
   C. Very loosely to prevent interfering with movement
   D. Only once a day and be removed only during AM care

70. When heat is first applied to the skin
   A. Blood vessels in the area dilate
   B. Tissues receive less oxygen
   C. Blood flow decreases
   D. Blood vessels constrict

71. When heat is applied for too long, a complication that occurs is
   A. Blood vessels dilate
   B. Blood flow increases
   C. Blood vessels constrict
   D. More nutrients reach the area

72. Moist heat applications have lower temperatures than dry heat applications because
   A. Dry heat penetrates more deeply
   B. Dry heat cannot cause burns
   C. Moist heat has greater and faster effects than dry heat
   D. Moist heat has a slower effect than dry heat

73. Heat and cold applications are applied for no longer than
   A. 1 hour
   B. 30 minutes
   C. 15 to 20 minutes
   D. 4 hours

74. When a warm or cold application is in place, you should check the area
   A. Every 15 to 20 minutes
   B. Every 5 minutes
   C. About every 30 minutes
   D. Once an hour

75. When giving a sitz bath
   A. Give the person privacy for the entire time
   B. Observe for signs of weakness, faintness, or fatigue
   C. Observe for signs of swelling in the perineal area
   D. Check the person every 15 minutes

76. You should remove warm or cold applications at once if
   A. The skin is warm and red with a heat application
   B. The person tells you the cold application has relieved some of the pain
   C. The skin appears pale, white, gray, or bluish in color
   D. The person is slightly chilled and asks for an extra blanket

77. When a person has hyperthermia, ice packs are applied to
   A. The abdomen
   B. The extremities
   C. The head, neck, and underarms
   D. The back

FILL IN THE BLANKS

78. Write out the meaning of each abbreviation.
   A. C _____
   B. F _____
   C. GI _____
   D. ID _____
   E. PPE _____

79. What are common causes of wounds?
   A. _____
   B. _____
   C. _____
   D. _____
   E. _____

80. You can cause a skin tear when moving, re-positioning, and transferring by holding on to a person's arm or leg _____.

81. List ways to prevent skin tears in the following.
   A. Improve hydration by offering the person
   _____.

   B. What kind of clothing would be helpful?
   _____
   _____

   C. Nail care of the person _____
   _____

   D. Lift and turn the person with a
   _____.

   E. Support the arms and legs with

    _____.

   F. Pad _____.

   G. Keep your fingernails _____

    and _____. Do not wear

    rings with _____.

82. Skin tears are portals _____.

83. When the person has vascular ulcers, report any

   _____.

84. You are caring for a person with a disease that affects venous circulation. You notice her toenails

   are long and sharp. You should _____

   _____.

85. Compression (anti-embolism, AE, or TED) stockings help prevent the development of thrombi

   because they _____

   _____.

86. When you are delegated to apply compression (AE, TED) stockings, what observations should you report and record?

   A. _____

   B. _____

   C. _____

   D. _____

   E. _____

   F. _____

   G. _____

   H. _____

   I. _____

87. When you apply elastic bandages, the fingers or

   toes are exposed to allow _____.

88. After applying elastic bandages, you should check

   the fingers or toes for _____.

   Also ask about _____.

   If any of these are noted, you should

   _____.

89. What 2 diseases are common causes of arterial

   ulcers? _____.

90. When a person has diabetes, what complications can occur with the following?

   A. Nerves – Person may not feel

    _____. Can develop

    _____.

   B. Blood vessels – Blood flow _____.

    What can occur? _____

91. Explain what can happen if a person with diabetes has these foot problems.

   A. Corns and calluses _____

   B. Ingrown toenails _____

   C. Hammer toes _____

   D. Dry and cracked skin _____

92. With primary intention healing, the wound edges

   are held together with _____

   _____.

93. Secondary intention healing is used for

   _____

   wounds. Because healing takes longer, the threat of

   _____ is great.

94. What should you do if you find a person's wound

   has dehiscence or evisceration? _____

   _____.

95. What observations would you make about wound appearance?

   A. _____

   B. _____

   C. _____

   D. _____

   E. _____

96. When you are delegated to change a dressing, what may the nurse tell you to do if the old dressings

   stick to the wound? _____

   _____

97. If the person has drainage from a wound, how is it measured?

   A. _____

    _____

    _____

   B. _____

98. What are purposes of a transparent adhesive film dressing?

    A. _____

    B. _____

    C. _____

    D. _____

99. What is the difference between wet-to-dry dressings and wet-to-wet dressings? _____

    _____

100. When taping a dressing in place, the tape should not encircle the entire body part because _____

    _____.

101. When delegated to apply dressings, what observations should be reported and recorded?

    A. _____

    B. _____

    C. _____

    D. _____

    E. _____

    F. _____

    G. _____

    H. _____

    I. _____

    J. _____

    K. _____

    L. _____

    M. _____

102. What are the uses of warm applications?

    A. _____

    B. _____

    C. _____

    D. _____

    E. _____

103. When you are caring for a confused person and heat or cold is applied, how can you know if the person is in pain? _____

104. When you prepare an ice bag, collar, or glove, remove the excess air by _____

    _____.

105. When heat or cold applications are in place, you can help promote comfort and safety and maintain quality of life by

    A. _____

    B. _____

    C. _____

    D. _____

OPTIONAL LEARNING EXERCISES

You are assigned to care for Mrs. Stevens. She is 87 years old and has diabetes and high blood pressure. She walks with difficulty and spends most of her day sitting in her chair. She is somewhat over-weight and tells you she had a knee replacement 5 years ago and had phlebitis after surgery. The nurse tells you to watch carefully for signs of vascular ulcers.

106. What risk factors does Mrs. Stevens have that may make her develop vascular ulcers?

    A. _____

    B. _____

    C. _____

    D. _____

    E. _____

107. If arterial ulcers develop, they are usually found

    _____

    _____.

Mr. Hawkins, age 74, was in an automobile accident and has a wound on his leg that is large and open. It has become infected and he is being treated with antibiotics. When you are talking with him, he tells you he has smoked for 55 years and has poor circulation in his legs. He lives alone and generally eats takeout foods or eats cereal when he is at home.

108. Why is he receiving antibiotics?

    _____

109. What side effect of the antibiotics can cause a problem that could interfere with healing?

    _____

    _____

110. What factors would increase Mr. Hawkins's risk for complications?

    A. _____

    B. _____

    C. _____

    D. _____

111. What is missing in Mr. Hawkins's diet that is needed to help in healing the wound? _____

_____

The nurse instructs you to apply a cold pack to Mrs. Wilson, a resident who has twisted her ankle. Use the information you learned in this chapter to answer the following questions.

112. What is the purpose of the cold application for this injury? _____

_____

113. What can you use to make a cold pack if no commercial cold packs are available? _____

_____

114. How will you protect Mrs. Wilson's skin?

_____

115. How often should you check the area under the cold pack? _____

116. How long should the cold pack remain in place?

_____

117. Mrs. Wilson tells you the cold pack is helping reduce the pain. She asks you to leave it in place when you start to remove it. What should you tell her? _____

_____

INDEPENDENT LEARNING ACTIVITIES

- Role-play this situation with a classmate. One of you should act as the person and the other should act as the nursing assistant. Work together to answer the questions for each role.

Situation: Mr. Chavez is 45 years old and has a reddened area on his left calf. The doctor has ordered moist warm compresses to the area and the nurse has delegated this task to you.

- As the nursing assistant:
  - What questions would you ask the nurse before you applied the compresses?
  - How will you check the temperature of the compresses?
  - How will you keep the compresses at the correct temperature?
  - How often will you check the compresses? What will you observe when you check the area?
- As Mr. Chavez:
  - How was the treatment explained to you?
  - How were you positioned? What did the nursing assistant do to make sure you were comfortable?
  - How did the compresses feel? Was the temperature maintained? How?
  - How often were the compresses checked?

CROSSWORD

Fill in the crossword by choosing words from this list.

Abrasion
Compress
Constrict
Contusion
Dehiscence

Dilate
Edema
Embolus
Evisceration

Gangrene
Hypothermia
Incision
Phlebitis

Thrombus
Trauma
Ulcer
Wound

Across

1. Accident or violent act that injures the skin, mucous membranes, bones, and organs
5. Separation of the wound along with the protrusion of abdominal organs
6. Inflammation of a vein
9. Partial-thickness wound caused by scraping away or rubbing of the skin
10. Soft pad applied over a body area
15. Closed wound caused by a blow to the body
16. Blood clot
17. Swelling caused by fluid collecting in tissues

Down

2. Shallow or deep crater-like sore of the skin or mucous membranes
3. Separation of wound layers
4. To narrow
7. Very low body temperature
8. Blood clot that travels through the vascular system until it lodges in a distant vessel
11. Condition where there is death of tissue
12. Break in the skin or mucous membrane
13. To expand or open wider
14. Cut produced surgically by a sharp instrument

31 PRESSURE ULCERS

FILL IN THE BLANKS: KEY TERMS

Avoidable pressure ulcer
Bedfast
Bony prominence
Chairfast

Colonized
Eschar
Friction
Pressure ulcer

Shear
Slough
Unavoidable pressure ulcer

1. _____ is the presence of bacteria on the wound surface or in wound tissue; the person does not have signs and symptoms of an infection.

2. Dead tissue that is shed from the skin is

_____.

3. A pressure ulcer that develops from the improper

use of the nursing process is an _____

_____.

4. A _____ is an area where the bone sticks out or projects from the flat surface of the body.

5. Thick, leathery dead tissue that may be loose or

adhered to the skin is _____.

6. _____ occurs when layers of the skin rub against each other, or when the skin remains in place and underlying tissues move and stretch and tear underlying capillaries and blood vessels causing tissue damage.

7. _____ means confined to bed.

8. The rubbing of one surface against another is

_____.

9. An _____ is a pressure ulcer that occurs despite efforts to prevent one through proper use of the nursing process.

10. A localized injury to the skin and/or underlying tissue, usually over a bony prominence, resulting from pressure or pressure in combination with

shear is a _____.

11. _____ means confined to a chair.

CIRCLE THE BEST ANSWER

12. A pressure ulcer occurs because
    A. The person repositions himself or herself in the bed or chair
    B. The person drinks too many fluids
    C. Skin and underlying tissue is damaged by unrelieved pressure
    D. The person is repositioned too frequently

13. Older and disabled persons are at great risk for pressure ulcers because of
    A. Acute illnesses
    B. Increased activity
    C. Age-related skin changes
    D. Good nutrition

14. The first sign of a pressure ulcer in an area would be
    A. Skin color over a bony area is reddened or a different color than surrounding tissue
    B. Swelling in the area
    C. A break in the skin
    D. Exposed tissue and some drainage from the area

15. Mrs. Greene keeps sliding down in bed. The nurse tells you to raise the head of the bed no more than 30 degrees. This position will prevent tissue damage caused by
    A. Pressure over hard surfaces
    B. Shearing
    C. Poor body mechanics
    D. Poor fluid balance

16. According to the CMS, the most common site of pressure ulcers is
    A. The ears
    B. Underneath the breasts
    C. Between abdominal folds
    D. The sacrum

17. A Stage 3 pressure ulcer would have
    A. Intact skin with redness or different skin coloring over a bony prominence
    B. Exposed subcutaneous fat and slough
    C. Full-thickness tissue loss with muscle, tendon, and bone exposure
    D. A blister or shallow ulcer

18. When there is a purple or maroon localized area of discolored intact skin or a blood-filled blister, this is
    A. A Stage 2 pressure ulcer
    B. A suspected deep tissue injury
    C. An unstageable pressure ulcer
    D. A Stage 4 pressure ulcer
19. When following a repositioning schedule, a bedfast person should be repositioned
    A. According to the schedule in the person's care plan
    B. Three times a day
    C. Every 15 minutes
    D. As often as you have time
20. One way to prevent friction in the bed is to
    A. Use soap when cleansing the skin
    B. Rub or massage reddened areas
    C. Use pillows and blankets to prevent skin from being in contact with skin
    D. Powder sheets lightly
21. Bed cradles are used to
    A. Position the person in good body alignment
    B. Prevent pressure on the legs, feet, and toes
    C. Keep the heels off the bed
    D. Distribute body weight evenly
22. When the person is using an eggcrate-type mattress, it is covered with a special cover and
    A. Only a bottom sheet
    B. A bottom sheet and a drawsheet
    C. Waterproof materials, a lift sheet, and a bottom sheet
    D. A bottom sheet and a waterproof pad

FILL IN THE BLANKS

23. Name the stage of pressure ulcer described in each of the following.

    A. The skin is gone and subcutaneous fat may be exposed. _____

    B. Full-thickness tissue loss occurs and the ulcer is covered by slough and/or eschar.

    _____

    C. The skin is red with light skin or red, blue, or purple with dark skin. The color does not return to normal when the skin is relieved of pressure.

    _____

D. Muscle, tendon, and bone are exposed and damaged. Eschar may be present. _____

    _____

E. Usually this pressure ulcer is due to damage of underlying soft tissue from pressure and/or shear. _____

F. The wound may involve an abrasion, blister, or shallow crater. _____

24. You can help prevent shearing by raising the head of the bed only _____. The care plan tells you
    A. _____
    B. _____
    C. _____

25. Explain how the following conditions place a person at risk for pressure ulcers.
    A. Urinary or fecal incontinence _____
    B. Poor nutrition _____
    C. Poor fluid balance _____
    D. Lowered mental awareness _____
    E. Circulatory problems _____
    F. Older person _____

26. Explain how these protective devices help prevent pressure ulcers.
    A. Bed cradle prevents pressure on

    _____ .

    B. Heel and elbow protectors prevent

    _____ and _____ .

    C. Heel and foot elevators raise _____ .

    D. Gel or fluid-filled pads and cushions

    _____ .

    E. Eggcrate-type pads distribute _____

    _____ .

    F. Special beds distribute _____ .

    There is little pressure on _____

    _____ .

OPTIONAL LEARNING EXERCISES

27. After admission to a nursing center, many pressure ulcers develop with the first _____ after admission.

28. A person at risk can develop a pressure ulcer within _____ after the onset of pressure.

29. When handling, moving, and positioning a person, it is important to follow the _____ _____ in the person's care plan.

 A. How often should a bedfast person be repositioned? _____

 B. How often should a chairfast person be repositioned? _____

 C. Remind a person sitting in a chair to shift their position every _____.

30. What are 2 ways pressure ulcers can occur on the ears?

 A. _____

 B. _____

31. If you are interviewed by the CMS staff about pressure ulcers, what questions may be asked?

 A. _____

 B. _____

 C. _____

 D. _____

 E. _____

INDEPENDENT LEARNING ACTIVITIES

- Take turns with a classmate and carry out these exercises. They will help you understand how a person who cannot move without assistance feels when pressure is unrelieved. NOTE: These exercises work best if the person wears thin clothes so the discomfort is more noticeable.
  - Place a pencil or similar hard object on the seat of a chair and have a classmate sit on the object for 10 minutes. Keep time and remind the person not to move, to make it more uncomfortable. Remember, persons at risk for pressure ulcers often are unable to change position without assistance.
  - Position a classmate in bed, making sure the bed linens are wrinkled to form lumps under bony pressure points. (For example, place a wrinkle under the sacrum in the supine position or under the hip or shoulder in the lateral position.)
- *Answer the following questions about the exercises done.*
  - How long did it *seem* when you waiting for 10 minutes to pass?
  - How many times did you begin to re-position yourself without thinking about it?
  - How did the pressure areas feel when you completed the 10 minutes? What color was the area?
  - How will this exercise affect your care of persons who cannot move?

32 HEARING, SPEECH, AND VISION PROBLEMS

FILL IN THE BLANKS: KEY TERMS

Aphasia
Blindness
Braille
Broca's aphasia
Cerumen
Deafness

Expressive aphasia
Expressive-receptive aphasia
Global aphasia
Hearing loss
Low vision
Mixed aphasia

Motor aphasia
Receptive aphasia
Tinnitus
Vertigo
Wernicke's aphasia

1. _____ is a touch reading and writing system that uses raised dots for each letter of the alphabet.

2. Another name for receptive aphasia is

_____.

3. Another name for earwax is

_____.

4. _____ is dizziness.

5. A ringing, roaring, hissing, or buzzing sound in the

ears is _____.

6. The total or partial loss of the ability to use or understand language; a language disorder resulting from damage to parts of the brain

responsible for language is _____.

7. _____ is not being able to hear the normal range of sounds associated with normal hearing.

8. _____ is difficulty expressing or sending out thoughts.

9. Eyesight that cannot be corrected with eyeglasses,

contact lenses, medicine, or surgery is

_____.

10. _____ is also called expressive aphasia or Broca's aphasia.

11. A hearing loss in which it is impossible for the person to understand speech through hearing

alone is _____.

12. Another name for expressive aphasia or motor

aphasia is _____.

13. _____ is also called expressive-receptive aphasia or mixed aphasia.

14. The absence of sight is _____.

15. Difficulty expressing or sending out thought

and difficulty understanding language is

_____.

16. Another name for expressive-receptive aphasia or

global aphasia is _____.

17. Difficulty understanding language is

_____. Also called

Wernicke's aphasia.

CIRCLE THE BEST ANSWER

18. If a person has chronic otitis media, the person may develop
    A. Vertigo
    B. Permanent hearing loss
    C. Diarrhea
    D. Nausea and vomiting

19. How would you know a person with dementia has otitis media?
    A. The person would tell you he or she has pain.
    B. The person would not be able to hear you.
    C. You might notice the person tugging or pulling at one or both ears.
    D. The person would have tinnitus.

20. If you are caring for a person who has Meniere's disease, it is important to
    A. Prevent falls
    B. Assist the person to move quickly
    C. Keep the lights in the room very bright
    D. Encourage the person to be active

21. Which of these is a preventable cause of hearing loss?
    A. Aging
    B. Heredity
    C. Exposure to very loud music
    D. Birth defects
22. When you are caring for a person with a hearing loss, which of these would help communication?
    A. Gain the person's attention by lightly touching the person's arm.
    B. Speak as loudly as possible.
    C. Make sure the radio or TV are playing in the room.
    D. Sit next to the person out of his or her line of sight.
23. When you are caring for a person with a hearing aid, follow the nurse's directions and the manufacturer instructions before
    A. Turning the hearing aid off at night
    B. Inserting a new battery if needed
    C. Cleaning the hearing aid
    D. Removing the battery at night
24. If a person has expressive aphasia, he or she
    A. Would not understand simple language
    B. Would speak in complete sentences
    C. Would have difficulty hearing what was said
    D. Might speak in single words or put words in the wrong order
25. When a person is speech-impaired, he or she
    A. Speaks rapidly in long sentences
    B. Often becomes angry and depressed
    C. Usually does not understand what is being said
    D. Needs to have his or her speech corrected
26. An effective measure to use when caring for a speech-impaired person is to
    A. Speak in a child-like way
    B. Ask the person questions to which you know the answer
    C. Use long, involved sentences
    D. Make sure the TV and radio are loud
27. When a person has glaucoma, he or she may have difficulty seeing objects
    A. That are far away
    B. To the right or left of him or her
    C. Directly in front of him or her
    D. That are bright colors
28. A risk factor for glaucoma is
    A. Everyone over 40 years of age
    B. Caucasian and Asians over 40 years of age
    C. Those with a family history of glaucoma
    D. Those who have poor nutrition
29. Cataracts most commonly are caused by
    A. Aging
    B. Injury
    C. Increased pressure in the eye
    D. Surgery
30. When a person has had eye surgery for cataracts, the care includes
    A. Removing the eye shield or patch for naps and at night
    B. Explaining the location of food on the food tray
    C. Reminding the person not to rub or press the affected eye
    D. Placing the over-bed table on the operative side
31. After cataract surgery, report to the nurse if
    A. The person complains of eye pain or has eye drainage
    B. Glasses need to be cleaned
    C. The person needs help with his or her food tray
    D. The person asks for help with basic needs
32. If a person has dry age-related macular degeneration (AMD)
    A. It can be treated with surgery
    B. The person will need to use eye drops for the rest of his or her life
    C. The person will eventually be blind
    D. The person will need to wear corrective glasses to see clearly
33. Which of these measures can reduce the risk of AMD?
    A. Exposing the eyes to sunlight
    B. Eating a healthy diet high in green leafy vegetables and fish
    C. Eating a diet high in red meats
    D. Decreasing the amount of exercise
34. Diabetic retinopathy is the result of
    A. High blood pressure
    B. Tiny blood vessels in the retina being damaged as a complication of diabetes
    C. Pressure increasing in the eye
    D. The lens becoming cloudy
35. A person with low vision
    A. Can be fitted with glasses that will improve vision to normal
    B. Can have corrective surgery to improve the vision
    C. Learns to use one or more visual and adaptive devices
    D. Is unable to see anything
36. A person who is legally blind
    A. Sees at 20 feet what a person with normal vision sees at 20 feet
    B. Is always totally blind
    C. Is usually blind from birth
    D. Sees at 20 feet what a person with normal vision sees at 200 feet
37. When you enter the room of a blind person, you should first
    A. Touch the person to let him or her know you are there
    B. Speak loudly to make sure the person knows you are there
    C. Make sure the lights are bright
    D. Identify yourself by giving your name, title, and reason for being there

38. When a person is blind, you should avoid
   A. Rearranging furniture and equipment
   B. Using words such as "see," "look," or "read"
   C. Letting the person move about
   D. Letting the person perform self-care
39. When you offer to assist a blind person to walk, it is best if you
   A. Walk slightly behind the person
   B. Walk 1 step ahead of the person
   C. Grasp the person's arm firmly to guide him or her
   D. Walk very slowly to allow the person to take small steps
40. If a blind person uses a cane, you can assist by
   A. Grasping the person by the arm holding the cane
   B. Coming up behind the person and grasping his or her elbow
   C. Giving the person verbal cues to avoid objects in the way
   D. Asking if you can assist before trying to help
41. If a blind person uses a guide dog, you
   A. Take the person by the arm on the side opposite the dog
   B. May pet, feed, or distract the dog
   C. May give the dog commands to avoid danger
   D. Understand that the dog sees for the person and is trained to keep the person safe
42. Eyeglasses should be cleaned with
   A. Cleaning solution or warm water
   B. Boiling water
   C. Detergent
   D. Dry cleansing tissues
43. When cleaning an ocular prosthesis (artificial eye), you should
   A. Wash the prosthesis with strong soap and hot water
   B. Wash the eyelid and eyelashes using sterile water and sterile wipes
   C. Use a small brush to remove any debris from the artificial eye
   D. Rinse the eye with sterile water before the person inserts the eye

FILL IN THE BLANKS

44. Write out the meaning of each abbreviation.
   A. AFB _____
   B. AMD _____
   C. ASL _____
   D. HOH _____
45. Otitis media often begins with _____.
   _____
46. If a person has chronic otitis media, it can cause permanent _____.

47. When a person has Meniere's disease, symptoms or attacks can occur _____
   or just _____.
48. With Meniere's disease, the person should not walk alone in case _____.
49. What are examples of noises that can cause hearing loss?
   A. _____
   B. _____
   C. _____
   D. _____
50. When persons are 75 years of age or older, about _____ have a hearing loss.
51. Symptoms of hearing loss include
   A. _____
   B. _____
   C. _____
   D. _____
   E. _____
   F. _____
   G. _____
   H. _____
   I. _____
   J. _____
   K. _____
52. If a woman is speaking to a hearing-impaired person, why should she adjust the pitch of her voice? _____
   _____
53. Why is it important for a person with a hearing loss to see your face when you are speaking to him or her? _____
   _____
54. What are common causes of speech disorders?
   A. _____
   B. _____
   C. _____
55. If a person has apraxia, the brain
   _____
   _____

56. Measures you can use to communicate with a speech-impaired person are

    A. Listen and give _____

    B. Repeat _____

    C. Write down _____

    D. Allow the person _____

    E. Watch _____

57. When a person has expressive aphasia, the person knows what _____

    _____.

    Thinking is _____.

58. When a person has receptive aphasia, the person may speak in _____

    _____ that have no

    _____.

59. Symptoms of glaucoma include

    A. Peripheral _____ and the

    person sees through _____

    B. Blurred _____

    C. Halos _____

60. Medications and surgery are used with glaucoma

    to _____.

61. Most cataracts are caused by _____.
    Other risk factors are

    A. _____

    B. _____

    C. _____

    D. _____

    E. _____

62. When you are caring for a person after cataract surgery, an eye shield is worn as directed and is

    worn for _____.

63. When assisting a blind or visually impaired person, what can be done to provide a consistent meal time setting?

    A. _____

    B. _____

    C. _____

    D. _____

    E. _____

    F. _____

64. A person with age-related macular degeneration (AMD) would develop a blind spot _____

    _____.

65. Everyone with diabetes is at risk for _____

    _____.

66. How can a person with low vision use a computer as an adaptive device?

    A. _____

    B. _____

67. When you orient a person with low or no vision to the room, why do you let the person move about the room?

    _____

OPTIONAL LEARNING EXERCISES

Mr. Herman is an 85-year-old man with hearing loss that has developed as he has become older. Answer the following questions about his care.

68. Two nursing assistants are caring for Mr. Herman—a male and a female. They notice that he answers questions asked by the male nursing assistant more quickly. What is the likely reason

    for this? _____

    _____

69. The nursing assistants have found that Mr. Herman is alert and oriented. They are surprised when Joan, another nursing assistant, tells them he is "senile." Why would Joan make this statement?

    _____

70. Mr. Herman says he is too tired to go to the game room for a party. He says no one likes him. What are some reasons for his actions and statements?

    A. Tired because _____

    _____

    B. No one likes him because _____

    _____

71. When giving care, the nursing assistant turns off the TV and radio in Mr. Herman's room. Why is

    this done? _____

You are caring for Mrs. Sanchez, who is legally blind because of glaucoma. Answer the following questions about her care.

72. When you enter the room, you notice that Mrs. Sanchez is looking at her mail with a magnifying glass. How is this possible, since you thought she was blind? _____

_____

73. When you enter the room, Mrs. Sanchez asks you to adjust the blinds. Why? _____

_____

74. When you are helping Mrs. Sanchez to move about the room, you allow her to touch the furniture and equipment. Why? _____

_____

INDEPENDENT LEARNING ACTIVITIES

- Cover your ears so you cannot hear clearly. Use one of these methods or one that you devise:
  - Commercial earplugs
  - Cotton plugs in ears
  - Cover ears with earmuffs or similar devices
- Keep your ears covered and your hearing muffled for at least 1 hour as you go about your daily activities. A wise student will not wear earplugs during class time! Answer the following questions about the experience.
  - How did you find yourself compensating for the hearing loss? Turning up the TV or radio? Asking others to write out information? Staying away from others? Getting angry or frustrated?
  - When you could not understand someone, what did you do? Ask them to repeat? Ask them to speak louder? Answer even if you were unsure of what was said? Not respond at all?
  - If you answered when unsure, what was your response? Did you tend to agree or disagree with the speaker? Why?
  - What methods listed in the chapter were helpful? What other methods did you use to understand what was being said? Watching the speaker? Cupping a hand around an ear?
  - How will this experience assist you when you care for a person with a hearing loss?
- Cover your eyes with a blindfold so you cannot see. Keep the blindfold on for at least 1 hour as you go about your normal activities. Have someone act as a guide during this time. In addition to your normal activities, include the activities listed.
  - Go outside with your guide and cross a street.
  - Visit a store or restaurant with your guide.
  - Eat a simple snack or meal.
  - Go to the toilet, wash your hands, and comb your hair.
  - Have your guide take you to a public area, place you in a chair or on a bench, and leave you alone for 5 to 10 minutes.

Note: You may wish to carry out this exercise using the blindfold and using this alternate method. If you wear glasses, cover the lenses with a heavy coating of petroleum jelly. This will simulate the vision experienced by a person with cataracts. Answer the following questions for either or both experiences.

  - How did you feel when you were unable to see what was going on around you? What noises or other sensory stimulants did you notice?
  - When you were crossing the street, how did you feel? Safe? Frightened?
  - When you were in a public area, what did you notice? How did you feel? How did others respond to you?
  - How comfortable did you feel about eating when you could not see the food? How were you able to locate the food? What problems did you have?
  - How did you manage in the bathroom? Were you able to find the equipment you needed? How competent did you feel about carrying out hand washing and grooming without being able to see?
  - What were your feelings when left alone in a public area for 5 to 10 minutes? How long did it *seem* to be before your guide returned? What concerns did you have? Safety? Fear of injury? Desertion?
  - How will this experience assist you when caring for a person with a vision loss?
- *Have a group discussion with your classmates after they have all carried out the exercises to simulate vision and hearing problems. Answer the following questions.*
  - Which disability did you find the most difficult to tolerate? Why?
  - If you had to live with one of these disabilities, which one would you choose? Why?
  - What happened during these exercises that surprised you about being unable to see or hear? How does this discovery change your attitude about the disabilities?

33 CANCER, IMMUNE SYSTEM, AND SKIN DISORDERS

FILL IN THE BLANKS: KEY TERMS

Benign tumor   Metastasis   Stomatitis

Cancer   Port   Tumor

Malignant tumor

1. A _____ is a tumor that invades and destroys nearby tissue and can spread to other body parts.

2. Inflammation of the mouth is

    _____.

3. A tumor that does not spread to other body parts

    is a _____.

4. A new growth of abnormal cells that may be

    benign or malignant is a _____.

5. The spread of cancer to other body parts is

    _____.

6. Another name for a malignant tumor is

    _____.

7. An implanted device in the body that allows medications or fluids to be given into a vein is a

    _____.

CIRCLE THE BEST ANSWER

8. Benign tumors
   A. Do not spread to other body parts
   B. Invade healthy tissue
   C. Are always very small
   D. Divide in an orderly and controlled way

9. A factor that increases the risk of cancer is
   A. Limiting exposure to sun
   B. Smoking and drinking alcohol
   C. A diet high in fresh fruits and vegetables
   D. Taking multivitamins and minerals

10. When surgery is done to treat cancer
    A. It always cures the cancer
    B. It often relieves pain from advanced cancer
    C. The person will continue to have pain
    D. The person loses body hair

11. When you care for a person receiving radiation therapy, you might expect the person to
    A. Need physical therapy
    B. Need special skin care measures
    C. Have dressings over the site
    D. Have weight gain

12. Chemotherapy involves
    A. X-ray beams aimed at the tumor
    B. Giving medications that prevent the production of certain hormones
    C. Therapy to help the immune system
    D. Giving medications that kill cells

13. While caring for a person receiving chemotherapy, she tells you she is upset because her hair is falling out. You know that
    A. The hair often falls out when a person receives chemotherapy
    B. This is symptom of her disease
    C. You should report this to the nurse at once
    D. You should change the subject so she will not be so upset

14. When hormone therapy is used to treat cancer, a woman may experience
    A. Stomatitis
    B. Flu-like symptoms
    C. Weight gain, hot flashes, and fluid retention
    D. Burns and skin breakdown

15. A person with cancer may complain of constipation because of
    A. The side effects of pain-relief medication
    B. Pain
    C. The side effects from cancer treatments
    D. Fluid and nutrition intake

16. When a person has cancer and expresses anger, fear, and depression, you can help most by
    A. Telling the person not to worry or get upset
    B. Giving the person privacy and time alone
    C. Being there when needed and listening to the person
    D. Changing the subject to distract the person

17. Treatment for autoimmune disorders is aimed at
    A. Curing the illness
    B. Controlling the autoimmune response
    C. Removing the affected organs
    D. Preventing metastasis
18. HIV is *not* spread by
    A. Blood
    B. Semen
    C. Sneezing or coughing
    D. Breast milk
19. To protect yourself from HIV and AIDS, you should
    A. Avoid all body fluids when giving care
    B. Refuse to give care to persons diagnosed with these diseases
    C. Follow Standard Precautions and the Bloodborne Pathogen Standard when giving care
    D. Always use sterile technique when giving any care
20. Shingles is caused by the same virus that causes
    A. HIV
    B. Measles
    C. Chicken pox
    D. Mumps

FILL IN THE BLANKS

21. Write out the abbreviations.

    A. AIDS _____

    B. HIV _____

    C. IV _____

22. Cancer is the _____ most common cause of death in the United States.

23. The goals of cancer treatment are

    A. _____

    B. _____

    C. _____

24. Some signs and symptoms of cancer are

    A. _____

    B. _____

    C. _____

    D. _____

E. _____

F. _____

G. _____

H. _____

I. _____

J. _____

25. With radiation therapy, skin care measures are needed at the treatment site because

    _____ and _____ can occur.

26. When chemotherapy is used, it affects

    _____ cells and _____ cells.

27. When a person is receiving chemotherapy, what side effects might occur?

    A. _____

    _____

    B. _____

    _____

    C. _____

    _____

28. When a person has an autoimmune disorder, it means the _____ system can cause disease by _____.

29. Acquired immunodeficiency syndrome (AIDS) is caused by a _____ that attacks the _____.

30. How does the human immunodeficiency virus (HIV) enter the bloodstream? _____

    _____

31. When caring for a person with HIV, the main threat to health care workers is from _____.

32. Those at risk for developing shingles are

    A. _____

    B. _____

    C. _____

OPTIONAL LEARNING EXERCISES

Mrs. Myers is a 62-year-old woman who is having chemotherapy to treat cancer. She has not been eating well and complains of feeling very tired. When you assist her with personal care, you notice a large amount of hair on her pillow. Answer the following questions about Mrs. Myers and her care.

33. Mrs. Myers may not be eating well because

    the chemotherapy _____ the

    gastrointestinal tract and causes _____,

    _____, _____,

    and _____.

34. She may also have _____,
    which is called stomatitis. You can help relieve the
    discomfort from this side effect when you provide

    _____.

35. What is causing Mrs. Myers to lose her hair?

    _____ This condition is

    called _____.

Answer this question about HIV.

36. What are reasons that many older persons do not
    consider themselves at risk for HIV?

    A. _____

    B. _____

    C. _____

INDEPENDENT LEARNING ACTIVITIES

- Interview a person who has been treated for cancer
  and ask the following questions.
  - How was the person told about the diagnosis
    of cancer? What kind of reaction did the person
    have? Was he or she frightened, angry,
    depressed, etc.?
  - What treatment was used to treat the cancer? What
    side effects did the person have? Did any of the
    treatment affect body image? Did the treatment
    leave any permanent disfigurement?
  - How did the cancer and the treatment affect the
    person's life? How able was the person to carry
    on normal activities, such as caring for family
    members or working?
  - How long ago did this occur? How is the person
    feeling now? What long-term effects have the
    cancer and treatments had on the person?

- If you have cared for a person with HIV/AIDS,
  answer the following questions about the experience.
  If you have not, think about how you might feel in
  that situation.
  - How did you react when you knew the person
    had HIV? What questions did you ask the nurse?
    The person?
  - What special precautions did you take when you
    were caring for the person?
  - How would you feel if you found out a person
    you had been caring for was diagnosed with HIV?
    How would this diagnosis affect the care you
    give?
  - When you use Standard Precautions and the
    Bloodborne Pathogen Standard for *all* persons you
    care for, how does that affect your reaction to an
    HIV patient?

34 NERVOUS SYSTEM AND MUSCULO-SKELETAL DISORDERS

FILL IN THE BLANKS: KEY TERMS

Amputation
Arthritis
Arthroplasty
Closed fracture
Compound fracture

Fracture
Gangrene
Hemiplegia
Open fracture
Paralysis

Paraplegia
Quadriplegia
Simple fracture
Tetraplegia

1. An open fracture is also called a

   _____

2. Another name for quadriplegia is

   _____

3. The removal of all or part of an extremity is

   _____

4. A _____ is when the bone is broken but the skin is intact.

5. _____ is paralysis and loss of sensory function in the arms, legs, and trunk. It can also be called tetraplegia.

6. Paralysis on one side of the body is

   _____

7. Joint inflammation is _____.

8. A closed fracture can also be called

   _____

9. A _____ is a broken bone.

10. An _____ occurs when the broken bone has come through the skin. It is also called a compound fracture.

11. An _____ is the surgical replacement of a joint.

12. Paralysis and loss of sensory function in the legs is

    _____

13. A condition in which there is death of tissue is

    _____

14. _____ is loss of motor function, loss of sensation, or both.

CIRCLE THE BEST ANSWER

15. The leading cause of disability in adults in the United States is
    A. Heart disease
    B. Cancer
    C. Stroke
    D. Diabetes

16. If a person has symptoms of a stroke that last a few minutes, it means that
    A. The person has had a transient ischemic attack (TIA)
    B. It is not a dangerous situation because it was temporary
    C. The person needs to lie down at once
    D. No further treatment is needed

17. Which of these persons has the most risk factors for stroke?
    A. A 70-year-old white man with hypertension and diabetes
    B. A 50-year-old white woman who smokes and is slightly over-weight
    C. A 70-year-old African-American man who has hypertension and diabetes
    D. A 75-year-old Asian woman who is inactive and has normal blood pressure and diabetes

18. If a person who has had a stroke ignores and forgets about the weaker side of the body, it is called
    A. Paralysis
    B. Incontinence
    C. Aphasia
    D. Neglect

19. When you are caring for a person who has had a stroke, the call light and other objects
    A. Should be removed from the room
    B. Are placed on the weak side of the body
    C. Are placed on the strong side of the body
    D. Are given to a family member to use for the person

20. Safety measures are needed for a person with Parkinson's disease to prevent
    A. Problems with communication
    B. Elimination difficulties
    C. Falls and injury
    D. Emotional changes
21. Multiple sclerosis (MS) is a disease that
    A. Is an acute illness from which the person recovers completely
    B. Always follows the same course with the same symptoms
    C. May have long periods without symptoms before a flare-up occurs
    D. Is easily treated with medications
22. When a person has secondary-progressive MS
    A. The symptoms gradually disappear with partial or complete recovery
    B. The person has no remissions
    C. More symptoms appear with each flare-up and the person's condition declines
    D. This stage follows relapsing-remitting MS
23. A person with amyotrophic lateral sclerosis (ALS) would be
    A. Confused and disoriented
    B. Able to walk with assistance even as the disease progresses
    C. Incontinent of bladder and bowel functions
    D. Unable to move the arms, legs, and body
24. If a person is in a persistent vegetative state after a traumatic brain injury, he or she
    A. Is unconscious and unaware and cannot be aroused
    B. Is unconscious and has sleep-wake cycles and alert periods
    C. Is unresponsive but can be aroused briefly
    D. Is unconscious and has sleep-wake cycles and alert periods. These symptoms last longer than 1 month
25. A person who has a spinal cord injury in the lumbar region will likely have
    A. Quadriplegia
    B. Paraplegia
    C. Hemiplegia
    D. Tetraplegia
26. When caring for a person with paralysis, it is important to
    A. Turn and re-position the person at least every 4 hours
    B. Check bath water, heat applications, and food for proper temperature
    C. Encourage the person to do as much as he or she can to maintain mobility
    D. Encourage deep-breathing and coughing exercises to prevent pneumonia

27. Autonomic dysreflexia occurs in a person who has paralysis
    A. Of any kind
    B. Above the mid-thoracic level
    C. In the lumbar region
    D. That is incomplete
28. If you are caring for a person with autonomic dysreflexia, report to the nurse at once if
    A. The person has sweating above the level of the injury
    B. The blood pressure is low
    C. The person complains of pain below the level of the injury
    D. The person has sweating below the level of the injury
29. If a person is at risk for autonomic dysreflexia, it is best if only the nurse
    A. Gives basic care
    B. Makes sure the catheter is draining properly
    C. Checks for fecal impactions or gives an enema
    D. Re-positions the person at least every 2 hours
30. Osteoarthritis differs from rheumatoid arthritis because osteoarthritis
    A. Is an inflammatory disease
    B. Occurs with aging
    C. Means that the person does not feel well
    D. Occurs on both sides of the body
31. When you are caring for a person with osteoarthritis, which of these would be most helpful to the person?
    A. Allow the person to stay in bed as much as desired.
    B. Keep the room cool, as osteoarthritis improves with cold temperatures.
    C. Help the person use good body mechanics and good posture and get regular rest.
    D. Tell the person not to exercise, as the exercise will prevent healing.
32. If you are caring for a person who has rheumatoid arthritis and the person has a flare-up of the disease, you should
    A. Make sure the person exercises more often
    B. Position the person in good alignment
    C. Encourage the person to rest in bed as much as possible
    D. Instruct the person to avoid any type of exercise that affects the joints
33. When caring for a person who has had a total hip replacement, it is correct to
    A. Have a high, firm chair for the person to use when out of bed
    B. Remove the abductor splint or pillow when turning the person in bed
    C. Remind the person to cross his or her legs when sitting in a chair
    D. Instruct the person that he or she should only use a bedpan for elimination

34. Which of these will help strengthen bones in a person at risk for osteoporosis?
    A. Bedrest
    B. Decreased calcium intake
    C. Exercise of weight-bearing joints
    D. Increased alcohol and caffeine intake
35. When a closed reduction and external fixation is done following a fracture
    A. The bone is moved back into place and is not exposed
    B. Surgery is used to expose the bone and move it into alignment
    C. Pins, screws, or wires are attached to keep the bones in place
    D. A cast is applied without moving the bone ends into alignment
36. When a person has a newly applied plaster cast, it will dry in
    A. 2 to 4 hours
    B. 3 to 4 days
    C. 24 to 48 hours
    D. 12 to 24 hours
37. You can prevent flat spots on a cast by
    A. Positioning the cast on a hard, flat surface
    B. Supporting the entire cast with pillows
    C. Using your fingertips to lift the cast
    D. Covering the cast with a blanket
38. If a person complains of numbness in a part that is in a cast, you should
    A. Tell the person to move the limb a little to relieve the numbness
    B. Re-position the person to help the numbness
    C. Gently rub the exposed toes or fingers
    D. Tell the nurse at once
39. When giving care to a person in traction, you should
    A. Put bottom linens on the bed from the top down
    B. Remove the weights while you are giving care
    C. Turn the person from side to side to change the bed and to give care
    D. Assist the person to use the commode chair when needed
40. When caring for a person who has had surgery to repair a hip fracture, the operated leg should be
    A. Abducted at all times
    B. Adducted at all times
    C. Exercised with range-of-motion exercises every 4 hours
    D. Positioned to keep the leg in external rotation
41. When you assist a person to get up in a chair after hip surgery
    A. Place the chair on the affected side
    B. Place the chair on the unaffected side
    C. Have a low, soft chair for the person to use
    D. Remind the person to cross the legs

42. If a person complains of pain in the amputated part
    A. Report this to the nurse at once
    B. Assume that the person is confused or disoriented
    C. Reassure the person that this is a normal reaction
    D. Tell the person that this a temporary sensation that will go away shortly

FILL IN THE BLANKS

43. Write out the meaning of each abbreviation.
    A. ADL _____
    B. AKA _____
    C. ALS _____
    D. BKA _____
    E. CVA _____
    F. MS _____
    G. RA _____
    H. ROM _____
    I. TBI _____
    J. TIA _____
44. What risk factors for stroke cannot be controlled?
    A. _____
    B. _____
    C. _____
    D. _____
45. What are the warning signs of stroke?
    A. _____
    B. _____
    C. _____
    D. _____
    E. _____
46. What are signs and symptoms of Parkinson's disease?
    A. _____
    B. _____
    C. _____
    D. _____
    E. _____

47. Which type of multiple sclerosis causes the person's condition to gradually decline with more and more symptoms and no remissions?

_____

48. What effect does amyotrophic lateral sclerosis have on

    A. Mind, intelligence, and memory

    _____

    B. Senses _____

    C. Bowel and bladder functions

    _____

    D. Motor nerve cells

    _____

49. If a person survives traumatic brain injury,

    some _____. Disabilities

    depend on the _____ and

    _____ of the injury.

50. When caring for a person with paralysis, you must check the person often if he or she is unable to use

    _____.

51. Range-of-motion exercises are important when caring for a person with paralysis because they will

    maintain _____ and prevent

    _____.

52. Raising the head of the bed 45 degrees or more for a person with a spinal cord injury may relieve signs and symptoms of _____.

53. If you are caring for a person with osteoarthritis, exercise is important because it

    A. Decreases _____

    B. Increases _____

    C. Improves _____

    D. Also helps with _____

       and promotes _____

54. Rest and joint care are also used to treat osteoarthritis. Explain how these treatments help.

    A. Regular rest _____

    B. Canes and walkers _____

    C. Splints _____

55. Which type of arthritis generally develops between the ages of 20 and 50? _____

56. What are the treatment goals for rheumatoid arthritis?

    A. _____

    B. _____

    C. _____

    D. _____

57. When caring for a person who has had a hip replacement, what measures are used to protect the hip?

    A. _____

    B. _____

    C. _____

    D. _____

    E. _____

    F. _____

    G. _____

    H. _____

58. List how these risk factors affect developing osteoporosis.

    A. Women's risk increases after _____

    B. Family _____

    C. Weight _____

59. Calcium is lost from bone if it does not

    _____. What happens to the

    bone when calcium is lost? _____

    _____

60. What joints are exercised to help prevent

    osteoporosis? _____ What

    exercises are often used on these joints? _____

    _____

61. When a person has a cast on a fracture, what do these symptoms mean?

    A. Pain _____

    B. Odor _____

    C. Numbness _____

    D. Cool skin _____

    E. Hot skin _____

62. When caring for a person in traction, what would you do in these situations?

    A. Weights are touching the floor _____

    _____

    B. Rope is frayed _____

    _____

    C. Perform ROM exercises on _____

    _____

    D. Usual position allowed _____

    _____

    E. Redness, drainage, and odor noted at pin site

    _____

    F. Person complains of numbness _____

    _____

63. After hip surgery, what positions of the hip are avoided?

    A. _____

    B. _____

    C. _____

    D. _____

64. When turning and positioning a person after hip surgery, usually the person is not positioned on

    _____.

65. If the person has an internal fixation device, the operative leg is not elevated when sitting in a chair

    because _____.

66. _____ is a common cause of vascular changes that can lead to an amputation.

OPTIONAL LEARNING EXERCISES

You are caring for Mrs. Huber, who has had a stroke. Questions 67 to 71 relate to Mrs. Huber and her care. Explain the reasons why the care plan gives each of the following instructions.

67. Position Mrs. Huber in a side-lying position.

    _____

68. Approach Mrs. Huber from the unaffected side.

    _____

69. Give Mrs. Huber a dysphagia diet. _____

    _____

70. Apply elastic stockings as part of her care. _____

    _____

71. Perform range-of-motion exercises. _____

    _____

72. List the ages when the following diseases are most likely to occur.

    A. Parkinson's disease _____

    _____

    B. Multiple sclerosis _____

    _____

    C. Amyotrophic lateral sclerosis _____

    _____

You are caring for 2 persons who have arthritis. Read the information about each of them and answer Questions 73 to 75 about these 2 persons.

- *Mr. Miller is 78 years old. He worked in construction for many years and did heavy physical work. He complains about pain in his hips and right knee. His fingers are deformed by arthritis and interfere with good range of motion.*

- *Mrs. Haxton is 40 years old. She has swelling, warmth, and tenderness in her wrists, several finger joints on both hands, and both knees. She tells you that she has had arthritis for about 10 years and it "comes and goes." At present, Mrs. Haxton has a temperature of 100.2°F and she states that she is tired and does not feel well.*

73. Which type of arthritis does Mr. Miller probably

    have? _____ At what time of day is he likely to have more joint stiffness?

    _____

74. Mrs. Haxton most likely has _____ arthritis. She complains of not feeling well because the arthritis affects _____ as well as the joints.

75. It is cold and raining today. Which of these persons is more likely to be affected by the weather?

    _____

INDEPENDENT LEARNING EXERCISES

- Many people have had a fracture at some time. If you have had a broken bone, answer these questions about your experience.
  - When did you know the bone was broken? Immediately? Several hours or days later? How did you find out?
  - What signs and symptoms did you have? Describe these signs and symptoms.
  - What treatment was done? Cast? Surgery? Pins, plates, screws, or traction? Describe the treatment and how you felt about it.
  - How did the fracture affect your day-to-day life? Work? School? Leisure activities?
  - What changes were needed for you to carry out ADL? How much help did you need from others? How did the need for help make you feel?
  - How was your mobility affected? Walking? Getting out of bed or out of a chair? Driving?
  - What discomfort did you have during the healing process? With the cast or surgical site?
  - What permanent or long-term problems happened? Periodic pain? Limited mobility?
- Try this experiment to have a "fractured leg." It will help you understand how a fracture interferes with normal activities. Make an immobilizer for your leg. Use one of the methods suggested or devise one of your own.
  - Find 4 pieces of sturdy cardboard that are long enough to reach from the ankle to mid-thigh. Place them on the front, back, and sides of the leg and secure them with elastic bandages or cloth strips. You should not be able to bend the knee.
  - Use several layers of newspaper or magazines and wrap them around the leg from the ankle to above the knee. Secure them with elastic bandages or cloth strips. You should not be able to bend the knee.
- After the "cast" is in place, leave it on for 1 to 2 hours and go about your normal routine. Answer these questions about the experience.
  - How much did the cast interfere with your routine?
  - How did the cast affect ADL? Driving? Walking?
  - What other problems did you have with the cast?
  - How did you feel when you were in the cast? Awkward? Embarrassed?
  - How do you think this short experience may help you when you care for a person with a cast?
- Try this experiment to understand how osteoporosis affects bone.
  - Fold a piece of standard 8½ x 11-inch paper in half length-wise 3 times. (It will now be about 1 inch x 11 inches). Try to tear it in half along the fold and along the 1-inch edge.
  - What happens? Unfold the paper once (it will be 2 inches x 11 inches) and cut pieces out along all of the edges. This step will make the paper porous, much like the bone becomes with osteoporosis.
  - Refold the paper to the 1 x 11-inch size and try to tear it again. What happens now?

35 CARDIOVASCULAR AND RESPIRATORY DISORDERS

FILL IN THE BLANKS: KEY TERMS

High blood pressure
Hypertension
Pre-hypertension

1. When the systolic pressure is 140 mm Hg or higher or the diastolic pressure is 90 mm Hg or higher, it is _____.

2. _____ is another name for hypertension.

3. _____ is when the systolic pressure is between 120 and 139 mm Hg or the diastolic pressure is between 80 and 89 mm Hg.

CIRCLE THE BEST ANSWER

4. The leading cause of death in the United States is
   A. Cardiovascular and respiratory disorders
   B. Cancer
   C. Strokes
   D. Accidents
5. Hypertension (high blood pressure) would be indicated by a reading of
   A. 120/70 mm Hg
   B. 100/60 mm Hg
   C. 140/90 mm Hg
   D. 130/60 mm Hg
6. A risk factor for hypertension that cannot change is
   A. Stress
   B. Being over-weight
   C. Age
   D. Lack of exercise
7. The most common cause of coronary artery disease is
   A. Lack of exercise
   B. Atherosclerosis
   C. Family history
   D. Stress
8. When a person has angina pectoris, the chest pain occurs when
   A. Oxygen does not reach the lungs
   B. The heart needs more oxygen
   C. The blood pressure is too high
   D. Heart muscle dies
9. If a person has angina pain, it usually will be relieved by
   A. Resting for 3 to 15 minutes
   B. Taking narcotic medications
   C. Using oxygen therapy
   D. Getting up and walking for exercise

10. If a person takes a nitroglycerin tablet for angina, you should
    A. Give them a large glass of water to swallow the pill
    B. Take the pills back to the nurses' station
    C. Make sure the person tells the nurse that a pill was taken
    D. Encourage the person to walk around the room
11. When a myocardial infarction occurs, it means that
    A. A part of the heart muscle dies
    B. The heart muscle is not receiving enough oxygen
    C. Pain can be relieved by rest
    D. Blood backs up into the lungs
12. If a person complains of pain or numbness in the back, neck, jaw, or stomach, you should tell the nurse at once because the person
    A. Is having an angina attack
    B. May be having a stroke
    C. May be having a myocardial infarction
    D. Has symptoms of COPD
13. When heart failure occurs, you may assist in the person's care by
    A. Encouraging increased exercise
    B. Promoting a diet high in sodium
    C. Assisting with self-care activities
    D. Giving the person plenty of fluids
14. An older person with heart failure is at risk for
    A. Contractures
    B. Skin breakdown
    C. Fractures
    D. Urinary tract infections
15. The most common risk factor for chronic obstructive pulmonary disease (COPD) is
    A. Family history
    B. Respiratory infections
    C. Cigarette smoking
    D. Exercise
16. When caring for a person who has COPD, you should
    A. Make sure the person has increased activity
    B. Encourage the person to sleep or rest in the supine position
    C. Encourage the person to stop smoking and to avoid second-hand smoke
    D. Complete all ADL for the person

17. If a person has chronic bronchitis, one of the first symptoms is
    A. Wheezing and tightening in the chest
    B. Shortness of breath on exertion
    C. A smoker's cough in the morning
    D. A high temperature for several days
18. When a person has an asthma attack, it is treated with
    A. Medications, including inhalers
    B. Oxygen therapy
    C. Cold air
    D. Increased fluid intake
19. If an older person has influenza, he or she may
    A. Have a very high body temperature
    B. Have an increased appetite
    C. Feel more energy than usual
    D. Not have signs and symptoms usually seen in influenza
20. Which of these symptoms is more likely to be from a cold rather than the flu?
    A. Sinus congestion (stuffy nose)
    B. High fever (100°F to 102°F)
    C. Fatigue for 2 to 3 weeks
    D. Bronchitis or pneumonia
21. When a person has pneumonia, fluid intake is increased because of fever and to
    A. Decrease the amount of bacteria in the lungs
    B. Dilute medication given to treat the disease
    C. Thin secretions
    D. Decrease inflammation of the breathing passages
22. Breathing is easier for a person with pneumonia when the person is positioned in
    A. Semi-Fowler's position
    B. Side-lying position
    C. Supine position
    D. A soft chair
23. When you care for a person with tuberculosis (TB), you should
    A. Use Standard Precautions and isolation precautions when caring for the person
    B. Avoid the person when possible
    C. Ask the facility to provide you with medication to prevent contracting TB
    D. Increase the person's fluid intake

FILL IN THE BLANKS

24. Write out the meaning of each abbreviation.
    A. CAD _____
    B. CDC _____
    C. CO_2 _____
    D. COPD _____
    E. MI _____
    F. mm Hg _____
    G. O_2 _____
    H. TB _____
25. What risk factors that you cannot change increase blood pressure?
    A. _____
    B. _____
    C. _____
    D. _____
26. The most common cause of coronary artery disease (CAD) is _____. When this occurs, _____ collects on the _____.
27. What activities or other factors can cause angina?
    A. _____
    B. _____
    C. _____
    D. _____
    E. _____
    F. _____
28. Where is nitroglycerin (tablets or spray) kept?
    _____
29. Signs and symptoms of a myocardial infarction may be chest pain that is
    A. _____
    B. _____
    C. _____
    D. _____
30. The goals of cardiac rehabilitation after a myocardial infarction are
    A. _____
    B. _____
    C. _____
31. When left-sided heart failure occurs, blood backs up into _____. What effect does this have on these areas and features of the body?
    A. Brain _____
    B. Kidneys _____

C. Skin _____

D. Blood pressure _____

32. When the person has right-sided heart failure, what happens to these areas?

   A. Feet and ankles _____

   B. Liver _____

   C. Abdomen _____

33. Older persons with heart failure are at risk for skin breakdown because of

   A. _____

   B. _____

   C. _____

34. How can you help prevent skin breakdown in

   older persons with heart failure? _____

   _____

35. What changes occur in the lungs when a person has chronic obstructive pulmonary disease (COPD)?

   A. _____

   B. _____

   C. _____

   D. _____

36. If a person has chronic bronchitis, the person must

   stop _____.

37. A common complication of influenza is _____

   _____.

38. If an older person has pneumonia, typical signs

   and symptoms may be masked by _____

   and other _____.

39. What signs and symptoms may be present if a person has active tuberculosis (TB)?

   A. _____

   B. _____

   C. _____

   D. _____

   E. _____

   F. _____

   G. _____

   H. _____

40. Why does TB sometimes become active as a person

   ages? _____

MATCHING

Match the symptom listed with disorders of coronary artery disease.

   A. Angina
   B. Myocardial infarction
   C. Heart failure

41. _____ Chest pain occurs with exertion

42. _____ Blood flow to the heart is suddenly blocked

43. _____ Blood backs up into the venous system

44. _____ Fluid occurs in the lungs

45. _____ Rest and nitroglycerin often relieve the symptoms

46. _____ Pain is described as crushing, stabbing, or squeezing

Match the form of chronic obstructive pulmonary disorder (COPD) with the related symptom.

   A. Chronic bronchitis
   B. Emphysema
   C. Asthma

47. _____ Person develops a barrel chest

48. _____ Mucus and inflamed breathing passages obstruct airflow

49. _____ Alveoli become less elastic

50. _____ Air passages narrow

51. _____ First symptom is often a smoker's cough in the morning

52. _____ Normal O_2 and CO_2 exchange cannot occur in affected alveoli

53. _____ Allergies and air pollutants are common triggers

OPTIONAL LEARNING EXERCISES

54. Why is hypertension called "the silent killer?"

   _____

55. When a person has CAD, what life-style changes are needed?

   A. Quit _____

   B. Increase regular _____

   D. Reduce _____

   E. Healthy diet to reduce _____,

   _____, and

   _____

   F. If overweight, _____

INDEPENDENT LEARNING ACTIVITIES

- If possible, visit a cardiac rehabilitation center. Observe and ask the staff the following questions.
  - What exercises are included for a person recovering from an MI? Cardiac surgery?
  - How is the person monitored while exercising?
  - How long does the person need to continue the program?
  - How often does the person come to the rehabilitation center? How much time is spent on each visit?
- Get permission from the staff to ask the following questions of one of the persons exercising.
  - What condition do you have that needed this program?
  - When did your rehabilitation begin after your diagnosis?
  - How long will you need to continue the rehabilitation program?
  - What benefits do you feel you are getting from the program?
  - What exercise will you continue after the rehabilitation program is completed?
  - What other life-style changes have you made?

36 DIGESTIVE AND ENDOCRINE DISORDERS

FILL IN THE BLANKS: KEY TERMS

Emesis   Hyperglycemia   Jaundice
Heartburn   Hypoglycemia   Vomitus

1. High sugar in the blood is _____.

2. _____ is when food and fluids are expelled from the stomach through the mouth.

3. Low sugar in the blood is _____.

4. Another word for vomitus is _____.

5. _____ is yellowish color of the skin or whites of the eyes.

6. A burning sensation in the chest and sometimes the throat is _____.

CIRCLE THE BEST ANSWER

7. A risk factor for gastro-esophageal reflux disease (GERD) is
   A. Eating small, frequent meals
   B. Lying down after eating a large meal
   C. Maintaining normal weight
   D. Respiratory illnesses

8. If you are caring for a person with GERD, the person may be
   A. Encouraged to eat large meals 2 or 3 times a day
   B. Instructed not to lay down for 3 hours after eating
   C. Told to sleep in a bed with no pillow
   D. Told to drink a glass of wine at bedtime

9. Vomiting can be life-threatening when it
   A. Is caused by an infection
   B. Is aspirated and obstructs an airway
   C. Contains undigested food
   D. Has a bitter taste

10. If vomitus looks like coffee grounds, you should report this to the nurse at once because
    A. It signals bleeding
    B. The person may need a diet change
    C. This indicates an infection
    D. The person may need pain medication

11. Diverticular disease may occur because of
    A. A high-fiber diet
    B. Regular bowel movements
    C. Aging
    D. Infections

12. Gallstones are
    A. Needed for digestion of fats
    B. Formed in the small intestine
    C. Formed when bile hardens into stone-like pieces
    D. Passed easily through the kidneys

13. A symptom of gallstones is
    A. Pain radiating down one or both arms
    B. Diarrhea
    C. Constipation
    D. Pain located between the shoulder blades

14. When hepatitis is contracted by eating or drinking food or water contaminated by feces, it is
    A. Hepatitis A
    B. Hepatitis B
    C. Hepatitis C
    D. Hepatitis D

15. When caring for a person with cirrhosis, itching may be decreased by
    A. Using very hot water when bathing
    B. Using warm water and baking soda for bathing
    C. Reminding the person not to scratch the skin
    D. Increasing fluid intake

16. An obese 50-year-old woman with hypertension is diagnosed with diabetes. She most likely has
    A. Type 1
    B. Type 2
    C. Gestational
    D. None of the above

17. A diabetic complains of thirst and frequent urination. You notice the person has a flushed face and slow, deep respirations. You know these are signs and symptoms of
    A. Hyperglycemia
    B. Hypoglycemia
    C. Diabetic coma
    D. An infection

MATCHING

Match the type of hepatitis with the correct statement.

  A. Hepatitis A
  B. Hepatitis B
  C. Hepatitis C
  D. Hepatitis D

18. _____ Occurs in persons infected with hepatitis B
19. _____ Occurs in international travelers (especially to developing countries)
20. _____ Caused by HBV
21. _____ Ingested when eating food or water contaminated with feces
22. _____ Person may have virus but no symptoms
23. _____ Serious liver damage shows up years later

Match the symptom with either hypoglycemia or hyperglycemia.

  A. Hypoglycemia
  B. Hyperglycemia

24. _____ Trembling, shakiness
25. _____ Sweet breath odor
26. _____ Tingling around the mouth
27. _____ Cold, clammy skin
28. _____ Slow, deep, and labored respirations
29. _____ Headache
30. _____ Flushed face
31. _____ Frequent urination

FILL IN THE BLANKS

32. Write out the meaning of each abbreviation.
  A. GERD _____
  B. HBV _____
  C. I&O _____
  D. IV _____

33. What life-style changes may be needed for a person with GERD?
  A. _____
  B. _____
  C. _____
  D. _____
  E. _____
  F. _____
  G. _____

34. What measures will help the person who is vomiting?
  A. Turn _____
  B. Place _____
  C. Move _____
  D. Provide _____
  E. Eliminate _____

35. The following are risk factors for diverticular disease. What is the specific risk for each of these related to the disease?
  A. Age _____
  B. Diet _____
  C. Bowel function _____

36. If a person with gallstones has jaundice, the skin and whites of the eyes will appear _____.

37. A gallbladder attack often follows a _____.

38. List the characteristics of the types of hepatitis.
  A. Hepatitis A is spread by the _____ route.
  B. Hepatitis B is present in the _____ of infected persons.
  C. Hepatitis C can be transmitted even when the person has _____.
  D. Hepatitis D occurs only in people with _____.
  E. Hepatitis E is not common in _____.

39. Cirrhosis is caused by
  A. Chronic _____ abuse
  B. Chronic _____ and _____
  C. _____ is becoming a common cause.

40. A person with _____ diabetes will be treated with healthy eating, exercise, and sometimes oral medications.

41. A person with _____ diabetes will be treated with daily insulin therapy as well as healthy diet and exercise.

OPTIONAL LEARNING EXERCISES

You are caring for several persons with diabetes. Answer Questions 42 to 47 about these persons.

Mr. Jones, a 75-year-old African-American man
Ms. Miller, a 45-year-old white, over-weight woman
Mrs. Thorpe, a 32-year-old pregnant woman
Ms. Hernandez, a 60-year-old Hispanic woman with hypertension

42. Three of these persons are most likely to have type 2 diabetes. They are

    A. _____

    B. _____

    C. _____

43. Mrs. Thorpe probably has

    _____ diabetes. She is at risk

    for developing _____ later in life.

44. Which type of diabetes develops rapidly?

    _____

45. Mrs. Hernandez has an open wound on her ankle. Why is this wound a concern? _____

    _____

46. Why is Ms. Miller instructed to decrease her food

    intake? _____

47. Mr. Jones tells you he feels shaky and dizzy and has a headache when he misses a meal.

    He probably is experiencing _____.

Edward P. has been diagnosed with cirrhosis. Answer the following questions about his disease and care.

48. Abdominal pain and bloating occur with cirrhosis

    when _____.

49. What skin changes may be observed?

    A. _____

    B. _____

50. Edward P. is likely to have dietary restrictions. These will include

    A. Healthy diet limited in _____

    B. _____ diet to reduce edema and ascites

INDEPENDENT LEARNING ACTIVITIES

- Talk with a person who has gastro-esophageal reflux disease (GERD) and ask the following questions.
  - What symptoms does the person have related to GERD?
  - What risk factors does the person have that may have caused the GERD?
  - What life-style changes has the person made since the diagnosis?
- Talk with a person who has had gallstones and ask the following questions.
  - What risk factors does the person have related to gallstone formation?
  - What signs and symptoms did the person have that helped the doctor diagnose gallstones?
  - What treatment did the person have to relieve the symptoms?
  - After treatment, what signs or symptoms have changed?
- Talk with a person with diabetes and ask the following questions.
  - What type of diabetes does the person have: type 1 or type 2?
  - How old was the person when diabetes was diagnosed?
  - What life-style changes have been made to treat the diabetes?
  - What complications of diabetes have occurred?
- Ask your instructor to help you arrange to attend a diabetic education class, if these are available at your agency. After attending, answer the following questions.
  - What are the ages of the members of the class? Were family members included in the class?
  - What information is given to the class about diet?
  - What exercise programs are recommended to the class?
  - What information is given about medications used to treat diabetes?

37 URINARY AND REPRODUCTIVE DISORDERS

FILL IN THE BLANKS: KEY TERMS

Cystocele	Hematuria	Suprapubic
Dialysis	Oliguria	Urinary diversion
Diuresis	Pyuria	Urostomy
Dysuria	Retocele	Uterine prolapse

1. Scant urine is _____.

2. Difficult or painful urination is _____.

3. A _____ is a surgically created opening between the ureter and the abdomen.

4. _____ is the process of passing urine; large amounts of urine are produced—1000 to 5000 mL a day.

5. A new pathway for urine to exit the body is a

_____.

6. Blood in the urine is _____.

7. _____ is pus in the urine.

8. _____ is the process of removing waste products from the blood.

9. An area above the pubic bone is _____.

10. _____ occurs when the bladder drops down.

11. When the uterus shifts downward into the vaginal

canal it is called _____.

12. A _____ occurs when the rectum shifts downward.

CIRCLE THE BEST ANSWER

13. Women have a higher risk of urinary tract infections because of
    A. Hormone levels in the body
    B. The short female urethra
    C. Bacteria
    D. Prostrate gland secretions

14. If a person has cystitis, the care plan will include
    A. Restricting fluid intake
    B. Assisting the person to ambulate frequently
    C. Straining the urine
    D. Encouraging the person to drink 2000 mL of fluid a day

15. If a man has benign prostatic hyperplasia (BPH), he will probably
    A. Be incontinent of urine
    B. Have frequent voiding at night
    C. Have increased urine output
    D. Have renal failure

16. After surgery to correct BPH, the care plan may include
    A. A balanced diet to prevent constipation
    B. Increased activity with an exercise plan
    C. Restricted fluid intake
    D. Care of the surgical incision

17. When caring for a person with a urinary diversion, the pouch is changed
    A. Each time the person voids
    B. Anytime it leaks
    C. Only once a week
    D. When the pouch is full

18. When caring for a person with a stoma, the nursing assistant knows
    A. The stoma does not have sensation
    B. Sterile technique is used when cleaning the area
    C. Pain medication is given before caring for the stoma
    D. The person is never allowed to help with the care

19. If you are caring for a person with renal calculi (kidney stones), your care will include
    A. Restricting fluids
    B. Keeping the person on strict bedrest
    C. Straining all urine
    D. Maintaining a strict diet

20. When you care for a person with acute renal failure, the care plan will include
    A. Increasing fluid intake to 2000 to 3000 mL per day
    B. Measuring and recording urine output every hour
    C. Making sure the person does not drink any fluids
    D. Measuring weight weekly

21. Chronic renal failure
    A. Occurs suddenly
    B. Generally improves and kidney function returns to normal within 1 year
    C. Occurs when nephrons of the kidney are destroyed over many years
    D. Has very little effect on the person's over-all health
22. If a person has chronic renal failure, which of these would be included in the care plan?
    A. A diet high in protein, potassium, and sodium
    B. Plenty of exercise
    C. Measures to prevent itching
    D. Frequent bathing with soap
23. When a person is receiving hemodialysis, you will
    A. Make sure the person drinks about 2000 mL each day
    B. Never take the blood pressure on the arm with the fistula
    C. Assist the person to ambulate several times a day
    D. Allow the person to eat whatever he or she wants to maintain weight
24. A woman with pelvic organ prolapse may be encouraged to
    A. Drink plenty of fluids
    B. Perform Kegel exercises several times a day
    C. Exercise vigorously each day
    D. Remain on complete bedrest
25. A woman who complains about frothy, thick, foul-smelling vaginal discharge most likely has
    A. Gonorrhea
    B. Genital warts
    C. Syphilis
    D. Trichomoniasis

MATCHING

Match the sexually transmitted disease with the correct statement.
    A. Herpes
    B. Genital warts
    C. Gonorrhea
    D. Chlamydia
    E. Syphilis
    F. Trichomoniasis
26. _____ Surgical removal if ointment is not effective
27. _____ Sores may have a watery discharge
28. _____ No symptoms in men, only in women
29. _____ May have vaginal bleeding
30. _____ Urinary urgency and frequency is present
31. _____ Treated with anti-viral medications
32. _____ Painless sores appear on genitals 10 to 90 days after exposure
33. _____ May not show symptoms

FILL IN THE BLANKS

34. Write out the meaning of the abbreviations.
    A. AIDS _____
    B. BPH _____
    C. HIV _____
    D. mL _____
    E. STD _____
    F. UTI _____
35. Why are older persons at high risk for urinary tract infections?
    A. _____
    B. _____
    C. _____
    D. _____
36. After a transurethral resection of the prostate (TURP), the person's care plan may include
    A. _____
    B. _____
    C. _____
    D. _____
    E. _____
37. When you care for a person with a urinary diversion, you should follow_____ for safety.
38. What are the risk factors for developing renal calculi?
    A. Age, race, sex _____
    B. _____
    C. _____
    D. _____
39. A person with renal calculi needs to drink 2000 to 3000 mL of fluid a day to help _____
    _____.
40. When acute renal failure occurs, there are 2 phases. Name and explain each phase.
    A. At first, _____ occurs.
       Urine output is _____.
       This phase lasts _____.
    B. Then _____ occurs.
       Urine output is _____.
       This phase lasts _____.

41. When caring for a person with acute renal failure, report to the nurse at once if the person has

_____.

42. Signs and symptoms of chronic renal failure appear when _____ is lost.

43. You may need to assist a person in chronic renal failure with nutritional needs. List what the care plan is likely to include for the following.

    A. Diet _____

    B. Fluids _____

44. Sexually transmitted diseases are transmitted by

_____.

45. Using _____ can help prevent the spread of STDs.

46. When caring for a person with an STD, you should

    follow _____

    and _____.

OPTIONAL LEARNING EXERCISES

You give home care to Mrs. Eunice Weber twice a week. She is 92 years old and lives alone. She has severe osteoporosis and uses a walker to move about in her home. She receives Meals on Wheels and spends most of the day sitting on the sofa. She has periods of incontinence or dribbling because of poor bladder control. When you arrive to care for her, she tells you she is not feeling well. She tells you it burns when she urinates, and when she needs to urinate, the urge comes on suddenly and she often does not get to the toilet in time. Answer the following questions about Mrs. Weber.

47. You should tell the _____ because these symptoms may mean Mrs. Weber

    has _____.

48. What is the urge to void called?

_____

49. How does Mrs. Weber's immobility affect the following?

    A. Fluid intake _____

    B. Perineal care _____

50. The doctor will probably order _____ to treat the condition.

51. The care plan will probably include "Encourage

    fluids to _____ per day."

Two weeks later you notice that Mrs. Weber has chills. When you take her temperature, it is 102°F. She tells you she has been vomiting since yesterday. You observe her urine and see that it is very cloudy.

52. You report these symptoms to the nurse because it can indicate that Mrs. Weber now has

    _____. This means the

    infection has moved from the _____

    to the _____.

INDEPENDENT LEARNING ACTIVITIES

- Talk with someone who has had urinary tract infections (UTIs). If you have had a UTI, answer these questions about your own experience.
  - What signs and symptoms were present?
  - How many UTIs have occurred?
  - What risk factors may have placed the person (or you) at risk for developing UTIs?
  - What treatment was used to treat the UTI?
  - What life-style changes were recommended to prevent a recurrence of the UTI?
- Talk with someone who has had renal calculi and ask the following questions.
  - What signs and symptoms were present?
  - How was the problem treated?
  - What dietary changes have been prescribed to prevent future attacks?

38 MENTAL HEALTH DISORDERS

FILL IN THE BLANKS: KEY TERMS

Affect
Anxiety
Compulsion
Defense mechanism
Delusion
Delusion of grandeur
Delusion of persecution
Emotional illness
Flashback

Hallucination
Mental
Mental disorder
Mental health
Mental illness
Obsession
Panic
Paranoia
Phobia

Psychiatric disorder
Psychosis
Stress
Stressor
Suicide
Suicide contagion
Withdrawal syndrome

1. Exposure to suicide or suicidal behaviors within one's family, one's peer group, or media reports of suicide is _____.

2. _____ is reliving a trauma in thoughts during the day and in nightmares during sleep.

3. When a person has an exaggerated belief about one's own importance, wealth, power, or talents, it is called _____.

4. A mental disorder, emotional disorder, or psychiatric disorder is also called a _____.

5. A _____ is any emotional, physical, social, or economic factor that causes stress.

6. The person's physical and mental response after stopping or severely reducing the intake of a substance that was used regularly is _____.

7. _____ means relating to the mind. It is something that exists in the mind or is performed by the mind.

8. A recurrent, unwanted thought, idea, or image is an _____.

9. The response or change in the body caused by any emotional, physical, social, or economic factor is _____.

10. _____ is a vague, uneasy feeling that occurs in response to stress.

11. _____ is another name for mental illness, mental disorder, or psychiatric disorder.

12. A _____ is an intense fear.

13. A false belief is a _____.

14. _____ is a disturbance in the ability to cope or adjust to stress; behavior and functioning are impaired. This condition is also called a mental disorder, emotional illness, or psychiatric disorder.

15. A state of severe mental impairment is _____.

16. A _____ is seeing, hearing, or feeling something that is not real.

17. _____ is a disorder of the mind. The person has false beliefs and suspicion about a person or situation.

18. Repeating an act over and over again is a _____.

19. _____ is when the person copes with and adjusts to the stresses of every-day living in ways accepted by society.

20. _____ is a false belief that one is being mistreated, abused, or harassed.

21. An intense and sudden feeling of fear, anxiety, terror, or dread is _____.

22. _____ is another name for mental illness, mental disorder, or emotional disorder.

23. A _____ is an unconscious reaction that blocks unpleasant or threatening feelings.

24. To kill oneself is _____.

25. Feelings and emotions are _____.

CIRCLE THE BEST ANSWER

26. Which of these statements about anxiety is *true*?
    A. Anxiety often occurs when needs are not met.
    B. Anxiety is always abnormal.
    C. The body does not respond to anxiety with physical symptoms.
    D. The level of anxiety is the same regardless of the cause.

27. An unhealthy coping mechanism would be
    A. Talking about the problem
    B. Playing music
    C. Smoking
    D. Exercising

28. Panic is
    A. The highest level of anxiety
    B. A disorder that occurs gradually
    C. A psychosis
    D. Vague, normal response to stress

29. When a person with obsessive-compulsive disorder is unable to perform his or her ritual (compulsion), the person
    A. Will become less anxious
    B. Will gradually forget about performing the ritual
    C. Will have more anxiety
    D. Will learn to use good coping mechanisms

30. Flashbacks occur in persons with
    A. Panic attacks
    B. Post-traumatic stress disorder (PTSD)
    C. Schizophrenia
    D. Depression

31. A person you are caring for tells you he is the president of the United States. He has a delusion of grandeur, which is a part of
    A. Obsessive-compulsive disorder
    B. Phobias
    C. Bipolar disorders
    D. Schizophrenia

32. During a manic phase, a person with bipolar disorder may
    A. Be sad, anxious, or have an empty mood
    B. Complain of chronic pain not caused by physical illness or injury
    C. Have an unrealistic belief in his or her abilities and powers
    D. Startle easily

33. A major risk of a depressive episode is that the person
    A. Is very sad
    B. May attempt suicide
    C. Has depressed body functions
    D. Cannot concentrate

34. If an older person is depressed, it may be wrongly diagnosed as a
    A. Cognitive disorder
    B. Physical problem
    C. Hormonal change
    D. Side effect of medications

35. A person with an antisocial personality disorder may
    A. Be suspicious and distrust others
    B. Have violent behavior
    C. See, hear, or feel something that is not real
    D. Blame others for actions and behaviors

36. An adult is considered an alcoholic if
    A. He or she enjoys a glass of wine with dinner
    B. He or she becomes "high" or drunk after 1 or 2 drinks
    C. He or she cannot stop drinking once drinking has begun
    D. He or she drinks only liquor with a high alcohol content

37. Alcohol can be more dangerous for an older person because
    A. The person has been drinking for a long period of time
    B. The person eats a poor diet
    C. Older people tend to take more medications that may be harmful when taken with alcohol
    D. The person is more likely to lie about alcohol intake than a young person

38. When a person is addicted to medications or drugs, he or she
    A. Takes the medication only as prescribed
    B. Takes smaller and smaller amounts to get the same effect
    C. Is only taking illegal drugs
    D. Continues to use the substance even when he or she knows it makes a situation worse

39. If a resident you are caring for tells you he has thoughts of suicide, you should
    A. Promise him you will not tell anyone
    B. Ignore him, as he often says this and nothing has happened before
    C. Tell the nurse at once
    D. Report this conversation when you give a report at the end of the shift

FILL IN THE BLANKS

40. Write out the meaning of each abbreviation.

    A. BPD _____

    B. NIAAA _____

    C. NIMH _____

    D. OCD _____

    E. PTSD _____

41. What are causes of mental health disorders?

    A. _____

    B. _____

    C. _____

    D. _____

    E. _____

    F. _____

    G. _____

42. Name the defense mechanism being used in the following situations.

    A. A girl fails a test. She blames another girl for not helping her study. _____

    B. A man does not like his boss. He buys the boss an expensive Christmas present.

    _____

    C. A girl complains of a stomach ache so she will

    not have to read aloud. _____

    D. A child is angry with his teacher. He hits his

    brother. _____

    E. A woman misses work frequently and is often late. She gets a bad job evaluation. She says that

    the boss does not like her. _____

43. When a person is having a panic attack, what changes would you expect to find when assessing the vital signs?

    A. Pulse _____

    B. Respirations _____

    C. Blood pressure _____

44. If a person has an intense fear of being in an open, crowded, or public place, this is called

    _____.

45. After a terrifying ordeal, a person may develop

    _____. Signs and symptoms of this disorder usually develop about _____ after the harmful event.

46. Below are examples of problems that occur with schizophrenia. Name each one.

    A. A man believes his neighbor is poisoning his

    water. _____

    B. A woman says that voices told her to set fire to

    her apartment. _____

    C. A man believes he can fly like a bird.

    _____

    D. A woman tells you she owns 3 BMW cars and is

    the president of MacDonald's. _____

    _____

47. What disorders of movement may occur when a person has schizophrenia?

    A. _____

    B. _____

    C. _____

    D. _____

    E. _____

48. The following are signs and symptoms of bipolar disorder. Name the episode (mania or depression) for each sign or symptom listed.

    A. Extreme irritability _____

    B. Thoughts of death or suicide _____

    C. Denial that anything is wrong _____

    D. Loss of interest in sex _____

    E. Jumping from one idea to another

    _____

    F. Feelings of guilt, worthlessness, or helplessness

    _____

    G. Unrealistic beliefs in one's abilities or powers

    _____

49. What losses in older persons may cause depression?

    A. _____

    B. _____

    C. _____

    D. _____

50. A person with antisocial personality disorder will display thinking and behaviors that show no

    regard for _____.

51. A person who greatly admires and loves family members and friends but suddenly shifts to intense

    anger and dislike may have a _____

    _____.

52. Describe the following symptoms of alcoholism.

    A. Craving _____

    B. Loss of control _____

    C. Physical dependence _____

    D. Tolerance _____

53. According to the NIAAA, a person needs help for alcohol abuse if he or she has the following problems.

    A. _____

    B. _____

    C. _____

    D. _____

    E. _____

    F. _____

    G. _____

    H. _____

    I. _____

    J. _____

54. When the person is in withdrawal from an addictive substance, what signs and symptoms occur?

    A. _____

    B. _____

    C. _____

    D. _____

    E. _____

    F. _____

55. It is important to identify depression in elderly men because the highest rate of suicide is among

    _____.

56. When interacting with persons with mental disorders, you should:

    A. _____

    B. _____

    C. _____

    D. _____

    E. _____

    F. _____

57. When a person has mental health disorders, quality of life must be met. Which right is being protected in each of these examples?

    A. All harmful items are removed from the

       person's setting. _____

    B. When the person says or does something, you share it only with the nurse.

       _____

    C. The person is given very simple choices so that

       he or she still feels in control. _____

       _____

    D. You report bruises or other signs that the

       person is not well cared for. _____

       _____

OPTIONAL LEARNING EXERCISES

58. Mr. Johnson is very worried about his surgery tomorrow. You notice that he is talking very fast and is sweating. You give him directions to collect a urine specimen. Five minutes later, he turns on his call light to ask you to repeat the directions. He tells you he is using the toilet "all the time" because he has diarrhea and frequent urination. The nurse says that all of these things are signs and symptoms of

_____.

59. You are assigned to care for Mrs. Grand, a new resident. She is getting ready to go to the dining room. You assist her to get dressed and she tells you she wants to wash her hands before going to the dining room. She goes to the bathroom and washes her hands for several minutes. As she leaves the room, she stops to turn off the light. Then she tells you she must wash her hands again. She repeats washing her hands and turning the lights on and off 4 or 5 times. You report this to the nurse, who tells you Mrs. Grand has _____

_____.

INDEPENDENT LEARNING ACTIVITIES

- Try this experiment with a group of classmates. Make labels with various roles for "staff members" and "mentally ill persons." A list is provided but you may add or subtract according to the size of your group. Make sure the group includes a mix of people with mental health diseases and staff or visitors.

Doctor	A person with bipolar disorder
Nurse	A person with delusions of grandeur
Visitor	A person with obsessive-compulsive disorder
Nursing assistant	A person with schizophrenia with paranoia
Recreational therapist	A person with hallucinations
Dietitian	A person with anorexia nervosa

Attach a label to each person so that he or she cannot read it. (It may be placed on the back or the forehead.) Have everyone move about the group and talk to each other based on how the person thinks he or she should approach the person with a certain "label." Continue the experiment for about 15 minutes and then use the following questions to guide a group discussion.
- How did you feel talking to a person with a mental health disorder?
- How were the people with a mental health disorder approached? How quickly were the "mentally ill persons" able to sense that this was their label? What cues did they receive from others?
- How quickly did "staff members" recognize the label they had? What cues did they receive from others?

- In what ways did the approach of others cause people to respond in a way that was expected? Did the people with mental health disorders show signs of the illness based on the reaction of others?
- What did the group learn about approaching a person with a mental health disorder?
- Consider this situation and answer the following questions concerning how you would feel about caring for a person with a mental health disorder.
  Situation: Marion Cross, age 65, is a patient in an acute care hospital with a diagnosis of pneumonia. The nurse tells you Mrs. Cross has a history of schizophrenia. You are assigned to provide AM care for Mrs. Cross.
  - How would you approach Mrs. Cross when you enter her room? How would your knowledge about her mental health disorder affect your initial contact with her?
  - What would you do if Mrs. Cross told you she sees an elephant in the room? What would you say to her?
  - How would you react if Mrs. Cross told you that she owns Disney World and goes there free anytime she wants? How would you respond?
  - How would you provide good oral hygiene if Mrs. Cross refuses to cooperate because she is sure the staff is trying to poison her? What could you try that might be helpful?
  - What would you do if Mrs. Cross curls up in a tight ball and refuses to talk or cooperate during AM care? What could you do to maintain her hygiene?
  - How would you feel about caring for a person with abnormal behavior? Why?

39 CONFUSION AND DEMENTIA

FILL IN THE BLANKS: KEY TERMS

Cognitive function   Dementia   Paranoia
Delirium   Elopement   Pseudodementia
Delusion   Hallucination   Sundowning

1. When the person has false beliefs and suspicions about a person or situation, it is called

   _____.

2. A false belief is a _____.

3. Seeing, hearing, or feeling something that is not

   real is _____.

4. Increased signs, symptoms, and behaviors of AD

   during hours of darkness is _____.

5. _____ is a state of temporary but acute mental confusion that comes on suddenly.

6. The loss of cognitive function and social function caused by changes in the brain is

   _____.

7. _____ is a false disorder of the mind.

8. _____ involves memory, thinking, reasoning, ability to understand, judgment, and behavior.

9. When a person leaves the center without staff

   knowledge, it is _____.

CIRCLE THE BEST ANSWER

10. Confusion caused by physical changes
    A. Occurs suddenly
    B. Cannot be cured
    C. Is cured by aiming treatment at the cause
    D. Is usually temporary

11. When a person is confused, it is helpful if you
    A. Repeat the date and time as often as needed
    B. Change the routine each day to stimulate the person
    C. Keep the drapes pulled during the day
    D. Give complex answers to questions

12. Hearing and vision decrease with confusion, so you should
    A. Speak in a loud voice
    B. Write out directions for the person
    C. Face the person and speak clearly
    D. Keep the lighting dim in the room

13. Dementia
    A. Is a normal part of aging
    B. Causes the person to have difficulty with routine personal, social, and occupational activities
    C. Is always temporary and can be cured
    D. Affects most older people

14. The most common type of permanent dementia is
    A. Alzheimer's disease
    B. Dementia
    C. Depression
    D. Delirium

15. The classic sign of Alzheimer's disease (AD) is
    A. Forgetting simple tasks
    B. Gradual loss of short-term memory
    C. Acute confusion and delirium
    D. Wandering and sundowning

16. In stage 1 of AD (mild), the person may
    A. Walk slowly with a shuffling gait
    B. Be totally incontinent
    C. Blame others for mistakes
    D. Become agitated and may be violent

17. In stage 2 of AD (moderate), the person may
    A. Have difficulty performing every-day tasks
    B. Need assistance with activities of daily living
    C. Be disoriented to time and place
    D. Have seizures

18. In stage 3 of AD (severe), the person may
    A. Forget recent events
    B. Lose impulse control and use foul language or have poor table manners
    C. Be less interested in things or be less outgoing
    D. Be disoriented to person, time, and place

19. When a person wanders, the major concern is
    A. The person's comfort
    B. The person is at risk for life-threatening accidents
    C. Inconvenience for the family or facility
    D. Making sure the person gets enough rest and sleep

20. When sundowning occurs, it may be related to
    A. Being tired or hungry
    B. Having poor judgment
    C. Impaired vision or hearing
    D. The person looking for something or someone
21. When you are caring for a person with paranoia and the person accuses you of stealing an item, you should
    A. Argue with the person and say you are not a thief
    B. Help the person search for the item and talk about what is found
    C. Leave the room immediately and report to the nurse
    D. Refuse to care for the person as long as the item is missing
22. Too much stimuli from being asked too many questions at once can overwhelm a person and cause
    A. Delusions
    B. Catastrophic reactions
    C. Hallucinations
    D. Sundowning
23. A caregiver may cause agitation and restlessness by
    A. Calling the person by name
    B. Selecting tasks and activities specific to the person's cognitive abilities and interests
    C. Encouraging activity early in the day
    D. Making the person hurry in order to complete care quickly
24. When you are caring for a person with AD, it is helpful if you
    A. Give simple, step-by-step instructions
    B. Play loud, familiar TV programs during meals and care activities
    C. Encourage late afternoon or early evening exercise and activity
    D. Restrain a person who insists on going outside
25. If a person with AD displays sexual behaviors, the nurse may tell you to
    A. Tell the person this behavior is not acceptable
    B. Make sure the person has good hygiene to prevent itching
    C. Avoid caring for the person
    D. Ignore the behavior because the disease causes it
26. What should you do when a person repeats the same motions or repeats the same words over and over?
    A. Remind the person to stop the repeating behavior
    B. Report this to the nurse immediately
    C. Take the person for a walk or distract the person with music or picture books
    D. Isolate the person in his or her room until the repeating behavior stops

27. A person with AD is encouraged to take part in therapies and activities that
    A. Increase the level of confusion
    B. Help the person to feel useful, worthwhile, and active
    C. Will prevent aggressive behaviors
    D. Improve physical problems such as incontinence and contractures
28. How do AD special care units differ from other areas of a care facility?
    A. Complete care is provided.
    B. Entrances and exits are locked.
    C. Meals are served in the person's room.
    D. No activities are provided.
29. A person with AD no longer stays in a secured unit when
    A. The condition improves
    B. The family requests a move to another unit
    C. The person cannot sit or walk
    D. Aggressive behaviors disrupt the unit
30. A family that cares for a person with dementia at home
    A. Usually does not need any help
    B. Cannot afford to have the person cared for in a nursing facility
    C. Needs assistance from others to cope with the person
    D. Must have special training to care for the person

FILL IN THE BLANKS

31. Write out the meaning of each abbreviation.
    A. AD _____
    B. ADL _____
    C. NIA _____
32. Cognitive function involves
    A. _____
    B. _____
    C. _____
    D. _____
    E. _____
    F. _____
33. When caring for a confused person, how can you help the person know the date and time?
    A. _____
    _____
    B. _____
    _____

34. How can you help the confused person maintain the day-night cycle?

    A. _____

    B. _____

    C. _____

35. What senses decrease with changes in the nervous system from aging? _____

36. Give examples of how early warnings signs of dementia may be seen in these areas.

    A. Memory _____

    B. Doing tasks _____

    C. Language _____

    D. Judgment _____

37. What substances can cause dementia?

    _____

38. Pseudodementia can occur with _____

    and _____.

39. The most common mental health disorder in older persons is _____.

40. A person with mild cognitive impairment has problems with _____.

    These problems do not interfere with _____.

41. Alzheimer's disease (AD) damages brain cells that control these functions.

    A. _____

    B. _____

    C. _____

    D. _____

    E. _____

    F. _____

    G. _____

    H. _____

42. Which of the seven stages of AD are described in the following examples?

    A. The person cannot walk without help.

    _____

    B. The person may need help choosing correct clothes to wear. _____

    C. The person shows no signs of memory problems. _____

D. Family, friends, and others notice problems.

    _____

E. The person has problems with shopping, paying bills, and managing money.

    _____

F. The person may forget names but recognizes faces. _____

G. The person does not know where to find keys, eyeglasses, or other objects. _____

43. The *MedicAlert + Safe Return* program will help an AD person who has the behavior of _____.

44. Which behavior of AD is described in the following examples?

    A. Confusion and restlessness increase after dark.

    _____

    B. Too much stimulation may trigger this behavior.

    _____

    C. The person may use this behavior to communicate as the disease progresses.

    _____

    D. The person may walk into traffic or go out not properly dressed for the weather.

    _____

    E. The person repeats the same words or motions over and over. _____

    F. The person may have false beliefs about who he or she is or who the caregiver may be.

    _____

    G. The person may pace, hit, or yell.

    _____

    H. The person touches himself or others in a sexual way that is inappropriate.

    _____

    I. The person complains of feeling bugs crawling or seeing animals that are not there.

    _____

    J. The person hits, pinches, grabs, bites, or swears at others. _____

    K. The person hides her dentures in a wastebasket.

45. When a person has dementia or AD, what is the reason the following items may be part of the care plan?

   A. Approach the person from the front.

   _____

   B. Provide plastic eating and drinking utensils.

   _____

   C. Respond to door alarms at once.

   _____

   D. Do not argue with a person who wants to leave.

   _____

   E. Do not ask a person to tell you what is

   bothering him or her. _____

   _____

   F. Turn off TV or movies when violent or

   disturbing programs are on. _____

   _____

   G. Use night-lights so the person can see.

   _____

   H. Promote exercise and activity during the day.

   _____

   I. Have equipment ready for any procedure.

   _____

46. Validation therapy is based on these principles.

   A. _____

   B. _____

   C. _____

   D. _____

   E. _____

   F. _____

OPTIONAL LEARNING EXERCISES

You are caring for Mr. Harris, a 78-year-old who is confused. You know there are ways to help a person to be more oriented. Answer the following questions about ways to help a confused person.

47. How can you help orient Mr. Harris to who he is every time you are in contact with him?

   _____

48. What are 2 ways you can help orient Mr. Harris to time?

   A. _____

   B. _____

49. How can you help maintain the day-night cycle

   when dressing Mr. Harris? _____

   _____

You are caring for Mrs. Matthews, an 82-year-old resident. The nurse tells you she lived with her daughter for the last 2 years but the family is now concerned for her safety. She left home when the temperature was 35°F and was found 2 miles away wearing a light sweater. On another occasion, she turned on the gas stove and could not remember how to turn it off. Sometimes, she did not recognize her daughter and resisted getting a bath or changing her clothes. Since admission to the care facility, she tells everyone she must leave to go to her birthday party. Answer these questions about Mrs. Matthews and her care.

50. Why would Mrs. Matthews most likely be in a special care unit in the nursing facility?

   _____

51. What disease is it likely that Mrs. Matthew has?

   _____

52. Mrs. Matthews is probably in stage _____ of the disease. What activities would indicate she is in this stage?

   A. _____

   B. _____

   C. _____

   D. _____

   E. _____

53. How often will the health team review Mrs. Matthews's need to stay on this unit?

   _____ Why is this done?

   _____

54. The nurse may encourage Mrs. Matthews's

   daughter to join a _____

   group. How can this be helpful to the daughter?

   _____

   _____

INDEPENDENT LEARNING ACTIVITIES

- Consider the situation and answer the following questions about how you would feel.

Situation: Imagine you are in a strange country where people talk to you but you do not understand what they are saying. They use strange tools to eat and you cannot figure out how to use them. They try to feed you food you do not recognize. Sometimes these people seem friendly and caring but at other times they become angry because you are not doing what they ask you to do. You become frightened when they try to remove your clothes and take you in a room to shower you. You become frightened and upset because you do not know what will happen next. At times other strangers come to your room and bring gifts. They talk kindly to you but you do not know them. They seem upset when you do not respond to their gifts and gestures. The doors and windows in this country are all locked and you cannot find a way out so you can go home.

- How does this situation relate to the information in this chapter?
- How would you react if you were the person in this situation? Why?
- What methods might you use to try to communicate with the person in this situation?
- Why would the person want to go home? What does "home" mean to him or her?
- How will this exercise help you when you care for a person who is confused?

- Consider the situation and answer the following questions about how you would care for a person who has dementia.

Situation: You are assigned to care for Ronald Myers, age 85, who has Alzheimer's disease. He often wanders from room to room and tries to open the outside doors. He frequently becomes agitated and restless, especially in the evenings. Most of the time Mr. Myers is unable to feed himself and he is often incontinent. He keeps repeating all day: "Help me, help me."

- How do you feel about caring for a person like this? Frightened? Angry? Impatient? How do you deal with your feelings so you can give care to the person?
- At what stage of Alzheimer's disease is Mr. Myers? What signs and symptoms support your answer?
- Why would it be ineffective to remind Mr. Myers of the date and time during your shift? Why is this a good technique with some confused persons and not with others?
- Why does Mr. Myers become more agitated toward evening? What is this called?
- What methods could you use to make sure Mr. Myers receives the care needed to maintain good personal hygiene? How could you get him to cooperate or participate in his care?
- What parts of Mr. Myers behavior would be most difficult for you to tolerate? What would you do if you found yourself becoming irritated and angry with Mr. Myers?
- What information in this chapter has helped you understand persons like Mr. Myers better? How will this information help you give better care to these persons and maintain their quality of life?

40 DEVELOPMENTAL DISABILITIES

FILL IN THE BLANKS: KEY TERMS

Birth defect
Developmental disability
Diplegia

Disability
Inherited

Intellectual disability
Spastic

1. _____ involves severe limits in intellectual function and adaptive behavior occurring before age 18.

2. An abnormality present at birth that can involve a body structure or function is a _____.

3. When similar body parts are affected on both sides of the body, it is called _____.

4. The uncontrolled contractions of skeletal muscles are _____.

5. A disability that occurs before 22 years of age is _____.

6. A _____ is any lost, absent, or impaired physical or mental function.

7. That which is passed down from parents to children is _____.

CIRCLE THE BEST ANSWER

8. A developmental disability (DD)
   A. Always occurs at birth
   B. Is usually temporary
   C. Limits function in 3 or more life skills
   D. Is present before the age of 12

9. Developmentally disabled adults
   A. Need life-long assistance, support, and special services
   B. Usually can live independently after they become adults
   C. Always need to be in long-term care in special centers
   D. Generally outgrow the problems as they mature

10. A person with intellectual disabilities would not usually have
    A. An IQ score about 70 or below
    B. Difficulty with interpersonal skills
    C. Limited skills needed to live, work, and play
    D. Mental health disorders

11. The Arc of the United States is a national organization
    A. Related to Alzheimer's disease
    B. That deals with intellectual and related developmental disabilities
    C. That provides care for people with physical disabilities
    D. For persons with cerebral palsy

12. The Arc beliefs about sexuality for those with DD include
    A. The right to have control over their own bodies
    B. Encouraging persons with DD to be sterilized
    C. Preventing persons with DD from learning about sex, marriage, and family
    D. Denying interaction with members of the opposite sex

13. Down syndrome (DS) is caused by
    A. An extra 21st chromosome
    B. Head injury during birth
    C. Diseases of the mother during pregnancy
    D. Lack of oxygen to the brain

14. A person with Down syndrome is at risk for
    A. Cerebral palsy
    B. Diplegia
    C. Leukemia
    D. Poor nutrition

15. Fragile X syndrome (FXS) occurs because of
    A. An extra 21st chromosome
    B. An inherited intellectual disability
    C. Lack of oxygen to the brain during birth
    D. A traumatic brain injury

16. Cerebral palsy is a group of disorders involving
    A. Intellectual disabilities
    B. Muscle weakness or poor muscle control
    C. Abnormal genes from one or both parents
    D. An increased risk of developing leukemia

17. When a person has spastic cerebral palsy, the symptoms include
    A. Constant slow weaving or writhing motions
    B. Uncontrolled contractions of skeletal muscles
    C. Using little or no eye contact
    D. A strong attachment to a single item, idea, activity, or person
18. A person with autism may
    A. Dislike being held or cuddled
    B. Have bladder and bowel control problems
    C. Have generalized seizures
    D. Have diplegia or hemiplegia
19. A person with autism
    A. Needs to develop social and work skills
    B. Will outgrow the condition
    C. Will always live in group homes or residential care centers
    D. Will have severe physical problems
20. Spina bifida occurs
    A. At birth due to injury during delivery
    B. Because of traumatic injury in childhood
    C. During the first month of pregnancy
    D. As a result of child abuse
21. Which of these types of spina bifida cause the person to have leg paralysis and lack of bowel and bladder control?
    A. Spina bifida cystica
    B. Myelomeningocele
    C. Spina bifida occulta
    D. Meningocele
22. A shunt placed in the brain of a child with hydrocephalus will
    A. Increase pressure on the brain
    B. Drain fluid from the brain to the abdomen or heart chamber
    C. Cause intellectual disabilities or neurological damage
    D. Cure the hydrocephalus
23. A person with a developmental disability will
    A. Always need to live with family or in a nursing care center
    B. Have his or her rights protected by the Americans with Disabilities Act of 1990 and the Developmental Disabilities Assistance and Bill of Rights Act of 2000
    C. Not be admitted to a nursing facility until he or she is past 60 years of age
    D. Outgrow the disability as he or she ages

FILL IN THE BLANKS

24. Write out the meaning of each abbreviation.
    A. ADA ___
    B. CP ___
    C. DD ___
    D. DS ___
    E. FXS ___
    F. IQ ___
    G. SB ___
25. A developmental disability is present when function is limited in 3 or more of these life skills.
    A. ___
    B. ___
    C. ___
    D. ___
    E. ___
    F. ___
    G. ___
26. What genetic conditions can cause intellectual disabilities?
    A. ___
    B. ___
    C. ___
    D. ___
    E. ___
27. Intellectual disabilities may be caused after birth by childhood diseases such as
    A. ___
    B. ___
    C. ___
    D. ___
    E. ___
    F. ___
28. Intellectual disabilities involve the condition being present before ___.
29. The Arc belief about sexuality for persons with intellectual disabilities includes the right to
    A. ___
    B. ___
    C. ___
    D. ___
    E. ___
    F. ___
    G. ___

H. _____

I. _____

J. _____

K. _____

30. If a child has Down syndrome (DS), what features are present in the following areas?

A. Head _____

B. Eyes _____

C. Tongue _____

D. Nose _____

E. Hands and fingers _____

31. Persons with Down syndrome need therapy in these areas.

A. _____

B. _____

C. _____

D. _____

32. What problems will boys with Fragile X syndrome have in the areas listed?

A. Social and emotional _____

B. Speech and language _____

_____

33. The usual cause of cerebral palsy is a lack of

_____.

34. Which type of cerebral palsy is described in each example?

A. Arm and leg on one side are paralyzed.

_____

B. Muscles contract or shorten. They are stiff and cannot relax. _____

_____

C. Both arms and both legs are paralyzed.

_____

D. Person has constant, slow, weaving, or writhing motions. _____

E. Both arms _or_ both legs are paralyzed.

_____

35. The goal for a person with cerebral palsy is to be

_____.

36. A person with autism has

A. _____

B. _____

C. _____

37. Spina bifida is a defect of the _____.

38. Children with spina bifida may having difficulty with learning problems because of problems with

A. _____

B. _____

C. _____

D. _____

39. Which type of spina bifida would cause the problems in each of the examples given?

A. The person has leg paralysis and a lack of bowel and bladder control. _____

_____

B. The person may have no symptoms.

_____

C. Nerve damage usually does not occur and surgery corrects the defect. _____

_____

40. If hydrochephalus is not treated, pressure increases in the head and causes _____ and _____.

OPTIONAL LEARNING EXERCISES

Mr. Murphy is one of the residents you care for. He has Down syndrome. Answer Questions 41 to 43, which relate to this person.

41. Mr. Murphy is 40 years old. What disease may appear in adults with Down syndrome?

    _____.

42. Mr. Murphy is encouraged to eat a well-balanced diet and to attend regular exercise classes. Including these in the care plan will help prevent

    the problems of _____ and

    _____.

43. What 2 therapies may help Mr. Murphy to

    communicate more clearly? _____

    and _____

You care for Mary Reynolds, who has cerebral palsy. Answer Questions 44 and 45 about Ms. Reynolds.

44. It is difficult to feed Ms. Reynolds because she drools, grimaces, and moves her head constantly. You know that she does this because she has a type

    of cerebral palsy called _____.

45. Because Ms. Reynolds remains in bed or a special chair all the time, she is at special risk for

    _____ because of immobility.

    She needs to be repositioned at least every

    _____

INDEPENDENT LEARNING ACTIVITIES

- Many communities have services available for families with children and adults who are developmentally disabled. Some communities have sheltered workshops, day care, sheltered living centers, or physical and occupational therapy programs available. If your community has these services, ask permission to visit them and observe the persons being served there. Answer the following questions when you observe in the agency.
  - What age-groups are served in this program?
  - What activities are available to the group?
  - What training is required for the people who work there?
  - How do the persons in the program act? Happy? Bored? Withdrawn? Other reactions?
  - What other services are available to these individuals in the agency? In the community?
  - Where do the persons in this program live? With family? Group homes? Other?

- Do you know a family who has a developmentally disabled family member? Ask the family if they will answer the following questions about living with this person.
  - How old is the developmentally disabled person? Where does the person live?
  - What abilities does the person have? What disabilities interfere with the activities of daily living for the person?
  - What therapies are being done to help the person reach his or her highest level of function?
  - What community programs have been helpful for the person?
  - How does this person's disability affect the family? Physical? Emotional? Financial? Day-to-day activities?

41 REHABILITATION AND RESTORATIVE NURSING CARE

FILL IN THE BLANKS: KEY TERMS

Activities of daily living
Disability

Prosthesis
Rehabilitation

Restorative aide
Restorative nursing care

1. A nursing assistant with special training in restorative nursing and rehabilitation skills is a

   _____.

2. _____ are activities usually done during a normal day in a person's life.

3. An artificial replacement for a missing body part is a

   _____.

4. Care that helps persons regain their health, strength, and independence is

   _____.

5. A _____ is any lost, absent, or impaired physical or mental function.

6. The process of restoring the disabled person to the highest possible level of physical, psychological, social, and economic functioning is

   _____.

CIRCLE THE BEST ANSWER

7. The focus of rehabilitation is on
   A. Improving abilities
   B. Restoring function to normal
   C. Helping the person regain health and strength
   D. Preventing injury

8. Restorative nursing will
   A. Cure the problem
   B. Allow the person to be independent
   C. Maintain the highest level of function
   D. Teach family members to care for the person

9. If you are a restorative aide, it means you have
   A. Special training in restorative nursing and rehabilitation skills
   B. Taken required classes for restorative aides
   C. Passed a special test to show you can perform these duties
   D. The most seniority at the facility

10. When assisting with rehabilitation and restorative care, it is important to
    A. Give complete care to prevent exertion by the person
    B. Make sure you do everything for the person
    C. Encourage the person to perform ADL to the extent possible
    D. Complete care quickly

11. Which of these would be most helpful for a person receiving rehabilitative care?
    A. Give the person pity or sympathy when tasks are difficult.
    B. Remind the person not to try new skills or those that are difficult.
    C. Give praise when even a little progress is made.
    D. Encourage the person to perform ADL quickly.

12. Complications can be prevented by
    A. Doing all ADL for the person
    B. Allowing the person to decide if he or she wants to move or exercise
    C. Making sure the person is in good alignment, is turned and re-positioned, and performs range-of-motions exercises
    D. Making sure rehabilitation is fast-paced

13. Rehabilitation begins
    A. After the person has recovered
    B. When the person first seeks health care
    C. When the person asks for help
    D. When a discharge date has been set

14. Self-help devices help meet the goal of
    A. Recovery of all normal abilities
    B. Self-care
    C. Living alone
    D. Dependence on others

15. When dysphagia occurs after a stroke, a person
    A. May learn exercises to improve swallowing
    B. Must be fed by the staff
    C. Will always need enteral nutrition
    D. Will be given a clear liquid diet to prevent choking

16. A rehabilitation plan includes information to meet
    A. Only physical care needs
    B. Only ambulation needs
    C. Physical, psychological, social, and economic needs
    D. Only psychological and social needs

17. The rehabilitation team meets to evaluate the person's progress
    A. Every 90 days
    B. Often, to change the plan as needed
    C. Every week
    D. Only when requested by the family or person
18. OBRA requires that nursing centers
    A. Have a full-time physical therapist
    B. Provide rehabilitation services
    C. Provide physical care only
    D. Employ full-time occupational and speech therapists

FILL IN THE BLANKS

19. Write out the meaning of the abbreviations.

    A. ADL _____

    B. ROM _____

20. Restorative nursing programs do the following.

    A. _____

    B. _____

21. A person in rehabilitation needs to adjust in these areas.

    A. _____

    B. _____

    C. _____

    D. _____

22. Rehabilitation takes longer in which age-group?

    _____ What are reasons for this?

    A. Changes affect _____

    B. Chronic _____

    C. Risk for _____

23. What are some self-help devices that will assist in self-feeding?

    A. _____

    B. _____

    C. _____

24. The goal for a prosthesis is to have the device

    _____

    _____.

25. When you are assisting with rehabilitation and restorative nursing care, why is it helpful to listen to how the nurse or therapist guides and directs the

    person? _____

    _____

26. When assisting with rehabilitation and restorative nursing care, what complications can be prevented if you report early signs and symptoms?

    _____

    _____

27. What can you do to promote the person's quality of life?

    A. _____

    B. _____

    C. _____

    D. _____

    E. _____

    F. _____

    G. _____

OPTIONAL LEARNING EXERCISES

Mrs. Mercer is 82 years old. She is a resident in a rehabilitation unit because she had a stroke that has caused weakness on her left side. Although she is right-handed, she needs to learn to use several self-help devices as she re-learns ways to carry out ADL. She often becomes angry or depressed. Answer Questions 28 to 33 about Mrs. Mercer and her care. (You will need to use information learned in previous chapters.)

28. Mrs. Mercer is having difficulty with controlling urinary and bowel elimination. What would be the

    goal of her care for these problems? _____

    _____ Her plan of care would include

    programs for _____.

29. What should you do to prepare Mrs. Mercer's food at meal time so she can feed herself? _____ _____

30. Mrs. Mercer can brush her teeth but needs help getting prepared. What should you do to get her ready to brush her teeth? _____ _____

31. Why does she need help at meal time and to brush her teeth? _____ _____

32. Mrs. Mercer needs help to get in and out of bed. When helping her to transfer, you remember to position the chair on her _____ side.

33. When Mrs. Mercer becomes discouraged because progress is slow, how can you help her? You can stress _____ and focus on _____.

INDEPENDENT LEARNING ACTIVITIES

- Role-play the following situation with a classmate. Answer the questions about how you felt when you played Mrs. Leeds to understand how a person with a disability feels. Use your non-dominant hand to attempt the activities Mrs. Leeds must do.
Situation: Mary Leeds is 62 years old and had a stroke last month. She has weakness on her dominant side and has been admitted to a rehabilitation unit to re-learn activities of daily living (ADL). She is practicing eating by using a spoon to place fluids and food in her mouth. She is also learning to button clothing.
  - How well could you hold the spoon with your non-dominant hand?
  - What problems did you having controlling the spoon?
  - How rapidly could you eat? What type of food was easier to eat?
  - How well were you able to button your clothing? What techniques did you find that made you more successful?
  - How did this experience make you feel? How will it affect the way you interact with persons who have similar disabilities?

- With your instructor's permission, borrow a wheelchair from your school to use for 1 to 2 hours. Have a classmate push you around in the chair in a grocery store, mall, or your school. *Stay in the chair for the entire time to experience the feelings of a person who must use a wheelchair.* Use a handicap-equipped bathroom during this experience.
  - How comfortable was the wheelchair? Did you use any special padding or cushion in the seat?
  - What difficulties were encountered while moving about? Doorways? Steps? Aisles? Crowds? How did you deal with any difficulties?
  - How accessible was the handicap-equipped bathroom? How much room was available for you to transfer from the wheelchair to the toilet?
  - How did other people treat you? How many spoke to you? How many talked to your classmate and avoided you?
  - How did this experience make you feel? How will it affect the way you interact with a person in a wheelchair?

42 ASSISTED LIVING

FILL IN THE BLANKS: KEY TERMS

Assisted living
Medication reminder
Service plan

1. A _____ is reminding the person to take medications, observing that they were taken as prescribed, and charting that they were taken.

2. A written plan that lists the services needed by the person and who provides them is a

_____.

3. _____ provides housing, support services, and health care to persons needing help with activities of daily living.

CIRCLE THE BEST ANSWER

4. Which of these persons *would not* be living in an ALR?
   A. Someone who needs help taking medications at certain times
   B. A person who has problems with thinking, reasoning, and judgment
   C. A person who needs constant care
   D. Someone who is lonely and wants to live with people

5. When a person lives in an ALR, one requirement of the facility would be
   A. The person has at least 2 rooms and a bath
   B. Both a bathtub and a shower are provided
   C. A door that locks; the person keeps the key
   D. A double or queen-sized bed

6. Environmental requirements in an ALR include
   A. Common bathrooms have toilet paper, soap, and cloth towels or a dryer
   B. Pets or animals must be kept in kennels
   C. Hot water temperatures are between 110°F and 130°F
   D. Garbage is stored in covered containers lined with plastic bags that are removed at least once a day

7. According to the Assisted Living Residents' Rights, the resident
   A. Is required to participate in activities to avoid isolation
   B. Knows that all correspondence, communication, visits, and financial and personal matters will be observed by the staff
   C. Has a doctor or pharmacist assigned by the facility
   D. Make choices about how to receive care

8. A staff member in an ALR would need additional training to
   A. Provide nutrition and menu planning
   B. Know early signs of illness and the need for health care
   C. Know how to prevent and report abuse and neglect
   D. Allow him or her to help with administration of medications

9. Which of these is often a requirement of a resident in an ALR?
   A. The person must be able to leave the building in an emergency.
   B. The person requires skilled nursing services.
   C. The person has complex nursing problems.
   D. The person needs 24-hour nursing care.

10. A service plan for a person in an ALR
    A. Is reviewed every 90 days
    B. Lists the services needed by the person and who provides them
    C. States the medications that the person takes each day
    D. Remains the same as long as the person lives in the ALR

11. Which of these is a required service in an ALR?
    A. Clean bed linens every day
    B. A garage for cars owned by residents
    C. A 24-hour emergency communication system
    D. A bank in the facility

12. Meals in an ALR
    A. Are always served in the person's room
    B. Include the noon meal only
    C. Are posted in a menu for residents to see
    D. Cannot meet special dietary needs

13. When you assist with housekeeping, you will be expected to
    A. Clean the tub or shower after each use
    B. Put out clean towels and washcloths every week
    C. Use a disinfectant or water and detergent to clean bathroom surfaces once a week
    D. Dust furniture every day

14. A measure you should follow when handling, preparing, or storing foods is
    A. Use left-over food within 4 or 5 days
    B. Wash all pots and pans in a dishwasher
    C. Date and refrigerate containers of left-overs and refrigerate as soon as possible
    D. Clean kitchen appliances, counters, tables, and other surfaces once a day

15. When practicing food safety, which of these is *incorrect*?
    A. Use a garbage disposer for food and liquid garbage.
    B. Place left-over food in the refrigerator as soon as possible.
    C. Empty garbage at least once a week.
    D. Place washed eating and cooking items in a drainer to dry.

16. When assisting with laundry, a guideline to follow is
    A. Sort items according to the amount of soil on the items
    B. Wear gloves when handling soiled laundry
    C. Use hot water to wash all items
    D. Use the highest setting on the dryer to sanitize the items

17. When you assist a person with medication, it may involve
    A. Opening containers for a person who cannot do so
    B. Measuring medications for the person
    C. Explaining to a person the action of a medication
    D. Preparing a pill organizer for the person each week

18. If a medication error occurs, you should
    A. Tell the person not to do it again
    B. Make sure the person takes the correct medication at the next scheduled time
    C. Report the error to the nurse
    D. Take all medications away from the person immediately

19. An attendant is needed in an ALR 24 hours a day to
    A. Give care to those who need it
    B. Make sure medications are dispensed when ordered
    C. Assist those who need assistance if an emergency occurs
    D. Provide activities for the residents

20. Which of these is *not* a right of a resident in the ALR?
    A. The right to have financial and other records kept in confidence
    B. The right to have overnight guests whenever the resident wishes.
    C. The right to perform work or refuse to perform work for the facility
    D. The right to request to relocate or refuse to relocate within the ALR

FILL IN THE BLANKS

21. Write out the meaning of each abbreviation.
    A. AD _____
    B. ADL _____
    C. ALR _____

22. When working in an assisted living setting, you should follow _____ _____ when contact with blood, body fluids, secretions, excretions, or potentially contaminated items is likely.

23. Persons in assisted living settings usually need help with one or more ADL such as
    A. _____
    B. _____
    C. _____
    D. _____
    E. _____
    F. _____

24. A bathroom in an ALR must provide privacy and
    A. _____
    B. _____
    C. _____
    D. _____
    E. _____

25. The ALR cannot employ a person with a _____.

26. The service plan lists
    A. _____
    B. _____
    C. _____

27. The service plan also relates to
    A. _____
    B. _____
    C. _____
    D. _____
    E. _____
    F. _____

28. How many meals are provided in an ALR?

   _____

   A. Usually there are no more than _____ hours allowed between the evening meal and breakfast.

   B. The time between the evening meal and breakfast can be longer if there is a

   _____ .

29. When providing housekeeping, bathroom surfaces are cleaned every _____ with a

   _____ or _____

   and _____ .

30. When you wash eating and cooking items by hand, what is the order in which they are washed?

   A. _____

   B. _____

   C. _____

   D. _____

   E. _____

31. If you are assisting the person with taking medications, you should know the 6 rights of medication administration. They are

   A. _____

   B. _____

   C. _____

D. _____

E. _____

F. _____

32. If a person is taking his or her medications and states that a pill looks different, what should you do?

   _____

33. If a person needs a medication reminder, it means reminding _____, observing

   _____, and charting

   _____ .

34. If you are assisting in medication administration, you should report any medication error to the RN. Errors would include:

   A. _____

   B. _____

   C. _____

   D. _____

   E. _____

   F. _____

   G. _____

   H. _____

   I. _____

OPTIONAL LEARNING EXERCISES

You are working in an assisted living facility. What would you do in the following situations?

35. You are providing housekeeping assistance to Mrs. Miller, who lives alone. The stove is on and a pan has burning food in it. Mrs. Miller tells you she did not put the pan on the stove. What should you do?

   _____

   _____

   What is a likely reason for her behavior?

   _____

36. A resident in the facility has lived there for 2 years and has needed little assistance. He recently had a stroke and now needs care for all of his ADL. Why is he being moved to a nursing facility?

   _____

   _____

37. Mrs. Jenkins tells you she is expecting an important phone call and wants to eat lunch in her room. What should you do?

   _____

   _____

38. Mr. Shante asks you to get his medications ready for him to take. What assistance are you allowed to give when the nurse has trained you?

A. _____

B. _____

C. _____

D. _____

E. _____

F. _____

G. _____

H. _____

39. When you are assisting Mrs. Clyde with her medications, you notice that 2 of the labels have an expired date. What should you do?

_____

_____

40. Mrs. Johnson asks you when the next meeting of the quilting group will be held. She also asks on what days the community crafts fair is planned. Where would you direct her to find this information?

_____

_____

INDEPENDENT LEARNING ACTIVITIES

- Find out if your community has any assisted living facilities. They may be part of another facility or may be an independent facility. Visit the facility to answer the following questions.
  - What services are offered in the facility? Who provides the services? Nursing assistants? Other assistants? What training is required?
  - What kinds of living quarters are provided? What belongings can the person bring from home?
  - What activities are scheduled? How are residents given information about these activities?
  - How do the residents act? Happy? Withdrawn? Sad? How do the staff members act?

- Find out what laws in your state apply to assisted living facilities. Answer the following questions about the laws.
  - What type of license is required for an assisted living facility? Do the laws apply to independent facilities as well as to those attached to other facilities?
  - What laws apply to staff training for these facilities? Does the state require workers to be nursing assistants with special training?
  - What does the state law state about assisting with medications? What non-licensed persons can assist with medications? What training is required?

43 BASIC EMERGENCY CARE

FILL IN THE BLANKS: KEY TERMS

Anaphylaxis   Fainting   Respiratory arrest   Shock
Cardiac arrest   First aid   Seizure   Sudden cardiac arrest
Convulsion   Hemorrhage

1. In _____ breathing stops but the heart still pumps for several minutes.

2. The sudden loss of consciousness from an inadequate blood supply to the brain is

   _____.

3. When the heart and breathing stop suddenly and without warning, it is _____.

4. _____ is a condition that results when there is not enough blood supply to organs and tissues.

5. Emergency care given to an ill or injured person before medical help arrives is

   _____.

6. A convulsion may also be called a

   _____.

7. _____ is the excessive loss of blood in a short period of time.

8. Violent and sudden contractions or tremors of muscles are a seizure or a _____.

9. A life-threatening sensitivity to an antigen is

   _____.

10. Another name for sudden cardiac arrest is

    _____.

CIRCLE THE BEST ANSWER

11. When an emergency occurs in nursing centers, the nurse determines when to
    A. Call the doctor for orders
    B. Activate the EMS system
    C. Call the supervisor
    D. Assist the person to bed

12. If you find a person lying on the floor, you should
    A. Keep the person lying down
    B. Help the person back to bed
    C. Elevate the head
    D. Help the person to a chair

13. If the nurse instructs you to activate the EMS system, you should
    A. Tell the operator your name and title
    B. Explain to the operator what seems to have happened
    C. Give the victim's name and age
    D. Hang up as soon as you have finished giving the information

14. It is important to restore breathing and circulation quickly because
    A. The lungs will be damaged
    B. The person will lose consciousness
    C. Heart, brain, and other organ damage occurs within minutes
    D. Hemorrhage will occur

15. Which of these is *not* a major sign of sudden cardiac arrest (SCA)?
    A. Complaints of chest pain
    B. No pulse
    C. No breathing
    D. No response

16. The purpose of the head tilt–chin lift maneuver is to
    A. Make the person more comfortable
    B. Keep the airway open
    C. Practice Standard Precautions
    D. Stimulate the heart to beat

17. When you use mouth-to-mouth breathing, you should
    A. Allow the person's chin to relax against the neck
    B. Place your mouth loosely over the person's mouth
    C. Blow into the person's mouth. You should see the chest rise
    D. Apply pressure on the chin to close the mouth

18. Mouth-to-nose breathing is used when
    A. You cannot ventilate through the person's mouth
    B. You want to avoid contact with body fluids
    C. You need to give rescue breaths to a child
    D. Chest compressions are not needed

19. Before starting chest compressions
    A. Make sure the person is breathing
    B. Check for a pulse
    C. Wait 30 seconds to see if the person regains consciousness
    D. Turn the person to the side

20. When chest compressions are started, you give compressions at a rate of
    A. 5 compressions, then check for a pulse
    B. 60 compressions per minute
    C. 100 compressions per minute
    D. 15 compressions per minute

21. The purpose of chest compressions is to
    A. Deflate the lungs
    B. Increase oxygen in the blood
    C. Force blood through the circulatory system
    D. Help the heart work more effectively

22. In order for chest compressions to be effective, the person must be
    A. In prone position
    B. On a soft surface
    C. Supine on a hard, flat surface
    D. In a semi-Fowler's position

23. When preparing to give chest compressions, locate the heel of the hands
    A. On the sternum between the nipples
    B. On the lower half of the sternum
    C. Side by side over the sternum
    D. Slightly below the end of the sternum

24. When giving chest compressions to an adult, depress the sternum
    A. About 1 to 1½ inches
    B. About ½ to 1 inch
    C. About 1½ inches
    D. At least 2 inches

25. CPR is done only when the person
    A. Does not respond when you shout, "Are you okay?"
    B. Is not breathing
    C. Is unconscious
    D. Does not respond, is not breathing, and has no pulse

26. Hands-only CPR is useful for persons who
    A. Have taken a BLS course
    B. Are not sure the victim is in cardiac arrest
    C. Have not been trained in BLS
    D. Do not like to do mouth-to-mouth resuscitation

27. If the person is not breathing or not breathing adequately, give 2 breaths that
    A. Last about 1 second each
    B. Last about 5 seconds each
    C. Last 5 to 10 seconds each
    D. Last 15 seconds each

28. When performing one rescuer CPR, chest compressions are at a rate of
    A. 15 compressions per minute
    B. 100 compressions per minute
    C. 60 compressions per minute
    D. 12 compressions per minute

29. When performing one rescuer CPR, a rescue breath is given after
    A. 5 minutes
    B. 100 compressions
    C. 30 compressions
    D. 4 cycles of 15 compressions and 2 breaths

30. Side-lying position is the recovery position when the person is breathing and has a pulse but is not responding because
    A. The position helps keep the airway open and prevents aspiration
    B. It makes the person respond more quickly
    C. You can observe the person more easily
    D. The person will be more comfortable

31. When an automated external defibrillator (AED) is used, it
    A. Stops the heart
    B. Slows the heartbeat down
    C. Stops ventricular fibrillation (VF) and restores a regular heartbeat
    D. Starts the heartbeat

32. Which of these is a sign of internal hemorrhage?
    A. Steady flow of blood from a wound
    B. Pain, shock, vomiting blood, or coughing up blood
    C. Bleeding that occurs in spurts
    D. Dried blood at the site of an injury

33. To control external bleeding, you should
    A. Remove any objects that have pierced or stabbed the person
    B. Keep the injured part flat or below the level of the body
    C. Apply pressure with your hand directly over the bleeding site
    D. Give the person warm or cool fluids to drink

34. If a person tells you she feels faint
    A. Have the person lie down in a supine position
    B. Let the person walk around to increase circulation
    C. Have the person sit or lie down before fainting occurs
    D. Raise the head with pillows if the person is already lying down

35. If a person is in shock, it is helpful if you
    A. Have the person sit in a chair
    B. Keep the person cool by removing some of his or her clothing
    C. Keep the person lying down, maintain an open airway, and control bleeding
    D. Give the person something to drink or eat

36. Anaphylactic shock occurs because of
    A. Hemorrhage
    B. An allergy to foods, insects, chemicals, or medications
    C. Sudden cardiac arrest
    D. Seizures

37. When a stroke occurs, position the person in the recovery position
    A. On the affected side
    B. On the unaffected side
    C. In the supine position
    D. In a semi-Fowler's position

38. If a person has a seizure, you should
    A. Place an object between the teeth
    B. Distract the person to stop the seizure
    C. Position the person in bed
    D. Move furniture, equipment, and sharp objects away from the person
39. If you are assisting a person with burns
    A. Remove burned clothing
    B. Cover the burn wounds with a sterile or clean, cool, moist covering
    C. Give the person plenty of fluids
    D. Apply oils or ointments to the burns

FILL IN THE BLANKS

40. Write the meaning of each abbreviation
    A. AED _____
    B. AHA _____
    C. BLS _____
    D. CPR _____
    E. DNR _____
    F. EMS _____
    G. SCA _____
    H. VF or V-fib _____
41. If you activate the EMS system, what information should you give to the operator?
    A. _____
    B. _____
    C. _____
    D. _____
    E. _____
    F. _____
42. Chain of Survival actions for adults are:
    A. _____
    B. _____
    C. _____
    D. _____
    E. _____
43. Cardiopulmonary resuscitation has 4 parts. They are
    A. C _____
    B. A _____
    C. B _____
    D. D _____

44. When opening the airway with the head tilt–chin lift maneuver, explain the steps needed
    A. Place _____
    B. Tilt _____
    C. Place _____
    D. Lift _____
    E. Do not _____
45. When you perform mouth-to-mouth breathing, it is likely you will have contact with _____.
46. If a person has a mouth that is severely injured and you need to perform rescue breathing, you will use _____.
47. To find the carotid pulse, place _____. Slide your fingers down _____.
48. When giving one rescuer CPR, give _____ compressions followed by _____ rescue breaths.
49. When giving 2-person CPR, change positions every _____ minutes or after _____ cycles of _____ compressions and _____ breaths.
50. If direct pressure does not stop hemorrhage, apply pressure over the artery _____.
51. Common causes of fainting are
    A. _____
    B. _____
    C. _____
    D. _____
52. List the signs and symptoms of shock.
    A. _____
    B. _____
    C. _____
    D. _____
    E. _____
    F. _____
    G. _____
53. Anaphylaxis is an emergency because it occurs within _____.

54. What signs or symptoms will be present on the affected side with a stroke?

    A. _____

    B. _____

55. Describe the 2 phases of a generalized tonic-clonic seizure.

    A. Tonic phase _____

    _____

    B. Clonic phase _____

    _____

56. The following relate to the emergency care of a person having a seizure.

    A. How do you protect the person's head?

    _____

    B. How is the person positioned?

    _____

    C. Why is furniture moved?

    _____

    D. What times are noted?

    _____

57. Partial-thickness burns involve the _____

    _____.

58. Full-thickness burns involve _____

    _____.

59. A _____ burn is very painful

    because _____.

OPTIONAL LEARNING EXERCISES

You are visiting a neighbor and she is washing dishes. As she washes a glass, it shatters and she sustains a deep cut on her wrist. Answer Questions 60 to 65 about how you would respond.

60. How would you determine whether the bleeding

    was from an artery or vein? _____

    _____.

61. Your neighbor is crying and walking around the room. What is the best thing you can do to help her?

    A. Stay _____.

    B. Position the arm in an _____.

    C. Instead of walking around, she should be kept

    _____ until help arrives.

62. Clean rubber gloves are on the counter. How can

    they be useful to you? _____

    _____

63. What materials in the home could be used to place

    over the wound? _____

    _____

64. Your neighbor is restless and has a rapid and weak pulse. You notice her skin is cold, moist, and pale. These signs indicate she may be in

    _____.

65. Her wound is still bleeding and she loses consciousness. What should you do before you continue to give first aid? _____

    _____

INDEPENDENT LEARNING ACTIVITIES

- You have learned some basic emergency care in this chapter. Find out where in your community a more advanced first aid course is available. Answer the following questions about the course.
  - What agency or agencies offer a course in first aid?
  - How long does the course last? How much does it cost?
  - Who may take the course? The public? Medical personnel? Others, such as police, firefighters, etc.?
  - What subjects are covered in the course?
  - Would taking this course help you in your job? In your family? In your community?
- Most health care facilities require that employees take a course in basic CPR. You may be required to take CPR as part of this course. Answer these questions about CPR training in your community.
  - What agency or agencies offer CPR courses?
  - How long does the course take? How much does it cost?
  - Who can take the courses? The public? Medical personnel? Are different classes offered to medical personnel? If so, what is the difference?
  - How often does the person need to be re-certified? How does the re-certification course differ from the beginning class?

44 END-OF-LIFE CARE

FILL IN THE BLANKS: KEY TERMS

Advance directive
Autopsy
End-of-life care

Palliative care
Post-mortem care
Reincarnation

Rigor mortis
Terminal illness

1. The support and care given during the time surrounding death is _____.

2. _____ involves relieving or reducing the intensity of uncomfortable symptoms without producing a cure.

3. The stiffness or rigidity of skeletal muscles that occurs after death is _____.

4. An _____ is a document stating a person's wishes about health care when that person cannot make his or her own decisions.

5. Care of the body after death is

_____

6. An illness or injury for which there is no reasonable expectation of recovery is a _____.

7. _____ is the belief that the spirit or soul is reborn in another human body or in another form of life.

8. The examination of the body after death is an

_____

CIRCLE THE BEST ANSWER

9. When a person has a terminal illness
   A. The doctor is able to accurately predict when the person will die
   B. Modern medicine can cure the disease
   C. The person may live longer than expected or die sooner than expected
   D. He or she will die when expected

10. When a person is receiving palliative care, he or she will
    A. Not receive any pain medications
    B. Probably recover from the illness
    C. Receive care to relieve symptoms
    D. Not be allowed to live at home

11. A person generally receives hospice care when
    A. He or she has less than 6 months to live
    B. Life-saving measures can cure the disease
    C. The family can no longer care for the person
    D. The doctor refuses to treat the person and the illness any longer

12. Death rite practices among people from India include
    A. Placing small pillows under the body's neck, feet, and wrists
    B. Wearing white clothing for mourning
    C. Using prayer to help them deal with anxiety and conflict
    D. Having an aversion to death

13. Children between ages 2 and 6 years see death as
    A. Final
    B. Punishment for being bad
    C. Suffering and pain
    D. A reunion with those who have died

14. Older persons see death as
    A. A temporary state
    B. Freedom from pain, suffering, and disability
    C. Something that happens to other people
    D. Something that affects plans, hopes, dreams, and ambitions

15. In which stage of dying does the person make promises and make "just one more" requests?
    A. Acceptance
    B. Anger
    C. Depression
    D. Bargaining

16. If a dying person begins to talk about worries and concerns, you should
    A. Call a spiritual leader
    B. Tell the nurse
    C. Be there and listen quietly
    D. Change the subject to more pleasant topics

17. When a person is dying, care should be given
    A. Only if the person requests it
    B. To meet basic needs
    C. Often, to keep the person active
    D. Only while the person is conscious

18. Because vision fails as death approaches, you should
    A. Explain what you are doing to the person when you are in the room
    B. Have the room lit very brightly
    C. Turn out all lights
    D. Keep the eyes covered at all times
19. Hearing is one of the last functions lost, so it is important to
    A. Speak in whispers
    B. Give care without talking to avoid disturbing the person
    C. Ask family and friends to speak loudly in the person's room
    D. Provide reassurance and explanations about care
20. As death nears, oral hygiene is
    A. Given during regular care
    B. Given frequently because taking oral fluids is difficult
    C. Given very infrequently to avoid disturbing the person
    D. Never given because the person cannot swallow
21. Which of these does *not* occur as death nears?
    A. Body temperature rises.
    B. The skin is cool, pale, and mottled.
    C. Perspiration decreases.
    D. Circulation fails.
22. Because of breathing difficulties, the dying person is generally more comfortable in
    A. The supine position
    B. A side-lying position
    C. A prone position
    D. A semi-Fowler's position
23. When a person is dying, you can help the family by
    A. Allowing the family to stay for as long as they wish
    B. Staying away from the room and delaying care
    C. Telling the family that they need to leave so you can give care
    D. Telling the family that the person dying is not in pain
24. If a person has a living will, it instructs doctors
    A. To start measures that will save the person's life
    B. To start CPR whenever necessary
    C. To not start measures that prolong dying
    D. To activate the EMS system for a person
25. If the doctor writes a "Do Not Resuscitate" (DNR) order it means that
    A. The person will not be resuscitated
    B. The person will be resuscitated if it is an emergency
    C. The doctor will decide whether or not to resuscitate
    D. The RN may decide that in a particular situation resuscitation is needed
26. A sign that death is near would be
    A. Deep, rapid respirations
    B. The blood pressure starts to fall
    C. Muscles tense and contract in spasms
    D. Peristalsis increases

27. An ID tag is attached to the right big toe or
    A. Wrist
    B. Ankle
    C. Upper arm
    D. Upper leg
28. The dying patient's bill of last rights includes
    A. The right to freedom from restraint
    B. The right to laugh
    C. The right to have a private room
    D. The right to be in denial

FILL IN THE BLANKS

29. Write out the meaning of these abbreviations.
    A. DNR _____
    B. ID _____
    C. POLST _____
30. It is important to examine your own feelings about death because they will affect _____ _____.
31. When you understand the dying process, you can approach the dying person with _____ _____.
32. The intent of palliative care is to _____ _____.
33. List the services that hospice provides to these persons or groups.
    A. Dying person _____
    B. Survivors _____
    C. Health team _____
34. Religious beliefs strengthen when dying and often provide _____.
35. Adults fear death because they fear
    A. _____
    B. _____
    C. _____
    D. _____
    E. _____
    F. _____
    G. _____

36. Name the 5 stages of dying.

    A. _____

    B. _____

    C. _____

    D. _____

    E. _____

37. When caring for a dying person, comfort goals are

    A. _____

    B. _____

38. By listening to the dying person, it lets the person

    _____ in his or

    her own way.

39. Touch shows _____.

40. Signs and symptoms of pain should be reported at

    once because _____
    is easier than relieving pain.

41. Where can you find measures used to prevent and

    control pain? _____

42. Ways to help a person with breathing problems
    include the following.

    A. Position the person in _____

    B. The doctor may order _____

    C. Open a _____

    D. Circulate air with a _____

43. Because hearing is one of the last functions lost, do

    not _____ the person.

44. When caring for a dying person, do not ask
    questions that need long answers because

    _____

    _____

45. Because crusting and irritation of the nostrils can

    occur, you should _____

    _____

46. If the person refuses to eat, you should

    _____

47. What kinds of elimination problems are common in

    the dying person? _____

48. The Patient Self-Determination Act and OBRA give
    2 rights that affect the rights of a dying person.
    They are:

    A. _____

    B. _____

49. A living will instructs doctors

    A. _____

    B. _____

50. When a person cannot make health care decisions,
    the authority to do so is given to the person with

    _____.

51. What are the signs that death is near?

    A. _____

    B. _____

    C. _____

    D. _____

    E. _____

    F. _____

52. The signs of death include no _____,

    no _____, and no _____.

    The pupils are _____ and

    _____.

53. Post-mortem care is not done when an

    _____ is to be done.

54. When assisting with post-mortem care, you need
    this information from the nurse.

    A. _____

    B. _____

    C. _____

    D. _____

    E. _____

55. The right to confidentiality before and after death

    provides that _____

    _____

OPTIONAL LEARNING EXERCISES

You are assigned to care for Mrs. Adams, who is dying.
Answer Questions 56 to 63 regarding this situation.

56. You find Mrs. Adams crying in her room. When you ask her what is wrong, she tells you no one gave her fresh water this morning and she has not had her bath yet. She tells you to just go away. What stage of dying is she displaying?

_____

57. Later in the day, Mrs. Adams tells you she can't wait until she is better so she can go home and plant her garden. She states that she knows the tests done last week were wrong and she will recover quickly from her illness. Now what stage is she displaying? _____ Why is she displaying 2 different stages so rapidly?

_____

58. A minister comes to visit Mrs. Adams while you are giving care. What should you do?

_____

59. You are working overnight and find Mrs. Adams awake during the night. She asks you to sit with her. She begins to talk about her fears, worries, and anxieties. What are 2 things you can do to convey caring to her? _____

_____

60. As Mrs. Adams becomes weaker, a family member is always at her bedside. When they ask to assist with her care, you know that this is acceptable because _____.

61. Mrs. Adams has very noisy breathing. This occurs as death nears and is called the

_____. It is due to

_____.

62. Mrs. Adams dies while you are working and the nurse asks you to assist with post-mortem care. As you clean soiled areas, you assist the nurse to turn the body and air is expelled. This occurs because

_____

_____

63. You wear gloves during post-mortem care because they will _____

_____

INDEPENDENT LEARNING ACTIVITIES

- It is important to explore your own beliefs about death and dying before you care for persons who are dying. Answer the following questions to understand your own feelings.
  - Have you attended a funeral or visited a funeral home? How did you feel?
  - Has anyone close to you died? How did you assist with any of the funeral arrangements? What kinds of preparation did the family do?
  - What cultural or religious practices in your family affect death and funeral arrangements? How do you think these practices will affect you when you care for those who are dying?

- Have you ever been present when someone died? In your personal life? As a student? At your job? How did you respond? What were you asked to do in this situation?
- What is your personal belief about a living will? How will you respond if a person or family refuses a feeding tube or a ventilator? How will you respond if they ask to have these measures discontinued and the person dies?
- What is your personal belief about a "Do Not Resuscitate" order? How would you feel if a person you are caring for has this order? How will you respond when the person dies and no effort is made to help the person?

Relieving Choking—Adult or Child (Over 1 Year of Age)

Name: _____   Date: _____

Procedure	S	U	Comments
1. Asked the person if he or she was choking.	___	___	_____
2. If indicated yes (did not talk), called for help:			
a. *In public area:* Activated the Emergency Medical Services (EMS) system and sent someone for automated external defibrillator (AED).	___	___	_____
b. *In a center:* Called emergency response team and sent for AED and emergency cart.	___	___	_____
3. Gave abdominal thrusts (if person was sitting or standing):			
a. Stood or kneeled behind the person.	___	___	_____
b. Wrapped your arms around the person's waist.	___	___	_____
c. Made a fist with one hand.	___	___	_____
d. Placed thumb side of fist against the abdomen. The fist was in the middle, above the navel and below the end of the sternum (breastbone).	___	___	_____
e. Grasped the fist with other hand.	___	___	_____
f. Pressed fist and hand into the person's abdomen with a quick, upward thrust.	___	___	_____
g. Repeated thrusts until the object was expelled or the person became un-responsive.	___	___	_____
4. *If person was lying down*, gave abdominal thrusts:			
a. Straddled the person's thighs.	___	___	_____
b. Placed heel of one hand against abdomen, in the middle above the navel and below the end of the sternum (breastbone).	___	___	_____
c. Placed second hand on top of first hand.	___	___	_____
d. Pressed both hands into the abdomen with a quick, upward thrust.	___	___	_____
e. Repeated thrusts until the object was expelled or the person became un-responsive.	___	___	_____
5. *If person was obese or pregnant*, gave chest thrusts:			
a. Stood behind the person.	___	___	_____
b. Placed your arms under the person's underarms. Wrapped your arms around the person's chest.	___	___	_____
c. Made a fist and placed the thumb side of fist on the middle of the sternum (breastbone).	___	___	_____
d. Grasped the fist with other hand.	___	___	_____
e. Gave thrusts to the chest until object was expelled or the person became unresponsive.	___	___	_____
6. *If object was dislodged*, person was encouraged to go to the hospital.	___	___	_____

Date of Satisfactory Completion _____   Instructor's Initials _____

Procedure—cont'd	S	U	Comments

7. *If person was unresponsive,* lowered person to the floor or ground. Positioned the person supine. Called EMS or emergency response system. *If alone,* provided 5 cycles (2 minutes) of cardiopulmonary resuscitation (CPR), then called EMS or emergency response system.

8. Started CPR:
   a. Did not check for a pulse. Began compressions. Gave 30 compressions.
   b. Used the head tilt–chin lift method to open the airway. Opened the person's mouth. Mouth was wide open. Looked for an object. Removed the object if seen and removed it easily. Used your fingers.
   c. Gave 2 breaths.

9. If choking was relieved in the unresponsive person:
   a. Checked for a response, breathing, and pulse.
      1. *If no response, normal breathing, or pulse,* continued CPR. Attached an AED.
      2. *If no response and no normal breathing but there was a pulse,* gave rescue breaths. For adult, gave 1 breath every 5 to 6 seconds (10 to 12 breaths per minute). For child, gave 1 breath every 3 to 5 seconds (12 to 20 breaths per minute). Checked pulse every 2 minutes. If no pulse, began CPR.
      3. *If person had normal breathing and a pulse,* placed the person in recovery position, if no response. Continued to check the person until help arrived. Encouraged the person to go to hospital when he or she responded.

Date of Satisfactory Completion _____   Instructor's Initials _____

Using a Fire Extinguisher

Name: _____   Date: _____

Procedure	S	U	Comments
1. Pulled the fire alarm.	___	___	_____
2. Got the nearest fire extinguisher.	___	___	_____
3. Carried it upright.	___	___	_____
4. Took it to the fire.	___	___	_____
5. Followed the word *PASS*:			
a. P—*Pulled* the safety pin.	___	___	_____
b. A—*Aimed* low. Directed the hose or nozzle at the base of the fire. Did not try to spray the tops of flames.	___	___	_____
c. S—*Squeezed* the lever. Squeezed or pushed down on the lever, handle, or button to start and stop the stream. Released the level, handle, or button to stop the stream.	___	___	_____
d. S—*Swept* back and forth. Swept the stream of water back and forth (side to side) at the base of the fire.	___	___	_____

Date of Satisfactory Completion _____   Instructor's Initials _____

Applying a Transfer/Gait Belt

Name: _____ Date: _____

	S	U	Comments
Quality of Life			
Remembered to:			
• Knock before entering the person's room	___	___	_____
• Address the person by name	___	___	_____
• Introduce yourself by name and title	___	___	_____
• Explain the procedure to the person before beginning and during the procedure	___	___	_____
• Protect the person's rights during the procedure	___	___	_____
• Handle the person gently during the procedure	___	___	_____

Procedure

	S	U	Comments
1. Saw *Promoting Safety and Comfort: Transfer/Gait Belts.*	___	___	_____
2. Practiced hand hygiene.	___	___	_____
3. Identified the person. Checked the identification (ID) bracelet against the assignment sheet. Called the person by name.	___	___	_____
4. Provided for privacy.	___	___	_____
5. Assisted the person to a sitting position.	___	___	_____
6. Applied the belt around the person's waist over clothing. Did not apply it over bare skin.	___	___	_____
7. Secured the buckle. The buckle was in front.	___	___	_____
8. Tightened the belt so it was snug. It did not cause discomfort or impaired breathing. You were able to slide your open, flat hand under the belt.	___	___	_____
9. Made sure that a woman's breasts were not caught under the belt.	___	___	_____
10. Turned the belt so the quick-release buckle was at the person's back. The buckle was not over the spine.	___	___	_____
11. Tucked any excess strap under the belt.	___	___	_____

Date of Satisfactory Completion _____ Instructor's Initials _____

Helping the Falling Person

Name: _____   Date: _____

Procedure	S	U	Comments
1. Stood behind the person with your feet apart. Kept your back straight.	___	___	_____
2. Brought the person close to your body as fast as possible. Used the transfer/gait belt. Or wrapped your arms around the person's waist. If necessary (but not preferred), you held the person under the arms.	___	___	_____
3. Moved your leg so the person's buttocks rested on it. Moved the leg near the person.	___	___	_____
4. Lowered the person to the floor. The person slid down your leg to the floor. You were bent at your hips and knees as you lowered the person.	___	___	_____
5. Called a nurse to check the person. Stayed with the person.	___	___	_____
6. Helped the nurse return the person to bed. Asked other staff to help if needed.	___	___	_____

Post-Procedure

	S	U	Comments
7. Provided for comfort.	___	___	_____
8. Placed the call light within reach.	___	___	_____
9. Raised or lowered the bed rails. Followed the care plan.	___	___	_____
10. Completed a safety check of the room.	___	___	_____
11. Reported and recorded the following:			
a. How the fall occurred.	___	___	_____
b. How far the person walked.	___	___	_____
c. How activity was tolerated before the fall.	___	___	_____
d. Complaints before the fall.	___	___	_____
e. How much help the person needed while walking.	___	___	_____
12. Completed an incident report.	___	___	_____

Date of Satisfactory Completion _____ Instructor's Initials _____

VIDEO CLIP **VIDEO** **Applying Restraints**

Name: _____   Date: _____

	S	U	Comments

Quality of Life
Remembered to:
- Knock before entering the person's room
- Address the person by name
- Introduce yourself by name and title
- Explain the procedure to the person before beginning and during the procedure
- Protect the person's rights during the procedure
- Handle the person gently during the procedure

Pre-Procedure
1. Followed *Delegation Guidelines: Applying Restraints*. Saw *Promoting Safety and Comfort: Applying Restraints.*
2. Collected the following as instructed by the nurse:
   a. Correct type and size of restraints
   b. Padding for skin and bony areas
   c. Bed rail pads or gap protectors (if needed)
3. Practiced hand hygiene.
4. Identified the person. Checked the identification (ID) bracelet against the assignment sheet. Called the person by name.
5. Provided for privacy.

Procedure
6. Made sure the person was comfortable and in good alignment.
7. Put the bed rail pads or gap protectors (if needed) on the bed if the person was in bed. Followed the manufacturer instructions.
8. Padded bony areas. Followed the nurse's instructions and the care plan.
9. Read the manufacturer instructions. Noted the front and back of the restraint.
10. *For wrist restraints:*
    a. Applied the restraint following the manufacturer instructions. Placed the soft part toward the skin.
    b. Secured the restraint so it was snug but not tight. Made sure you could slide 1 finger under the restraint. Followed the manufacturer instructions. Adjusted the straps if the restraint was too loose or too tight. Checked for snugness again.
    c. Buckled or tied the straps to the movable part of the bed frame out of the person's reach. Used a center-approved tie.
    d. Repeated steps for the other wrist.
       1. Applied the restraint following the manufacturer instructions. Placed the soft part toward the skin.
       2. Secured the restraint so it was snug but not tight. Made sure you could slide 1 finger under the restraint. Followed the manufacturer instructions. Adjusted the straps if the restraint was too loose or too tight. Checked for snugness again.

Date of Satisfactory Completion _____   Instructor's Initials _____

Procedure—cont'd	S	U	Comments
3. Buckled or tied the straps to the movable part of the bed frame out of the person's reach. Used a center-approved tie.	___	___	_____
11. *For mitt restraints:*			
a. Made sure the person's hands were clean and dry.	___	___	_____
b. Applied the mitt restraint. Followed the manufacturer instructions.	___	___	_____
c. Secured the restraint to the bed if directed by the nurse. Buckled or tied the straps to the movable part of the bed frame. Used a center-approved tie.	___	___	_____
d. Made sure the restraint was snug. Slid 1 finger between the restraint and the wrist. Followed the manufacturer instructions. Adjusted the straps if the restraint was too loose or too tight. Checked for snugness again.	___	___	_____
e. Repeated steps for the other hand.			
1. Applied the mitt restraint. Followed the manufacturer instructions.	___	___	_____
2. Secured the restraint to the bed if directed by the nurse. Buckled or tied the straps to the movable part of the bed frame. Used a center-approved tie.	___	___	_____
3. Made sure the restraint was snug. Slid 1 finger between the restraint and the wrist. Followed the manufacturer instructions. Adjusted the straps if the restraint was too loose or too tight. Checked for snugness again.	___	___	_____
12. *For a belt restraint:*			
a. Assisted the person to a sitting position.	___	___	_____
b. Applied the restraint with your free hand. Followed the manufacturer instructions.	___	___	_____
c. Removed wrinkles or creases from the front and back of the restraint.	___	___	_____
d. Brought the ties through the slots in the belt.	___	___	_____
e. Helped the person lie down if he or she was in bed.	___	___	_____
f. Made sure the person was comfortable and in good alignment.	___	___	_____
g. Buckled or tied the straps to the movable part of the bed frame out of the person's reach or to the chair or wheelchair. Used a center-approved tie.	___	___	_____
h. Made sure the belt was snug. Slid an open hand between the restraint and the person. Adjusted the restraint if it was too loose or too tight. Checked for snugness again.	___	___	_____
13. *For a vest restraint:*			
a. Assisted the person to a sitting position.	___	___	_____
b. Applied the restraint with your free hand. Followed the manufacturer instructions. The "V" part of the vest crossed in front.	___	___	_____
c. Brought the straps through the slots.	___	___	_____
d. Made sure the vest was free of wrinkles in the front and back.	___	___	_____
e. Helped the person to lie down if he or she was in bed.	___	___	_____
f. Made sure the person was comfortable and in good alignment.			

Date of Satisfactory Completion _____   Instructor's Initials _____

	S	U	Comments
Procedure—cont'd			

g. Buckled or tied the straps underneath the chair seat or to the movable part of the bed frame. Used a center-approved tie. If secured to the bed frame, the straps were secured at waist level out of the person's reach.

h. Made sure the vest was snug. Slid an open hand between the restraint and the person. Adjusted the restraint if it was too loose or too tight. Checked for snugness again.

14. *For a jacket restraint:*
   a. Assisted the person to a sitting position.
   b. Applied the restraint with your free hand. Followed the manufacturer instructions. The jacket opening was in the back.
   c. Closed the back with the zipper, ties, or hook and loop closures.
   d. Made sure the side seams were under the arms. Removed any wrinkles in the front and back.
   e. Helped the person lie down if he or she was in bed.
   f. Made sure the person was comfortable and in good alignment.
   g. Buckled or tied the straps to the chair or to the movable part of the bed frame. Used a center-approved knot. If secured to the bed frame, the straps were secured at waist level out of the person's reach.
   h. Made sure the jacket was snug. Slid an open hand between the restraint and the person. Adjusted the restraint if it was too tight. Checked for snugness again.

Post-Procedure
15. Positioned the person as the nurse directed.
16. Provided for comfort
17. Placed the call light within the person's reach.
18. Raised or lowered bed rails. Followed the care plan and the manufacturer instructions for the restraint.
19. Unscreened the person.
20. Completed a safety check of the room.
21. Decontaminated your hands.
22. Checked the person and the restraint at least every 15 minutes. Reported and recorded your observations:
   a. For wrist and mitt restraints: checked the pulse, color, and temperature of the restrained parts.
   b. For vest, jacket, and belt restraints: checked the person's breathing. *Called for the nurse at once if the person was not breathing or was having problems breathing.* Made sure the restraint was properly positioned in the front and back.
23. Did the following at least every 2 hours:
   a. Removed or released the restraint.
   b. Measured vital signs.
   c. Repositioned the person.
   d. Met food, fluid, hygiene, and elimination needs.

Date of Satisfactory Completion _____   Instructor's Initials _____

	S	U	Comments
Post-Procedure—cont'd			
e. Gave skin care.	___	___	_____
f. Performed range-of-motion exercises or helped the person walk. Followed the care plan.	___	___	_____
g. Provided for physical and emotional comfort.	___	___	_____
h. Reapplied the restraints.	___	___	_____
24. Completed a safety check of the room.	___	___	_____
25. Reported and recorded your observations and the care given.	___	___	_____

Date of Satisfactory Completion _____ Instructor's Initials _____

NNAAP™ Skill   CD-ROM   VIDEO   **Hand Washing**

Name: _____   Date: _____

Procedure

	S	U	Comments
1. Saw *Promoting Safety and Comfort: Hand Hygiene.*	___	___	_____
2. Made sure you had soap, paper towels, an orangewood stick or nail file, and a wastebasket. Collected missing items.	___	___	_____
3. Pushed your watch up your arm 4 to 5 inches. If your uniform sleeves were long, pushed them up.	___	___	_____
4. Stood away from the sink so your clothes did not touch the sink. Stood so the soap and faucet were easy to reach. Did not touch the inside of the sink at any time.	___	___	_____
5. Turned on and adjusted the water until it felt warm.			
6. Wet your wrists and hands. Kept your hands lower than your elbows. Was sure to wet the area 3 to 4 inches above your wrists.	___	___	_____
7. Applied about 1 teaspoon of soap to your hands.	___	___	_____
8. Rubbed your palms together and interlaced your fingers to work up a good lather. This step lasted at least 20 seconds or the amount of time required by your state competency test.	___	___	_____
9. Washed each hand and wrist thoroughly. Cleaned between the fingers.	___	___	_____
10. Cleaned under the fingernails. Rubbed your fingertips against your palms.	___	___	_____
11. Cleaned under fingernails with a nail file or orangewood stick. This step was done for the first hand washing of the day and when hands were highly soiled.	___	___	_____
12. Rinsed your wrists and hands well. Water flowed from the arms to the hands.	___	___	_____
13. Repeated, if needed:			
a. Applied about 1 teaspoon of soap to your hands.	___	___	_____
b. Rubbed your palms together and interlaced your fingers to work up a good lather. This step lasted at least 20 seconds or the amount of time required by your state competency test.	___	___	_____
c. Washed each hand and wrist thoroughly. Cleaned well between the fingers.	___	___	_____
d. Cleaned under the fingernails. Rubbed your fingertips against your palms.	___	___	_____
e. Cleaned under the fingernails with a nail file or orangewood stick. This step was done for the first hand washing of the day and when your hands were highly soiled.	___	___	_____
f. Rinsed your wrists and hands well. Water flowed from the arms to the hands.	___	___	_____
14. Dried your wrists and hands well with clean, dry paper towels. Patted dry. Started at fingertips.	___	___	_____
15. Discarded the paper towels in wastebasket.	___	___	_____
16. Turned off faucets with clean, dry paper towels. This prevented you from contaminating your hands. Used a clean paper towel for each faucet.	___	___	_____
17. Discarded the paper towels in the wastebasket.	___	___	_____

Date of Satisfactory Completion _____   Instructor's Initials _____

VIDEO CLIP   VIDEO   **Using an Alcohol-Based Hand Rub**

Name: _____   Date: _____

Procedure	S	U	Comments
1. Saw *Promoting Safety and Comfort: Hand Hygiene.*			
2. Applied the product to the palm of one hand. Follow the manufacturer instructions for the amount to use.			
3. Rubbed palms together in a circular manner.			
4. Interlaced fingers to spread hand rub on all surfaces of fingers.			
5. Rubbed tips of fingers up and down on palm of opposite hand.			
6. Coated surface of each thumb with hand rub.			
7. Rubbed fingertips in palm of opposite hand using circular motions.			
8. Continued rubbing in product until hands were dry (at least 15 seconds or followed to manufacturer recommendation). Did not use water or paper towels when using alcohol-based hand rubs.			
9. Applied hand lotion or cream after hand hygiene. Helped prevent the skin from chapping and drying.			

Date of Satisfactory Completion _____   Instructor's Initials _____

NNAAP™ Skill · CD-ROM · VIDEO CLIP · VIDEO · **Removing Gloves**

Name: _____   Date: _____

Procedure	S	U	Comments
1. Saw *Promoting Safety and Comfort: Gloves.*	___	___	_____
2. Made sure that glove touched only glove.	___	___	_____
3. Grasped a glove just below the cuff. Grasped it on the outside.	___	___	_____
4. Pulled the glove down over your hand so it was inside out.	___	___	_____
5. Held the removed glove with your other gloved hand.	___	___	_____
6. Reached inside the other glove. Used the first two fingers of the ungloved hand.	___	___	_____
7. Pulled the glove down (inside out) over your hand and the other glove.	___	___	_____
8. Discarded the gloves. Followed center policy.	___	___	_____
9. Decontaminated your hands.	___	___	_____

Date of Satisfactory Completion _____   Instructor's Initials _____

NNAAP™ Skill **CD-ROM** **VIDEO** **Donning and Removing a Gown**

Name: _____   Date: _____

Procedure	S	U	Comments
1. Removed your watch and all jewelry.	___	___	_____
2. Rolled up uniform sleeves.	___	___	_____
3. Practiced hand hygiene.	___	___	_____
4. Held a clean gown out in front of you. Allowed it to unfold. Did not shake the gown.	___	___	_____
5. Put your hands and arms through the sleeves.	___	___	_____
6. Made sure the gown covered you from your neck to your knees. It covered your arms to the end of your wrists.	___	___	_____
7. Tied the strings at the back of the neck.	___	___	_____
8. Overlapped the back of the gown. Made sure it covered your uniform. The gown was snug, not loose. (If gown did not cover your back, second gown was put on with the opening in the front.)	___	___	_____
9. Tied the waist strings. Tied them at the back or the side. Did not tie them in front.	___	___	_____
10. Put on other personal protective equipment (PPE).			
a. Mask or respirator, if needed.	___	___	_____
b. Goggles or face shield, if needed.	___	___	_____
c. Gloves. Made sure gloves covered the gown cuffs.	___	___	_____
11. Provided care.	___	___	_____
12. Removed and discarded the gloves.	___	___	_____
13. Removed and discarded the goggles or face shield if worn.	___	___	_____
14. Removed the gown. Did not touch the outside of the gown.			
a. Untied the neck and waist strings.	___	___	_____
b. Pulled the gown down from each shoulder toward the same hand.	___	___	_____
c. Turned the gown inside out as it was removed. Held it at the inside shoulder seams and brought your hands together.	___	___	_____
15. Held and rolled up the gown away from you. Kept it inside out.	___	___	_____
16. Discarded the gown.	___	___	_____
17. Removed and discarded the mask if worn.	___	___	_____
18. Decontaminated your hands.	___	___	_____

Date of Satisfactory Completion _____   Instructor's Initials _____

VIDEO **Donning and Removing a Mask**

Name: _____   Date: _____

Procedure	S	U	Comments
1. Practiced hand hygiene.	___	___	___
2. Put on a gown if required.	___	___	___
3. Picked up a mask by its upper ties. Did not touch the part that covers your face.	___	___	___
4. Placed the mask over your nose and mouth.	___	___	___
5. Placed the upper strings above your ears. Tied them at the back in the middle of your head.	___	___	___
6. Tied the lower strings at the back of your neck. The lower part of the mask was under your chin.	___	___	___
7. Pinched the metal band around your nose. The top of the mask was snug over your nose. If you were wearing eyeglasses, the mask was snug under the bottom of the eyeglasses.	___	___	___
8. Made sure the mask was snug over your face and under your chin.	___	___	___
9. Put on goggles or a face shield if needed and not part of the mask.	___	___	___
10. Put on gloves.	___	___	___
11. Provided care. Avoided coughing, sneezing, and unnecessary talking.	___	___	___
12. Changed the mask if it became wet or contaminated.	___	___	___
13. Removed the mask.			
a. Removed the gloves.	___	___	___
b. Removed the goggles or face shield and gown if worn.	___	___	___
c. Untied the lower strings of the mask.	___	___	___
d. Untied the top strings.	___	___	___
e. Held the top strings. Removed the mask.	___	___	___
14. Discarded the mask.	___	___	___
15. Decontaminated your hands.	___	___	___

Date of Satisfactory Completion _____   Instructor's Initials _____

Sterile Gloving

Name: _____   Date: _____

Procedure	S	U	Comments
1. Followed *Delegation Guidelines: Assisting With Sterile Procedures*. Saw *Promoting Safety and Comfort:*			
a. *Assisting With Sterile Procedures*	____	____	_____
b. *Sterile Gloving*	____	____	_____
2. Practiced hand hygiene.	____	____	_____
3. Inspected the package of sterile gloves for sterility.	____	____	_____
a. Checked the expiration date.	____	____	_____
b. Saw if the package was dry.	____	____	_____
c. Checked for tears, holes, punctures, and watermarks.	____	____	_____
4. Arranged a work surface.	____	____	_____
a. Made sure you had enough room.	____	____	_____
b. Arranged the work surface at waist level and within your vision.	____	____	_____
c. Cleaned and dried the work surface.	____	____	_____
d. Did not reach over or turn your back on the work surface.	____	____	_____
5. Opened the package. Grasped the flaps. Gently peeled them back.	____	____	_____
6. Removed the inner package. Placed it on the work surface.	____	____	_____
7. Read the manufacturer instructions on the inner package. It may be labeled with *left*, *right*, *up*, and *down*.	____	____	_____
8. Arranged the inner package for left, right, up, and down. The left glove was on your left. The right glove was on your right. The cuffs were near you with the fingers pointing away from you.	____	____	_____
9. Grasped the folded edges of the inner package. Used the thumb and index finger of each hand.	____	____	_____
10. Folded back the inner package to expose the gloves. Did not touch or otherwise contaminate the inside of the package or the gloves. The inside of the inner package is a sterile field.	____	____	_____
11. Noted that each glove had a cuff about 2 to 3 inches wide. The cuffs and insides of the gloves are *not considered sterile*.	____	____	_____
12. Put on the right glove, if you are right-handed. Put on the left glove, if you are left-handed.			
a. Picked up the glove with your other hand. Used your thumb, index, and middle fingers.	____	____	_____
b. Touched only the cuff and inside of the glove.	____	____	_____
c. Turned the hand to be gloved palm side up.	____	____	_____
d. Lifted the cuff up. Slid your fingers and hand into the glove.	____	____	_____
e. Pulled the glove up over your hand. If some fingers got stuck, left them that way until the other glove was on. *Did not use your ungloved hand to straighten the glove. Did not let the outside of the glove touch any non-sterile surface.*			
f. Left the cuff turned down.	____	____	_____

Date of Satisfactory Completion _____   Instructor's Initials _____

Procedure—cont'd

	S	U	Comments
13. Put on the other glove. Used your gloved hand.			
a. Reached under the cuff of the second glove. Used the four fingers of your gloved hand. Kept your gloved thumb close to your gloved palm.	_____	_____	_____
b. Pulled on the second glove. Your gloved hand did not touch the cuff or any surface. Held the thumb of your first gloved hand away from the gloved palm.	_____	_____	_____
14. Adjusted each glove with the other hand. The gloves were smooth and comfortable.	_____	_____	_____
15. Slid your fingers under the cuffs to pull them up.	_____	_____	_____
16. Touched only sterile items.	_____	_____	_____
17. Removed the gloves.	_____	_____	_____
18. Decontaminated your hands.	_____	_____	_____

Date of Satisfactory Completion _____   Instructor's Initials _____

Raising the Person's Head and Shoulders

Name: _____   Date: _____

	S	U	Comments

Quality of Life
Remembered to:
- Knock before entering the person's room
- Address the person by name
- Introduce yourself by name and title
- Explain the procedure to the person before beginning and during the procedure
- Protect the person's rights during the procedure
- Handle the person gently during the procedure

Pre-Procedure
1. Followed Delegation Guidelines:
   a. *Preventing Work-Related Injuries*
   b. *Moving Persons in Bed*
   Saw *Promoting Safety and Comfort:*
   a. *Safe Resident Handling, Moving, and Transfers*
   b. *Preventing Work-Related Injuries*
2. Asked a co-worker to assist if needed help.
3. Practiced hand hygiene.
4. Identified the person. Checked the identification (ID) bracelet against the assignment sheet. Called the person by name.
5. Provided for privacy.
6. Locked the bed wheels.
7. Raised the bed for body mechanics. Bed rails were up if used.

Procedure
8. Asked your co-worker to stand on the other side of the bed. Lowered the bed rail if up.
9. Asked the person to put the near arm under your near arm and behind your shoulder. His or her hand rested on top of your shoulder. If you stood on the right side, the person's right hand rested on your shoulder. The person did the same with your co-worker. The person's left hand rested on your co-worker's left shoulder.
10. Put your arm nearest to the person under his or her arm. Your hand was on the person's shoulder. Your co-worker did the same.
11. Put your free arm under the person's neck and shoulders. Your co-worker did the same. Supported the neck.
12. Helped the person raise to a sitting or semi-sitting position on the "count of 3."
13. Used the arm and hand that supported the person's neck and shoulders to give care. Your co-worker supported the person.
14. Helped the person lie down. Provided support with your locked arm. Supported the person's neck and shoulders with your other arm. Your co-worker did the same.

Date of Satisfactory Completion _____   Instructor's Initials _____

Post-Procedure

	S	U	Comments
15. Provided for comfort.	___	___	_____
16. Placed the call light within reach.	___	___	_____
17. Lowered the bed to its lowest position.	___	___	_____
18. Raised or lowered bed rails. Followed the care plan.	___	___	_____
19. Unscreened the person.	___	___	_____
20. Completed a safety check of the room.	___	___	_____
21. Decontaminated your hands.	___	___	_____
22. Reported and recorded your observations.	___	___	_____

Date of Satisfactory Completion _____   Instructor's Initials _____

VIDEO   **Moving the Person up in Bed**

Name: _____   Date: _____

	S	U	Comments
Quality of Life			
Remembered to:			
• Knock before entering the person's room	___	___	_____
• Address the person by name	___	___	_____
• Introduce yourself by name and title	___	___	_____
• Explain the procedure to the person before beginning and during the procedure	___	___	_____
• Protect the person's rights during the procedure	___	___	_____
• Handle the person gently during the procedure	___	___	_____

Pre-Procedure

1. Followed *Delegation Guidelines:*
   a. *Preventing Work-Related Injuries*   ___ ___ _____
   b. *Moving Persons in Bed*   ___ ___ _____
   Saw *Promoting Safety and Comfort:*
   a. *Safe Resident Handling, Moving, and Transfers*   ___ ___ _____
   b. *Preventing Work-Related Injuries*   ___ ___ _____
   c. *Moving the Person Up in Bed*   ___ ___ _____
2. Asked a co-worker to help you.   ___ ___ _____
3. Practiced hand hygiene.   ___ ___ _____
4. Identified the person. Checked the identification (ID) bracelet against the assignment sheet.
   Called the person by name.   ___ ___ _____
5. Provided for privacy.   ___ ___ _____
6. Locked the bed wheels.   ___ ___ _____
7. Raised the bed for body mechanics. Bed rails were up if used.   ___ ___ _____

Procedure

8. Lowered the head of the bed to a level appropriate for the person. It was as flat as possible.   ___ ___ _____
9. Stood on one side of the bed. Your co-worker stood on the other side.   ___ ___ _____
10. Lowered the bed rails if up.   ___ ___ _____
11. Removed pillows as directed by the nurse. Placed a pillow upright against the head-board if the person could be without it.   ___ ___ _____
12. Stood with a wide base of support. Pointed the foot near the head of the bed toward the head of the bed. Faced the head of the bed.   ___ ___ _____
13. Bent your hips and knees. Kept your back straight.   ___ ___ _____
14. Placed one arm under the person's shoulders and one arm under the thighs. Your co-worker did the same. Grasped each other's forearms.   ___ ___ _____
15. Asked the person to grasp the trapeze.   ___ ___ _____
16. Had the person flex both knees.   ___ ___ _____
17. Explained the following:
    a. You will count "1, 2, 3."   ___ ___ _____
    b. The move will be on "3."   ___ ___ _____
    c. On "3," the person will push against the bed with their feet if able. And the person will pull up with the trapeze.   ___ ___ _____

Date of Satisfactory Completion _____   Instructor's Initials _____

Procedure—cont'd	S	U	Comments

18. Moved the person to the head of the bed on the count of "3." Shifted your weight from your rear leg to your front leg. Your co-worker did the same.

19. Repeated steps 12 through 18 if necessary.
    a. Stood with a wide base of support. Pointed the foot near the head of the bed toward the head of the bed. Faced the head of the bed.
    b. Bent your hips and knees. Kept your back straight.
    c. Placed one arm under the person's shoulder and one arm under the thighs. Your co-worker did the same. Grasped each other's forearms.
    d. Asked the person to grasp the trapeze.
    e. Had the person flex both knees.
    f. Explained the following:
        i. You will count "1, 2, 3."
        ii. The move will be on "3."
        iii. On "3," the person will push against the bed with the feet if able. And the person will pull up with the trapeze.
    g. Moved the person to the head of the bed on the count of "3." Shifted your weight from your rear leg to your front leg. Your co-worker did the same.

Post-Procedure

20. Put the pillow under the person's head and shoulders. Straightened linens.

21. Positioned the person in good alignment. Raised the head of the bed to a level appropriate for the person.

22. Provided for comfort.

23. Placed the call light within reach.

24. Lowered the bed to its lowest position.

25. Raised or lowered bed rails. Followed the care plan.

26. Unscreened the person.

27. Completed a safety check of the room.

28. Decontaminated your hands.

29. Reported and recorded your observations.

Date of Satisfactory Completion _____   Instructor's Initials _____

VIDEO CLIP **VIDEO** **Moving the Person up in Bed with an Assist Device**

Name: _____   Date: _____

Quality of Life	S	U	Comments
Remembered to:			
• Knock before entering the person's room	___	___	_____
• Address the person by name	___	___	_____
• Introduce yourself by name and title	___	___	_____
• Explain the procedure to the person before beginning and during the procedure	___	___	_____
• Protect the person's rights during the procedure	___	___	_____
• Handle the person gently during the procedure	___	___	_____

Pre-Procedure

	S	U	Comments
1. Followed *Delegation Guidelines:*			
a. *Preventing Work-Related Injuries*	___	___	_____
b. *Moving Persons in Bed*	___	___	_____
Saw *Promoting Safety and Comfort:*			
a. *Safe Resident Handling, Moving, and Transfers*	___	___	_____
b. *Preventing Work-Related Injuries*	___	___	_____
c. *Moving the Person Up in Bed*	___	___	_____
d. *Moving the Person Up in Bed With an Assist Device*	___	___	_____
2. Asked a co-worker to help you.	___	___	_____
3. Practiced hand hygiene.	___	___	_____
4. Identified the person. Checked the identification (ID) bracelet against the assignment sheet. Called the person by name.	___	___	_____
5. Provided for privacy.	___	___	_____
6. Locked the bed wheels.	___	___	_____
7. Raised the bed for body mechanics. Bed rails were up if used.	___	___	_____

Procedure

	S	U	Comments
8. Lowered the head of the bed to a level appropriate for the person. It was as flat as possible.	___	___	_____
9. Stood on one side of the bed. Your co-worker stood on the other side.	___	___	_____
10. Lowered the bed rails if up.	___	___	_____
11. Removed pillows as directed by the nurse. Placed a pillow upright against the head-board if the person could be without it.	___	___	_____
12. Stood with a wide base of support. Pointed the foot near the head of the bed toward the head of the bed. Faced that direction.	___	___	_____
13. Rolled the sides of the assist device up close to the person. (NOTE: Omitted this step if the device had handles.)	___	___	_____
14. Grasped the rolled-up assist device firmly near the person's shoulders and hips. Or grasped it by the handles. Supported the head.	___	___	_____
15. Bent your hips and knees.	___	___	_____
16. Moved the person up in bed on the count of "3." Shifted your weight from your rear leg to your front leg.	___	___	_____

Date of Satisfactory Completion _____   Instructor's Initials _____

	S	U	Comments

Procedure—cont'd

17. Repeated steps 12 through 16 if necessary.
    a. Stood with a wide base of support. Pointed the foot near the head of the bed toward the head of the bed. Faced that direction.
    b. Rolled the sides of the assist device up close to the person. (NOTE: Omitted this step if the device had handles.)
    c. Grasped the rolled-up assist device firmly near the person's shoulders and hips. Or grasped it by the handles.
    d. Bent your hips and knees.
    e. Moved the person up in bed on the count of "3." Shifted your weight from your rear leg to your front leg.
18. Unrolled the assist device. (NOTE: Omitted this step if the device had handles.)

Post-Procedure

19. Put the pillow under the person's head and shoulders.
20. Positioned the person in good alignment. Raised the head of the bed to a level appropriate for the person
21. Provided for comfort.
22. Placed the call light within reach.
23. Lowered the bed to its lowest position.
24. Raised or lowered bed rails. Followed the care plan.
25. Unscreened the person.
26. Completed a safety check of the room.
27. Decontaminated your hands.
28. Reported and recorded your observations.

Date of Satisfactory Completion _____   Instructor's Initials _____

VIDEO   **Moving the Person to the Side of the Bed**

Name: _____   Date: _____

	S	U	Comments

Quality of Life

Remembered to:

- Knock before entering the person's room
- Address the person by name
- Introduce yourself by name and title
- Explain the procedure to the person before beginning and during the procedure
- Protect the person's rights during the procedure
- Handle the person gently during the procedure

Pre-Procedure

1. Followed *Delegation Guidelines:*
   a. *Preventing Work-Related Injuries*
   b. *Moving Persons in Bed*
   Saw *Promoting Safety and Comfort:*
   a. *Safe Resident Handling, Moving, and Transfers*
   b. *Preventing Work-Related Injuries*
   c. *Moving the Person to the Side of the Bed*
2. Asked a co-worker to assist if using an assist device.
3. Practiced hand hygiene.
4. Identified the person. Checked the identification (ID) bracelet against the assignment sheet. Called the person by name.
5. Provided for privacy.
6. Locked the bed wheels.
7. Raised the bed for body mechanics. Bed rails were up if used.

Procedure

8. Lowered the head of the bed to a level appropriate for the person. It was as flat as possible.
9. Stood on the side of the bed to which the person was moved.
10. Lowered the bed rails if bed rails were used. (Both bed rails were lowered for step 15).
11. Removed pillows as directed by the nurse.
12. Stood with your feet about 12 inches apart. One foot was in front of the other. Flexed your knees.
13. Crossed the person's arms over his or her chest.
14. *Method 1: Moving the person in segments:*
    (If back or spinal injury, did not use this method.)
    a. Placed your arm under the person's neck and shoulders. Grasped the far shoulder.
    b. Placed your other arm under the mid-back.
    c. Moved the upper part of the person's body toward you. Rocked backward and shifted your weight to your rear leg.
    d. Placed one arm under the person's waist and one under the thighs.
    e. Rocked backward to move the lower part of the person toward you.

Date of Satisfactory Completion _____   Instructor's Initials _____

Procedure—cont'd	S	U	Comments

Procedure—cont'd

    f. Repeated the procedure for the legs and feet.
       Your arms were under the person's thighs and calves.

15. *Method 2: Moving the person with a drawsheet:*

    a. Rolled up the drawsheet close to the person.

    b. Grasped the rolled-up drawsheet near the person's
       shoulders and hips. Your co-worker did the same.
       Supported the person's head.

    c. Rocked backward on the count of "3" and moved
       the person toward you. Your co-worker rocked
       backward slightly and then forward toward you
       with arms kept straight.

    d. Unrolled the drawsheet. Removed any wrinkles.

Post-Procedure

16. Positioned the person in good alignment.

17. Provided for comfort.

18. Placed the call light within reach.

19. Lowered the bed to its lowest position.

20. Raised or lowered bed rails. Followed the care plan.

21. Unscreened the person.

22. Completed a safety check of the room.

23. Decontaminated your hands.

24. Reported and recorded your observations.

Date of Satisfactory Completion _____   Instructor's Initials _____

NNAAP™ Skill   CD-ROM   VIDEO CLIP   VIDEO   **Turning and Repositioning the Person**

Name: _____   Date: _____

	S	U	Comments
Quality of Life			
Remembered to:			
• Knock before entering the person's room	___	___	_____
• Address the person by name	___	___	_____
• Introduce yourself by name and title	___	___	_____
• Explain the procedure to the person before beginning and during the procedure	___	___	_____
• Protect the person's rights during the procedure	___	___	_____
• Handle the person gently during the procedure	___	___	_____
Pre-Procedure			
1. Followed *Delegation Guidelines:*			
a. *Preventing Work-Related Injuries*	___	___	_____
b. *Moving Persons in Bed*	___	___	_____
c. *Turning Persons*			
Saw *Promoting Safety and Comfort:*			
a. *Safe Resident Handling, Moving, and Transfers*	___	___	_____
b. *Preventing Work-Related Injuries*	___	___	_____
c. *Moving the Person to the Side of the Bed*	___	___	_____
d. *Turning Persons*	___	___	_____
2. Practiced hand hygiene.	___	___	_____
3. Identified the person. Checked the identification (ID) bracelet against the assignment sheet. Called the person by name.			
4. Provided for privacy.	___	___	_____
5. Locked the bed wheels.	___	___	_____
6. Raised the bed for body mechanics. Bed rails were up.	___	___	_____
Procedure			
7. Lowered the head of the bed to a level appropriate for the person. It was as flat as possible.	___	___	_____
8. Stood on the side of the bed opposite to where you turned the person.	___	___	_____
9. Lowered the bed rails near you.	___	___	_____
10. Moved the person to the side near you.	___	___	_____
11. Crossed the person's arms over his or her chest. Crossed the leg near you over the far leg.	___	___	_____
12. *Turned the person away from you:*			
a. Stood with a wide base of support. Flexed the knees.	___	___	_____
b. Placed one hand on the person's shoulder. Placed the other on the hip near you.	___	___	_____
c. Rolled the person gently away from you toward the raised bed rail. Shifted your weight from your rear leg to your front leg.	___	___	_____
13. *Turned the person toward you:*			
a. Raised the bed rail.	___	___	_____
b. Went to the other side of the bed. Lowered the bed rail.	___	___	_____
c. Stood with a wide base of support. Flexed your knees.	___	___	_____
d. Placed one hand on the person's far shoulder. Placed the other on the far hip.	___	___	_____
e. Rolled the person toward you gently.	___	___	_____

Date of Satisfactory Completion _____   Instructor's Initials _____

Procedure—cont'd	S	U	Comments
14. Positioned the person. Followed the nurse's directions, the care plan, and these common measures:			
a. Placed a pillow under the head and neck.	_____	_____	_____
b. Adjusted the shoulder. The person did not lie on an arm.	_____	_____	_____
c. Placed a pillow under the upper hand and arm.	_____	_____	_____
d. Positioned a pillow against the back.	_____	_____	_____
e. Flexed the upper knee. Positioned the upper leg in front of the lower leg.	_____	_____	_____
f. Supported the upper leg and thigh on pillows. Made sure the ankle was supported.	_____	_____	_____

Post-Procedure

	S	U	Comments
15. Provided for comfort.	_____	_____	_____
16. Placed the call light within reach.	_____	_____	_____
17. Lowered the bed to its lowest position.	_____	_____	_____
18. Raised or lowered bed rails. Followed the care plan.	_____	_____	_____
19. Unscreened the person.	_____	_____	_____
20. Completed a safety check of the room.	_____	_____	_____
21. Decontaminated your hands.	_____	_____	_____
22. Reported and recorded your observations.	_____	_____	_____

Date of Satisfactory Completion _____ Instructor's Initials _____

VIDEO Logrolling the Person

Name: _____   Date: _____

Quality of Life	S	U	Comments

Remembered to:

- Knock before entering the person's room
- Address the person by name
- Introduce yourself by name and title
- Explain the procedure to the person before beginning and during the procedure
- Protect the person's rights during the procedure
- Handle the person gently during the procedure

Pre-Procedure

1. Followed *Delegation Guidelines:*
   a. *Preventing Work-Related Injuries*
   b. *Moving Persons in Bed*
   c. *Turning Persons*
   Saw *Promoting Safety and Comfort:*
   a. *Safe Resident Handling, Moving, and Transfers*
   b. *Preventing Work-Related Injuries*
   c. *Turning Persons*
   d. *Logrolling*
2. Asked a co-worker to help you.
3. Practiced hand hygiene.
4. Identified the person. Checked the identification (ID) bracelet against the assignment sheet. Called the person by name.
5. Provided for privacy.
6. Locked the bed wheels.
7. Raised the bed for body mechanics. Bed rails were up if used.

Procedure

8. Made sure the bed was flat.
9. Stood on the side opposite to which you turned the person. Your co-worker stood on the other side.
10. Lowered the bed rails if used.
11. Moved the person as a unit to the side of the bed near you. Used the assist device. (If spinal cord injury, assisted the nurse as directed.)
12. Placed the person's arms across the chest. Placed a pillow between the knees.
13. Raised the bed rail if used.
14. Went to the other side.
15. Stood near the shoulders and chest. Your co-worker stood near the hips and thighs.
16. Stood with a broad base of support. One foot was in front of the other.
17. Asked the person to hold his or her body rigid.
18. Rolled the person toward you. Or used the assist device. Turned the person as a unit.

Date of Satisfactory Completion _____   Instructor's Initials _____

Procedure—cont'd	S	U	Comments

19. Positioned the person in good alignment. Used
pillows as directed by the nurse and the care plan.
Followed these common measures (unless the
spinal cord was involved):
   a. One pillow against the back for support.
   b. One pillow under the head and neck if allowed.
   c. One pillow or a folded bath blanket between the legs.
   d. A small pillow under the upper arm and hand.

Post-Procedure

20. Provided for comfort.
21. Placed the call light within reach.
22. Lowered the bed to its lowest position.
23. Raised or lowered bed rails.
   Followed the care plan.
24. Unscreened the person.
25. Completed a safety check of the room.
26. Decontaminated your hands.
27. Reported and recorded your observations.

Date of Satisfactory Completion _____   Instructor's Initials _____

Sitting on the Side of the Bed (Dangling)

Name: _____   Date: _____

Quality of Life	S	U	Comments
Remembered to:			
• Knock before entering the person's room	_____	_____	_____
• Address the person by name	_____	_____	_____
• Introduce yourself by name and title	_____	_____	_____
• Explain the procedure to the person before beginning and during the procedure	_____	_____	_____
• Protect the person's rights during the procedure	_____	_____	_____
• Handle the person gently during the procedure	_____	_____	_____

Pre-Procedure

	S	U	Comments
1. Followed *Delegation Guidelines:*			
a. *Preventing Work-Related Injuries*	_____	_____	_____
b. *Dangling*	_____	_____	_____
Saw *Promoting Safety and Comfort:*			
a. *Safe Resident Handling, Moving, and Transfers*	_____	_____	_____
b. *Preventing Work-Related Injuries*	_____	_____	_____
c. *Dangling*	_____	_____	_____
2. Asked a co-worker to help you.	_____	_____	_____
3. Practiced hand hygiene.	_____	_____	_____
4. Identified the person. Checked the identification (ID) bracelet against the assignment sheet. Called the person by name.	_____	_____	_____
5. Provided for privacy.	_____	_____	_____
6. Decided what side of the bed to use.	_____	_____	_____
7. Moved furniture to provide moving space.	_____	_____	_____
8. Locked the bed wheels.	_____	_____	_____
9. Raised the bed for body mechanics. Bed rails were up if used.	_____	_____	_____

Procedure

	S	U	Comments
10. Lowered the bed rail if up.	_____	_____	_____
11. Positioned the person in a side-lying position facing you. The person lay on the strong side.	_____	_____	_____
12. Raised the head of the bed to a sitting position.	_____	_____	_____
13. Stood by the person's hips. Faced the foot of the bed.	_____	_____	_____
14. Stood with your feet apart. The foot near the head of the bed was in front of the other foot.	_____	_____	_____
15. Slid one arm under the person's neck and shoulders. Grasped the far shoulder. Placed your other hand over the thighs near the knees.	_____	_____	_____
16. Pivoted toward the foot of the bed while moving the person's legs and feet over the side of the bed. As the legs went over the edge of the mattress, the trunk was upright.	_____	_____	_____
17. Asked the person to hold on to the edge of the mattress. This supported the person in the sitting position. Raised half-length rail, if possible, for person to grasp on strong side. Co-worker supported person at all times.	_____	_____	_____
18. Did not leave the person alone. Provided support at all times.	_____	_____	_____

Date of Satisfactory Completion _____   Instructor's Initials _____

Procedure—cont'd	S	U	Comments
19. Checked the person's condition:			
a. Asked how the person felt. Asked if the person felt dizzy or light-headed.	———	———	———————
b. Checked pulse and respiration.	———	———	———————
c. Checked for difficulty breathing.	———	———	———————
d. Noted if the skin was pale or bluish in color (*cyanosis*).	———	———	———————
20. Reversed the procedure to return the person to bed. (Or prepared to transfer the person to a chair or wheelchair. Lowered the bed to its lowest position so the person's feet were flat on the floor. Supported the person at all times.)	———	———	———————
21. Lowered the head of the bed after the person returned to bed. Helped him or her move to the center of the bed.	———	———	———————
22. Positioned the person in good alignment.	———	———	———————
Post-Procedure			
23. Provided for comfort.	———	———	———————
24. Placed the call light within reach.	———	———	———————
25. Lowered the bed to its lowest position.	———	———	———————
26. Raised or lowered bed rails. Followed the care plan.	———	———	———————
27. Returned furniture to its proper place.	———	———	———————
28. Unscreened the person.	———	———	———————
29. Completed a safety check of the room.	———	———	———————
30. Decontaminated your hands.	———	———	———————
31. Reported and recorded your observations.	———	———	———————

Date of Satisfactory Completion _____   Instructor's Initials _____

| NNAAP™ Skill | CD-ROM | VIDEO CLIP | VIDEO | **Transferring a Person to a Chair or Wheelchair** |

Name: _____   Date: _____

	S	U	Comments
Quality of Life			
Remembered to:			
• Knock before entering the person's room	____	____	_____
• Address the person by name	____	____	_____
• Introduce yourself by name and title	____	____	_____
• Explain the procedure to the person before beginning and during the procedure	____	____	_____
• Protect the person's rights during the procedure	____	____	_____
• Handle the person gently during the procedure	____	____	_____
Pre-Procedure			
1. Followed *Delegation Guidelines:*			
a. *Preventing Work-Related Injuries*	____	____	_____
b. *Transferring Persons*	____	____	_____
Saw *Promoting Safety and Comfort:*			
a. *Transfer/Gait Belts*	____	____	_____
b. *Safe Resident Handling, Moving, and Transfers*	____	____	_____
c. *Preventing Work-Related Injuries*	____	____	_____
d. *Transferring Persons*	____	____	_____
e. *Bed to Chair or Wheelchair Transfers*	____	____	_____
2. Collected:			
a. Wheelchair or arm chair	____	____	_____
b. Bath blanket	____	____	_____
c. Lap blanket	____	____	_____
d. Robe and non-skid footwear	____	____	_____
e. Paper or sheet	____	____	_____
f. Transfer belt (if needed)	____	____	_____
g. Seat cushion (if needed)	____	____	_____
3. Practiced hand hygiene.			
4. Identified the person. Checked the identification (ID) bracelet against the assignment sheet. Called the person by name.	____	____	_____
5. Provided for privacy.	____	____	_____
6. Decided what side of the bed to use. Moved furniture for a safe transfer.	____	____	_____
Procedure			
7. Positioned the chair:			
a. The chair was near the head of bed on the person's strong side.	____	____	_____
b. The chair faced the foot of the bed.	____	____	_____
c. The arm of the chair almost touched the bed.	____	____	_____
8. Placed a folded bath blanket or cushion on the seat (if needed).	____	____	_____
9. Locked the wheelchair wheels. Raised the footplates. Removed or swung the front rigging out of the way.	____	____	_____
10. Lowered the bed to its lowest position. Locked the bed wheels.	____	____	_____
11. Fan-folded top linens to the foot of the bed.	____	____	_____

Date of Satisfactory Completion _____   Instructor's Initials _____

Procedure—cont'd	S	U	Comments

12. Placed the paper or sheet under the person's feet. Put footwear on the person.

13. Helped the person sit on the side of bed. His or her feet touched the floor.

14. Helped the person put on a robe.

15. Applied the transfer belt if needed.

16. *Method 1: Using a transfer belt:*
  a. Stood in front of the person.
  b. Had the person hold on to the mattress.
  c. Made sure the person's feet were flat on the floor.
  d. Had the person lean forward.
  e. Grasped the transfer belt at each side. Grasped the handles or grasped the belt from underneath.
  f. Prevented the person from sliding or falling by doing one of the following:
    1. Braced your knees against the person's knees. Blocked his or her feet with your feet.
    2. Used the knee and foot of one leg to block the person's weak leg or foot. Placed your other foot slightly behind your own for balance.
    3. Straddled your legs around the person's weak leg.
  g. Explained the following:
    1. You will count "1, 2, 3."
    2. The move will be on "3."
    3. On "3," the person pushes down on the mattress and stands.
  h. Asked the person to push down on the mattress and stand on the count of "3." Pulled the person to a standing position as you straightened your knees.

17. *Method 2: No transfer belt:* (NOTE: Used this method only if directed by the nurse and the care plan.)
  a. Followed steps 16, a–c
    1. Stood in front of the person.
    2. Had the person hold on to the mattress.
    3. Made sure the person's feet were flat on the floor.
  b. Placed your hands under the person's arms. Your hands were around the person's shoulder blades.
  c. Had the person lean forward.
  d. Prevented the person from sliding or falling by doing one of the following:
    1. Braced your knees against the person's knees. Blocked his or her feet with your feet.
    2. Used the knee and foot of one leg to block the person's weak leg or foot. Placed your other foot slightly behind you for balance.
    3. Straddled your legs around the person's weak leg.
  e. Explained the "count of 3."
    1. You will count "1, 2, 3."
    2. The move will be on "3."
    3. On "3," the person pushes down on the mattress and stands.
  f. Asked the person to push down on the mattress and stand on the count of "3." Pulled the person to a standing position as you straightened your knees.

Date of Satisfactory Completion _____   Instructor's Initials _____

Procedure—cont'd	S	U	Comments
18. Supported the person in the standing position. Held the transfer belt, or kept hands around the person's shoulder blades. Continued to prevent the person from sliding or falling.			
19. Turned the person so he or she could grasp the far arm of the chair. The legs touched the edge of the chair.			
20. Continued to turn the person until the other armrest was grasped.			
21. Lowered the person into the chair as you bent your hips and knees. The person assisted by leaning forward and bending his or her elbows and knees.			
22. Made sure the person's hips were to the back of the seat. Positioned person in good alignment.			
23. Attached the wheelchair front rigging. Positioned the person's feet on the wheelchair footplates.			
24. Covered the person's lap and legs with a lap blanket. Kept the blanket off the floor and the wheels.			
25. Removed the transfer belt if used.			
26. Positioned the chair as the person preferred. Locked the wheelchair wheels according to the care plan.			

Post-Procedure

	S	U	Comments
27. Provided for comfort.			
28. Placed the call light within reach.			
29. Unscreened the person.			
30. Completed a safety check of the room.			
31. Decontaminated your hands.			
32. Reported and recorded your observations.			

Date of Satisfactory Completion _____ Instructor's Initials _____

Transferring a Person from a Chair or Wheelchair to Bed

Name: _____   Date: _____

	S	U	Comments

Quality of Life

Remembered to:
- Knock before entering the person's room
- Address the person by name
- Introduce yourself by name and title
- Explain the procedure to the person before beginning and during the procedure
- Protect the person's rights during the procedure
- Handle the person gently during the procedure

Pre-Procedure
1. Followed *Delegation Guidelines:*
   a. *Preventing Work-Related Injuries*
   b. *Transferring Persons*
   Saw *Promoting Safety and Comfort:*
   a. *Transfer/Gait Belts*
   b. *Safe Resident Handling, Moving, and Transfers*
   c. *Preventing Work-Related Injuries*
   d. *Transferring Persons*
   e. Bed to Chair or Wheelchair Transfers
2. Collected a transfer belt if needed.
3. Practiced hand hygiene.
4. Identified the person. Checked the identification (ID) bracelet against the assignment sheet. Called the person by name.
5. Provided for privacy.

Procedure
6. Moved furniture for moving space.
7. Raised the head of the bed to a sitting position. The bed was in the lowest position.
8. Moved the call light so it was on the strong side for when the person was in bed.
9. Positioned the chair or wheelchair so the person's strong side was next to the bed. Had a co-worker help you if necessary.
10. Locked the wheelchair and the bed wheels.
11. Removed and folded the lap blanket.
12. Removed the person's feet from the footplates. Raised the footplates. Removed or swung the front rigging out of the way. (The person had on non-skid footwear.)
13. Applied the transfer belt (if needed).
14. Made sure the person's feet were flat on the floor.
15. Stood in front of the person.
16. Asked the person to hold on to the armrest. (If directed by the nurse, placed your hands under the person's arms and around the shoulder blades.)
17. Had the person lean forward.
18. Grasped the transfer belt on each side, if used. Grasped underneath the belt.

Date of Satisfactory Completion _____   Instructor's Initials _____

Procedure—cont'd	S	U	Comments

Procedure—cont'd

19. Prevented the person from sliding or falling by
doing one of the following:
   a. Braced your knees against the person's knees.
     Blocked his or her feet with your feet.
   b. Used the knee and foot of one leg to block the
     person's weak leg or foot. Placed your other foot
     slightly behind you for balance.
   c. Straddled your legs around the person's weak leg.
20. Explained the following:
   1. You will count "1, 2, 3."
   2. The move will be on "3."
   3. On "3," the person pushes down on the
     mattress and stands.
21. Asked the person to push down on the armrests on
the count of "3." Pulled the person to a standing
position as you straightened your knees.
22. Supported the person in the standing position.
Held the transfer belt, or kept hands around the
person's shoulder blades. Continued to
prevent the person from sliding or falling.
23. Turned the person so he or she could reach the edge
of the mattress. The person's legs touched the mattress.
24. Continued to turn the person until he or she reached
the mattress with both hands.
25. Lowered him or her to the bed as you bent your
hips and knees. The person assisted by leaning
forward and bending his or her elbows and knees.
26. Removed the transfer belt.
27. Removed the robe and footwear.
28. Helped the person lie down.

Post-Procedure

29. Provided for comfort.
30. Placed the call light and other needed items
within reach.
31. Raised or lowered bed rails. Followed the care plan.
32. Arranged furniture to meet the person's needs.
33. Unscreened the person.
34. Completed a safety check of the room.
35. Decontaminated your hands.
36. Reported and recorded your observations.

Date of Satisfactory Completion _____　Instructor's Initials _____

VIDEO CLIP   VIDEO   **Transferring the Person using a Mechanical Lift**

Name: _____   Date: _____

Quality of Life	S	U	Comments
Remembered to:			
• Knock before entering the person's room	___	___	_____
• Address the person by name	___	___	_____
• Introduce yourself by name and title	___	___	_____
• Explain the procedure to the person before beginning and during the procedure	___	___	_____
• Protect the person's rights during the procedure	___	___	_____
• Handle the person gently during the procedure	___	___	_____

Pre-Procedure

	S	U	Comments
1. Followed *Delegation Guidelines:*			
a. *Preventing Work-Related Injuries*	___	___	_____
b. *Transferring Persons*	___	___	_____
c. *Using Mechanical Lifts*	___	___	_____
Saw *Promoting Safety and Comfort:*			
a. *Safe Resident Handling, Moving, and Transfers*	___	___	_____
b. *Preventing Work-Related Injuries*	___	___	_____
c. *Transferring Persons*	___	___	_____
d. *Using Mechanical Lifts*	___	___	_____
2. Asked a co-worker to help you.	___	___	_____
3. Collected:			
a. Mechanical lift and sling	___	___	_____
b. Arm chair or wheelchair	___	___	_____
c. Footwear	___	___	_____
d. Bath blanket or cushion	___	___	_____
e. Lap blanket	___	___	_____
4. Practiced hand hygiene.	___	___	_____
5. Identified the person. Checked the identification (ID) bracelet against the assignment sheet. Called the person by name.	___	___	_____
6. Provided for privacy.	___	___	_____

Procedure

	S	U	Comments
7. Raised the bed for body mechanics. Bed rails were up if used.	___	___	_____
8. Lowered the head of the bed to a level appropriate for the person. It was as flat as possible.	___	___	_____
9. Stood on one side of the bed. Your co-worker stood on the other side.	___	___	_____
10. Lowered the bed rails if up.	___	___	_____
11. Centered the sling under the person. To position the sling, turned the person from side to side as if making an occupied bed. Positioned the sling according to the manufacturer instructions.	___	___	_____
12. Positioned the person in semi-Fowler's position.	___	___	_____
13. Placed the chair at the head of the bed. It was even with the head-board and about 1 foot away from the bed. Placed a folded bath blanket or cushion in the chair.	___	___	_____
14. Locked the bed wheels. Lowered the bed to its lowest position.	___	___	_____
15. Raised the lift so you could position it over the person.	___	___	_____

Date of Satisfactory Completion _____   Instructor's Initials _____

	S	U	Comments
Procedure—cont'd			
16. Positioned the lift over the person.	___	___	___
17. Locked the lift wheels in position.	___	___	___
18. Attached the sling to the sling hooks.	___	___	___
19. Raised the head of the bed to a sitting position.	___	___	___
20. Crossed the person's arms over the chest.	___	___	___
21. Raised the lift high enough until the person and the sling were free of the bed.	___	___	___
22. Had your co-worker support the person's legs as you moved the lift and the person away from the bed.	___	___	___
23. Positioned the lift so the person's back was toward the chair.	___	___	___
24. Positioned the chair so you could lower the person into it.	___	___	___
25. Lowered the person into the chair. Guided the person into the chair.	___	___	___
26. Lowered the spreader bar to unhook the sling. Removed the sling from under the person unless otherwise indicated.	___	___	___
27. Put footwear on the person. Positioned the person's feet on the wheelchair footplates.	___	___	___
28. Covered the person's lap and legs with a lap blanket. Kept it off the floor and wheels.	___	___	___
29. Positioned the chair as the person preferred. Locked the wheelchair wheels according to the care plan.	___	___	___
Post-Procedure			
30. Provided for comfort.	___	___	___
31. Placed the call light and other needed items within reach.	___	___	___
32. Unscreened the person.	___	___	___
33. Completed a safety check of the room.	___	___	___
34. Decontaminated your hands.	___	___	___
35. Reported and recorded your observations.	___	___	___
36. Reversed the procedure to return the person to bed.	___	___	___

Date of Satisfactory Completion _____   Instructor's Initials _____

Transferring the Person to and from the Toilet

Name: _____   Date: _____

	S	U	Comments
Quality of Life			
Remembered to:			
• Knock before entering the person's room	___	___	___
• Address the person by name	___	___	___
• Introduce yourself by name and title	___	___	___
• Explain the procedure to the person before beginning and during the procedure	___	___	___
• Protect the person's rights during the procedure	___	___	___
• Handle the person gently during the procedure	___	___	___

Pre-Procedure

1. Followed *Delegation Guidelines:*
   a. *Preventing Work-Related Injuries*
   b. *Transferring Persons*
   Saw *Promoting Safety and Comfort:*
   a. *Transfer/Gait Belts*
   b. *Safe Resident Handling, Moving, and Transfers*
   c. *Preventing Work-Related Injuries*
   d. *Transferring Persons*
   e. *Bed to Chair or Wheelchair Transfers*
   f. *Transferring the Person To and From the Toilet*
2. Practiced hand hygiene.

Procedure

3. Had the person wear non-skid footwear.
4. Positioned the wheelchair next to the toilet if there was enough room. If not, positioned the chair at a right angle (90 degrees) to the toilet. If possible, the person's strong side was near the toilet.
5. Locked the wheelchair wheels.
6. Raised the footplates. Removed or swung the front rigging out of the way.
7. Applied the transfer belt.
8. Helped the person unfasten clothing.
9. Used the transfer belt to help the person stand and turn to the toilet. The person used the grab bars to turn to the toilet.
10. Supported the person with the transfer belt while he or she lowered clothing. Or had the person hold on to the grab bars for support. Lowered the person's pants and undergarments.
11. Used the transfer belt to lower the person onto the toilet seat. Made sure he or she was properly positioned on the toilet.
12. Told the person you will stay nearby. Reminded the person to use the call light or call for you when help is needed. Stayed with the person if required by the care plan.
13. Closed the bathroom door to provide privacy.
14. Stayed near the bathroom. Completed other tasks in the person's room. Checked on the person every 5 minutes.
15. Knocked on the bathroom door when the person called for you.

Date of Satisfactory Completion _____   Instructor's Initials _____

	S	U	Comments
Procedure—cont'd			
16. Helped with wiping, perineal care, flushing, and hand washing as needed. Wore gloves and practiced hand hygiene after removing the gloves.			
17. Used the transfer belt to help the person stand.			
18. Helped the person raise and secure clothing.			
19. Used the transfer belt to transfer the person to the wheelchair.			
20. Made sure the person's buttocks were to the back of the seat. Positioned the person in good alignment.			
21. Positioned the person's feet on the footplates.			
22. Removed the transfer belt.			
23. Covered the person's lap and legs with a lap blanket. Kept the blanket off the floor and wheels.			
24. Positioned the chair as the person preferred. Locked the wheelchair wheels according to the care plan.			
Post-Procedure			
25. Provided for comfort.			
26. Placed the call light and other needed items within the person's reach.			
27. Unscreened the person.			
28. Completed a safety check of the room.			
29. Practiced hand hygiene.			
30. Reported and recorded your observations.			

Date of Satisfactory Completion _____   Instructor's Initials _____

VIDEO CLIP   VIDEO   **Moving the Person to a Stretcher**

Name: _____   Date: _____

	S	U	Comments

Quality of Life
Remembered to:
- Knock before entering the person's room
- Address the person by name
- Introduce yourself by name and title
- Explain the procedure to the person before beginning and during the procedure
- Protect the person's rights during the procedure
- Handle the person gently during the procedure

Pre-Procedure
1. Followed *Delegation Guidelines:*
   a. *Preventing Work-Related Injuries*
   b. *Transferring Persons*
   Saw *Promoting Safety and Comfort:*
   a. *Safe Resident Handling, Moving, and Transfers*
   b. *Preventing Work-Related Injuries*
   c. *Transferring Persons*
   d. *Moving the Person to a Stretcher*
2. Asked 1 or 2 staff members to help.
3. Collected:
   - Stretcher covered with a sheet or bath blanket
   - Bath blanket
   - Pillow(s) if needed
   - Slide sheet, slide board, drawsheet or other assist device
4. Practiced hand hygiene.
5. Identified the person. Checked the identification (ID) bracelet against the assignment sheet. Called the person by name.
6. Provided for privacy.
7. Raised the bed and stretcher for body mechanics.

Procedure
8. Positioned yourself and co-workers.
   a. One or two workers on the side of the bed where the stretcher was.
   b. One worker on the other side of the bed.
9. Lowered the head of the bed. It was as flat as possible.
10. Lowered the bed rails if used.
11. Covered the person with a bath blanket. Fan-folded top linens to the foot of the bed.
12. Positioned the assist device. Or loosened the drawsheet on each side.
13. Used the assist device to move the person to the side of the bed where the stretcher was.
14. Protected the person from falling. Held the far arm and leg.
15. Had your co-workers position the stretcher next to the bed. They stood behind the stretcher.
16. Locked the bed and stretcher wheels.
17. Grasped the assist device.
18. Transferred the person to the stretcher on the count of "3." Centered the person on the stretcher.

Date of Satisfactory Completion _____   Instructor's Initials _____

	S	U	Comments
Procedure—cont'd			
19. Placed a pillow or pillows under the person's head and shoulders if allowed. Raised the head of the stretcher if allowed.	———	———	———————
20. Covered the person. Provided privacy.	———	———	———————
21. Fastened the safety straps. Raised the side rails.	———	———	———————
22. Unlocked the stretcher wheels. Transported the person.	———	———	———————
Post-Procedure			
23. Decontaminated your hands.	———	———	———————
24. Reported and recorded:			
a. The time of the transport	———	———	———————
b. Where the person was transported to	———	———	———————
c. Who went with the person	———	———	———————
d. How the transfer was tolerated	———	———	———————
25. Reversed the procedure to return the person to bed.	———	———	———————

Date of Satisfactory Completion _____   Instructor's Initials _____

VIDEO CLIP   VIDEO   **Making a Closed Bed**

Name: _____   Date: _____

Quality of Life   S   U   **Comments**
Remembered to:
- Knock before entering the person's room   ____   ____   _____
- Address the person by name   ____   ____   _____
- Introduce yourself by name and title   ____   ____   _____
- Explain the procedure to the person before beginning   ____   ____   _____
  and during the procedure   ____   ____   _____
- Protect the person's rights during the procedure   ____   ____   _____
- Handle the person gently during the procedure   ____   ____   _____

Pre-Procedure
1. Followed *Delegation Guidelines:*
   Making Beds
   Saw *Promoting Safety and Comfort:*
   Making Beds   ____   ____   _____
2. Practiced hand hygiene.   ____   ____   _____
3. Collected clean linens: ____   ____   _____
   - Mattress pad (if needed)   ____   ____   _____
   - Bottom sheet (flat or fitted)   ____   ____   _____
   - Waterproof drawsheet or waterproof pad (if needed)   ____   ____   _____
   - Cotton drawsheet (if needed)   ____   ____   _____
   - Top sheet   ____   ____   _____
   - Blanket   ____   ____   _____
   - Bedspread   ____   ____   _____
   - Pillowcase for each pillow   ____   ____   _____
   - Bath towel(s)   ____   ____   _____
   - Hand towel   ____   ____   _____
   - Washcloth   ____   ____   _____
   - Gown or pajamas   ____   ____   _____
   - Bath blanket   ____   ____   _____
   - Gloves   ____   ____   _____
   - Laundry bag   ____   ____   _____
   - Paper towels if needed barrier for clean linens   ____   ____   _____
4. Placed linens on a clean surface. Used paper towels   ____   ____   _____
   as a barrier between the clean surface and clean
   linens if center policy.
5. Raised the bed for body mechanics.   ____   ____   _____
   Bed rails were down.

Procedure
6. Put on gloves.
7. Removed linens. Rolled each piece away from you.   ____   ____   _____
   Placed each piece in a laundry bag. (NOTE:
   Discarded incontinence products or disposable bed
   protectors in the trash. Did not put them in the
   laundry bag.)
8. Cleaned the bed frame and mattress (if this was   ____   ____   _____
   your job).
9. Removed and discarded gloves.   ____   ____   _____
   Decontaminated your hands.
10. Moved the mattress to the head of the bed.   ____   ____   _____
11. Put the mattress pad on the mattress. It was even   ____   ____   _____
    with the top of the mattress.

Date of Satisfactory Completion _____   Instructor's Initials _____

Procedure—cont'd	S	U	Comments
12. Placed the bottom sheet on the mattress pad. Unfolded it length-wise. Placed the center crease in the middle of the bed.	___	___	_____
If using a flat sheet:			
a. Positioned the lower edge even with the bottom of the mattress.	___	___	_____
b. Placed the large hem at the top and the small hem at the bottom.	___	___	_____
c. Faced hem-stitching downward, away from the person.	___	___	_____
13. Opened the sheet. Fan-folded it to the other side of the bed.	___	___	_____
14. Tucked the corners of a fitted sheet over the mattress at the top and then the foot of the bed. If using a flat sheet, tucked the top of the sheet under the mattress. The sheet was tight and smooth.	___	___	_____
15. Made a mitered corner if using a flat sheet.	___	___	_____
16. Placed the waterproof drawsheet on the bed. It was in the middle of the mattress. Or put the waterproof pad on the bed.			
17. Opened the waterproof drawsheet. Fan-folded it to the other side of the bed.	___	___	_____
18. Placed a cotton drawsheet over the waterproof drawsheet. It covered the entire waterproof drawsheet.	___	___	_____
19. Opened the cotton drawsheet. Fan-folded it to the other side of the bed.	___	___	_____
20. Tucked both drawsheets under the mattress. Or tucked each in separately.	___	___	_____
21. Went to the other side of the bed.	___	___	_____
22. Mitered the top corner of the flat bottom sheet.	___	___	_____
23. Pulled the bottom sheet tight so there were no wrinkles. Tucked in the sheet.	___	___	_____
24. Pulled the drawsheets tight so there were no wrinkles. Tucked both in together or separately.	___	___	_____
25. Went to the other side of the bed.	___	___	_____
26. Put the top sheet on the bed. Unfolded it length-wise. Placed the center crease in the middle.	___	___	_____
If using a flat sheet:			
a. Placed the large hem even with the top of the mattress.	___	___	_____
b. Opened the sheet. Fan-folded it to the other side.	___	___	_____
c. Faced hem-stitching outward, away from the person.	___	___	_____
d. Did not tuck the bottom in yet.	___	___	_____
e. Never tucked top linens in on the sides.	___	___	_____
27. Placed the blanket on the bed:			
a. Unfolded it so the center crease was in the middle.	___	___	_____
b. Put the upper hem about 6 to 8 inches from the top of the mattress.	___	___	_____
c. Opened the blanket. Fan-folded it to the other side.	___	___	_____
d. If no bedspread, turned the top sheet down over the blanket. Hem-stitching was down, away from the person.	___	___	_____

Date of Satisfactory Completion _____   Instructor's Initials _____

Procedure—cont'd   S   U   **Comments**

28. Placed the bedspread on the bed:
    a. Unfolded it so the center crease was in the middle.   _____   _____   _____
    b. Placed the upper hem even with the top of the mattress. _____   _____   _____
    c. Opened and fan-folded the spread to the other side.   _____   _____   _____
    d. Made sure the bedspread facing the door was even.   _____   _____   _____
       It covered all top linens.
29. Tucked in top linens together at the foot of the bed.   _____   _____   _____
    They were smooth and tight. Made a mitered corner.
30. Went to the other side.   _____   _____   _____
31. Straightened all top linens. Worked from the head   _____   _____   _____
    of the bed to the foot.
32. Tucked in top linens together at the foot of the bed.   _____   _____   _____
    Made a mitered corner.
33. Turned the top hem of the bedspread under the   _____   _____   _____
    blanket to make a cuff.
34. Turned the top sheet down over the bedspread.   _____   _____   _____
    Hem-stitching was down. (NOTE: Not done in
    some centers.) The bedspread covered the pillow,
    and it was tucked under the pillow.
35. Put the pillowcases on the pillow. Folded extra   _____   _____   _____
    material under the pillow at the seam end of the
    pillowcase.
36. Placed the pillow on the bed. The open end of the   _____   _____   _____
    pillowcase was away from the door. The seam
    was toward the head of the bed.

Post-Procedure
37. Provided for comfort. NOTE: Omitted this step if the   _____   _____   _____
    bed was prepared for a new person.
38. Attached the call light to the bed. Or placed it   _____   _____   _____
    within the person's reach.
39. Lowered bed to its lowest position. Locked the   _____   _____   _____
    bed wheels.
40. Put the towels, washcloth, gown or pajamas, and   _____   _____   _____
    bath blanket in the bedside stand.
41. Completed a safety check of the room.   _____   _____   _____
42. Followed center policy for dirty linens.   _____   _____   _____
43. Decontaminated your hands.   _____   _____   _____

Date of Satisfactory Completion _____   Instructor's Initials _____

Making an Open Bed

Name: _____   Date: _____

	S	U	Comments

Quality of Life

Remembered to:
- Knock before entering the person's room
- Address the person by name
- Introduce yourself by name and title
- Explain the procedure to the person before beginning and during the procedure
- Protect the person's rights during the procedure
- Handle the person gently during the procedure

Procedure

1. Followed *Delegation Guidelines:*
   Making Beds
   Saw *Promoting Safety and Comfort:*
   Making Beds
2. Practiced hand hygiene.
3. Collected linens for a closed bed:
   - Mattress pad (if needed)
   - Bottom sheet (flat or fitted)
   - Waterproof drawsheet or waterproof pad (if needed)
   - Cotton drawsheet (if needed)
   - Top sheet
   - Blanket
   - Bedspread
   - Pillowcase for each pillow
   - Bath towel(s)
   - Hand towel
   - Washcloth
   - Gown or pajamas
4. Made a closed bed:
   a. Placed linens on a clean surface.
   b. Raised the bed for body mechanics.
   c. Put on gloves.
   d. Removed linens. Rolled each piece away from you. Placed each piece in a laundry bag.
      (NOTE: Discarded incontinence products or disposable bed protectors in the trash. Did not put them in the laundry bag.)
   e. Cleaned the bed frame and mattress if this was part of your job.
   f. Removed and discarded gloves. Decontaminated your hands.
   g. Moved the mattress to the head of the bed.
   h. Put the mattress pad on the mattress. It was even with the top of the mattress.

Procedure—cont'd   S   U   **Comments**

    i. Placed the bottom sheet on the mattress pad.
       Unfolded it length-wise. Placed the center crease in
       the middle of the bed.
       If using a flat sheet:
       1) Positioned the lower edge even with the
          bottom of the mattress.   _____   _____   _____
       2) Placed the large hem at the top and the small
          hem at the bottom.   _____   _____   _____
       3) Faced hem-stitching downward, away from
          the person.   _____   _____   _____
    j. Opened the sheet. Fan-folded it to the other side of the bed.   _____   _____   _____
    k. Tucked the top of the sheet under the mattress.
       The sheet was tight and smooth.   _____   _____   _____
    l. Made a mitered corner if using a flat sheet.   _____   _____   _____
   m. Placed the waterproof drawsheet on the bed.   _____   _____   _____
       It was in the middle of the mattress. Or put the
       waterproof pad on the bed.
    n. Opened the waterproof drawsheet. Fan-folded it to   _____   _____   _____
       the other side of the bed.
    o. Placed a cotton drawsheet over the waterproof   _____   _____   _____
       drawsheet. It covered the entire waterproof drawsheet.
    p. Opened the cotton drawsheet. Fan-folded it to the   _____   _____   _____
       other side of the bed.
    q. Tucked both drawsheets under the mattress.   _____   _____   _____
       Or tucked each in separately.
    r. Went to the other side of the bed.   _____   _____   _____
    s. Mitered the top corner of the flat bottom sheet.   _____   _____   _____
    t. Pulled the bottom sheet tight so there were no   _____   _____   _____
       wrinkles. Tucked in the sheet.
    u. Pulled the drawsheets tight so there were no   _____   _____   _____
       wrinkles. Tucked both in together or separately.
    v. Went to the other side of the bed.   _____   _____   _____
   w. Put the top sheet on the bed. Unfolded it length-wise.
       Placed the center crease in the middle.
       Did the following if using a flat sheet:
       1) Placed the large hem even with the top of the mattress.   _____   _____   _____
       2) Opened the sheet. Fan-folded it to the other side.   _____   _____   _____
       3) Faced hem-stitching outward, away from the person.   _____   _____   _____
       4) Did not tuck the bottom in yet.   _____   _____   _____
       5) Never tucked top linens in on the sides.   _____   _____   _____
    x. Placed the blanket on the bed:
       1) Unfolded it so the center crease was in the middle.   _____   _____   _____
       2) Put the upper hem about 6 to 8 inches from the top
          of the mattress.
       3) Opened the blanket. Fan-folded it to the other side. _____   _____   _____
       4) If no bedspread, turned the top sheet down over the
          blanket. Hem-stitching was down, away from the person.
       (NOTE: Followed center procedure.)
    y. Placed the bedspread on the bed:
       1) Unfolded it so the center crease was in the middle.   _____   _____   _____
       2) Placed the upper hem even with the top of the mattress.   _____   _____   _____
       3) Opened and fan-folded the spread to the other side.   _____   _____   _____
       4) Made sure the spread facing the door was even. It   _____   _____   _____
          covered all top linens.

Date of Satisfactory Completion _____   Instructor's Initials _____

Procedure—cont'd	S	U	Comments
z. Tucked in top linens together at the foot of the bed. They were smooth and tight. Made a mitered corner.	___	___	_____
aa. Went to the other side.	___	___	_____
bb. Straightened all top linens. Worked from the head of the bed to the foot.	___	___	_____
cc. Tucked in top linens together at the foot of the bed. Made a mitered corner.	___	___	_____
dd. Turned the top hem of the spread under the blanket to make a cuff. (NOTE: Followed center procedure.)	___	___	_____
ee. Turned the top sheet down over the spread.	___	___	_____
ff. Hem-stitching was down. (NOTE: Not done in some centers.) The bedspread covered the pillow and it was tucked under the pillow.	___	___	_____
gg. Put the pillowcases on the pillow. Folded extra material under the pillow at the seam end of the pillowcase.	___	___	_____
hh. Placed the pillow on the bed. The open end of the pillowcase was away from the door. The seam was toward the head of the bed.	___	___	_____
5. Fan-folded top linens to the foot of the bed.	___	___	_____
6. Attached the call light to the bed.	___	___	_____
7. Lowered bed to its lowest position.	___	___	_____
8. Put the towels, washcloth, gown or pajamas, and bath blanket in the bedside stand.	___	___	_____
Post-Procedure			
9. Provided for comfort.	___	___	_____
10. Placed the call light within the person's reach.	___	___	_____
11. Completed a safety check of the room.	___	___	_____
12. Followed center policy for dirty linens.	___	___	_____
13. Decontaminated your hands.	___	___	_____

Date of Satisfactory Completion _____   Instructor's Initials _____

CD-ROM   VIDEO CLIP   VIDEO   **Making an Occupied Bed**

Name: _____   Date: _____

	S	U	Comments
Quality of Life			
Remembered to:			
• Knock before entering the person's room	___	___	_____
• Address the person by name	___	___	_____
• Introduce yourself by name and title	___	___	_____
• Explain the procedure to the person before beginning and during the procedure	___	___	_____
• Protect the person's rights during the procedure	___	___	_____
• Handle the person gently during the procedure	___	___	_____

Pre-Procedure

1. Followed *Delegation Guidelines:*
   Making Beds
   Saw *Promoting Safety and Comfort:*
   a. *Making Beds*
   b. *The Occupied Bed*
2. Practiced hand hygiene.
3. Collected the following:
   a. Gloves
   b. Laundry bag
   c. Clean linens
   d. Paper towels, if clean linens barrier needed
4. Placed linens on a clean surface. Placed paper towels between the clean surface and clean linens if required by center policy.
5. Identified the person. Checked the identification (ID) bracelet against the assignment sheet.
   Called the person by name.
6. Provided for privacy.
7. Removed the call light.
8. Raised the bed for body mechanics.
   Bed rails were up if used.
   Bed wheels were locked.
9. Lowered the head of the bed. It was as flat as possible.

Procedure

10. Decontaminated your hands. Put on gloves.
11. Loosened top linens at the foot of the bed.
12. Lowered the bed rail near you.
13. Removed the bedspread. Then removed the blanket. Placed each over the chair.
14. Covered the person with a bath blanket.
    Used the blanket in the bedside stand.
    a. Unfolded a bath blanket over the top sheet.
    b. Asked the person to hold on to the bath blanket. If he or she could not, tucked the top part under the person's shoulders.
    c. Grasped the top sheet under the bath blanket at the shoulders. Brought the sheet down to the foot of the bed. Removed the sheet from under the blanket.
15. Positioned the person on the side of the bed away from you. Adjusted the pillow for comfort.

Date of Satisfactory Completion _____   Instructor's Initials _____

Procedure—cont'd	S	U	Comments

16. Loosened bottom linens from the head to the foot of the bed.
17. Fan-folded bottom linens one at a time toward the person. Started with the cotton drawsheet. If reusing the mattress pad, did not fan-fold it.
18. Placed a clean mattress pad on the bed Unfolded it length-wise. The center crease was in the middle. Fan-folded the top part toward the person. If reusing the mattress pad, straightened and smoothed any wrinkles.
19. Placed the bottom sheet on the mattress pad. Hem-stitching was away from the person. Unfolded the sheet so the crease was in the middle. The small hem was even with the bottom of the mattress. Fan-folded the top part toward the person.
20. Tucked the corners of a fitted sheet over the mattress. If using a flat sheet, made a mitered corner at the head of the bed. Tucked the sheet under the mattress from the head to the foot.
21. Pulled the waterproof drawsheet toward you over the bottom sheet. Tucked excess material under the mattress. Did the following for a clean waterproof drawsheet.
    a. Placed the waterproof drawsheet on the bed. It was in the middle of the mattress.
    b. Fan-folded the part toward the person.
    c. Tucked in excess fabric.
22. Placed the cotton drawsheet over the waterproof drawsheet. It covered the entire waterproof drawsheet. Fan-folded the top part toward the person. Tucked in excess fabric.
23. Explained to the person that he or she will roll over a "bump." Assured the person that he or she would not fall.
24. Helped the person turn to the other side. Adjusted the pillow for comfort.
25. Raised the bed rail if used. Went to the other side and lowered the bed rail.
26. Loosened bottom linens. Removed one piece at a time. Placed each piece in the laundry bag. (NOTE: Discarded disposable bed protectors and incontinence products in the trash. Did not put them in the laundry bag.)
27. Removed and discarded the gloves. Decontaminated your hands.
28. Straightened and smoothed the mattress pad.
29. Pulled the clean bottom sheet toward you. Tucked the corners of a fitted sheet over the mattress. If using a flat sheet, made a mitered corner at the top. Tucked the sheet under the mattress from the head to the foot of the bed.
30. Pulled the drawsheets tightly toward you. Tucked both under together or separately.

Date of Satisfactory Completion _____   Instructor's Initials _____

Procedure—cont'd

	S	U	Comments
31. Positioned the person supine in the center of the bed. Adjusted the pillow for comfort.			
32. Put the top sheet on the bed. Unfolded it length-wise. The crease was in the middle. The large hem was even with the top of the mattress. Hem-stitching was on the outside.			
33. Asked the person to hold on to the top sheet so you could remove the bath blanket. Or tucked the top sheet under the person's shoulders. Removed and discarded the bath blanket.			
34. Placed the blanket on the bed. Unfolded it so the center crease was in the middle and it covered the person. The upper hem was 6 to 8 inches from the top of the mattress.			
35. Placed the bedspread on the bed. Unfolded it so the center crease was in the middle and it covered the person. The top hem was even with the mattress top.			
36. Turned the top hem of the spread under the blanket to make a cuff.			
37. Brought the top sheet down over the spread to form a cuff.			
38. Went to the foot of the bed.			
39. Made a toe pleat. Made a 2-inch pleat across the foot of the bed. The pleat was about 6 to 8 inches from the foot of the bed.			
40. Lifted the mattress corner with one arm. Tucked all top linens under the mattress together. Made a mitered corner.			
41. Raised the bed rail. Went to the other side and lowered the bed rail.			
42. Straightened and smoothed top linens.			
43. Tucked the top linens under the bottom of the mattress. Made a mitered corner.			
44. Changed the pillowcase(s).			

Post-Procedure

	S	U	Comments
45. Provided for comfort.			
46. Placed the call light within reach.			
47. Lowered bed to its lowest position. Locked the bed wheels.			
48. Raised or lowered bed rails. Followed the care plan.			
49. Put the clean towels, washcloth, gown or pajamas, and bath blanket in the bedside stand.			
50. Unscreened the person.			
51. Completed a safety check of the room.			
52. Followed center policy for dirty linen.			
53. Decontaminated your hands.			

Date of Satisfactory Completion _____   Instructor's Initials _____

VIDEO CLIP   VIDEO   **Making a Surgical Bed**

Name: _____   Date: _____

Procedure	S	U	Comments
1. Followed *Delegation Guidelines: Making Beds*			
Saw *Promoting Safety and Comfort:*			
a. *Making Beds*			
b. *Surgical Bed*			
2. Practiced hand hygiene.			
3. Collected the following:			
a. Clean linens			
b. Gloves			
c. Laundry bag			
d. Equipment requested by the nurse.			
e. Paper towel, if barrier for clean linens needed			
4. Placed linens on a clean surface. Placed paper towels between the clean surface and clean linens if barrier required by center policy.			
5. Removed the call light.			
6. Raised the bed for body mechanics.			
7. Removed all linens from the bed. Wore gloves. Decontaminated hands after removed gloves.			
8. Made a closed bed. Did not tuck top linens under the mattress.			
a. Moved the mattress to the head of the bed.			
b. Put the mattress pad on the mattress. It was even with the top of the mattress.			
c. Placed the bottom sheet on the mattress pad:			
• Unfolded it length-wise.			
• Placed the center crease in the middle of the bed.			
• Positioned the lower edge even with the bottom of the mattress.			
• Placed the large hem at the top and the small hem at the bottom.			
• Faced hem-stitching downward			
d. Opened the sheet. Fan-folded it to the other side of the bed.			
e. Tucked the top of the sheet under the mattress. The sheet was tight and smooth.			
f. Made a mitered corner if using a flat sheet.			
g. Placed the waterproof drawsheet on the bed. It was in the middle of the mattress. Or put the waterproof pad on the bed.			
h. Opened the waterproof drawsheet. Fan-folded it to the other side of the bed.			
i. Placed a cotton drawsheet over the waterproof drawsheet. It covered the entire waterproof drawsheet.			
j. Opened the cotton drawsheet. Fan-folded it to the other side of the bed.			
k. Tucked both drawsheets under the mattress. Or tucked each in separately.			
l. Went to the other side of the bed.			

Date of Satisfactory Completion _____   Instructor's Initials _____

Procedure—cont'd	S	U	Comments
m. Mitered the top corner of the flat bottom sheet.	_____	_____	_____
n. Pulled the bottom sheet tight so there were no wrinkles. Tucked in the sheet.	_____	_____	_____
o. Pulled the drawsheets tight so there were no wrinkles. Tucked both in together or separately.	_____	_____	_____
p. Went to the other side of the bed.	_____	_____	_____
q. Put the top sheet on the bed:			
Unfolded it length-wise.	_____	_____	_____
Placed the center crease in the middle.	_____	_____	_____
Placed the large hem even with the top of the mattress.	_____	_____	_____
Opened the sheet. Fan-folded it to the other side.	_____	_____	_____
Faced hem-stitching outward, away from the person.	_____	_____	_____
9. Folded all top linens at the foot of the bed back onto the bed. The fold was even with the edge of the mattress.	_____	_____	_____
10. Fan-folded linens lengthwise to the side of the bed farthest from the door.	_____	_____	_____
11. Put the pillowcase(s) on the pillow(s).	_____	_____	_____
12. Placed the pillow(s) on a clean surface.	_____	_____	_____
13. Left the bed in its highest position.	_____	_____	_____
14. Left both bed rails down.	_____	_____	_____
15. Put the clean towels, washcloth, gown or pajamas, and bath blanket in the bedside stand.	_____	_____	_____
16. Moved furniture away from the bed. Allowed room for the stretcher and staff.	_____	_____	_____
17. Did not attach the call light to the bed.	_____	_____	_____
18. Completed a safety check of the room.	_____	_____	_____
19. Followed center policy for dirty linens.	_____	_____	_____
20. Decontaminated your hands.	_____	_____	_____

Date of Satisfactory Completion _____   Instructor's Initials _____

VIDEO Assisting the Person to Brush and Floss the Teeth

Name: _____   Date: _____

Quality of Life	S	U	Comments

Remembered to:
- Knock before entering the person's room
- Address the person by name
- Introduce yourself by name and title
- Explain the procedure to the person before beginning and during the procedure
- Protect the person's rights during the procedure
- Handle the person gently during the procedure

Pre-Procedure
1. Followed *Delegation Guidelines:*
   Oral Hygiene
   Saw *Promoting Safety and Comfort: Oral Hygiene*
2. Practiced hand hygiene.
3. Collected the following:
   - Toothbrush
   - Toothpaste
   - Mouthwash (or solution noted in care plan)
   - Dental floss (if used)
   - Water glass with cool water
   - Straw
   - Kidney basin
   - Hand towel
   - Paper towels
   - Gloves
4. Placed the paper towels on the over-bed table.
   Arranged items on top of them.
5. Identified the person. Checked the identification (ID) bracelet against the assignment sheet.
   Called the person by name.
6. Provided for privacy.
7. Lowered the bed rail near you if up.

Procedure
8. Positioned the person so he or she could brush with ease.
9. Placed the towel over the person's chest.
   This protected garments and linens from spills.
10. Adjusted the over-bed table in front of the person.
11. Allowed the person to perform oral hygiene.
    This included brushing the teeth and tongue, rinsing the mouth, flossing, and using mouthwash or other solution.
12. Removed the towel when the person was done.
13. Moved the over-bed table to the side of the bed.

Post-Procedure
14. Provided for comfort.
15. Placed the call light within reach.
16. Raised or lowered bed rails. Followed the care plan.
17. Cleaned and returned items to their proper place.
    Wore gloves.

Date of Satisfactory Completion _____   Instructor's Initials _____

Post-Procedure—cont'd   S   U   Comments

18. Wiped off the over-bed table with the paper towels.   _____   _____   _____
    Discarded the paper towels.

19. Removed the gloves.   _____   _____   _____
    Decontaminated your hands.

20. Unscreened the person.   _____   _____   _____

21. Completed a safety check of the room.   _____   _____   _____

22. Followed center policy for dirty linens.   _____   _____   _____

23. Decontaminated your hands.   _____   _____   _____

24. Reported and recorded your observations.   _____   _____   _____

Date of Satisfactory Completion _____   Instructor's Initials _____

NNAAP™ Skill   CD-ROM   VIDEO CLIP   VIDEO   **Brushing and Flossing the Person's Teeth**

Name: _____   Date: _____

	S	U	Comments
Quality of Life			
Remembered to:			
• Knock before entering the person's room	___	___	_____
• Address the person by name	___	___	_____
• Introduce yourself by name and title	___	___	_____
• Explain the procedure to the person before beginning and during the procedure	___	___	_____
• Protect the person's rights during the procedure	___	___	_____
• Handle the person gently during the procedure	___	___	_____

Pre-Procedure

	S	U	Comments
1. Followed *Delegation Guidelines: Oral Hygiene*	___	___	_____
Saw *Promoting Safety and Comfort: Oral Hygiene*	___	___	_____
2. Practiced hand hygiene.	___	___	_____
3. Collected the following:			
a. Toothbrush with soft bristles	___	___	_____
b. Toothpaste	___	___	_____
c. Mouthwash (or solution noted in care plan)	___	___	_____
d. Dental floss (if used)	___	___	_____
e. Water glass with cool water	___	___	_____
f. Straw	___	___	_____
g. Kidney basin	___	___	_____
h. Hand towel	___	___	_____
i. Paper towels	___	___	_____
j. Gloves	___	___	_____
4. Placed the paper towels on the over-bed table. Arranged items on top of them.	___	___	_____
5. Identified the person. Checked the identification (ID) bracelet against the assignment sheet. Called the person by name.	___	___	_____
6. Provided for privacy.	___	___	_____
7. Raised the bed for body mechanics. Bed rails were up if used.	___	___	_____

Procedure

	S	U	Comments
8. Lowered the bed rail near you if up.	___	___	_____
9. Assisted the person to a sitting position or to a side-lying position near you.	___	___	_____
10. Placed the towel across the person's chest.	___	___	_____
11. Adjusted the over-bed table so you could reach it with ease.	___	___	_____
12. Decontaminated your hands. Put on gloves.	___	___	_____
13. Held the toothbrush over the kidney basin. Poured some water over the brush.	___	___	_____
14. Applied toothpaste to the toothbrush.	___	___	_____
15. Brushed the teeth gently.	___	___	_____
16. Brushed the tongue gently.	___	___	_____
17. Let the person rinse the mouth with water. Held the kidney basin under the person's chin. Repeated as needed.	___	___	_____

Date of Satisfactory Completion _____   Instructor's Initials _____

Procedure—cont'd	S	U	Comments
18. Flossed the person's teeth (optional):			
a. Broke off an 18-inch piece of floss from the dispenser.	_____	_____	_____
b. Held the floss between the middle fingers of each hand.	_____	_____	_____
c. Stretched the floss with your thumbs.	_____	_____	_____
d. Started at the upper back tooth on the right side. Worked around to the left side.	_____	_____	_____
e. Moved the floss gently up and down between the teeth. Moved the floss up and down against the side of the tooth. Worked from the top of the crown to the gum line.	_____	_____	_____
f. Moved to a new section of floss after every second tooth.	_____	_____	_____
g. Flossed the lower teeth. Used up and down motions for the upper teeth. Started on the right side. Worked around to the left side.	_____	_____	_____
19. Allowed the person to use mouthwash or other solution. Held the kidney basin under the chin.	_____	_____	_____
20. Wiped the person's mouth. Removed the towel.	_____	_____	_____
21. Removed and discarded the gloves. Decontaminated your hands.	_____	_____	_____
Post-Procedure			
22. Provided for comfort.	_____	_____	_____
23. Placed the call light within reach.	_____	_____	_____
24. Lowered the bed to its lowest position.	_____	_____	_____
25. Raised or lowered bed rails. Followed the care plan.	_____	_____	_____
26. Cleaned and returned equipment to its proper place. Wore gloves.	_____	_____	_____
27. Wiped off the over-bed table with the paper towels. Discarded the paper towels.	_____	_____	_____
28. Unscreened the person.	_____	_____	_____
29. Completed a safety check of the room.	_____	_____	_____
30. Followed center policy for dirty linens.	_____	_____	_____
31. Removed the gloves. Decontaminated your hands.	_____	_____	_____
32. Reported and recorded your observations.	_____	_____	_____

Date of Satisfactory Completion _____   Instructor's Initials _____

CD-ROM VIDEO Providing Mouth Care for the Unconscious Person

Name: _____   Date: _____

	S	U	Comments
Quality of Life			
Remembered to:			
• Knock before entering the person's room	___	___	_____
• Address the person by name	___	___	_____
• Introduce yourself by name and title	___	___	_____
• Explain the procedure to the person before beginning and during the procedure	___	___	_____
• Protect the person's rights during the procedure	___	___	_____
• Handle the person gently during the procedure	___	___	_____
Pre-Procedure			
1. Followed *Delegation Guidelines:* *Oral Hygiene* Saw *Promoting Safety and Comfort:*	___	___	_____
a. *Oral Hygiene*	___	___	_____
b. *Mouth Care for the Unconscious Person*	___	___	_____
2. Practiced hand hygiene.	___	___	_____
3. Collected the following:			
a. Cleaning agent (checked the care plan)	___	___	_____
b. Sponge swabs	___	___	_____
c. Padded tongue blade	___	___	_____
d. Water glass or cup with cool water	___	___	_____
e. Hand towel	___	___	_____
f. Kidney basin	___	___	_____
g. Lip lubricant	___	___	_____
h. Paper towels	___	___	_____
i. Gloves	___	___	_____
4. Placed the paper towels on the over-bed table. Arranged items on top of them.	___	___	_____
5. Identified the person. Checked the identification (ID) bracelet against the assignment sheet. Called the person by name.	___	___	_____
6. Provided for privacy.	___	___	_____
7. Raised the bed for body mechanics. Bed rails were up if used.	___	___	_____
Procedure			
8. Lowered the bed rail near you if up.	___	___	_____
9. Decontaminated your hands. Put on gloves.	___	___	_____
10. Positioned the person in a side-lying position near you. Turned his or her head well to the side.	___	___	_____
11. Placed the towel under the person's face.	___	___	_____
12. Placed the kidney basin under the chin.	___	___	_____
13. Separated the upper and lower teeth. Used the padded tongue blade. Was gentle. Never used force. If you had problems, asked the nurse for help.	___	___	_____
14. Cleaned the mouth using sponge swaps moistened with the cleaning agent.	___	___	_____
a. Cleaned the chewing and inner surfaces of the teeth.	___	___	_____
b. Cleaned the gums and outer surfaces of the teeth.	___	___	_____
c. Swabbed the roof of the mouth, inside of the cheeks, and lips.	___	___	_____

Date of Satisfactory Completion _____   Instructor's Initials _____

	S	U	Comments
Procedure—cont'd			
d. Swabbed the tongue.	_____	_____	_____
e. Moistened a clean swab with water. Swabbed the mouth to rinse.	_____	_____	_____
f. Placed used swabs in the kidney basin.	_____	_____	_____
15. Removed the kidney basin and supplies.	_____	_____	_____
16. Wiped the person's mouth. Removed the towel.	_____	_____	_____
17. Applied lubricant to the lips.	_____	_____	_____
18. Removed and discarded the gloves. Decontaminated your hands.	_____	_____	_____
Post-Procedure			
19. Provided for comfort.	_____	_____	_____
20. Placed the call light within reach.	_____	_____	_____
21. Lowered the bed to its lowest position.	_____	_____	_____
22. Raised or lowered bed rails. Followed the care plan.	_____	_____	_____
23. Cleaned and returned equipment to its proper place. Discarded disposable items. (Wore gloves.)	_____	_____	_____
24. Wiped off the over-bed table with the paper towels. Discarded the paper towels.	_____	_____	_____
25. Unscreened the person.	_____	_____	_____
26. Completed a safety check of the room.	_____	_____	_____
27. Told the person you were leaving the room. Told him or her when you would return.	_____	_____	_____
28. Followed center policy for dirty linens.	_____	_____	_____
29. Removed the gloves. Decontaminated your hands.	_____	_____	_____
30. Reported and recorded your observations.	_____	_____	_____

Date of Satisfactory Completion _____   Instructor's Initials _____

NNAAP™ Skill **CD-ROM** **VIDEO CLIP** **VIDEO** **Providing Denture Care**

Name: _____   Date: _____

	S	U	Comments
Quality of Life			

Remembered to:
- Knock before entering the person's room
- Address the person by name
- Introduce yourself by name and title
- Explain the procedure to the person before beginning and during the procedure
- Protect the person's rights during the procedure
- Handle the person gently during the procedure

Pre-Procedure
1. Followed *Delegation Guidelines:*
   Oral Hygiene
   Saw *Promoting Safety and Comfort:*
   a. *Oral Hygiene*
   b. *Denture Care*
2. Practiced hand hygiene.
3. Collected the following:
   - Denture brush or toothbrush (for cleaning dentures)
   - Denture cup labeled with the person's name and room and bed number
   - Denture cleaning agent
   - Soft-bristled toothbrush or sponge swabs (for oral hygiene)
   - Toothpaste
   - Water glass with cool water
   - Straw
   - Mouthwash (or other noted solution)
   - Kidney basin
   - Two hand towels
   - Gauze squares
   - Paper towels
   - Gloves
4. Placed the paper towels on the over-bed table. Arranged items on top of them.
5. Identified the person. Checked the identification (ID) bracelet against the assignment sheet. Called the person by name.
6. Provided for privacy.
7. Raised the bed for body mechanics.

Procedure
8. Lowered the bed rail near you if up.
9. Decontaminated your hands. Put on gloves.
10. Placed the towel over the person's chest.
11. Asked the person to remove the dentures. Carefully placed them in the kidney basin.
12. Removed the dentures if the person could not do so. Used gauze square to get a good grip on the slippery dentures.
    a. Grasped the upper denture with your thumb and index finger. Moved it up and down slightly to break the seal. Gently removed the denture. Placed it in the kidney basin.

Date of Satisfactory Completion _____   Instructor's Initials _____

Procedure—cont'd   S   U   Comments

    b. Grasped and removed the lower denture with
       thumb and index finger. Turned it slightly and
       lifted it out of the person's mouth.
       Placed it in the kidney basin.

13. Followed the care plan for raising side rails.

14. Took the kidney basin, denture cup, denture brush,
    and denture cleaning agent to the sink.

15. Lined the sink with a towel. Filled the sink
    half-way with water.

16. Rinsed each denture under cool or warm running
    water. Followed center policy for water temperature.

17. Returned dentures to the kidney basin or denture cup.

18. Applied the denture cleaning agent to the brush.

19. Brushed the dentures.

20. Rinsed the dentures under running water.
    Used warm or cool water as directed by the
    cleaning agent manufacturer. (Some state
    competency tests require cool water.)

21. Rinsed the denture cup. Placed dentures in the
    denture cup. Covered the dentures with cool or
    warm water. Followed center policy for water
    temperature.

22. Cleaned the kidney basin.

23. Took the denture cup and kidney basin to the
    over-bed table.

24. Lowered the bed rail if up.

25. Positioned the person for oral hygiene.

26. Cleaned the person's gums and tongue, used
    toothpaste and the toothbrush (or sponge swab).

27. Had the person use mouthwash (or noted solution).
    Held the kidney basin under the chin.

28. Asked the person to insert the dentures.
    Inserted them if the person could not:
    a. Held the upper denture firmly with your
       thumb and index finger. Raised the upper lip
       with the other hand. Inserted the denture.
       Gently pressed on the denture with your index
       fingers to make sure it was in place.
    b. Held the lower denture with your thumb and
       index finger. Pulled the lower lip down slightly.
       Inserted the denture. Gently pressed down
       on it to make sure it was in place.

29. Placed the denture cup in the top drawer of the
    bedside stand if the dentures were not worn.
    If not worn, the dentures were in water or a
    denture soaking solution.

30. Wiped the person's mouth. Removed the towel.

31. Removed the gloves.
    Decontaminated your hands.

32. Assisted with hand washing.

33. Provided for comfort.

34. Placed the call light within reach.

35. Lowered the bed to its lowest position.

Date of Satisfactory Completion _____   Instructor's Initials _____

Procedure—cont'd	S	U	Comments
36. Raised or lowered bed rails. Followed the care plan.	___	___	_____
37. Removed the towel from the sink. Drained the sink.	___	___	_____
38. Cleaned and returned equipment to its proper place. Discarded disposable items. (Wore gloves.)	___	___	_____
39. Wiped off the over-bed table with the paper towels. Discarded the paper towels.	___	___	_____
40. Unscreened the person.	___	___	_____
41. Completed a safety check of the room.	___	___	_____
42. Followed center policy for dirty linens.	___	___	_____
43. Removed the gloves. Decontaminated your hands.	___	___	_____
44. Reported and recorded your observations.	___	___	_____

Date of Satisfactory Completion _____   Instructor's Initials _____

NNAAP™ Skill   CD-ROM   VIDEO CLIP   VIDEO   **Giving a Complete Bed Bath**

Name: _____   Date: _____

	S	U	Comments

Quality of Life
Remembered to:
- Knock before entering the person's room
- Address the person by name
- Introduce yourself by name and title
- Explain the procedure to the person before beginning and during the procedure
- Protect the person's rights during the procedure
- Handle the person gently during the procedure

Pre-Procedure
1. Followed *Delegation Guidelines: Bathing*
   Saw *Promoting Safety and Comfort: Bathing*
2. Practiced hand hygiene.
3. Identified the person. Checked the identification (ID) bracelet against the assignment sheet. Called the person by name.
4. Collected clean linens for a closed bed and placed linens on a clean surface:
   - Mattress pad (if needed)
   - Bottom sheet
   - Plastic drawsheet or waterproof pad (if used)
   - Cotton drawsheet (if needed)
   - Top sheet
   - Blanket
   - Bedspread
   - Two pillowcases
   - Gloves
   - Laundry bag
5. Collected the following:
   - Wash basin
   - Soap
   - Bath thermometer
   - Orangewood stick or nail file
   - Washcloth
   - Two bath towels and two hand towels
   - Bath blanket
   - Clothing or sleepwear
   - Lotion
   - Powder
   - Deodorant or antiperspirant
   - Brush and comb
   - Other grooming items as requested
   - Paper towels
   - Gloves
6. Covered the over-bed table with paper towels. Arranged items on the over-bed table. Adjusted the height as needed.
7. Provided for privacy.
8. Raised the bed for body mechanics. Bed rails were up if used.

Date of Satisfactory Completion _____   Instructor's Initials _____

Procedure

9. Removed the call light.
10. Decontaminated your hands.
    Put on gloves.
11. Covered the person with a bath blanket.
    Removed top linens.
12. Lowered the head of the bed. It was as flat as possible.
    The person had at least one pillow.
13. Filled the wash basin ⅔ (two-thirds) full with water.
    Followed the care plan for water temperature.
    Water temperature was 110°F–115°F (43.3°C–46.1°C)
    for adults. Measured water temperature. Used the bath
    thermometer. Or tested the water by dipping your
    elbow or inner wrist into the basin.
14. Lowered the bed rail near you if up.
15. Asked the person to check the water temperature.
    Adjusted the water temperature if too hot or
    too cold. Raised the bed rail before leaving the bedside.
    Lowered the bed rail when you returned.
16. Placed the basin on the over-bed table.
17. Removed the sleepwear. Did not expose the person.
18. Placed a hand towel over the person's chest.
19. Made a mitt with the washcloth. Used a mitt for
    the entire bath.
20. Washed around the person's eyes with water.
    Did not use soap.
    a. Cleaned the far eye. Gently wiped from the inner
       to the outer aspect of the eye with a corner of the mitt.
    b. Cleaned the eye near you. Used a clean part of
       the washcloth for each stroke.
21. Asked the person if you should use soap to wash the face.
22. Washed the face, ears, and neck. Rinsed and patted
    dry with the towel on the chest.
23. Helped the person move to the side of the bed near you.
24. Exposed the far arm. Placed a bath towel length-wise
    under the arm. Applied soap to the washcloth.
25. Supported the arm with your palm under the person's
    elbow. His or her forearm rested on your forearm.
26. Washed the arm, shoulder, and underarm.
    Used long, firm strokes. Rinsed and patted dry.
27. Placed the basin on the towel. Put the person's hand
    into the water. Washed it well. Cleaned under the
    fingernails with an orangewood stick or nail file.
28. Had the person exercise the hand and fingers.
29. Removed the basin. Dried the hand well.
    Covered the arm with the bath blanket.
30. Repeated for the near arm:
    a. Placed a bath towel length-wise under the near arm.
    b. Supported the arm with your palm under the person's
       elbow. His or her forearm rested on your forearm.
    c. Washed the arm, shoulder, and underarm.
       Used long, firm strokes. Rinsed and patted dry.
    d. Placed the basin on the towel. Put the person's
       hand into the water. Washed it well. Cleaned under
       the fingernails with an orangewood stick or nail file.

Date of Satisfactory Completion _____   Instructor's Initials _____

Procedure—cont'd   S   U   Comments

    e. Had the person exercise the hand and fingers.   _____ _____ _____

    f. Removed the basin. Dried the hand well.   _____ _____ _____
      Covered the arm with the bath blanket.

31. Placed a bath towel over the chest cross-wise.   _____ _____ _____
    Held the towel in place. Pulled the bath blanket
    from under the towel to the waist.
    Applied soap to the washcloth.

32. Lifted the towel slightly and washed the chest.   _____ _____ _____
    Did not expose the person. Rinsed and patted dry,
    especially under the breasts.

33. Moved the towel length-wise over the chest and   _____ _____ _____
    abdomen. Did not expose the person. Pulled the
    bath blanket down to the pubic area. Applied soap
    to the washcloth.

34. Lifted the towel slightly and washed the abdomen.   _____ _____ _____
    Rinsed and patted dry.

35. Pulled the bath blanket up to the shoulders.   _____ _____ _____
    Covered both arms. Removed the towel.

36. Changed soapy or cool water. Measured water   _____ _____ _____
    temperature. Followed the person's care plan. Water
    temperature usually 110°F–115°F (43.3°C–46.1°C)
    for adults. Used the bath thermometer. Or tested the
    water by dipping your elbow or inner wrist into
    the basin. If bed rails used, raised the bed rail
    near you before you left the bedside.
    Lowered it when you returned.

37. Uncovered the far leg. Did not expose the genital area.   _____ _____ _____
    Placed a towel length-wise under the foot and
    leg. Applied soap to the washcloth.

38. Bent the knee and supported the leg with your   _____ _____ _____
    arm. Washed it with long, firm strokes.
    Rinsed and patted dry.

39. Placed the basin on the towel near the foot.   _____ _____ _____

40. Lifted the leg slightly. Slid the basin under the foot.   _____ _____ _____

41. Placed the foot in the basin. Used an orangewood stick
    or nail file to clean under toenails if necessary.
    If the person could not bend the knees:

    a. Washed the foot. Carefully separated the toes.   _____ _____ _____
      Rinsed and patted dry.

    b. Cleaned under the toenails with the orangewood   _____ _____ _____
      stick or nail file if necessary.

42. Removed the basin. Dried the leg and foot.   _____ _____ _____
    Applied lotion to the foot if directed by the nurse
    and care plan. Covered the leg with the bath
    blanket. Removed the towel.

43. Repeated for the near leg:

    a. Uncovered the near leg. Did not expose the   _____ _____ _____
      genital area. Placed a towel length-wise under
      the foot and leg.

    b. Bent the knee and supported the leg with your arm.   _____ _____ _____
      Washed it with long, firm strokes. Rinsed and
      patted dry.

    c. Placed the basin on the towel near the foot.   _____ _____ _____

Date of Satisfactory Completion _____ Instructor's Initials _____

Procedure—cont'd	S	U	Comments
d. Lifted the leg slightly. Slid the basin under the foot.	___	___	_____
e. Placed the foot in the basin. Used an orangewood stick or nail file to clean under toenails if necessary. If the person could not bend the knee: Washed the foot. Carefully separated the toes. Rinsed and patted dry. Cleaned under the toenails with an orangewood stick or nail file if necessary.	___	___	_____
f. Removed the basin. Dried the leg and foot. Applied lotion to the foot if directed by the nurse and care plan. Covered the leg with the bath blanket. Removed the towel.	___	___	_____
44. Changed the water. Measured water temperature. Followed the care plan. Water temperature is usually 110°F–115°F (43.3°C–46.1°C) for adults. Used the bath thermometer. Or tested the water by dipping your elbow or inner wrist into the basin. If bed rails used, raised the bed rail near you before you left the bedside. Lowered it when you returned.	___	___	_____
45. Turned the person onto the side away from you. The person was covered with the bath blanket.	___	___	_____
46. Uncovered the back and buttocks. Did not expose the person. Placed a towel length-wise on the bed along the back. Applied soap to the washcloth.	___	___	_____
47. Washed the back. Worked from the back of the neck to the lower end of the buttocks. Used long, firm, continuous strokes. Rinsed and dried well.	___	___	_____
48. Gave a back massage. The person may have wanted the back massage after the bath.	___	___	_____
49. Turned the person onto his or her back.	___	___	_____
50. Changed the water for perineal care. Measured water temperature. Followed the care plan. Water temperature is usually 110°F–115°F (43.3°C–46.1°C) for adults. Used the bath thermometer. Or tested the water by dipping your elbow or inner wrist into the basin. (Some state competency tests require changing gloves and hand hygiene at this time.) If bed rails used, raised the bed rail near you before you left the bedside. Lowered it when you returned.	___	___	_____
51. Allowed the person to wash the genital area. Adjusted the over-bed table so he or she could reach the wash basin, soap, and towels with ease. Placed the call light within reach. Asked the person to signal when finished. Made sure the person understood what to do.	___	___	_____
52. Removed the gloves. Decontaminated your hands.	___	___	_____
53. Answered the call light promptly. Knocked before entering the room. Provided perineal care if the person could not do so. (Decontaminated your hands and wore gloves for perineal care.)	___	___	_____

Date of Satisfactory Completion _____   Instructor's Initials _____

Procedure—cont'd   **S**   **U**   **Comments**

54. Gave a back massage if you had not already done so.

55. Applied deodorant or antiperspirant.
    Applied lotion and powder as requested.
    Saw *Promoting Safety and Comfort: Bathing.*

56. Put clean garments on the person.

57. Combed and brushed the hair.

58. Made the bed.

Post-Procedure

59. Provided for comfort.

60. Placed the call light within reach.

61. Lowered the bed to its lowest position.

62. Raised or lowered bed rails. Followed the care plan.

63. Put on clean gloves.

64. Emptied and cleaned the wash basin.
    Returned it and other supplies to their proper place.

65. Wiped off the over-bed table with the paper towels.
    Discarded the paper towels.

66. Unscreened the person.

67. Completed a safety check of the room.

68. Followed center policy for dirty linens.

69. Removed the gloves.
    Decontaminated your hands.

70. Reported and recorded your observations.

Date of Satisfactory Completion _____   Instructor's Initials _____

VIDEO   **Assisting with the Partial Bath**

Name: _____   Date: _____

	S	U	Comments
Quality of Life			
Remembered to:			
• Knock before entering the person's room	___	___	_____
• Address the person by name	___	___	_____
• Introduce yourself by name and title	___	___	_____
• Explain the procedure to the person before beginning and during the procedure	___	___	_____
• Protect the person's rights during the procedure	___	___	_____
• Handle the person gently during the procedure	___	___	_____

Pre-Procedure

1. Followed *Delegation Guidelines:*
   Bathing   ___   ___   _____

   Saw *Promoting Safety and Comfort:*
   Bathing   ___   ___   _____

2. Did the following:

   a. Practiced hand hygiene.   ___   ___   _____

   b. Identified the person. Checked the identification (ID) bracelet against the assignment sheet. Called the person by name.   ___   ___   _____

   c. Collected clean linens for a closed bed and placed linens on a clean surface:
   - Mattress pad (if needed)   ___   ___   _____
   - Bottom sheet   ___   ___   _____
   - Waterproof drawsheet or waterproof pad (if used)   ___   ___   _____
   - Cotton drawsheet (if needed)   ___   ___   _____
   - Top sheet   ___   ___   _____
   - Blanket   ___   ___   _____
   - Bedspread   ___   ___   _____
   - Two pillowcases   ___   ___   _____
   - Gloves   ___   ___   _____
   - Laundry bag   ___   ___   _____

   d. Collected the following:
   - Wash basin   ___   ___   _____
   - Soap   ___   ___   _____
   - Bath thermometer   ___   ___   _____
   - Orangewood stick or nail file   ___   ___   _____
   - Washcloth   ___   ___   _____
   - Two bath towels and two hand towels   ___   ___   _____
   - Bath blanket   ___   ___   _____
   - Clothing or sleepwear   ___   ___   _____
   - Lotion   ___   ___   _____
   - Powder   ___   ___   _____
   - Deodorant or antiperspirant   ___   ___   _____
   - Brush and comb   ___   ___   _____
   - Other grooming items as requested   ___   ___   _____
   - Paper towels   ___   ___   _____
   - Gloves   ___   ___   _____

Date of Satisfactory Completion _____   Instructor's Initials _____

Pre-Procedure—cont'd   S   U   Comments

    e. Covered the over-bed table with paper towels.
       Arranged items on the over-bed table.
       Adjusted the height as needed.

    f. Provided for privacy.

    g. Raised the bed for body mechanics.
       Bed rails were up if used.

Procedure

3. Made sure the bed was in the lowest position.

4. Decontaminated your hands.
    Put on gloves.

5. Covered the person with a bath blanket.
    Removed top linens.

6. Filled the wash basin ⅔ (two-thirds) full
    with water. Water temperature was 110°F–115°F
    (43.3°C–46.1°C) for adults or as directed by the nurse.
    Measured water temperature with the bath
    thermometer. Or tested the water by dipping
    your elbow or inner wrist into the basin.

7. Asked the person to check the water temperature.
    Adjusted if too hot or too cold.

8. Placed the basin on the over-bed table.

9. Positioned the person in Fowler's position.
    Or assisted him or her to sit at the bedside.

10. Adjusted the over-bed table so the person could
    reach the basin and supplies.

11. Helped the person undress. Provided for privacy
    and warmth with a bath blanket.

12. Asked the person to wash easy-to-reach body parts.
    Explained that you would wash the back and areas
    the person could not reach.

13. Placed the call light within reach. Asked the person to
    signal when help was needed or bathing was complete.

14. Decontaminated your hands. Left the room.

15. Returned when the call light was on.
    Knocked before entering. Decontaminated your hands.

16. Changed the bath water. Measured bath water
    temperature: 110°F–115°F (43.3°C–46.1°C) for adults
    or as directed by the nurse. Used the bath
    thermometer. Or tested the water by dipping your
    elbow or inner wrist into the basin.

17. Raised the bed for body mechanics.
    The far bed rail was up if used.

18. Asked what was washed. Put on gloves.
    Washed and dried areas the person could not reach.
    The face, hands, underarms, back, buttocks,
    and perineal area were washed for the partial bath.

19. Removed the gloves.
    Decontaminated your hands.

20. Gave a back massage.

21. Applied lotion, powder, and deodorant or
    antiperspirant as requested.

22. Helped the person put on clean garments.

23. Assisted with hair care and other grooming needs.

Date of Satisfactory Completion _____   Instructor's Initials _____

Procedure—cont'd	S	U	Comments
24. Assisted the person to a chair. (Lowered the bed if the person transferred to a chair.) Or turned the person onto the side away from you.	___	___	_____
25. Made the bed. (Raised the bed for body mechanics.)	___	___	_____
Post-Procedure			
26. Provided for comfort.	___	___	_____
27. Placed the call light within reach.	___	___	_____
28. Lowered the bed to its lowest position.	___	___	_____
29. Raised or lowered bed rails. Followed the care plan.	___	___	_____
30. Put on clean gloves.	___	___	_____
31. Emptied, cleaned, and dried the bath basin. Returned it and other supplies to their proper place.	___	___	_____
32. Wiped off the over-bed table with the paper towels. Discarded the paper towels.	___	___	_____
33. Unscreened the person.	___	___	_____
34. Completed a safety check of the room.	___	___	_____
35. Followed center policy for dirty linens.	___	___	_____
36. Removed your gloves. Decontaminated your hands.	___	___	_____
37. Reported and recorded your observations.	___	___	_____

Date of Satisfactory Completion _____   Instructor's Initials _____

VIDEO CLIP   VIDEO   **Assisting with a Tub Bath or Shower**

Name: _____   Date: _____

	S	U	Comments

Quality of Life

Remembered to:
- Knock before entering the person's room
- Address the person by name
- Introduce yourself by name and title
- Explain the procedure to the person before beginning and during the procedure
- Protect the person's rights during the procedure
- Handle the person gently during the procedure

Pre-Procedure

1. Followed *Delegation Guidelines:*
   a. *Bathing*
   b. *Tub Baths and Showers*
   Saw *Promoting Safety and Comfort:*
   a. *Bathing*
   b. *Tub Baths and Showers*
2. Reserved the bathtub or shower.
3. Practiced hand hygiene.
4. Identified the person. Checked the identification (ID) bracelet against the assignment sheet. Called the person by name.
5. Collected the following:
   - Two washcloths and two bath towels
   - Soap
   - Bath thermometer (for tub both)
   - Clothing or sleepwear
   - Grooming items as requested
   - Robe and non-skid footwear
   - Rubber bath mat if needed
   - Disposable bath mat
   - Gloves
   - Wheelchair, shower chair, transfer bench, and so on as needed.

Procedure

6. Placed items in the tub or shower room. Used the space provided or a chair.
7. Cleaned and disinfected the tub or shower.
8. Placed a rubber bath mat in the tub or on the shower floor. Did not block the drain.
9. Placed the disposable bath mat on the floor in front of the tub or shower.
10. Placed the OCCUPIED sign on the door.
11. Returned to the person's room. Provided for privacy. Decontaminated your hands.
12. Helped the person sit on the side of the bed.
13. Helped the person put on a robe and non-skid footwear. Or the person left on clothing.
14. Assisted or transported the person to the tub room or shower.
15. Had the person sit on a chair if he or she walked to the tub or shower room.

Date of Satisfactory Completion _____   Instructor's Initials _____

Procedure—cont'd	S	U	Comments
16. Provided for privacy.	___	___	___
17. *For a tub bath:*			
a. Filled the tub half-way with warm water (usually 105°F [40.5°C]). Followed the care plan for water temperature.	___	___	___
b. Measured water temperature with bath thermometer. Or checked the digital display.	___	___	___
18. *For a shower:*			
a. Turned on the shower.	___	___	___
b. Adjusted water temperature and pressure. Checked the digital display.	___	___	___
c. Asked the person to check the water temperature. Adjusted the water if too hot or too cold.	___	___	___
19. Helped the person undress and removed footwear.	___	___	___
20. Helped the person into the tub or shower. Positioned the shower chair and locked the wheels.	___	___	___
21. Asked the person if he or she wanted hair shampooed. If yes, performed this before washing the body. Covered the head with towel after shampooing to prevent chilling.	___	___	___
22. Assisted with washing as necessary. Wore gloves.	___	___	___
23. Asked the person to use the call light when done or when help was needed. Reminded the person that a tub bath lasts no longer than 20 minutes.	___	___	___
24. Placed a towel across the chair.	___	___	___
25. Left the room if the person could bathe alone. If not, stayed in the room or nearby. Removed the gloves and decontaminated your hands if you left the room.	___	___	___
26. Checked the person at least every 5 minutes.			
27. Returned when the person signaled for you. Knocked before entering. Decontaminated your hands.	___	___	___
28. Turned off the shower or drained the tub. Covered the person while the tub drained.	___	___	___
29. Helped the person out of the shower or tub and onto a chair.	___	___	___
30. Helped the person dry off. Patted gently. Dried under the breasts and between skin folds, in the perineal area, and between the toes.	___	___	___
31. Assisted with lotion and other grooming items as needed.	___	___	___
32. Helped the person dress and put on footwear.	___	___	___
33. Helped the person return to the room. Provided for privacy.	___	___	___
34. Assisted the person to a chair or into bed.	___	___	___
35. Provided a back massage if the person returned to bed.	___	___	___
36. Assisted with hair care and other grooming needs.	___	___	___
Post-Procedure			
37. Provided for comfort.	___	___	___
38. Placed the call light within reach.	___	___	___
39. Raised or lowered bed rails. Followed the care plan.	___	___	___
40. Unscreened the person.	___	___	___

Date of Satisfactory Completion _____ Instructor's Initials _____

Post-Procedure—cont'd

	S	U	Comments
41. Completed a safety check of the room.	_____	_____	_____
42. Cleaned and disinfected the tub or shower. Removed soiled linens. Wore gloves.	_____	_____	_____
43. Discarded disposable items. Put the UNOCCUPIED sign on the door. Returned supplies to their proper place.	_____	_____	_____
44. Followed center policy for dirty linens.	_____	_____	_____
45. Removed the gloves. Decontaminated your hands.	_____	_____	_____
46. Reported and recorded your observations.	_____	_____	_____

Date of Satisfactory Completion _____   Instructor's Initials _____

VIDEO CLIP VIDEO **Giving a Back Massage**

Name: _____   Date: _____

	S	U	Comments

Quality of Life

Remembered to:
- Knock before entering the person's room
- Address the person by name
- Introduce yourself by name and title
- Explain the procedure to the person before beginning and during the procedure
- Protect the person's rights during the procedure
- Handle the person gently during the procedure

Pre-Procedure

1. Followed *Delegation Guidelines:*
   The Back Massage.
   Saw *Promoting Safety and Comfort: The Back Massage.*
2. Practiced hand hygiene.
3. Identified the person. Checked the identification (ID) bracelet against the assignment sheet.
   Called the person by name.
4. Collected the following:
   - Bath blanket
   - Bath towel
   - Lotion
5. Provided for privacy.
6. Raised the bed for body mechanics.
   Bed rails were up if used.

Procedure

7. Lowered the bed rail near you if up.
8. Positioned the person in the prone or side-lying position. The back was toward you.
9. Exposed the back, shoulders, upper arms, and buttocks. Covered the rest of the body with the bath blanket. Exposed the buttocks if person gave consent.
10. Laid the towel on the bed along the back (if the person was in the side-lying position).
11. Warmed the lotion.
12. Explained that the lotion may feel cool and wet.
13. Applied lotion to the lower back area.
14. Stroked up from the buttocks to the shoulders.
    Then stroked down over the upper arms.
    Stroked up the upper arms, across the shoulders, and down the back to the buttocks. Used firm strokes.
    Kept your hands in contact with the person's skin.
    If the person did not want the buttocks exposed, stroked down the back to the waist and up the back to the shoulders.
15. Repeated stroking up from the buttocks to the shoulders. Then stroked down over the upper arms.
    Stroked up the upper arms, across the shoulders, and down the back to the buttocks. Used firm strokes.
    Kept your hands in contact with the person's skin.
    Did not stroke down to the buttocks without permission.
    Continued this for at least 3 minutes.

Date of Satisfactory Completion _____   Instructor's Initials _____

Procedure—cont'd

	S	U	Comments
16. Kneaded the back:			
a. Grasped the skin between your thumb and fingers.	___	___	_____
b. Kneaded half of the back. Started at the buttocks and moved up to the shoulder. Then kneaded down from the shoulder to the buttocks.	___	___	_____
c. Repeated on the other half of the back.	___	___	_____
17. Applied lotion to bony areas. Used circular motions with the tips of your fingers. (Did not massage reddened bony areas.)	___	___	_____
18. Used fast movements to stimulate. Used slow movements to relax the person.	___	___	_____
19. Stroked with long, firm movements to end the massage. Told the person you were finishing.	___	___	_____
20. Straightened and secured clothing or sleepwear.	___	___	_____
21. Covered the person. Removed the towel and bath blanket.	___	___	_____

Post-Procedure

	S	U	Comments
22. Provided for comfort.	___	___	_____
23. Placed the call light within reach.	___	___	_____
24. Lowered the bed to its lowest position.	___	___	_____
25. Raised or lowered bed rails. Followed the care plan.	___	___	_____
26. Returned lotion to its proper place.	___	___	_____
27. Unscreened the person.	___	___	_____
28. Completed a safety check of the room.	___	___	_____
29. Followed center policy for dirty linens.	___	___	_____
30. Decontaminated your hands.	___	___	_____
31. Reported and recorded your observations.	___	___	_____

Date of Satisfactory Completion _____ Instructor's Initials _____

Giving Female Perineal Care

NNAAP™ Skill CD-ROM VIDEO CLIP VIDEO

Name: _____   Date: _____

	S	U	Comments

Quality of Life

Remembered to:
- Knock before entering the person's room
- Address the person by name
- Introduce yourself by name and title
- Explain the procedure to the person before beginning and during the procedure
- Protect the person's rights during the procedure
- Handle the person gently during the procedure

Pre-Procedure

1. Followed *Delegation Guidelines:*
   Perineal Care.
   Saw *Promoting Safety and Comfort:*
   Perineal Care.
2. Practiced hand hygiene.
3. Collected the following:
   - Soap or other cleaning agent as directed
   - At least 4 washcloths
   - Bath towel
   - Bath blanket
   - Bath thermometer
   - Wash basin
   - Waterproof pad
   - Gloves
   - Paper towels
4. Covered the over-bed table with paper towels. Arranged items on top of them.
5. Identified the person. Checked the identification (ID) bracelet against the assignment sheet. Called her by name.
6. Provided for privacy.
7. Raised the bed for body mechanics. Bed rails were up if used.

Procedure

8. Lowered the bed rail near you if up.
9. Decontaminated your hands. Put on gloves.
10. Covered the person with a bath blanket. Moved top linens to the foot of the bed.
11. Positioned the person on her back.
12. Draped the person.
13. Raised the bed rail if used.
14. Filled the wash basin. Water temperature was 105°F–109°F (40.5°C–42.7°C) or followed the care plan for water temperature. Measured water temperature according to center policy.
15. Asked the person to check the water temperature. Adjusted if it was too hot or too cold. Raised the bed rail before leaving the bedside. Lowered it when returned.
16. Placed the basin on the over-bed table.

Date of Satisfactory Completion _____   Instructor's Initials _____

Procedure—cont'd   **S**   **U**   **Comments**

17. Lowered the bed rail if up.
18. Helped the person flex her knees and spread her legs.
    Or helped her spread her legs as much as possible
    with the knees straight.
19. Placed a waterproof pad under her buttocks.
    Protected her and dry linens.
20. Folded the corner of the bath blanket between her legs
    onto her abdomen.
21. Wet the washcloths.
22. Squeezed out water from a washcloth.
    Made a mitted washcloth. Applied soap.
23. Spread the labia. Cleaned downward from front to
    back with one stroke.
24. Repeated until area clean. Used a clean part of the
    washcloth for each stroke. Used more than one
    washcloth if needed.
    a. Squeezed out water from washcloth.
       Made a mitted washcloth. Applied soap.
    b. Separated the labia. Cleaned downward from
       front to back with one stroke.
25. Rinsed the perineum with a clean washcloth.
    Separated the labia. Stroked downward from front
    to back. Repeated as necessary. Used a clean part of
    the washcloth for each stroke. Used more than one
    washcloth if needed.
26. Patted the area dry with the towel. Dried from front
    to back.
27. Folded the blanket back between her legs.
28. Helped her lower her legs and turn onto her side
    away from you.
29. Applied soap to a mitted washcloth.
30. Cleaned the rectal area. Cleaned from the vagina to
    the anus with one stroke.
31. Repeated until the area was clean. Used a clean part
    of the washcloth for each stroke. Used more than one
    washcloth if needed.
    a. Applied soap to a mitted washcloth.
    b. Cleaned the rectal area. Cleaned from the vagina
       to the anus with one stroke.
32. Rinsed the rectal area with a washcloth. Stroked from
    the vagina to the anus. Repeated as necessary.
    Used a clean part of the washcloth for each stroke.
    Used more than one washcloth if needed.
33. Patted the area dry with the towel. Dried from front to back.
34. Removed any wet or soiled incontinence product.
    Removed the waterproof pad.
35. Removed and discarded the gloves.
    Decontaminated your hands.
    Put on clean gloves.
36. Provided clean and dry linens and incontinence
    products as needed.

Date of Satisfactory Completion _____   Instructor's Initials _____

Post-Procedure	**S**	**U**	**Comments**
37. Covered the person. Removed the bath blanket.	———	———	———————
38. Provided for comfort.	———	———	———————
39. Placed the call light within reach.	———	———	———————
40. Lowered the bed to its lowest position.	———	———	———————
41. Raised or lowered bed rails. Followed the care plan.	———	———	———————
42. Emptied, cleaned, and dried the wash basin.	———	———	———————
43. Returned the basin and supplies to their proper place.	———	———	———————
44. Wiped off the over-bed table with the paper towels. Discarded the paper towels.	———	———	———————
45. Unscreened the person.	———	———	———————
46. Completed a safety check of the room.	———	———	———————
47. Followed center policy for dirty linens.	———	———	———————
48. Removed the gloves. Decontaminated your hands.	———	———	———————
49. Reported and recorded your observations.	———	———	———————

Date of Satisfactory Completion _____ Instructor's Initials _____

CD-ROM VIDEO CLIP VIDEO **Giving Male Perineal Care**

Name: _____   Date: _____

	S	U	Comments

Quality of Life

Remembered to:
- Knock before entering the person's room
- Address the person by name
- Introduce yourself by name and title
- Explain the procedure to the person before beginning and during the procedure
- Protect the person's rights during the procedure
- Handle the person gently during the procedure

Procedure

1. Followed steps 1 through 17 in *Giving Female Perineal Care.*
   a. Followed *Delegation Guidelines: Perineal Care.*
      Saw *Promoting Safety and Comfort: Perineal Care.*
   b. Practiced hand hygiene.
   c. Collected the following:
      - Soap or other cleaning agent as directed
      - At least 4 washcloths
      - Bath towel
      - Bath blanket
      - Bath thermometer
      - Wash basin
      - Waterproof pad
      - Gloves
      - Paper towels
   d. Covered the over-bed table with paper towels. Arranged items on top of them.
   e. Identified the person. Checked the identification (ID) bracelet against the assignment sheet. Called him by name.
   f. Provided for privacy.
   g. Raised the bed for body mechanics. Bed rails were up if used.
   h. Lowered the bed rail near you if up.
   i. Decontaminated your hands. Put on gloves.
   j. Covered the person with a bath blanket. Moved top linens to the foot of the bed.
   k. Positioned the person on his back.
   l. Draped the person.
   m. Raised the bed rail if used.
   n. Filled the wash basin. Water temperature was 105°F–109°F (40.5°C–42.7°C). Followed the care plan for water temperature. Measured water temperature according to center policy.
   o. Asked the person to check the water temperature. Adjusted the water temperature if too hot or too cold. Raised the bed rail before leaving bedside. Lowered it when returned.
   p. Placed the basin on the over-bed table.
   q. Lowered the bed rail if up.

Date of Satisfactory Completion _____   Instructor's Initials _____

	S	U	Comments
Procedure—cont'd			
2. Placed a waterproof pad under his buttocks. Protected the person and dry linens from the wet or soiled incontinence product.	____	____	_____
3. Retracted the foreskin if he was not circumcised.	____	____	_____
4. Grasped the penis.	____	____	_____
5. Cleaned the tip. Used a circular motion. Started at the meatus of the urethra and worked outward. Repeated as needed. Used a clean part of the washcloth each time.	____	____	_____
6. Rinsed the area with another washcloth.	____	____	_____
7. Returned the foreskin immediately after rinsing to its natural position.	____	____	_____
8. Cleaned the shaft of the penis. Used firm downward strokes. Rinsed the area.	____	____	_____
9. Helped the person flex his knees and spread his legs. Or helped him spread his legs as much as possible with his knees straight.	____	____	_____
10. Cleaned the scrotum. Rinsed well. Observed for redness and irritation of the skin folds.	____	____	_____
11. Patted dry the penis and the scrotum. Used the towel.	____	____	_____
12. Folded the bath blanket back between his legs.	____	____	_____
13. Helped the person lower his legs and turn onto his side away from you.	____	____	_____
14. Cleaned the rectal area:			
a. Applied soap to a mitted washcloth.	____	____	_____
b. Cleaned from behind scrotum to the anus with one stroke.	____	____	_____
c. Repeated until the area was clean. Used a clean part of the washcloth for each stroke. Used more than one washcloth if needed.	____	____	_____
d. Rinsed the rectal area with a washcloth. Stroked from the scrotum to the anus. Repeated as necessary. Used a clean part of the washcloth for each stroke. Used more than one washcloth if needed.	____	____	_____
e. Rinsed and dried well.	____	____	_____
15. Removed any wet or soiled incontinence product. Removed the waterproof pad.	____	____	_____
16. Removed and discarded the gloves. Decontaminated your hands. Put on clean gloves.	____	____	_____
17. Provided clean and dry linens and incontinence products.	____	____	_____
Post-Procedure			
18. Covered the person. Removed the bath blanket.	____	____	_____
19. Provided for comfort.	____	____	_____
20. Placed call light within reach.	____	____	_____
21. Lowered the bed to its lowest position.	____	____	_____
22. Raised or lowered bed rails. Followed the care plan.	____	____	_____
23. Emptied, cleaned, and dried the wash basin.	____	____	_____
24. Returned the basin and supplies to their proper place.	____	____	_____
25. Wiped off the over-bed table with the paper towels. Discarded the paper towels.	____	____	_____
26. Unscreened the person.	____	____	_____
27. Completed a safety check of the room.	____	____	_____
28. Followed center policy for dirty linens.	____	____	_____
29. Removed the gloves. Decontaminated your hands.	____	____	_____
30. Reported and recorded your observations.	____	____	_____

Date of Satisfactory Completion _____   Instructor's Initials _____

CD-ROM　VIDEO CLIP　VIDEO　**Brushing and Combing the Person's Hair**

Name: _____　Date: _____

	S	U	Comments
Quality of Life Remembered to:			
• Knock before entering the person's room	___	___	_____
• Address the person by name	___	___	_____
• Introduce yourself by name and title	___	___	_____
• Explain the procedure to the person before beginning and during the procedure			
• Protect the person's rights during the procedure	___	___	_____
• Handle the person gently during the procedure	___	___	_____

Pre-Procedure

1. Followed *Delegation Guidelines:*
   Brushing and Combing Hair.
   Saw *Promoting Safety and Comfort:*
   Brushing and Combing Hair.
2. Practiced hand hygiene.
3. Identified the person. Checked the identification (ID) bracelet against the assignment sheet.
   Called the person by name.
4. Asked the person how to style hair.
5. Collected the following:
   • Comb and brush
   • Bath towel
   • Other hair items as requested
6. Arranged items on the bedside stand.
7. Provided for privacy.

Procedure

8. Lowered the bed rail if up.
9. Helped the person to the chair. The person put on a robe and non-skid footwear while up. (If the person was in bed, raised the bed for body mechanics. Bed rails were up if used. Lowered the bed rail near you. Assisted the person to a semi-Fowler's position if allowed.)
10. Placed a towel across the person's back and shoulders or across the pillow.
11. Asked the person to remove eyeglasses. Put them in the eyeglass case. Put the case inside the bedside stand.
12. *Brushed and combed hair that was not matted or tangled:*
    a. Used the comb to part the hair.
       1. Parted hair down the middle into two sides.
       2. Divided one side into two smaller sections.
    b. Brushed one of the small sections of hair. Started at the scalp and brushed toward the hair ends. Did the same for the other small section of hair.
    c. Repeated for the other side:
       1. Divided other side into two smaller sections. Used comb for this step.
       2. Brushed one of the small sections of hair. Started at the scalp and brushed toward the hair ends. Did the same for the other small section of hair.

Date of Satisfactory Completion _____　Instructor's Initials _____

Procedure—cont'd	S	U	Comments
13. *Brushed and combed matted and tangled hair:*			
a. Took a small section of hair near the ends.	___	___	___
b. Combed or brushed through to the hair ends.	___	___	___
c. Added small sections of hair as you worked up to the scalp.	___	___	___
d. Combed or brushed through each longer section to the hair ends.	___	___	___
e. Brushed or combed from the scalp to the hair ends.	___	___	___
14. Styled the hair as the person preferred.	___	___	___
15. Removed the towel.	___	___	___
16. Allowed the person to put on the eyeglasses.	___	___	___
Post-Procedure			
17. Provided for comfort.	___	___	___
18. Placed the call light within reach.	___	___	___
19. Lowered the bed to its lowest position.	___	___	___
20. Raised or lowered bed rails. Followed the care plan.	___	___	___
21. Cleaned and returned hair care items to their proper place.	___	___	___
22. Unscreened the person.	___	___	___
23. Completed a safety check of the room.	___	___	___
24. Followed center policy for dirty linens.	___	___	___
25. Decontaminated your hands.	___	___	___

Date of Satisfactory Completion _____   Instructor's Initials _____

CD-ROM   VIDEO CLIP   VIDEO   **Shampooing the Person's Hair**

Name: _____   Date: _____

	S	U	Comments
Quality of Life			
Remembered to:			
• Knock before entering the person's room	___	___	_____
• Address the person by name	___	___	_____
• Introduce yourself by name and title	___	___	_____
• Explain the procedure to the person before beginning and during the procedure	___	___	_____
• Protect the person's rights during the procedure	___	___	_____
• Handle the person gently during the procedure	___	___	_____
Pre-Procedure			
1. Followed *Delegation Guidelines: Shampooing.*	___		_____
Saw *Promoting Safety and Comfort: Shampooing.*	___		_____
2. Practiced hand hygiene.	___	___	_____
3. Collected the following:			
• Two bath towels	___	___	_____
• Washcloth	___	___	_____
• Shampoo	___	___	_____
• Hair conditioner (if requested)	___	___	_____
• Bath thermometer	___	___	_____
• Pitcher or hand-held nozzle (if needed)	___	___	_____
• Shampoo tray (if needed)	___	___	_____
• Basin or pan (if needed)	___	___	_____
• Waterproof pad (if needed)	___	___	_____
• Gloves (if needed)	___	___	_____
• Comb and brush	___	___	_____
• Hair dryer	___	___	_____
4. Arranged items nearby.	___	___	_____
5. Identified the person. Checked the identification (ID) bracelet against the assignment sheet. Called the person by name.	___	___	_____
6. Provided for privacy.	___	___	_____
7. Removed any hearing aids and eyeglasses.	___	___	_____
8. Raised the bed for body mechanics for a shampoo in bed. Bed rails were up if used.	___	___	_____
9. Decontaminated your hands.	___	___	_____
Procedure			
10. Lowered the bed rail near you if up.	___	___	_____
11. Covered the person's chest with a bath towel.	___	___	_____
12. Brushed and combed hair to remove snarls and tangles.	___	___	_____
13. Positioned the person for the method you used.			
To shampoo the person in bed:			
a. Lowered the head of the bed and removed the pillow.	___	___	_____
b. Placed the waterproof pad and shampoo tray under the head and shoulders.	___	___	_____
c. Supported the head and neck with a folded towel if necessary.	___	___	_____
14. Raised the bed rail if used.	___	___	_____
15. Obtained water. Water temperature usually 105°F (40.5°C). Tested water temperature according to center policy.	___	___	_____

Date of Satisfactory Completion _____   Instructor's Initials _____

Procedure—cont'd	**S**	**U**	**Comments**
16. Lowered the bed rail near you if up.	___	___	_____
17. Put on gloves (if needed).	___	___	_____
18. Asked the person to hold a washcloth over the eyes. It did not cover the nose and mouth. (NOTE: A damp washcloth is easier to hold. It will not slip. However, some state competency tests require a dry washcloth.)	___	___	_____
19. Used the pitcher or nozzle to wet the hair.	___	___	_____
20. Applied a small amount of shampoo.	___	___	_____
21. Worked up a lather with both hands. Started at the hairline. Worked toward the back of the head.	___	___	_____
22. Massaged the scalp with your fingertips. Did not scratch the scalp.	___	___	_____
23. Rinsed the hair until the water ran clear.	___	___	_____
24. Repeated:			
a. Applied a small amount of shampoo.	___	___	_____
b. Worked up a lather with both hands. Started at the hairline. Worked toward the back of the head.	___	___	_____
c. Massaged the scalp with your fingertips. Did not scratch the scalp.	___	___	_____
d. Rinsed the hair until the water ran clear.	___	___	_____
25. Applied conditioner. Followed directions on the container.	___	___	_____
26. Squeezed water from the person's hair.	___	___	_____
27. Covered the hair with a bath towel.	___	___	_____
28. Removed the shampoo tray and waterproof pad.	___	___	_____
29. Dried the person's face with the towel. Used the towel on the person's chest.	___	___	_____
30. Helped the person raise the head if appropriate. For the person in bed, raised the head of the bed.	___	___	_____
31. Rubbed the hair and scalp with the towel. Used the second towel if the first one was wet.	___	___	_____
32. Combed the hair to remove snarls and tangles.	___	___	_____
33. Dried and styled hair as quickly as possible.	___	___	_____
34. Removed and discarded the gloves if used. Decontaminated your hands.	___	___	_____
Post-Procedure			
35. Provided for comfort.	___	___	_____
36. Assisted person to replace hearing aids and eyeglasses.	___	___	_____
37. Placed the call light within reach.	___	___	_____
38. Lowered the bed to its lowest position.	___	___	_____
39. Raised or lowered bed rails. Followed the care plan.	___	___	_____
40. Unscreened the person.	___	___	_____
41. Completed a safety check of the room.	___	___	_____
42. Cleaned, dried, and returned equipment to its proper place. Remembered to clean the brush and comb. Discarded disposable items.	___	___	_____
43. Followed center policy for dirty linens.	___	___	_____
44. Decontaminated your hands.	___	___	_____
45. Reported and recorded your observations.	___	___	_____

Date of Satisfactory Completion _____ Instructor's Initials _____

VIDEO CLIP **VIDEO** ## Shaving the Person's Face with a Safety Razor

Name: _____   Date: _____

	S	U	Comments

Quality of Life
Remembered to:
- Knock before entering the person's room
- Address the person by name
- Introduce yourself by name and title
- Explain the procedure to the person before beginning and during the procedure
- Protect the person's rights during the procedure
- Handle the person gently during the procedure

Pre-Procedure
1. Followed *Delegation Guidelines: Shaving.* Saw *Promoting Safety and Comfort: Shaving.*
2. Practiced hand hygiene.
3. Collected the following:
   - Wash basin
   - Bath towel
   - Hand towel
   - Washcloth
   - Safety razor
   - Mirror
   - Shaving cream, soap, or lotion
   - Shaving brush
   - After-shave or lotion
   - Tissues
   - Paper towels
   - Gloves
4. Arranged paper towels and supplies on the over-bed table.
5. Identified the person. Checked the identification (ID) bracelet against the assignment sheet. Called the person by name.
6. Provided for privacy.
7. Raised the bed for body mechanics. Bed rails were up if used.

Procedure
8. Filled the wash basin with warm water.
9. Placed the basin on the over-bed table.
10. Lowered the bed rail near you if up.
11. Decontaminated your hands. Put on gloves.
12. Assisted the person to semi-Fowler's position if allowed or to the supine position.
13. Adjusted lighting to clearly see the person's face.
14. Placed the bath towel over the person's chest and shoulders.
15. Adjusted the over-bed table for easy reach.
16. Tightened the razor blade to the shaver.
17. Washed the person's face. Did not dry.

Date of Satisfactory Completion _____   Instructor's Initials _____

Procedure—cont'd	S	U	Comments
18. Wet the washcloth or towel. Wrung it out.	___	___	___
19. Applied the washcloth or towel to the face for a few minutes.	___	___	___
20. Applied shaving cream with your hands or used a shaving brush to apply lather.	___	___	___
21. Held the skin taut with one hand.	___	___	___
22. Shaved in the direction of hair growth. Used shorter strokes around the chin and lips.			
23. Rinsed the razor often. Wiped it with tissues or paper towels.	___	___	___
24. Applied direct pressure to any bleeding areas.	___	___	___
25. Washed off any remaining shaving cream or soap. Patted dry with a towel.	___	___	___
26. Applied after-shave or lotion if requested. Did not apply if there were nicks or cuts.	___	___	___
27. Removed the towel and gloves. Decontaminated your hands.	___	___	___
Post-Procedure			
28. Provided for comfort.	___	___	___
29. Placed the call light within reach.	___	___	___
30. Lowered the bed to its lowest position.	___	___	___
31. Raised or lowered bed rails. Followed the care plan.	___	___	___
32. Cleaned and returned equipment and supplies to their proper place. Discarded razor blade or disposable razor into the sharps container. Discarded disposable items. Wore gloves.	___	___	___
33. Wiped off the over-bed table with paper towels. Discarded the paper towels.	___	___	___
34. Unscreened the person.	___	___	___
35. Completed a safety check of the room.	___	___	___
36. Followed center policy for dirty linens.	___	___	___
37. Removed the gloves. Decontaminated your hands.	___	___	___
38. Reported nicks, cuts, irritation, or bleeding to the nurse at once. Also reported and recorded other observations.			

Date of Satisfactory Completion _____ Instructor's Initials _____

VIDEO **Shaving the Person's Face with an Electric Razor**

Name: _____   Date: _____

	S	U	Comments

Quality of Life
Remembered to:
- Knock before entering the person's room
- Address the person by name
- Introduce yourself by name and title
- Explain the procedure to the person before beginning and during the procedure
- Protect the person's rights during the procedure
- Handle the person gently during the procedure

Pre-Procedure
1. Followed *Delegation Guidelines:*
   Shaving.
   Saw *Promoting Safety and Comfort:*
   Shaving.
2. Practiced hand hygiene.
3. Collected the following:
   - Wash basin
   - Bath towel
   - Hand towel
   - Washcloth
   - Person's own electric razor
   - Mirror
   - Soap
   - Pre-shave or after-shave lotion
   - Tissues
   - Paper towels
   - Gloves
4. Arranged paper towels and supplies on the over-bed table.
5. Identified the person. Checked the identification (ID) bracelet against the assignment sheet. Called the person by name.
6. Provided for privacy.
7. If worn, dentures were in person's mouth.
8. Did not use electric shaver if person was using oxygen. (NOTE: Could use shaver on battery power.)
9. Raised the bed for body mechanics Bed rails were up if used.

Procedure
10. Filled the wash basin with warm water.
11. Placed the basin on the over-bed table.
12. Lowered the bed rail near you if up.
13. Decontaminated your hands. Put on gloves.
14. Assisted the person to semi-Fowler's position if allowed or to the supine position.
15. Adjusted lighting to clearly see the person's face.
16. Placed the bath towel over the person's chest and shoulders.
17. Adjusted the over-bed table for easy reach.

Date of Satisfactory Completion _____   Instructor's Initials _____

Procedure—cont'd	S	U	Comments
18. Washed the person's face and rinsed. The beard may have been softened by leaving a moist, warm washcloth or towel in place for a few minutes. Patted dry.	___	___	___
19. Applied pre-shave lotion or talcum powder, if desired.	___	___	___
20. Held the skin taut with one hand as you shaved in circular motions.	___	___	___
21. Shaved the cheek area first, then around the mouth.	___	___	___
22. Shaved the neck area last. Had the person tilt head back if able.	___	___	___
23. Applied direct pressure to any bleeding areas.	___	___	___
24. Applied after-shave lotion if requested. (Did not apply if there were nicks or cuts.)	___	___	___
25. Removed the towel and gloves. Decontaminated your hands.	___	___	___
Post-Procedure			
26. Provided for comfort.	___	___	___
27. Placed the call light within reach.	___	___	___
28. Lowered the bed to its lowest position.	___	___	___
29. Raised or lowered bed rails. Followed the care plan.	___	___	___
30. Cleaned equipment and put in proper place. Cleaned shaver by removing head and using a soft brush to remove the whiskers. Wiped off head of shaver with alcohol prep. Put shaver back in case.	___	___	___
31. Wiped off the over-bed table with paper towels. Discarded the paper towels.	___	___	___
32. Unscreened the person.	___	___	___
33. Completed a safety check of the room.	___	___	___
34. Followed center policy for dirty linens.	___	___	___
35. Removed the gloves. Decontaminated your hands.	___	___	___
36. Reported nicks, cuts, irritation, or bleeding to the nurse at once. Also reported and recorded other observations.			

Date of Satisfactory Completion _____   Instructor's Initials _____

NNAAP™ Skill   CD-ROM   VIDEO CLIP   VIDEO   **Giving Nail and Foot Care**

Name: _____   Date: _____

Quality of Life	S	U	Comments
Remembered to:			
• Knock before entering the person's room	____	____	_____
• Address the person by name	____	____	_____
• Introduce yourself by name and title	____	____	_____
• Explain the procedure to the person before beginning and during the procedure	____	____	_____
• Protect the person's rights during the procedure	____	____	_____
• Handle the person gently during the procedure	____	____	_____

Pre-Procedure	S	U	Comments
1. Followed *Delegation Guidelines: Nail and Foot Care.* Saw *Promoting Safety and Comfort: Nail and Foot Care.*	____	____	_____
2. Practiced hand hygiene.	____	____	_____
3. Collected the following:			
• Wash basin or whirlpool foot bath	____	____	_____
• Soap	____	____	_____
• Bath thermometer	____	____	_____
• Bath towel	____	____	_____
• Hand towel	____	____	_____
• Washcloth	____	____	_____
• Kidney basin	____	____	_____
• Nail clippers	____	____	_____
• Orangewood stick	____	____	_____
• Emery board or nail file	____	____	_____
• Lotion for the hands	____	____	_____
• Lotion or petroleum jelly for the feet	____	____	_____
• Paper towels	____	____	_____
• Bath mat	____	____	_____
• Gloves	____	____	_____
4. Arranged paper towels and items on the over-bed table.	____	____	_____
5. Identified the person. Checked the identification (ID) bracelet against the assignment sheet. Called the person by name.	____	____	_____
6. Provided for privacy.	____	____	_____
7. Assisted the person to the bedside chair. Placed the call light within reach.	____	____	_____

Procedure	S	U	Comments
8. Placed the bath mat under the feet.	____	____	_____
9. Filled the wash basin or whirlpool foot bath ⅔ (two-thirds) full with water. The nurse indicated what water temperature to use. (Measured water temperature with a bath thermometer. Or tested it by dipping your elbow or inner wrist into the basin. Followed center policy.) Also asked the person to check the water temperature. Adjusted the water temperature as needed.	____	____	_____
10. Placed the basin or foot bath on the bath mat.	____	____	_____

Date of Satisfactory Completion _____   Instructor's Initials _____

Procedure—cont'd	S	U	Comments
11. Put on gloves.	___	___	_____
12. Helped the person put the feet into the basin or foot bath. Made sure both feet were completely covered by water.	___	___	_____
13. Adjusted the over-bed table in front of the person.	___	___	_____
14. Filled the kidney basin ⅔ (two-thirds) full with water. The nurse told you what water temperature to use. (Measured water temperature with a bath thermometer. Or tested it by dipping your elbow or inner wrist into the basin. Followed center policy.) Also asked the person to check the water temperature. Adjusted the water temperature as needed.	___	___	_____
15. Placed the kidney basin on the over-bed table.	___	___	_____
16. Placed the person's fingers into the basin. Positioned the arms for comfort.	___	___	_____
17. Allowed the fingers to soak for 5–10 minutes. Allowed the feet to soak for 15–20 minutes. Re-warmed water as needed.	___	___	_____
18. Removed the kidney basin.	___	___	_____
19. Cleaned under the fingernails with the flat end of the orangewood stick. Used a towel to wipe the orangewood stick after each nail.	___	___	_____
20. Dried the hands and between the fingers thoroughly.	___	___	_____
21. Shaped nails with an emery board or nail file. Nails were smooth with no rough edges. Checked each nail for smoothness. Filed as needed.	___	___	_____
22. Applied lotion to the hands. Warmed the lotion before applying it.	___	___	_____
23. Moved the over-bed table to the side.	___	___	_____
24. Lifted a foot out of the water. Supported the foot and ankle with one hand. With the other hand, washed the foot and between the toes with soap and a washcloth. Returned the foot to the water for rinsing. Rinsed between the toes.	___	___	_____
25. Repeated for the other foot: Lifted a foot out of the water. Supported the foot and ankle with one hand. With the other hand, washed the foot and between the toes with soap and a washcloth. Returned the foot to the water for rinsing. Rinsed between the toes.	___	___	_____
26. Removed the feet from the basin or foot bath. Dried thoroughly, especially between the toes.	___	___	_____
27. Applied lotion or petroleum jelly to the tops and soles of the feet. Did not apply between the toes. Warmed lotion or petroleum jelly before applying it. Removed excess lotion or petroleum jelly with a towel.	___	___	_____
28. Removed and discarded the gloves. Decontaminated your hands.	___	___	_____
29. Assisted the person to put on stockings.	___	___	_____
30. Helped the person put on non-skid footwear.	___	___	_____

Post-Procedure

	S	U	Comments
31. Provided for comfort.	___	___	_____
32. Placed the call light within reach.	___	___	_____
33. Raised or lowered bed rails. Followed the care plan.	___	___	_____

Date of Satisfactory Completion _____   Instructor's Initials _____

Post-Procedure—cont'd	**S**	**U**	**Comments**
34. Cleaned, dried, and returned equipment and supplies to their proper place. Discarded disposable items. Wore gloves.			
35. Unscreened the person.			
36. Completed a safety check of the room.			
37. Followed center policy for dirty linens.			
38. Removed the gloves. Decontaminated your hands.			
39. Reported and recorded your observations.			

Date of Satisfactory Completion _____   Instructor's Initials _____

CD-ROM   VIDEO CLIP   VIDEO   **Undressing the Person**

Name: _____   Date: _____

	S	U	Comments

Quality of Life

Remembered to:

- Knock before entering the person's room
- Address the person by name
- Introduce yourself by name and title
- Explain the procedure to the person before beginning and during the procedure
- Protect the person's rights during the procedure
- Handle the person gently during the procedure

Pre-Procedure

1. Followed *Delegation Guidelines: Dressing and Undressing.*
2. Practiced hand hygiene.
3. Collected a bath blanket and clothing requested by the person.
4. Identified the person. Checked the identification (ID) bracelet against the assignment sheet. Called the person by name.
5. Provided for privacy.
6. Raised the bed for body mechanics. Bed rails were up if used.
7. Lowered the bed rail on the person's weak side.
8. Positioned the person supine.
9. Covered the person with a bath blanket. Fan-folded linens to the foot of the bed.

Procedure

10. Removed garments that opened in the back:
    a. Raised the head and shoulders. Or turned the person onto the side away from you.
    b. Undid buttons, zippers, ties, or snaps.
    c. Brought the sides of the garment to the sides of the person. If he or she was in a side-lying position, tucked the far side under the person. Folded the near side onto the chest.
    d. Positioned the person supine.
    e. Slid the garment off the shoulder on the strong side. Removed it from the arm.
    f. Removed the garment from the weak side.
11. Removed garments that opened in the front:
    a. Undid buttons, zippers, ties, or snaps.
    b. Slid the garment off the shoulder and arm on the strong side.
    c. Assisted the person to sit up or raised the head and shoulders. Brought the garment over to the weak side.
    d. Lowered the head and shoulders. Removed the garment from the weak side.
    e. If you could not raise the head and shoulders:
        1. Turned the person toward you. Tucked the removed part under the person.
        2. Turned him or her onto the side away from you.

Date of Satisfactory Completion _____   Instructor's Initials _____

Procedure—cont'd   S   U   Comments

3. Pulled the side of the garment out from under the person. Made sure he or she was not lying on it when supine.

4. Returned the person to the supine position.

5. Removed the garment from the weak side.

12. Removed pullover garments:
   a. Undid any buttons, zippers, ties, or snaps.
   b. Removed the garment from the strong side.
   c. Raised the head and shoulders. Or turned the person onto the side away from you. Brought the garment up to the person's neck.
   d. Removed the garment from the weak side.
   e. Brought the garment over the person's head.
   f. Positioned him or her in the supine position.

13. Removed pants or slacks:
   a. Removed footwear and socks.
   b. Positioned the person supine.
   c. Undid buttons, zippers, ties, snaps, or buckles.
   d. Removed the belt.
   e. Asked the person to lift the buttocks off the bed. Slid the pants down over the hips and buttocks. Had the person lower the hips and buttocks.
   f. If the person could not raise the hips off the bed:
      1. Turned the person toward you.
      2. Slid the pants off the hip and buttocks on the strong side.
      3. Turned the person away from you.
      4. Slid the pants off the hip and buttocks on the weak side.
   g. Slid the pants down the legs and over the feet.

14. Dressed the person.

Post-Procedure

15. Provided for comfort.

16. Placed the call light within reach.

17. Lowered the bed to its lowest position.

18. Raised or lowered bed rails. Followed the care plan.

19. Unscreened the person.

20. Completed a safety check of the room.

21. Followed center policy for soiled clothing.

22. Decontaminated your hands.

23. Reported and recorded your observations.

Date of Satisfactory Completion _____   Instructor's Initials _____

NNAAP™ Skill   CD-ROM   VIDEO   **Dressing the Person**

Name: _____   Date: _____

Quality of Life	S	U	Comments
Remembered to:			
• Knock before entering the person's room	___	___	_____
• Address the person by name	___	___	_____
• Introduce yourself by name and title	___	___	_____
• Explain the procedure to the person before beginning and during the procedure	___	___	_____
• Protect the person's rights during the procedure	___	___	_____
• Handle the person gently during the procedure	___	___	_____

Pre-Procedure

	S	U	Comments
1. Followed *Delegation Guidelines: Dressing and Undressing.*	___	___	_____
2. Practiced hand hygiene.	___	___	_____
3. Asked the person what he or she would like to wear.	___	___	_____
4. Got a bath blanket and clothing requested by the person.	___	___	_____
5. Identified the person. Checked the identification (ID) bracelet against the assignment sheet. Called the person by name.	___	___	_____
6. Provided for privacy.	___	___	_____
7. Raised the bed for body mechanics. Bed rails were up if used.	___	___	_____
8. Lowered the bed rail (if up) on the person's strong side.	___	___	_____
9. Positioned the person supine.	___	___	_____
10. Covered the person with a bath blanket. Fan-folded linens to the foot of the bed.	___	___	_____
11. Undressed the person.	___	___	_____

Procedure

	S	U	Comments
12. Put on garments that opened in the back:			
a. Slid the garment onto the arm and shoulder of the weak side.	___	___	_____
b. Slid the garment onto the arm and shoulder of the strong arm.	___	___	_____
c. Raised the person's head and shoulders.	___	___	_____
d. Brought the sides to the back.	___	___	_____
e. If you could not raise the person's head and shoulders:			
1. Turned the person toward you.	___	___	_____
2. Brought one side of the garment to the person's back.	___	___	_____
3. Turned the person away from you.	___	___	_____
4. Brought the other side to the person's back.	___	___	_____
f. Fastened buttons, ties, snaps, zippers, or other closures.	___	___	_____
g. Positioned the person supine.	___	___	_____
13. Put on garments that opened in the front:			
a. Slid the garment onto the arm and shoulder on the weak side.	___	___	_____
b. Raised the head and shoulders. Brought the side of the garment around to the back. Lowered the person down. Slid the garment arm onto the arm and shoulder of the strong arm.	___	___	_____
c. If the person could not raise the head and shoulders:			
1. Turned the person away from you.	___	___	_____
2. Tucked the garment under the person.	___	___	_____

Date of Satisfactory Completion _____   Instructor's Initials _____

Procedure—cont'd   S   U   **Comments**

    3. Turned the person toward you.

    4. Pulled the garment out from under the person.

    5. Turned the person back to the supine position.

    6. Slid the garment over the arm and shoulder of
       the strong arm.

  d. Fastened buttons, ties, snaps, zippers, or other closures.

14. Put on pullover garments:

  a. Positioned the person supine.

  b. Brought the neck of the garment over the head.

  c. Slid the arm and shoulder of the garment onto
    the weak side.

  d. Raised the person's head and shoulders.

  e. Brought the garment down.

  f. Slid the arm and shoulder of the garment onto the
    strong side.

  g. If the person could not assume a semi-sitting position:

    1. Turned the person away from you.

    2. Tucked the garment under the person.

    3. Turned the person toward you.

    4. Pulled the garment out from under the person.

    5. Positioned the person supine.

    6. Slid the arm and shoulder of the garment onto
      the strong side.

  h. Fastened buttons, ties, snaps, zippers, or other closures.

15. Put on pants or slacks:

  a. Slid the pants over the feet and up the legs.

  b. Asked the person to raise the hips and buttocks
    off the bed.

  c. Brought the pants up over the buttocks and hips.

  d. Asked the person to lower the hips and buttocks.

  e. If the person could not raise the hips and buttocks:

    1. Turned the person onto the strong side.

    2. Pulled the pants over the buttock and hip on the
      weak side.

    3. Turned the person onto the weak side.

    4. Pulled the pants over the buttock and hip on the
      strong side.

    5. Positioned the person supine.

  f. Fastened buttons, ties, snaps, the zipper, belt buckle,
    or other closure.

16. Put socks and non-skid footwear on the person. Made
    sure socks were up all the way and smooth.

17. Helped the person get out of bed. If the person stayed
    in bed, covered the person. Removed the bath blanket.

Post-Procedure

18. Provided for comfort.

19. Placed the call light within reach.

20. Lowered the bed to its lowest position.

21. Raised or lowered bed rails. Followed the care plan.

22. Unscreened the person.

23. Completed a safety check of the room.

24. Followed center policy for soiled clothing.

25. Decontaminated your hands.

26. Reported and recorded your observations.

Date of Satisfactory Completion _____   Instructor's Initials _____

CD-ROM **VIDEO CLIP** **VIDEO** ## Changing the Gown of the Person with an IV

Name: _____   Date: _____

Quality of Life	S	U	Comments

Quality of Life
Remembered to:
- Knock before entering the person's room
- Address the person by name
- Introduce yourself by name and title
- Explain the procedure to the person before beginning and during the procedure
- Protect the person's rights during the procedure
- Handle the person gently during the procedure

Pre-Procedure
1. Followed *Delegation Guidelines:*
   Changing Hospital Gowns.
   Saw *Promoting Safety and Comfort:*
   Changing Hospital Gowns.
2. Practiced hand hygiene.
3. Got a clean gown and a bath blanket.
4. Identified the person. Checked the identification (ID) bracelet against the assignment sheet. Called the person by name.
5. Provided for privacy.
6. Raised the bed for body mechanics. Bed rails were up if used.

Procedure
7. Lowered the bed rail near you (if up).
8. Covered the person with a bath blanket. Fan-folded linens to the foot of the bed.
9. Untied the gown. Freed parts the person was lying on.
10. Removed the gown from the arm with *no IV*.
11. Gathered up the sleeve of the arm *with the IV*. Slid it over the IV site and tubing. Removed the arm and hand from the sleeve.
12. Kept the sleeve gathered. Slid your arm along the tubing to the bag.
13. Removed the bag from the pole. Slid the bag and tubing through the sleeve. Did not pull on the tubing. Kept the bag above the person.
14. Hung the IV bag on the pole.
15. Gathered the sleeve of the clean gown that went on the arm with the IV infusion.
16. Removed the bag from the pole. Slipped the sleeve over the bag at the shoulder part of the gown. Hung the bag.
17. Slid the gathered sleeve over the tubing, hand, arm, and IV site. Then slid it onto the shoulder.
18. Put the other side of the gown on the person. Fastened the gown.
19. Covered the person. Removed the bath blanket.

Post-Procedure
20. Provided for comfort.
21. Placed the call light within reach.
22. Lowered the bed to its lowest position.
23. Raised or lowered bed rails. Followed the care plan.
24. Unscreened the person.

Date of Satisfactory Completion _____   Instructor's Initials _____

Post-Procedure—cont'd	S	U	Comments
25. Completed a safety check of the room.	_____	_____	_____
26. Followed center policy for dirty linens.	_____	_____	_____
27. Decontaminated your hands.	_____	_____	_____
28. Asked the nurse to check the flow rate.	_____	_____	_____
29. Reported and recorded your observations.	_____	_____	_____

Date of Satisfactory Completion _____   Instructor's Initials _____

NNAAP™ Skill   CD-ROM   VIDEO CLIP   VIDEO   **Measuring Intake and Output**

Name: _____   Date: _____

	S	U	Comments
Quality of Life			
Remembered to:			
• Knock before entering the person's room	____	____	_____
• Address the person by name	____	____	_____
• Introduce yourself by name and title	____	____	_____
• Explain the procedure to the person before beginning and during the procedure	____	____	_____
• Protect the person's rights during the procedure	____	____	_____
• Handle the person gently during the procedure	____	____	_____
Pre-Procedure			
1. Followed *Delegation Guidelines: Intake and Output.* Saw *Promoting Safety and Comfort: Intake and Output.*	____	____	_____
	____	____	_____
2. Practiced hand hygiene.	____	____	_____
3. Collected the following:			
• Intake and output (I&O) record	____	____	_____
• Graduates	____	____	_____
• Gloves	____	____	_____
Procedure			
4. Put on gloves.	____	____	_____
5. Measured intake as follows:			
a. Poured liquid remaining in the container into the graduate.	____	____	_____
b. Measured the amount at eye level or on a flat surface. Kept the container level.	____		_____
c. Checked the serving amount on the I&O record.	____	____	_____
d. Subtracted the remaining amount from the full serving amount. Noted the amount.	____	____	_____
e. Poured fluid in the graduate back into the container.	____	____	_____
f. Repeated steps for each liquid:			
1) Poured liquid remaining in the container into the graduate.	____		_____
2) Measured the amount at eye level. Kept the container level.	____	____	_____
3) Checked the serving amount on the I&O record.	____	____	_____
4) Subtracted the remaining amount from the full serving amount. Noted the amount.	____	____	_____
5) Poured fluid in the graduate back into the container.	____	____	_____
g. Added the amounts from each liquid together.	____	____	_____
h. Recorded the time and amount on the I&O record.	____	____	_____
6. Measured output as follows:			
a. Poured fluid into the graduate used to measure output.	____	____	_____
b. Measured the amount at eye level or on a flat surface. Kept the container level.	____	____	_____
c. Disposed of fluid in the toilet. Avoided splashes.			
7. Cleaned and rinsed the graduates. Disposed of rinse into the toilet. Returned the graduates to their proper place.	____	____	_____
8. Cleaned and rinsed voiding receptacle or drainage container. Disposed of the rinse into the toilet. Returned item to its proper place.	____	____	_____

Date of Satisfactory Completion _____   Instructor's Initials _____

Procedure—cont'd	S	U	Comments
9. Removed the gloves. Practiced hand hygiene.	___	___	_____
10. Recorded the output on the I&O record.	___	___	_____
Post-Procedure			
11. Provided for comfort.	___	___	_____
12. Made sure the call light was within reach.	___	___	_____
13. Completed a safety check of the room.	___	___	_____
14. Reported and recorded your observations.	___	___	_____

Date of Satisfactory Completion _____   Instructor's Initials _____

Preparing the Person for a Meal

Name: _____   Date: _____

	S	U	Comments
Quality of Life			
Remembered to:			
• Knock before entering the person's room	___	___	_____
• Address the person by name	___	___	_____
• Introduce yourself by name and title	___	___	_____
• Explain the procedure to the person before beginning and during the procedure	___	___	_____
• Protect the person's rights during the procedure	___	___	_____
• Handle the person gently during the procedure	___	___	_____

Pre-Procedure

1. Followed *Delegation Guidelines:*
   Preparing for Meals.   ___ ___ _____
   Saw *Promoting Safety and Comfort:*
   Preparing for Meals.   ___ ___ _____
2. Practiced hand hygiene.   ___ ___ _____
3. Collected the following:
   • Equipment for oral hygiene   ___ ___ _____
   • Bedpan and cover, urinal, commode, or specimen pan ___ ___ _____
   • Toilet tissue   ___ ___ _____
   • Wash basin   ___ ___ _____
   • Soap   ___ ___ _____
   • Washcloth   ___ ___ _____
   • Towel   ___ ___ _____
   • Gloves   ___ ___ _____
4. Provided for privacy.   ___ ___ _____

Procedure

5. Made sure eyeglasses and hearing aids were in place. ___ ___ _____
6. Assisted with oral hygiene. Made sure dentures were in place. Wore gloves and decontaminated your hands after removing gloves.
7. Assisted with elimination. Made sure the incontinent person was clean and dry. Wore gloves and practiced hand hygiene after removing gloves. ___ ___ _____
8. Assisted with hand washing. Wore gloves and practiced hand hygiene after removing your gloves. ___ ___ _____
9. Did the following if the person ate in bed:
   a. Raised the head of the bed to a comfortable position. (Fowler's position preferred.) ___ ___ _____
   b. Removed items from the over-bed table. Cleaned the over-bed table. ___ ___ _____
   c. Adjusted the over-bed table in front of the person. ___ ___ _____
10. Did the following if the person was sitting in a chair:
    a. Positioned the person in a chair or wheelchair. ___ ___ _____
    b. Removed items from the over-bed table. Cleaned the over-bed table. ___ ___ _____
    c. Adjusted the over-bed table in front of the person. ___ ___ _____
11. Assisted the person to the dining area, if person ate in dining area. ___ ___ _____

Date of Satisfactory Completion _____   Instructor's Initials _____

Post-Procedure

	S	U	Comments
12. Provided for comfort.	___	___	___
13. Placed the call light within reach.	___	___	___
14. Emptied, cleaned, and disinfected equipment. Returned equipment to its proper place. Wore gloves and practiced hand hygiene after removing gloves.	___	___	___
15. Straightened the room. Eliminated unpleasant noises, odors, or equipment.	___	___	___
16. Unscreened the person.	___	___	___
17. Completed a safety check of the room.	___	___	___
18. Decontaminated your hands.	___	___	___

Date of Satisfactory Completion _____   Instructor's Initials _____

VIDEO   Serving Meal Trays

Name: _____   Date: _____

	S	U	Comments

Quality of Life

Remembered to:
- Knock before entering the person's room
- Address the person by name
- Introduce yourself by name and title
- Explain the procedure to the person before beginning and during the procedure
- Protect the person's rights during the procedure
- Handle the person gently during the procedure

Pre-Procedure

1. Followed *Delegation Guidelines: Serving Meal Trays.*
   Saw *Promoting Safety and Comfort: Serving Meal Trays.*
2. Practiced hand hygiene.

Procedure

3. Made sure the tray was complete. Checked items on the tray with the dietary card. Made sure assist devices were included.
4. Identified the person. Checked the identification (ID) bracelet against the dietary card.
   Called person by name.
5. Placed the tray within the person's reach.
   Adjusted the over-bed table as needed.
6. Removed food covers. Opened cartons, cut meat into bite-sized pieces, buttered bread, and so on as needed. Seasoned food as person preferred and as allowed on the care plan.
7. Placed the napkin, clothes protector, assist devices, and eating utensils within reach.
8. Placed the call light within reach.
9. Did the following when the person was done eating:
   a. Measured and recorded intake if ordered.
   b. Noted the amount and type of foods eaten.
   c. Checked for and removed any food in the mouth (pocketing). Wore gloves. Decontaminated your hands after removing gloves.
   d. Removed the tray.
   e. Cleaned spills. Changed soiled linens and clothing.
   f. Helped the person return to bed if needed.
   g. Assisted with oral hygiene and hand washing. Wore gloves. Decontaminated your hands after removing the gloves.

Post-Procedure

10. Provided for comfort.
11. Placed the call light within reach.
12. Raised or lowered bed rails. Followed the care plan.
13. Completed a safety check of the room.
14. Followed center policy for soiled linens.
15. Decontaminated your hands.
16. Reported and recorded your observations.

Date of Satisfactory Completion _____   Instructor's Initials _____

NNAAP™ Skill   CD-ROM   VIDEO CLIP   VIDEO   **Feeding the Person**

Name: _____   Date: _____

	S	U	Comments

Quality of Life

Remembered to:
- Knock before entering the person's room
- Address the person by name
- Introduce yourself by name and title
- Explain the procedure to the person before beginning and during the procedure
- Protect the person's rights during the procedure
- Handle the person gently during the procedure

Pre-Procedure

1. Followed *Delegation Guidelines:*
   Feeding the Person.
   Saw *Promoting Safety and Comfort:*
   Feeding the Person.
2. Practiced hand hygiene.
3. Positioned the person in a comfortable position for eating (usually sitting or Fowler's).
4. Got the tray. Placed it on the over-bed table or dining table.

Procedure

5. Identified the person. Checked the identification (ID) bracelet with the dietary card.
   Called the person by name.
6. Draped a napkin across the person's chest and underneath the chin.
7. Told the person what foods and fluids were on the tray.
8. Prepared food for eating. Cut food into bite-sized pieces. Seasoned foods as the person preferred and was allowed on the care plan.
9. Placed a chair where you could sit comfortably. Sat facing the person.
10. Served foods in the order the person preferred. Identified foods as you served them. Alternated between solid and liquid foods. Used a spoon for safety. Allowed enough time for chewing and swallowing. Did not rush the person. Offered liquids on the person's tray.
11. Checked the person's mouth before offering more food or fluids. Made sure the person's mouth was empty between bites and swallows.
12. Used straws for liquids if person could not drink out of a glass or cup. Had one straw for each liquid. Provided short straws for weak persons.
13. Wiped the person's hands, face, and mouth as needed during the meal. Used a napkin.
14. Followed the care plan if the person had dysphagia (checked if person could use a straw). Gave thickened liquids with a spoon.
15. Conversed with the person in a pleasant manner.
16. Encouraged the person to eat as much as possible.
17. Wiped the person's mouth with a napkin. Discarded the napkin.

Date of Satisfactory Completion _____   Instructor's Initials _____

Procedure—cont'd	S	U	Comments
18. Noted how much and which foods were eaten.	___	___	_____
19. Measured and recorded intake if ordered.	___	___	_____
20. Removed the tray.	___	___	_____
21. Took the person back to his or her room, if in dining area.	___	___	_____
22. Assisted with oral hygiene and hand washing. Wore gloves. Provided for privacy. Decontaminated your hands after removing the gloves.	___	___	_____

Post-Procedure

	S	U	Comments
23. Provided for comfort.	___	___	_____
24. Placed the call light within reach.	___	___	_____
25. Raised or lowered bed rails. Followed the care plan.	___	___	_____
26. Completed a safety check of the room.	___	___	_____
27. Returned the food tray to the food cart.	___	___	_____
28. Decontaminated your hands.	___	___	_____
29. Reported and recorded your observations.	___	___	_____

Date of Satisfactory Completion _____ Instructor's Initials _____

Providing Drinking Water

Name: _____   Date: _____

	S	U	Comments
Quality of Life			
Remembered to:			
• Knock before entering the person's room	___	___	_____
• Address the person by name	___	___	_____
• Introduce yourself by name and title	___	___	_____
• Explain the procedure to the person before beginning and during the procedure	___	___	_____
• Protect the person's rights during the procedure	___	___	_____
• Handle the person gently during the procedure	___	___	_____

Pre-Procedure

1. Followed *Delegation Guidelines:*
   Providing Drinking Water.
   Saw *Promoting Safety and Comfort:*
   Providing Drinking Water.   ___ ___ _____
2. Obtained a list of persons who have special fluid
   orders from the nurse. Or used your assignment sheet.   ___ ___ _____
3. Practiced hand hygiene.   ___ ___ _____
4. Collected the following:
   • Cart   ___ ___ _____
   • Ice chest filled with ice   ___ ___ _____
   • Cover for ice chest   ___ ___ _____
   • Scoop   ___ ___ _____
   • Water cups   ___ ___ _____
   • Straws   ___ ___ _____
   • Paper towels   ___ ___ _____
   • Water pitcher for resident use   ___ ___ _____
   • Large water pitcher filled with cold water
     (optional, depending on center Procedure)   ___ ___ _____
   • Towel for the scoop   ___ ___ _____
5. Covered the cart with paper towels. Arranged
   equipment on top of the paper towels.   ___ ___ _____

Procedure

6. Took the cart to the person's room door.
   Did not take the cart into the room.   ___ ___ _____
7. Checked the person's fluid orders.
   Used the list obtained from the nurse.   ___ ___ _____
8. Identified the person. Checked the identification (ID)
   bracelet against the fluid order sheet or your
   assignment sheet. Called the person by name.   ___ ___ _____
9. Took the pitcher from the person's over-bed table.
   Emptied it into the bathroom sink.   ___ ___ _____
10. Determined if a new water pitcher was needed.   ___ ___ _____
11. Used the scoop to fill the pitcher with ice.
    Did not let the scoop touch the rim or inside
    of the pitcher. Did not place the person's
    pitcher on the cart.   ___ ___ _____
12. Placed the scoop on the towel.   ___ ___ _____
13. Filled the water pitcher with water. Got water from
    the bathroom or used the larger water pitcher
    on the cart.

Date of Satisfactory Completion _____   Instructor's Initials _____

	S	U	Comments

Procedure—cont'd

14. Placed the pitcher, cup, and straw (if used) on the over-bed table. Filled the cup with water. Did not let the water pitcher touch the rim or inside of the cup.

15. Made sure the pitcher, cup, and straw (if used) were within the person's reach.

Post-Procedure

16. Provided for comfort.
17. Placed the call light within reach.
18. Completed a safety check of the room.
19. Decontaminated your hands.
20. Repeated for each resident.
    - Took the cart to the person's room door. Did not take the cart into the room.
    - Checked the person's fluid orders. Used the list obtained from the nurse.
    - Identified the person. Checked the ID bracelet against the fluid order sheet or your assignment sheet. Called the person by name.
    - Took the pitcher from the person's over-bed table. Emptied it into the bathroom sink.
    - Determined if a new water pitcher was needed.
    - Used the scoop to fill the pitcher with ice. Did not let the scoop touch the rim or inside of the pitcher. Did not place the person's pitcher on the cart.
    - Placed the scoop on the towel.
    - Filled the water pitcher with water. Got water from the bathroom or used the larger water pitcher on the cart.
    - Placed the pitcher, cup, and straw (if used) on the over-bed table.
    - Filled the cup with water. Did not let the water pitcher touch the rim or inside of the cup.
    - Made sure the pitcher, cup, and straw (if used) were within the person's reach.
    - Provided for comfort.
    - Placed the call light within reach.
    - Completed a safety check of the room.
    - Decontaminated your hands.

Date of Satisfactory Completion _____ Instructor's Initials _____

Giving the Bedpan

NNAAP™ Skill · CD-ROM · VIDEO CLIP · VIDEO

Name: _____ Date: _____

	S	U	Comments

Quality of Life

Remembered to:
- Knock before entering the person's room
- Address the person by name
- Introduce yourself by name and title
- Explain the procedure to the person before beginning and during the procedure
- Protect the person's rights during the procedure
- Handle the person gently during the procedure

Pre-Procedure

1. Followed *Delegation Guidelines: Bedpans.* Saw *Promoting Safety and Comfort: Bedpans.*
2. Provided for privacy.
3. Practiced hand hygiene.
4. Put on gloves.
5. Collected the following:
   - Bedpan
   - Bedpan cover
   - Toilet tissue
   - Waterproof pad (if required by center)
6. Arranged equipment on the chair or bed.

Procedure

7. Lowered the bed rail near you if up.
8. Positioned the person supine. Raised the head of the bed slightly.
9. Folded the top linens and gown out of the way. Kept the lower body covered.
10. Asked the person to flex the knees and raise the buttocks by pushing against the mattress with his or her feet.
11. Slid a hand under the lower back. Helped raise the buttocks. If using waterproof pad, placed it under the person's buttocks.
12. Slid the bedpan under the person.
13. If the person did not assist in getting on the bedpan:
    a. Placed the waterproof pad under the person's buttocks if using one.
    b. Turned the person onto the side away from you.
    c. Placed the bedpan firmly against the buttocks.
    d. Pushed the bedpan down and toward the person.
    e. Held the bedpan securely. Turned the person onto his or her back.
    f. Made sure the bedpan was centered under the person.
14. Covered the person.
15. Raised the head of the bed so the person was in a sitting position (Fowler's) if using standard bedpan. (NOTE: Removed gloves and washed your hands before raising head of bed if required by the state competency test.)

Date of Satisfactory Completion _____ Instructor's Initials _____

Procedure—cont'd	S	U	Comments
16. Made sure the person was correctly positioned on the bedpan.			
17. Raised the bed rail if used.			
18. Placed the toilet tissue and call light within reach.			
19. Asked the person to signal when done or when help was needed.			
20. Removed the gloves. Practiced hand hygiene.			
21. Left the room and closed the door.			
22. Returned when the person signaled. Or checked on the person every 5 minutes. Knocked before entering.			
23. Decontaminated your hands. Put on gloves.			
24. Raised the bed for body mechanics. Lowered the bed rail (if used) and the head of the bed.			
25. Asked the person to raise the buttocks. Removed the bedpan. Or held the bedpan and turned the person onto the side away from you.			
26. Cleaned the genital area if the person did not do so. Cleaned from front (urethra) to back (anus) with toilet tissue. Used fresh tissue for each wipe. Provided perineal care if needed. Removed and discarded the waterproof pad if using.			
27. Covered the bedpan. Took it to the bathroom. Raised the bed rail (if used) before leaving the bedside.			
28. Noted the color, amount, and character of the urine or feces.			
29. Emptied the bedpan contents into the toilet and flushed.			
30. Rinsed the bedpan. Poured the rinse into the toilet and flushed.			
31. Cleaned the bedpan with a disinfectant.			
32. Removed soiled gloves. Practiced hand hygiene and put on clean gloves.			
33. Returned the bedpan and clean cover to the bedside stand.			
34. Helped the person with hand washing. Wore gloves.			
35. Removed the gloves. Practiced hand hygiene.			
Post-Procedure			
36. Provided for comfort.			
37. Placed the call light within reach.			
38. Lowered the bed to its lowest position.			
39. Raised or lowered bed rails. Followed the care plan.			
40. Unscreened the person.			
41. Completed a safety check of the room.			
42. Followed center policy for soiled linens.			
43. Practiced hand hygiene.			
44. Reported and recorded your observations.			

Date of Satisfactory Completion _____ Instructor's Initials _____

VIDEO CLIP **VIDEO** **Giving the Urinal**

Name: _____   Date: _____

Quality of Life	S	U	Comments
Remembered to:			
• Knock before entering the person's room	___	___	_____
• Address the person by name	___	___	_____
• Introduce yourself by name and title	___	___	_____
• Explain the procedure to the person before beginning and during the procedure	___	___	_____
• Protect the person's rights during the procedure	___	___	_____
• Handle the person gently during the procedure	___	___	_____

Pre-Procedure

	S	U	Comments
1. Followed *Delegation Guidelines: Urinals.* Saw *Promoting Safety and Comfort: Urinals.*	___	___	_____
2. Provided for privacy.	___	___	_____
3. Determined if the person will stand, sit, or lie in bed.	___	___	_____
4. Practiced hand hygiene.	___	___	_____
5. Put on gloves.	___	___	_____
6. Collected the following:			
• Urinal	___	___	_____
• Non-skid footwear if the person will stand to void	___	___	_____

Procedure

	S	U	Comments
7. Gave the person the urinal if he was in bed. Reminded him to tilt the bottom down to prevent spills.	___	___	_____
8. If he stood:			
a. Helped him sit on the side of the bed.	___	___	_____
b. Put non-skid footwear on him.	___	___	_____
c. Helped him stand. Provided support if he was unsteady.	___	___	_____
d. Gave him the urinal.	___	___	_____
9. Positioned the urinal if necessary. Positioned the penis in the urinal if he could not do so.	___	___	_____
10. Placed the call light within reach. Asked him to signal when done or when he needed help.	___	___	_____
11. Provided for privacy.	___	___	_____
12. Removed the gloves. Practiced hand hygiene.	___	___	_____
13. Left the room and closed the door.	___	___	_____
14. Returned when he signaled. Or checked on him every 5 minutes. Knocked before entering.	___	___	_____
15. Practiced hand hygiene. Put on gloves.	___	___	_____
16. Closed the cap on the urinal. Took it to the bathroom.	___	___	_____
17. Noted the color, amount, and clarity of the urine.	___	___	_____
18. Emptied the urinal into the toilet and flushed.	___	___	_____
19. Rinsed the urinal with cold water. Poured rinse into the toilet and flushed.	___	___	_____
20. Cleaned the urinal with a disinfectant.	___	___	_____
21. Returned the urinal to its proper place.	___	___	_____
22. Removed soiled gloves. Practiced hand hygiene and put on clean gloves.	___	___	_____
23. Assisted with hand washing.	___	___	_____
24. Removed the gloves. Practiced hand hygiene.	___	___	_____

Date of Satisfactory Completion _____   Instructor's Initials _____

Post-Procedure	S	U	Comments
25. Provided for comfort.	_____	_____	_____
26. Placed the call light within reach.	_____	_____	_____
27. Raised or lowered bed rails. Followed the care plan.	_____	_____	_____
28. Unscreened him.	_____	_____	_____
29. Completed a safety check of the room.	_____	_____	_____
30. Followed center policy for soiled linens.	_____	_____	_____
31. Practiced hand hygiene.	_____	_____	_____
32. Reported and recorded your observations.	_____	_____	_____

Date of Satisfactory Completion _____   Instructor's Initials _____

VIDEO CLIP **VIDEO** ## Helping the Person to the Commode

Name: _____   Date: _____

	S	U	Comments

Quality of Life
Remembered to:
- Knock before entering the person's room
- Address the person by name
- Introduce yourself by name and title
- Explain the procedure to the person before beginning and during the procedure
- Protect the person's rights during the procedure
- Handle the person gently during the procedure

Pre-Procedure
1. Followed *Delegation Guidelines: Commodes.*
   Saw *Promoting Safety and Comfort: Commodes*
2. Provided for privacy.
3. Practiced hand hygiene.
4. Put on gloves.
5. Collected the following:
   - Commode
   - Toilet tissue
   - Bath blanket
   - Transfer belt
   - Robe and non-skid footwear

Procedure
6. Brought the commode next to the bed. Removed the chair seat and container lid.
7. Helped the person sit on the side of the bed. Lowered the bed rail if used.
8. Helped the person put on a robe and non-skid footwear.
9. Assisted the person to the commode. Used the transfer belt.
10. Removed the transfer belt. Covered the person with a bath blanket for warmth.
11. Placed the toilet tissue and call light within reach.
12. Asked the person to signal when done or when help was needed. (Stayed with the person if necessary. Was respectful. Provided as much privacy as possible.)
13. Removed the gloves. Practiced hand hygiene.
14. Left the room. Closed the door.
15. Returned when the person signaled. Or checked on the person every 5 minutes. Knocked before entering.
16. Decontaminated your hands. Put on gloves.
17. Helped the person clean the genital area as needed. Removed the gloves and practiced hand hygiene.
18. Applied the transfer belt. Helped the person back to bed using the transfer belt. Removed the transfer belt, robe, and footwear. Raised the bed rail if used.
19. Put on clean gloves. Removed and covered the commode container. Cleaned the commode.
20. Took the container to the bathroom.
21. Observed urine and feces for color, amount, and character.
22. Emptied the container contents into the toilet and flushed.

Date of Satisfactory Completion _____   Instructor's Initials _____

Procedure—cont'd	S	U	Comments
23. Rinsed the container. Poured rinse into the toilet and flushed.	___	___	_____
24. Cleaned and disinfected the container.	___	___	_____
25. Returned the container to the commode. Returned other supplies to their proper place.	___	___	_____
26. Removed soiled gloves. Practiced hand hygiene and put on clean gloves.	___	___	_____
27. Assisted with hand washing.	___	___	_____
28. Removed the gloves. Practiced hand hygiene.	___	___	_____
Post-Procedure			
29. Provided for comfort.	___	___	_____
30. Placed the call light within reach.	___	___	_____
31. Raised or lowered bed rails. Followed the care plan.	___	___	_____
32. Unscreened the person.	___	___	_____
33. Completed a safety check of the room.	___	___	_____
34. Followed center policy for soiled linens.	___	___	_____
35. Practiced hand hygiene.	___	___	_____
36. Reported and recorded your observations.	___	___	_____

Date of Satisfactory Completion _____   Instructor's Initials _____

NNAAP™ Skill   CD-ROM   VIDEO CLIP   VIDEO   **Giving Catheter Care**

Name: _____   Date: _____

Quality of Life	S	U	Comments
Remembered to:			
• Knock before entering the person's room	_____	_____	_____
• Address the person by name	_____	_____	_____
• Introduce yourself by name and title	_____	_____	_____
• Explain the procedure to the person before beginning and during the procedure	_____	_____	_____
• Protect the person's rights during the procedure	_____	_____	_____
• Handle the person gently during the procedure	_____	_____	_____

Pre-Procedure

	S	U	Comments
1. Followed *Delegation Guidelines:*			
a. *Perineal Care.*	_____	_____	_____
b. *Catheters.*	_____	_____	_____
Saw *Promoting Safety and Comfort:*			
a. *Perineal Care.*	_____	_____	_____
b. *Catheters.*	_____	_____	_____
2. Practiced hand hygiene.	_____	_____	_____
3. Collected the following:			
• Items for perineal care:			
Soap or other cleaning agent as directed	_____	_____	_____
At least 4 washcloths	_____	_____	_____
Bath towel	_____	_____	_____
Bath thermometer	_____	_____	_____
Wash basin	_____	_____	_____
Waterproof pad	_____	_____	_____
Paper towels	_____	_____	_____
• Gloves	_____	_____	_____
• Bath blanket	_____	_____	_____
4. Covered the over-bed table with paper towels. Arranged items on top of paper towels.	_____	_____	_____
5. Identified the person. Checked the identification (ID) bracelet against the assignment sheet. Called the person by name.	_____	_____	_____
6. Provided for privacy.			
7. Filled the wash basin. Water temperature was 105°F (40.5°C). Measured water temperature according to center policy. Asked the person to check the water temperature. Adjusted water temperature as needed.	_____	_____	_____
8. Raised the bed for body mechanics. Bed rails were up if used.	_____	_____	_____

Procedure

	S	U	Comments
9. Lowered the bed rail near you if used.	_____	_____	_____
10. Decontaminated your hands. Put on gloves.	_____	_____	_____
11. Covered the person with a bath blanket. Fan-folded top linens to the foot of the bed.	_____	_____	_____
12. Draped the person for perineal care.	_____	_____	_____
13. Folded back the bath blanket to expose the genital area.	_____	_____	_____
14. Placed the waterproof pad under the buttocks. Asked the person to flex the knees and raise the buttocks off the bed.	_____	_____	_____

Date of Satisfactory Completion _____   Instructor's Initials _____

	S	U	Comments
Procedure—cont'd			
15. Separated the labia (female). With an uncircumcised male, retracted the foreskin. Checked for crusts, abnormal drainage, or secretions.	___	___	_____
16. Gave perineal care.	___	___	_____
17. Applied soap to clean, wet washcloth.	___	___	_____
18. Held the catheter near the meatus.	___	___	_____
19. Cleaned the catheter from the meatus down the catheter about 4 inches. Cleaned downward, away from the meatus with 1 stroke. Did not tug or pull on the catheter. Repeated as needed with a clean area of the washcloth. Used a clean washcloth if needed.	___	___	_____
20. Rinsed the catheter with a clean washcloth. Rinsed from the meatus down the catheter about 4 inches. Rinsed downward, away from the meatus with 1 stroke. Did not tug or pull on the catheter. Repeated as needed with a clean area of the washcloth. Used a clean washcloth if needed.	___	___	_____
21. Dried the catheter with a towel. Dried from the meatus down the catheter about 4 inches. Did not tug or pull on the catheter.	___	___	_____
22. Patted the perineal area dry. Dried from front to back.	___	___	_____
23. Returned the foreskin to its natural position.	___	___	_____
24. Secured the catheter. Coiled and secured tubing.	___	___	_____
25. Removed the waterproof pad.	___	___	_____
26. Covered the person. Removed the bath blanket.	___	___	_____
27. Removed the gloves. Practiced hand hygiene.	___	___	_____
Post-Procedure			
28. Provided for comfort.	___	___	_____
29. Placed the call light within reach.	___	___	_____
30. Lowered the bed to its lowest position.	___	___	_____
31. Raised or lowered bed rails. Followed the care plan.	___	___	_____
32. Cleaned, dried, and returned equipment to its proper place. Discarded disposable items. (Wore gloves for this step.)	___	___	_____
33. Unscreened the person.	___	___	_____
34. Completed a safety check of the room.	___	___	_____
35. Followed center policy for soiled linens.	___	___	_____
36. Removed the gloves. Practiced hand hygiene.	___	___	_____
37. Reported and recorded your observations.	___	___	_____

Date of Satisfactory Completion _____   Instructor's Initials _____

VIDEO CLIP **VIDEO** ## Changing a Leg Bag to a Drainage Bag

Name: _____   Date: _____

	S	U	Comments

Quality of Life
Remembered to:
- Knock before entering the person's room
- Address the person by name
- Introduce yourself by name and title
- Explain the procedure to the person before beginning and during the procedure
- Protect the person's rights during the procedure
- Handle the person gently during the procedure

Pre-Procedure
1. Followed *Delegation Guidelines: Drainage Systems.* Saw *Promoting Safety and Comfort: Drainage Systems.*
2. Practiced hand hygiene.
3. Collected the following:
   - Gloves
   - Drainage bag and tubing
   - Antiseptic wipes
   - Waterproof pad
   - Sterile cap and plug
   - Catheter clamp
   - Paper towels
   - Bedpan
   - Bath blanket
4. Arranged paper towels and equipment on the over-bed table.
5. Identified the person. Checked the identification (ID) bracelet against the assignment sheet. Called the person by name.
6. Provided for privacy.

Procedure
7. Had the person sit on the side of the bed.
8. Practiced hand hygiene. Put on gloves.
9. Exposed the catheter and leg bag.
10. Clamped the catheter. This prevented urine from draining from the catheter into the drainage tubing.
11. Allowed urine to drain from below the clamp into the drainage tubing. This emptied the lower end of the catheter.
12. Helped the person lie down.
13. Raised the bed rails if used. Raised the bed for body mechanics.
14. Lowered the bed rail near you if up.
15. Covered the person with a bath blanket. Fan-folded top linens to the foot of the bed. Exposed the catheter and leg bag.
16. Placed the waterproof pad under the person's leg.
17. Opened the antiseptic wipes. Put them on paper towels.

Date of Satisfactory Completion _____   Instructor's Initials _____

Procedure—cont'd	S	U	Comments
18. Opened the package with the sterile cap and plug. Placed the package on the paper towels. Did not let anything touch the sterile cap or plug.	___	___	___
19. Opened the package with the drainage bag and tubing.	___	___	___
20. Attached the drainage bag to the bed frame.	___	___	___
21. Disconnected the catheter from the drainage tubing. Did not allow anything touch the ends.	___	___	___
22. Inserted the sterile plug into the catheter end. Touched only the end of the plug. Did not touch the part that went inside the catheter. (If you contaminated the end of the catheter, wiped the end with an antiseptic wipe. Did so before you inserted the sterile plug.)	___	___	___
23. Placed the sterile cap on the end of the leg bag drainage tube. (If you contaminated the tubing end, wiped the end with an antiseptic wipe. Did so before you applied the sterile cap.)	___	___	___
24. Removed the cap from the new drainage tubing.	___	___	___
25. Removed the sterile plug from the catheter.	___	___	___
26. Inserted the end of the drainage tubing into the catheter.	___	___	___
27. Removed the clamp from the catheter.	___	___	___
28. Looped the drainage tubing on the bed. Secured the tubing to the bottom linens.	___	___	___
29. Removed the leg bag. Placed it in the bedpan.	___	___	___
30. Removed and discarded the waterproof pad.	___	___	___
31. Covered the person. Removed the bath blanket.	___	___	___
32. Took the bedpan to the bathroom.	___	___	___
33. Removed the gloves. Practiced hand hygiene.	___	___	___
Post-Procedure			
34. Provided for comfort.	___	___	___
35. Placed the call light within reach.	___	___	___
36. Lowered the bed to its lowest position.	___	___	___
37. Raised or lowered bed rails. Followed the care plan.	___	___	___
38. Unscreened the person.	___	___	___
39. Put on clean gloves. Discarded disposable items.	___	___	___
40. Emptied the drainage bag.	___	___	___
41. Discarded the drainage tubing and bag following center policy. Or cleaned the bag following center policy.	___	___	___
42. Cleaned and disinfected the bedpan. Placed it in a clean cover.	___	___	___
43. Returned the bedpan and other supplies to their proper place.	___	___	___
44. Removed the gloves. Practiced hand hygiene.	___	___	___
45. Completed a safety check of the room.	___	___	___
46. Followed center policy for soiled linens.	___	___	___
47. Practiced hand hygiene.	___	___	___
48. Reported and recorded your observations.	___	___	___

Date of Satisfactory Completion _____ Instructor's Initials _____

CD-ROM   VIDEO CLIP   VIDEO   **Emptying a Urinary Drainage Bag**

Name: _____   Date: _____

	S	U	Comments
Quality of Life			
Remembered to:			
• Knock before entering the person's room	___	___	_____
• Address the person by name	___	___	_____
• Introduce yourself by name and title	___	___	_____
• Explain the procedure to the person before beginning and during the procedure	___	___	_____
• Protect the person's rights during the procedure	___	___	_____
• Handle the person gently during the procedure	___	___	_____
Pre-Procedure			
1. Followed *Delegation Guidelines: Drainage Systems.* Saw *Promoting Safety and Comfort: Drainage Systems.*	___	___	_____
2. Collected the following:			
• Graduate (measuring container)	___	___	_____
• Waterproof pad or plastic bag to place on the floor under the graduate	___	___	_____
• Gloves	___	___	_____
• Paper towels	___	___	_____
• Antiseptic wipes (if used by your nursing center)	___	___	_____
3. Practiced hand hygiene.	___	___	_____
4. Identified the person. Checked the identification (ID) bracelet against the assignment sheet. Called the person by name.	___	___	_____
5. Provided for privacy.	___	___	_____
Procedure			
6. Put on the gloves.	___	___	_____
7. Placed paper towel on the floor. Placed graduate on top of it.	___	___	_____
8. Positioned the graduate under the collection bag.	___	___	_____
9. Opened the clamp on the drain.	___	___	_____
10. Allowed all urine to drain into the graduate. Did not let the drain touch the graduate.	___	___	_____
11. Closed and positioned the clamp.	___	___	_____
12. Wiped the drain with an antiseptic wipe. (Not all facilities include this step.)	___	___	_____
13. Measured the urine.	___	___	_____
14. Removed and discarded the paper towel.	___	___	_____
15. Emptied the contents of the graduate into the toilet and flushed.	___	___	_____
16. Rinsed the graduate. Emptied the rinse into the toilet and flushed.	___	___	_____
17. Cleaned and disinfected the graduate.	___	___	_____
18. Returned the graduate to its proper place.	___	___	_____
19. Removed the gloves. Practiced hand hygiene.	___	___	_____
20. Recorded the time and amount on the intake and output (I&O) record.	___	___	_____

Date of Satisfactory Completion _____   Instructor's Initials _____

Post-Procedure   S   U   **Comments**

21. Provided for comfort.

22. Placed the call light within reach.

23. Unscreened the person.

24. Completed a safety check of the room.

25. Reported and recorded the amount and other observations.

Date of Satisfactory Completion _____ Instructor's Initials _____

VIDEO CLIP   VIDEO   **Applying a Condom Catheter**

Name: _____   Date: _____

	S	U	Comments

Quality of Life
Remembered to:
- Knock before entering the person's room
- Address the person by name
- Introduce yourself by name and title
- Explain the procedure to the person before beginning and during the procedure
- Protect the person's rights during the procedure
- Handle the person gently during the procedure

Pre-Procedure
1. Followed *Delegation Guidelines:*
   a. *Perineal Care.*
   b. *Condom Catheters.*
   Saw *Promoting Safety and Comfort:*
   a. *Perineal Care.*
   b. *Condom Catheters.*
2. Practiced hand hygiene.
3. Collected the following:
   - Condom catheter
   - Elastic tape
   - Drainage bag or leg bag
   - Cap for the drainage bag
   - Basin of warm water
   - Soap
   - Towel and washcloth
   - Bath blanket
   - Gloves
   - Waterproof pad
   - Paper towels
4. Covered the over-bed table with paper towels. Arranged items on top of paper towels.
5. Identified the person. Checked the identification (ID) bracelet against the assignment sheet. Called the person by name.
6. Provided for privacy.
7. Filled the wash basin. Water temperature was 105°F (40.5°C). Measured water temperature according to center policy. Asked the person to check the water temperature. Adjusted water temperature as needed.
8. Raised the bed for body mechanics. Bed rails were up if used.

Procedure
9. Lowered the bed rail near you if up.
10. Practiced hand hygiene. Put on gloves.
11. Covered the person with a bath blanket. Lowered top linens to the knees.
12. Asked the person to raise his buttocks off the bed. Or turned him onto his side away from you.
13. Slid the waterproof pad under his buttocks.

Date of Satisfactory Completion _____   Instructor's Initials _____

Procedure—cont'd	S	U	Comments
14. Had the person lower his buttocks. Or turned him onto his back.	___	___	_____
15. Secured the drainage bag to the bed frame. Or had a leg bag ready. Closed the drain.	___	___	_____
16. Exposed the genital area.	___	___	_____
17. Removed the condom catheter:			
a. Removed the tape. Rolled the sheath off the penis.	___	___	_____
b. Disconnected the drainage tubing from the condom. Capped the drainage tube.	___	___	_____
c. Discarded the tape and condom.	___	___	_____
18. Provided perineal care. Observed the penis for reddened areas, skin breakdown, and irritations.	___	___	_____
19. Removed gloves and practiced hand hygiene. Put on clean gloves.	___	___	_____
20. Removed the protective backing from the condom. This exposed the adhesive strip.	___	___	_____
21. Held the penis firmly. Rolled the condom onto the penis. Left a 1-inch space between the penis and the end of the catheter.	___	___	_____
22. Secured the condom:			
a. For a self-adhering condom, pressed the condom to the penis.	___	___	_____
b. For a condom secured with elastic tape, applied elastic tape in a spiral. Did not apply tape completely around the penis.	___	___	_____
23. Made sure the penis tip did not touch the condom. Made sure the condom was not twisted.	___	___	_____
24. Connected the condom to the drainage tubing. Coiled and secured excess tubing on the bed. Or attached a leg bag.	___	___	_____
25. Removed the waterproof pad and gloves. Discarded them. Practiced hand hygiene.	___	___	_____
26. Covered the person. Removed the bath blanket.	___	___	_____
Post-Procedure			
27. Provided for comfort.	___	___	_____
28. Placed the call light within reach.	___	___	_____
29. Lowered the bed to its lowest position.	___	___	_____
30. Raised or lowered bed rails. Followed the care plan.	___	___	_____
31. Unscreened the person.	___	___	_____
32. Practiced hand hygiene. Put on clean gloves.	___	___	_____
33. Measured and recorded the amount of urine in the bag. Cleaned and discarded the collection bag.	___	___	_____
34. Cleaned, dried, and returned the wash basin and other equipment. Returned items to their proper place.	___	___	_____
35. Removed the gloves. Practiced hand hygiene.	___	___	_____
36. Completed a safety check of the room.	___	___	_____
37. Reported and recorded your observations.	___	___	_____

Date of Satisfactory Completion _____ Instructor's Initials _____

VIDEO CLIP **VIDEO** **Giving a Cleansing Enema**

Name: _____   Date: _____

	S	U	Comments

Quality of Life
Remembered to:
- Knock before entering the person's room
- Address the person by name
- Introduce yourself by name and title
- Explain the procedure to the person before beginning and during the procedure
- Protect the person's rights during the procedure
- Handle the person gently during the procedure

Pre-Procedure
1. Followed *Delegation Guidelines:*
   Enemas.
   Saw *Promoting Safety and Comfort:*
   Enemas.
2. Practiced hand hygiene.
3. Collected the following before going to the person's room:
   - Disposable enema kit as directed by the nurse (enema bag, tube, clamp, and waterproof pad)
   - Bath thermometer
   - Waterproof pad (if not part of the enema kit)
   - Water-soluble lubricant
   - 3 to 5 mL (1 teaspoon) castile soap or 1 to 2 teaspoons of salt
   - Intravenous (IV) pole
   - Gloves
4. Arranged items in the person's room and bathroom.
5. Decontaminated your hands.
6. Identified the person. Checked the identification (ID) bracelet against the assignment sheet. Called the person by name.
7. Put on gloves.
8. Collected the following:
   - Commode or bedpan and cover
   - Toilet tissue
   - Bath blanket
   - Robe and non-skid footwear
   - Paper towels
9. Provided for privacy.
10. Raised the bed for body mechanics. Bed rails were up if used.

Procedure
11. Removed the gloves and decontaminated your hands. Put on clean gloves.
12. Lowered the bed rail near you if up.
13. Covered the person with a bath blanket. Fan-folded top linens to the foot of the bed.
14. Positioned the IV pole so the enema bag was 12 inches above the anus. Or it was at the height directed by the nurse.
15. Raised the bed rail if used.

Date of Satisfactory Completion _____   Instructor's Initials _____

Procedure—cont'd	S	U	Comments
16. Prepared the enema:			
a. Closed the clamp on the tube.	___	___	___
b. Adjusted water flow until it was lukewarm.	___	___	___
c. Filled the enema bag for the amount ordered.	___	___	___
d. Measured water temperature with the bath thermometer. Followed the nurse's directions for water temperature.	___	___	___
e. Prepared the solution as directed by the nurse:			
1) Tap water: added nothing	___	___	___
2) Saline enema: added salt as directed	___	___	___
3) Soapsuds enema (SSE): added castile soap as directed.	___	___	___
f. Stirred the solution with the bath thermometer. If suds (SSE), scooped them off.	___	___	___
g. Sealed the bag.	___	___	___
h. Hung the bag on the IV pole.	___	___	___
17. Lowered the bed rail near you if up.	___	___	___
18. Positioned the person in Sims' position or in left side-lying position.	___	___	___
19. Placed a waterproof pad under the buttocks.	___	___	___
20. Exposed the anal area.	___	___	___
21. Placed the bedpan behind the person.	___	___	___
22. Positioned the enema tube in the bedpan. Removed the cap from the tubing.	___	___	___
23. Opened the clamp. Allowed solution to flow through the tube to remove air. Clamped the tube.	___	___	___
24. Lubricated the tube 2 to 4 inches from the tip.	___	___	___
25. Separated the buttocks to see the anus.	___	___	___
26. Asked the person to take a deep breath through the mouth.	___	___	___
27. Inserted the tube gently 2 to 4 inches into the adult's rectum. Did this when the person was exhaling. Stopped if the person complained of pain, you felt resistance, or bleeding occurred.	___	___	___
28. Checked the amount of solution in the bag.	___	___	___
29. Unclamped the tube. Gave the solution slowly.	___	___	___
30. Asked the person to take slow, deep breaths. This helped the person relax.	___	___	___
31. Clamped the tube if the person needed to have a bowel movement (BM), had cramping, or started to expel solution. Also clamped the tube if the person was sweating or complained of nausea or weakness. Unclamped when symptoms subsided.	___	___	___
32. Gave the amount of solution ordered. Stopped if the person did not tolerate the procedure.	___	___	___
33. Clamped the tube before it emptied. This prevented air from entering the bowel.	___	___	___
34. Held toilet tissue around the tube and against the anus. Removed the tube.	___	___	___
35. Discarded toilet tissue in the bedpan.	___	___	___
36. Wrapped the tubing tip with paper towels. Placed it inside the enema bag.	___	___	___

Date of Satisfactory Completion _____   Instructor's Initials _____

Procedure—cont'd   S   U   Comments

37. Assisted the person to the bathroom or commode.
    The person wore a robe and non-skid footwear
    while up. The bed was in the lowest position.
    Or helped the person onto the bedpan. Raised the
    head of the bed. Raised or lowered bed rail
    according to the care plan.

38. Placed the call light and toilet tissue within reach.
    Reminded the person not to flush the toilet.

39. Discarded disposable items.

40. Removed the gloves. Practiced hand hygiene.

41. Left the room if the person could be left alone.

42. Returned when the person signaled. Or checked
    on the person every 5 minutes. Knocked before
    entering room or bathroom.

43. Decontaminated your hands and put on gloves.
    Lowered the bed rail if up.

44. Observed enema results for amount, color, consistency,
    shape, and odor. Called the nurse to observe results.

45. Provided perineal care as needed.

46. Removed the waterproof pad.

47. Emptied, cleaned, and disinfected equipment.
    Flushed the toilet after the nurse observed the results.

48. Returned equipment to its proper place.

49. Removed the gloves and practiced hand hygiene.

50. Assisted with hand washing. Wore gloves for this step.

51. Covered the person. Removed the bath blanket.

Post-Procedure

52. Provided for comfort.

53. Placed the call light within reach.

54. Lowered the bed to its lowest position.

55. Raised or lowered bed rails. Followed the care plan.

56. Unscreened the person.

57. Completed a safety check of the room.

58. Followed center policy for dirty linens and used supplies.

59. Practiced hand hygiene.

60. Reported and recorded your observations.

Date of Satisfactory Completion _____   Instructor's Initials _____

VIDEO **Giving a Small-Volume Enema**

Name: _____   Date: _____

Quality of Life	S	U	Comments
Remembered to:			
• Knock before entering the person's room			
• Address the person by name			
• Introduce yourself by name and title			
• Explain the procedure to the person before beginning and during the procedure			
• Protect the person's rights during the procedure			
• Handle the person gently during the procedure			

Pre-Procedure

1. Followed *Delegation Guidelines: Enemas.*
   Saw *Promoting Safety and Comfort: Enemas.*
2. Practiced hand hygiene.
3. Collected the following before going to the person's room:
   • Small-volume enema
   • Waterproof pad
   • Gloves
4. Arranged items in the person's room.
5. Practiced hand hygiene.
6. Identified the person. Checked the identification (ID) bracelet against the assignment sheet. Called the person by name.
7. Put on gloves.
8. Collected the following:
   • Commode or bedpan
   • Waterproof pad
   • Toilet tissue
   • Robe and non-skid footwear
   • Bath blanket
9. Provided for privacy.
10. Raised the bed for body mechanics. Bed rails were up if used.

Procedure

11. Removed the gloves and practiced hand hygiene. Put on clean gloves.
12. Lowered the bed rail near you if up.
13. Covered the person with a bath blanket. Fan-folded top linens to the foot of the bed.
14. Positioned the person in Sims' position or in left side-lying position.
15. Placed a waterproof pad under the buttocks.
16. Exposed the anal area.
17. Placed the bedpan near the person.
18. Removed the cap from the enema tip.
19. Separated the buttocks to see the anus.
20. Asked the person to take a deep breath through the mouth.

Date of Satisfactory Completion _____   Instructor's Initials _____

Procedure—cont'd   S   U   **Comments**

21. Inserted the enema tip 2 inches into the rectum.   _____ _____ _____
    Did this when the person was exhaling.
    Inserted the tip gently. Stopped if the person
    complained of pain, you felt resistance,
    or bleeding occurred.
22. Squeezed and rolled the bottle gently.   _____ _____ _____
    Released pressure on the bottle after you removed
    the tip from the rectum.
23. Placed the bottle into the box, tip first.   _____ _____ _____
24. Assisted the person to the bathroom or commode   _____ _____ _____
    when he or she had the urge to have a bowel
    movement (BM). The person wore a robe and non-skid
    footwear while up. The bed was in the lowest
    position. Or helped the person onto the bedpan
    and raised the head of the bed. Raised or lowered
    bed rails according to the care plan.
25. Placed the call light and toilet tissue within reach. _____ _____ _____
    Reminded the person not to flush the toilet.
26. Discarded disposable items.   _____ _____ _____
27. Removed the gloves. Practiced hand hygiene.   _____ _____ _____
28. Left the room if the person could be left alone.   _____ _____ _____
29. Returned when the person signaled.   _____ _____ _____
    Or checked on the person every 5 minutes.
    Knocked before entering the room or bathroom.
30. Practiced hand hygiene. Put on gloves.   _____ _____ _____
31. Lowered the bed rail if up.   _____ _____ _____
32. Observed enema results for amount, color, consistency, _____ _____ _____
    shape, and odor. Called the nurse to observe results.
33. Provided perineal care as needed.   _____ _____ _____
34. Removed the waterproof pad.   _____ _____ _____
35. Emptied, cleaned, and disinfected equipment.   _____ _____ _____
    Flushed the toilet after the nurse observed the results.
36. Returned equipment to its proper place.   _____ _____ _____
37. Removed the gloves and practiced hand hygiene.   _____ _____ _____
38. Assisted with hand washing. Wore gloves for this step. _____ _____ _____
39. Covered the person. Removed the bath blanket.   _____ _____ _____

Post-Procedure
40. Provided for comfort.   _____ _____ _____
41. Placed the call light within reach.   _____ _____ _____
42. Lowered the bed to its lowest position.   _____ _____ _____
43. Raised or lowered bed rails. Followed the care plan. _____ _____ _____
44. Unscreened the person.   _____ _____ _____
45. Completed a safety check of the room.   _____ _____ _____
46. Followed center policy for dirty linens and used supplies. _____ _____ _____
47. Practiced hand hygiene.   _____ _____ _____
48. Reported and recorded your observations.   _____ _____ _____

Date of Satisfactory Completion _____   Instructor's Initials _____

VIDEO ## Giving an Oil-Retention Enema

Name: _____   Date: _____

	S	U	Comments

Quality of Life

Remembered to:
- Knock before entering the person's room
- Address the person by name
- Introduce yourself by name and title
- Explain the procedure to the person before beginning and during the procedure
- Protect the person's rights during the procedure
- Handle the person gently during the procedure

Pre-Procedure

1. Followed *Delegation Guidelines:*
   a. *Enemas.*
   b. *The Oil-Retention Enema.*
   Saw *Promoting Safety and Comfort:*
   a. *Enemas.*
   b. *The Oil-Retention Enema.*
2. Practiced hand hygiene.
3. Collected the following before going to the person's room:
   - Oil-retention enema
   - Waterproof pad
4. Arranged items in the person's room.
5. Practiced hand hygiene.
6. Identified the person. Checked the identification (ID) bracelet against the assignment sheet. Called the person by name.
7. Collected the following:
   - Gloves
   - Bath blanket
8. Put on gloves.
9. Provided for privacy.
10. Raised the bed for body mechanics. Bed rails were up if used.

Procedure

11. Followed these steps:
    a. Lowered the bed rail near you if up.
    b. Removed the gloves and practiced hand hygiene. Put on clean gloves.
    c. Covered the person with a bath blanket. Fan-folded top linens to the foot of the bed.
    d. Positioned the person in Sims' position or in left side-lying position.
    e. Placed a waterproof pad under the buttocks.
    f. Exposed the anal area.
    g. Positioned the bedpan near the person.
    h. Removed the cap from the enema tip.
    i. Separated the buttocks to see the anus.
    j. Asked the person to take a deep breath through the mouth.
    k. Inserted the enema tip 2 inches into the rectum. Did this when the person was exhaling. Inserted the tip gently. Stopped if the person complained of pain, you felt resistance, or bleeding occurred.

Date of Satisfactory Completion _____   Instructor's Initials _____

Procedure—cont'd	S	U	Comments
l. Squeezed and rolled the bottle gently. Released pressure on the bottle after you removed the tip from the rectum.	___	___	_____
m. Placed the bottle into the box, tip first.	___	___	_____
12. Covered the person. Left the person in the Sims' or left side-lying position.	___	___	_____
13. Encouraged the person to retain the enema for the time ordered.	___	___	_____
14. Placed more waterproof pads on the bed if needed.	___	___	_____
15. Removed the gloves. Practiced hand hygiene.	___	___	_____

Post-Procedure

	S	U	Comments
16. Provided for comfort.	___	___	_____
17. Placed the call light within reach.	___	___	_____
18. Lowered the bed to its lowest position.	___	___	_____
19. Raised or lowered bed rails. Followed the care plan.	___	___	_____
20. Unscreened the person.	___	___	_____
21. Completed a safety check of the room.	___	___	_____
22. Followed center policy for dirty linens and used supplies.	___	___	_____
23. Practiced hand hygiene.	___	___	_____
24. Reported and recorded your observations.	___	___	_____
25. Checked the person often.	___	___	_____

Date of Satisfactory Completion _____   Instructor's Initials _____

VIDEO CLIP   VIDEO   ## Changing an Ostomy Pouch

Name: _____   Date: _____

	S	U	Comments
Quality of Life			
Remembered to:			
• Knock before entering the person's room.	_____	_____	_____
• Address the person by name.	_____	_____	_____
• Introduce yourself by name and title.	_____	_____	_____
• Explain the procedure to the person before beginning and during the procedure.	_____	_____	_____
• Protect the person's rights during the procedure.	_____	_____	_____
• Handle the person gently during the procedure.	_____	_____	_____

	S	U	Comments
Pre-Procedure			
1. Followed *Delegation Guidelines: Ostomy Pouches.* Saw *Promoting Safety and Comfort: Ostomy Pouches.*	_____	_____	_____
2. Practiced hand hygiene.	_____	_____	_____
3. Collected the following before going to the person's room:			
• Clean pouch with skin barrier	_____	_____	_____
• Pouch clamp, clip, or wire closure	_____	_____	_____
• Clean ostomy belt (if used)	_____	_____	_____
• Gauze pads or washcloths	_____	_____	_____
• Adhesive remover wipes	_____	_____	_____
• Skin paste (optional)	_____	_____	_____
• Pouch deodorant	_____	_____	_____
• Disposable bag	_____	_____	_____
4. Arranged your work area.	_____	_____	_____
5. Practiced hand hygiene.	_____	_____	_____
6. Identified the person. Checked the ID bracelet against the assignment sheet. Also called the person by name.	_____	_____	_____
7. Put on gloves.	_____	_____	_____
8. Collected the following:			
• Bedpan with cover	_____	_____	_____
• Waterproof pad	_____	_____	_____
• Bath blanket	_____	_____	_____
• Wash basin with warm water	_____	_____	_____
• Paper towels	_____	_____	_____
• Gloves	_____	_____	_____
9. Provided for privacy.	_____	_____	_____
10. Raised the bed for body mechanics. Bed rails were up if used.	_____	_____	_____

	S	U	Comments
Procedure			
11. Removed the gloves and practiced hand hygiene. Put on clean gloves.	_____	_____	_____
12. Lowered the bed rail near you if up.	_____	_____	_____
13. Covered the person with a bath blanket. Fan-folded linens to the foot of the bed.	_____	_____	_____
14. Placed the waterproof pad under the buttocks.	_____	_____	_____
15. Disconnected the pouch from the belt if one is worn. Removed the belt.	_____	_____	_____
16. Removed and placed the pouch and skin barrier in the bedpan. Gently pushed the skin down and lifted up on the barrier. Used the adhesive remover wipes if necessary.	_____	_____	_____

Date of Satisfactory Completion _____   Instructor's Initials _____

Procedure—cont'd   S   U   Comments

17. Wiped the stoma and around it with a gauze pad.   ____   ____   _____
    This removed excess stool and mucous. Discarded
    the gauze pad into the disposable bag.
18. Wet the gauze pads or the washcloth.   ____   ____   _____
19. Washed the stoma and the skin around it with a gauze   ____ ____   _____
    pad or washcloth. Washed gently. Did not scrub
    or rub the skin.
20. Patted dry with a gauze pad or the towel.   ____   ____   _____
21. Observed the stoma and the skin around the stoma. ____   ____   _____
    Reported bleeding, skin irritation, or skin breakdown
    to the nurse.
22. Remove the backing from the new pouch.   ____   ____   _____
23. Applied a thin layer of paste around the pouch opening. ____ ____   _____
    Allowed it to dry. Followed the manufacturer instructions.
24. Pulled the skin around the stoma taut. The skin was ____ ____   _____
    wrinkle-free.
25. Centered the pouch over the stoma. The drain pointed ____ ____   _____
    downward.
26. Pressed around the pouch and skin barrier so it sealed to the ____ ____   _____
    skin. Applied gentle pressure with your fingers. Started at
    the bottom and work up around the sides to the top.
27. Maintained the pressure for 1 to 2 minutes.   ____   ____   _____
    Followed the manufacturer instructions.
28. Tugged downward on the pouch gently.   ____   ____   _____
    Made sure the pouch was secure.
29. Added deodorant to the pouch.   ____   ____   _____
30. Closed the pouch at the bottom. Used a clamp, clip, or ____ ____   _____
    wire closure.
31. Attached the ostomy belt if used. The belt was not ____ ____   _____
    too tight. You were able to slide 2 fingers under the belt.
32. Removed the waterproof pad.   ____   ____   _____
33. Discarded disposable supplies into the disposable bag. ____ ____   _____
34. Remove the gloves. Practiced hand hygiene.   ____   ____   _____
35. Covered the person. Removed the bath blanket.   ____   ____   _____

Post-Procedure
36. Provided for comfort.   ____   ____   _____
37. Placed the call light within reach.   ____   ____   _____
38. Lowered the bed to its lowest position.   ____   ____   _____
39. Raised or lowered bed rails. Followed the care plan. ____ ____   _____
40. Unscreened the person.   ____   ____   _____
41. Practiced hand hygiene. Put on gloves.   ____   ____   _____
42. Took the bedpan and disposable bag into the bathroom. ____ ____   _____
43. Emptied the pouch and bedpan into the toilet. Observed ____ ____   _____
    the color, amount, consistency, and odor of stools.
    Flushed the toilet.
44. Discarded the pouch into the disposable bag.   ____   ____   _____
    Discarded the disposable bag.
45. Emptied, cleaned, and disinfected equipment.   ____   ____   _____
    Returned equipment to its proper place.
46. Removed the gloves. Practiced hand hygiene.   ____   ____   _____
47. Completed a safety check of the room.   ____   ____   _____
48. Followed center policy for dirty linens.   ____   ____   _____
49. Practiced hand hygiene.   ____   ____   _____
50. Reported and recorded your observations.   ____   ____   _____

Date of Satisfactory Completion _____   Instructor's Initials _____

NNAAP™ Skill   CD-ROM   VIDEO CLIP   VIDEO   **Performing Range-of-Motion Exercises**

Name: _____   Date: _____

Quality of Life	S	U	Comments
Remembered to:			
• Knock before entering the person's room	___	___	_____
• Address the person by name	___	___	_____
• Introduce yourself by name and title	___	___	_____
• Explain the procedure to the person before beginning and during the procedure	___	___	_____
• Protect the person's rights during the procedure	___	___	_____
• Handle the person gently during the procedure	___	___	_____

Pre-Procedure

1. Followed *Delegation Guidelines: Range-of-Motion Exercises.*
   Saw *Promoting Safety and Comfort: Range-of-Motion Exercises.*   ___ ___ _____
2. Practiced hand hygiene.   ___ ___ _____
3. Identified the person. Checked the identification (ID) bracelet against the assignment sheet. Called the person by name.   ___ ___ _____
4. Obtained a bath blanket.   ___ ___ _____
5. Provided for privacy.   ___ ___ _____
6. Raised the bed for body mechanics. Bed rails were up if used.   ___ ___ _____

Procedure

7. Lowered the bed rail near you if up.   ___ ___ _____
8. Positioned the person supine.   ___ ___ _____
9. Covered the person with a bath blanket. Fan-folded top linens to the foot of the bed.   ___ ___ _____
10. Exercised the neck *if allowed by the center and if instructed to do so by the nurse:*
    a. Placed your hands over the person's ears to support the head. Supported the jaws with your fingers.   ___ ___ _____
    b. Flexion—brought the head forward. The chin touched the chest.   ___ ___ _____
    c. Extension—straightened the head.   ___ ___ _____
    d. Hyperextension—brought the head backward until the chin pointed up.   ___ ___ _____
    e. Rotation—turned the head from side to side.   ___ ___ _____
    f. Lateral flexion—moved the head to the right and to the left.   ___ ___ _____
    g. Repeated flexion, extension, hyperextension, rotation, and lateral flexion 5 times—or the number of times stated on the care plan.   ___ ___ _____
11. Exercised the shoulder:
    a. Grasped the wrist with one hand. Grasped the elbow with the other hand.   ___ ___ _____
    b. Flexion—raised the arm straight in front and over the head.   ___ ___ _____
    c. Extension—brought the arm down to the side.   ___ ___ _____
    d. Hyperextension—moved the arm behind the body. (Did this if the person was sitting in a straight-backed chair or was standing.)   ___ ___ _____

Date of Satisfactory Completion _____   Instructor's Initials _____

Procedure—cont'd	S	U	Comments
e. Abduction—moved the straight arm away from the side of the body.	_____	_____	_____
f. Adduction—moved the straight arm to the side of the body.	_____	_____	_____
g. Internal rotation—bent the elbow. Placed it at the same level as the shoulder. Moved the forearm down toward the body.	_____	_____	_____
h. External rotation—moved the forearm toward the head.	_____	_____	_____
i. Repeated flexion, extension, hyperextension, abduction, adduction, and internal and external rotation 5 times—or the number of times stated on the care plan.	_____	_____	_____
12. Exercised the elbow:			
a. Grasped the person's wrist with one hand. Grasped the elbow with the other hand.	_____	_____	_____
b. Flexion—bent the arm so the same-side shoulder was touched.	_____	_____	_____
c. Extension—straightened the arm.	_____	_____	_____
d. Repeated flexion and extension 5 times—or the number of times stated on the care plan.	_____	_____	_____
13. Exercised the forearm:			
a. Continue to support the wrist and elbow.	_____	_____	_____
b. Pronation—turned the hand so the palm was down.	_____	_____	_____
c. Supination—turned the hand so the palm was up.	_____	_____	_____
d. Repeated pronation and supination 5 times—or the number of times stated on the care plan.	_____	_____	_____
14. Exercised the wrist:			
a. Held the wrist with both of your hands.	_____	_____	_____
b. Flexion—bent the hand down.	_____	_____	_____
c. Extension—straightened the hand.	_____	_____	_____
d. Hyperextension—bent the hand back.	_____	_____	_____
e. Radial flexion—turned the hand toward the thumb.	_____	_____	_____
f. Ulnar flexion—turned the hand toward the little finger.	_____	_____	_____
g. Repeated flexion, extension, hyperextension, and radial and ulnar flexion 5 times—or the number of times stated on the care plan.	_____	_____	_____
15. Exercised the thumb:			
a. Held the person's hand with one hand. Held the thumb with your other hand.	_____	_____	_____
b. Abduction—moved the thumb out from the inner part of the index finger.	_____	_____	_____
c. Adduction—moved the thumb back next to the index finger.	_____	_____	_____
d. Opposition—touched each finger with the thumb.	_____	_____	_____
e. Flexion—bent the thumb into the hand.	_____	_____	_____
f. Extension—moved the thumb out to the side of the fingers.	_____	_____	_____
g. Repeated abduction, adduction, opposition, flexion, and extension 5 times—or the number of times stated on the care plan.	_____	_____	_____
16. Exercised the fingers:			
a. Abduction—spread the fingers and the thumb apart.	_____	_____	_____
b. Adduction—bought the fingers and thumb together.	_____	_____	_____
c. Flexion—made a fist.	_____	_____	_____

Date of Satisfactory Completion _____   Instructor's Initials _____

Procedure—cont'd	S	U	Comments
d. Extension —straightened the fingers so the fingers, hand, and arm were straight.	_____	_____	_____
e. Repeated abduction, adduction, flexion and extension 5 times—or the number of times stated on the care plan.	_____	_____	_____
17. Exercised the hip:			
a. Supported the leg. Placed one hand under the knee. Placed your other hand under the ankle.	_____	_____	_____
b. Flexion—raised the leg.	_____	_____	_____
c. Extension—straightened the leg.	_____	_____	_____
d. Abduction—moved the leg away from the body.	_____	_____	_____
e. Adduction—moved the leg toward the other leg.	_____	_____	_____
f. Internal rotation—turned the leg inward.	_____	_____	_____
g. External rotation—turned the leg outward.	_____	_____	_____
h. Repeated flexion, extension, abduction, adduction, and internal and external rotation 5 times—or the number of times stated on the care plan.	_____	_____	_____
18. Exercised the knee:			
a. Supported the knee. Placed one hand under the knee. Placed your other hand under the ankle.	_____	_____	_____
b. Flexion—bent the leg.	_____	_____	_____
c. Extension—straightened the leg.	_____	_____	_____
d. Repeated flexion and extension of the knee 5 times—or the number of times stated on the care plan.	_____	_____	_____
19. Exercised the ankle:			
a. Supported the foot and ankle. Placed one hand under the foot. Placed your other hand under the ankle.	_____	_____	_____
b. Dorsiflexion—pulled the foot forward. Pushed down on the heel at the same time.	_____	_____	_____
c. Plantar flexion—turned the foot down. Or pointed the toes.	_____	_____	_____
d. Repeated dorsiflexion and plantar flexion 5 times—or the number of times stated on the care plan.	_____	_____	_____
20. Exercised the foot:			
a. Continued to support the foot and ankle.	_____	_____	_____
b. Pronation—turned the outside of the foot up and the inside down.	_____	_____	_____
c. Supination—turned the inside of the foot up and the outside down.	_____	_____	_____
d. Repeated pronation and supination 5 times—or the number of times stated on the care plan.	_____	_____	_____
21. Exercised the toes:			
a. Flexion—curled the toes.	_____	_____	_____
b. Extension—straightened the toes.	_____	_____	_____
c. Abduction—spread the toes apart.	_____	_____	_____
d. Adduction—pulled the toes together.	_____	_____	_____
e. Repeated flexion, extension, abduction, and adduction 5 times—or the number of times stated on the care plan.	_____	_____	_____
22. Covered the leg. Raised the bed rail if used.	_____	_____	_____
23. Went to the other side. Lowered the bed rail near you if up.	_____	_____	_____

Date of Satisfactory Completion _____ Instructor's Initials _____

Procedure—cont'd   S   U   **Comments**

24. Repeated exercises:
    a. Exercised the shoulder:
       1. Grasped the wrist with one hand. Grasped the elbow with the other hand.   ___ ___ _____
       2. Flexion—raised the arm straight in front and over the head.   ___ ___ _____
       3. Extension—brought the arm down to the side.   ___ ___ _____
       4. Hyperextension—moved the arm behind the body. (Did this if the person was sitting in a straight-backed chair or was standing.)   ___ ___ _____
       5. Abduction—moved the straight arm away from the side of the body.   ___ ___ _____
       6. Adduction—moved the straight arm to the side of the body.   ___ ___ _____
       7. Internal rotation—bent the elbow. Placed it at the same level as the shoulder. Moved the forearm down toward the body.   ___ ___ _____
       8. External rotation—moved the forearm toward the head.   ___ ___ _____
       9. Repeated flexion, extension, hyperextension, abduction, adduction, and internal and external rotation 5 times—or the number of times stated on the care plan.   ___ ___ _____
    b. Exercised the elbow:
       1. Grasped the person's wrist with one hand. Grasped the elbow with your other hand.   ___ ___ _____
       2. Flexion—bent the arm so the same-side shoulder was touched.   ___ ___ _____
       3. Extension—straightened the arm.   ___ ___ _____
       4. Repeated flexion and extension 5 times—or the number of times stated on the care plan.   ___ ___ _____
    c. Exercised the forearm:
       1. Continued to support the wrist and elbow.   ___ ___ _____
       2. Pronation—turned the hand so the palm was down.   ___ ___ _____
       3. Supination—turned the hand so the palm was up.   ___ ___ _____
       4. Repeated pronation and supination 5 times—or the number of times stated on the care plan.   ___ ___ _____
    d. Exercised the wrist:
       1. Held the wrist with both of your hands.   ___ ___ _____
       2. Flexion—bent the hand down.   ___ ___ _____
       3. Extension—straightened the hand.   ___ ___ _____
       4. Hyperextension—bent the hand back.   ___ ___ _____
       5. Radial flexion—turned the hand toward the thumb.   ___ ___ _____
       6. Ulnar flexion—turned the hand toward the little finger.   ___ ___ _____
       7. Repeated flexion, extension, hyperextension, and radial and ulnar flexion 5 times—or the number of times stated on the care plan.   ___ ___ _____
    e. Exercised the thumb:
       1. Held the person's hand with one hand. Held the thumb with your other hand.   ___ ___ _____
       2. Abduction—moved the thumb out from the inner part of the index finger.   ___ ___ _____
       3. Adduction—moved the thumb back next to the index finger.   ___ ___ _____

Date of Satisfactory Completion _____   Instructor's Initials _____

Procedure—cont'd	S	U	Comments
4. Opposition—touched each finger with the thumb.	___	___	_____
5. Flexion—bent the thumb into the hand.	___	___	_____
6. Extension—moved the thumb out to the side of the fingers.	___	___	_____
7. Repeated abduction, adduction, opposition, flexion, and extension 5 times—or the number of times stated on the care plan.	___	___	_____
f. Exercised the fingers:			
1. Abduction—spread the fingers and the thumb apart.	___	___	_____
2. Adduction—bought the fingers and thumb together.	___	___	_____
3. Flexion—made a fist.	___	___	_____
4. Extension—straightened the fingers so the fingers, hand, and arm were straight.	___	___	_____
5. Repeated abduction, adduction, extension, and flexion 5 times—or the number of times stated on the care plan.	___	___	_____
g. Exercised the hip:			
1. Supported the leg. Placed one hand under the knee. Placed your other hand under the ankle.	___	___	_____
2. Flexion—raised the leg.	___	___	_____
3. Extension—straightened the leg.	___	___	_____
4. Abduction—moved the leg away from the body.	___	___	_____
5. Adduction—moved the leg toward the other leg.	___	___	_____
6. Internal rotation—turned the leg inward.	___	___	_____
7. External rotation—turned the leg outward.	___	___	_____
8. Repeated flexion, extension, abduction, adduction, and internal and external rotation 5 times—or the number of times stated on the care plan.	___	___	_____
h. Exercised the knee:			
1. Supported the knee. Placed one hand under the knee. Placed your other hand under the ankle.	___	___	_____
2. Flexion—bent the leg.	___	___	_____
3. Extension—straightened the leg.	___	___	_____
4. Repeated flexion and extension of the knee 5 times—or the number of times stated on the care plan.	___	___	_____
i. Exercised the ankle:			
1. Supported the foot and ankle. Placed one hand under the foot. Placed your other hand under the ankle.	___	___	_____
2. Dorsiflexion—pulled the foot forward. Pushed down on the heel at the same time.	___	___	_____
3. Plantar flexion—turned the foot down. Or pointed the toes.	___	___	_____
4. Repeated dorsiflexion and plantar flexion 5 times—or the number of times stated on the care plan.	___	___	_____
j. Exercised the foot:			
1. Continued to support the foot and ankle.	___	___	_____
2. Pronation—turned the outside of the foot up and the inside down.	___	___	_____
3. Supination—turned the inside of the foot up and the outside down.	___	___	_____
4. Repeated pronation and supination 5 times—or the number of times stated on the care plan.	___	___	_____

Date of Satisfactory Completion _____   Instructor's Initials _____

Procedure—cont'd	S	U	Comments
k. Exercised the toes:			
1. Flexion—curled the toes.	___	___	_____
2. Extension—straightened the toes.	___	___	_____
3. Abduction—spread the toes apart.	___	___	_____
4. Adduction—pulled the toes together.	___	___	_____
5. Repeated flexion, extension, abduction, and adduction 5 times—or the number of times stated on the care plan.	___	___	_____

Post-Procedure

	S	U	Comments
25. Provided for comfort.	___	___	_____
26. Removed the bath blanket.	___	___	_____
27. Placed the call light within reach.	___	___	_____
28. Lowered the bed to its lowest position.	___	___	_____
29. Raised or lowered bed rails. Followed the care plan.	___	___	_____
30. Folded and returned the bath blanket its proper place.	___	___	_____
31. Unscreened the person.	___	___	_____
32. Completed a safety check of the room.	___	___	_____
33. Decontaminated your hands.	___	___	_____
34. Reported and recorded your observations.	___	___	_____

Date of Satisfactory Completion _____   Instructor's Initials _____

Helping the Person Walk

VIDEO CLIP   VIDEO

Name: _____   Date: _____

	S	U	Comments
Quality of Life			

Quality of Life

Remembered to:

- Knock before entering the person's room
- Address the person by name
- Introduce yourself by name and title
- Explain the procedure to the person before beginning and during the procedure
- Protect the person's rights during the procedure
- Handle the person gently during the procedure

Pre-Procedure

1. Followed *Delegation Guidelines: Ambulation.*
   Saw *Promoting Safety and Comfort: Ambulation.*
2. Practiced hand hygiene.
3. Collected the following:
   - Robe and non-skid shoes
   - Paper or sheet to protect bottom linens
   - Gait (transfer) belt
4. Identified the person. Checked the identification (ID) bracelet against the assignment sheet.
   Called the person by name.
5. Provided for privacy.

Procedure

6. Lowered the bed to its lowest position. Locked the bed wheels. Lowered the bed rail near you if up.
7. Fan-folded top linens to the foot of the bed.
8. Placed the paper or sheet under the person's feet. Put the shoes on the person. Fastened the shoes.
9. Helped the person sit on the side of the bed.
10. Helped the person put on the robe.
11. Made sure the person's feet were flat on the floor.
12. Applied the gait belt.
13. Helped the person stand. Grasped the gait belt at each side. If no gait belt, placed your arms under the person's arms around to the shoulder blades.
14. Stood at the person's weak side while he or she gained balance. Held the belt at the side and back. If not using a gait belt, had one arm around the back and the other at the elbow to support the person.
15. Encouraged the person to stand erect with the head up and back straight.
16. Helped the person walk. Walked to the side and slightly behind the person on the person's weak side. Provided support with the gait belt. If not using a gait belt, had one arm around the back and the other at the elbow to support the person. Encouraged the person to use the hand rail on his or her strong side.

Date of Satisfactory Completion _____   Instructor's Initials _____

Procedure—cont'd	S	U	Comments
17. Encouraged the person to walk normally. The heel struck the floor first. Discouraged shuffling, sliding, or walking on tip-toes.			
18. Walked the required distance if the person tolerated the activity. Did not rush the person.			
19. Helped the person return to bed. Removed the gait belt.			
20. Lowered the head of the bed. Helped the person to the center of the bed.			
21. Removed the shoes. Removed the paper or sheet over the bottom sheet.			

Post-Procedure

	S	U	Comments
22. Provided for comfort.			
23. Placed the call light within reach.			
24. Raised or lowered bed rails. Followed the care plan.			
25. Returned the robe and shoes to their proper place.			
26. Unscreened the person.			
27. Completed a safety check of the room.			
28. Decontaminated your hands.			
29. Reported and recorded your observations.			

Date of Satisfactory Completion _____   Instructor's Initials _____

Using a Pulse Oximeter

Name: _____ Date: _____

	S	U	Comments

Quality of Life
Remembered to:
- Knock before entering the person's room
- Address the person by name
- Introduce yourself by name and title
- Explain the procedure to the person before beginning and during the procedure
- Protect the person's rights during the procedure
- Handle the person gently during the procedure

Pre-Procedure
1. Followed *Delegation Guidelines:*
   Pulse Oximetry.
   Saw *Promoting Safety and Comfort:*
   Pulse Oximetry.
2. Practiced hand hygiene.
3. Collected the following:
   - Oximeter and sensor
   - Tape
   - Towel
4. Arranged your work area.
5. Decontaminated your hands.
6. Identified the person. Checked the identification (ID) bracelet against the assignment sheet. Also called the person by name.
7. Provided for privacy.

Procedure
8. Provided for comfort.
9. Dried the site with a towel.
10. Clipped or taped the sensor to the site.
11. Turned on the oximeter.
12. Set the high and low alarm limits for saturation of peripheral oxygen (SpO$_2$) and pulse rate. Turned on audio and visual alarms. (This step was done for continuous monitoring.)
13. Checked the person's pulse (apical or radial) with the pulse on the display. The pulses should have been about the same. Noted both pulses on the assignment sheet.
14. Read the SpO$_2$ on the display. Noted the value on the flow sheet and the assignment sheet. Also recorded if the person received supplemental oxygen and the flow rate.
15. Left the sensor in place for continuous monitoring. Otherwise, turned off the device and removed the sensor. If continuous monitoring, the site sensor was changed at least every 2 hours.

Post-Procedure
16. Provided for comfort.
17. Placed the call light within reach.
18. Unscreened the person.
19. Completed a safety check of the room.

Date of Satisfactory Completion _____ Instructor's Initials _____

Post-Procedure—cont'd

	S	U	Comments
20. Returned the device to its proper place (unless monitoring was continuous).	___	___	_____
21. Decontaminated your hands.	___	___	_____
22. Reported and recorded the SpO_2, the pulse rate, and your other observations.	___	___	_____

Date of Satisfactory Completion _____   Instructor's Initials _____

VIDEO Assisting with Deep-Breathing and Coughing Exercises

Name: _____   Date: _____

	S	U	Comments

Quality of Life

Remembered to:

- Knock before entering the person's room
- Address the person by name
- Introduce yourself by name and title
- Explain the procedure to the person before beginning and during the procedure
- Protect the person's rights during the procedure
- Handle the person gently during the procedure

Pre-Procedure

1. Followed *Delegation Guidelines:*
   Deep Breathing and Coughing.
   Saw *Promoting Safety and Comfort:*
   Deep Breathing and Coughing.
2. Practiced hand hygiene.
3. Collected the following before going to the person's room:
   - Box of tissues
   - Gloves
   - Mask (needed for person with respiratory infections)
4. Identified the person. Checked the identification (ID) bracelet against the assignment sheet. Also called the person by name.
5. Provided for privacy.

Procedure

6. Lowered the bed rail if up.
7. Helped the person to a comfortable sitting position: sitting on the side of the bed, semi-Fowler's or Fowler's.
8. Put on gloves and mask, if required.
9. Had the person deep breathe:
   a. Had the person place the hands over the rib cage.
   b. Had the person take a deep breath. It was as deep as possible. Reminded the person to inhale through the nose.
   c. Asked the person to hold the breath for 2 to 3 seconds.
   d. Asked the person to exhale slowly through pursed lips. Asked the person to exhale until the ribs moved as far down as possible.
   e. Repeated 4 more times:
      1. Deep breathed in through the nose.
      2. Held 2 to 3 seconds.
      3. Exhaled slowly with pursed lips until the ribs moved as far down as possible.
10. Asked the person to cough:
    a. Had the person place both hands over the incision. One hand was on top of the other. The person could have held a pillow or folded towel over the incision.
    b. Had the person take a deep breath through the nose.
    c. Asked the person to cough strongly twice with the mouth open.
    d. Had box of tissues within person's reach for productive cough.

Date of Satisfactory Completion _____   Instructor's Initials _____

Post-Procedure

	S	U	Comments
11. Provided for comfort.	___	___	_____
12. Placed the call light within reach.	___	___	_____
13. Raised or lowered the bed rails. Followed the care plan.	___	___	_____
14. Unscreened the person.	___	___	_____
15. Completed a safety check of the room.	___	___	_____
16. Removed gloves and decontaminated your hands.	___	___	_____
17. Reported and recorded your observations.	___	___	_____

Date of Satisfactory Completion _____   Instructor's Initials _____

Assisting with Incentive Spirometry

VIDEO CLIP   VIDEO

Name: _____   Date: _____

	S	U	Comments
Quality of Life			
Remembered to:			
• Knock before entering the person's room	___	___	_____
• Address the person by name	___	___	_____
• Introduce yourself by name and title	___	___	_____
• Explain the procedure to the person before beginning and during the procedure	___	___	_____
• Protect the person's rights during the procedure	___	___	_____
• Handle the person gently during the procedure	___	___	_____
Pre-Procedure			
1. Followed *Delegation Guidelines: Spirometry.*	___	___	_____
2. Practiced hand hygiene.	___	___	_____
3. Collected the following before going into the person's room:			
• Box of tissues	___	___	_____
• Gloves	___	___	_____
• Spirometer	___	___	_____
4. Identified the person. Checked the identification (ID) bracelet against the assignment sheet. Also called the person by name.	___	___	_____
5. Provided for privacy.	___	___	_____
Procedure			
6. Lowered the bed rail if up.	___	___	_____
7. Helped the person to a comfortable sitting position: sitting on the side of the bed, semi-Fowler's, or Fowler's.	___	___	_____
8. Had the person hold the spirometer upright.	___	___	_____
9. Had the person exhale normally.	___	___	_____
10. Had the person seal his or her lips around the mouthpiece.	___	___	_____
11. Asked the person to take a slow, deep breath until the balls were raised to the desired height.	___	___	_____
12. Asked the person to hold the breath for 3 to 6 seconds to keep the balls floating.	___		_____
13. Had the person remove the mouthpiece and exhale slowly. The person coughed at this time, if necessary.	___	___	_____
14. Asked the person to take some normal breaths, then use device again.	___	___	_____
Post-Procedure			
15. Provided for comfort.	___	___	_____
16. Placed the call light within reach.	___	___	_____
17. Raised or lowered the bed rails. Followed the care plan.	___	___	_____
18. Unscreened the person.	___	___	_____
19. Completed a safety check of the room.	___	___	_____
20. Decontaminated your hands.	___	___	_____
21. Reported and recorded your observations.	___	___	_____

Date of Satisfactory Completion _____   Instructor's Initials _____

Setting up for Oxygen Administration

Name: _____   Date: _____

	S	U	Comments
Quality of Life			
Remembered to:			
• Knock before entering the person's room	___	___	_____
• Address the person by name	___	___	_____
• Introduce yourself by name and title	___	___	_____
• Explain the procedure to the person before beginning and during the procedure	___	___	_____
• Protect the person's rights during the procedure	___	___	_____
• Handle the person gently during the procedure	___	___	_____

Pre-Procedure

1. Followed *Delegation Guidelines:*
   Oxygen Administration Set-Up.
   Saw *Promoting Safety and Comfort:*
   Oxygen Administration Set-Up.   ___ ___ _____
2. Practiced hand hygiene.
3. Collected the following before going to the person's room:
   • Oxygen device with connection tubing   ___ ___ _____
   • Flowmeter   ___ ___ _____
   • Humidifier (if ordered)   ___ ___ _____
   • Distilled water (if using humidifier)   ___ ___ _____
4. Arranged your work area.   ___ ___ _____
5. Decontaminated your hands.   ___ ___ _____
6. Identified the person. Checked the identification (ID) bracelet against the assignment sheet. Also called the person by name.

Procedure

7. Made sure the flowmeter was in the *OFF* position.   ___ ___ _____
8. Attached the flowmeter to the wall outlet or to the tank. ___ ___ _____
9. Filled the humidifier with distilled water.   ___ ___ _____
10. Attached the humidifier to the bottom of the flowmeter. ___ ___ _____
11. Attached the oxygen device and connecting tubing to the humidifier. *Did not set the flowmeter. Did not apply the oxygen device on the person.*
12. Placed the cap securely on the distilled water. Stored the water according to center policy.   ___ ___ _____
13. Discarded the packaging from the oxygen device and connecting tubing.   ___ ___ _____

Post-Procedure

14. Provided for comfort.   ___ ___ _____
15. Placed the call light within reach.   ___ ___ _____
16. Decontaminated your hands.   ___ ___ _____
17. Completed a safety check of the room.   ___ ___ _____
18. Told the nurse when you were done.
    The nurse then:
    a. *Turned on the oxygen and set the flow rate.*   ___ ___ _____
    b. *Applied the oxygen device on the person.*   ___ ___ _____

Date of Satisfactory Completion _____   Instructor's Initials _____

Taking A Temperature with an Electronic Thermometer

CD-ROM   VIDEO CLIP   VIDEO

Name: _____   Date: _____

	S	U	Comments
Quality of Life			
Remembered to:			
• Knock before entering the person's room	___	___	_____
• Address the person by name	___	___	_____
• Introduce yourself by name and title	___	___	_____
• Explain the procedure to the person before beginning and during the procedure	___	___	_____
• Protect the person's rights during the procedure	___	___	_____
• Handle the person gently during the procedure	___	___	_____

Pre-Procedure

1. Followed *Delegation Guidelines:*
   Taking Temperatures.   ___ ___ _____
   Saw *Promoting Safety and Comfort:*
   Taking Temperatures.   ___ ___ _____
2. For an *oral temperature*, asked the person not to eat, drink, smoke, or chew gum for at least 15 to 20 minutes before measurement or as required by center policy.   ___ ___ _____
3. Practiced hand hygiene.   ___ _____
4. Collected the following:
   • Thermometer—electronic, tympanic membrane, or temporal   ___ ___ _____
   • Probe (Blue for an oral or ancillary temperature. Red for a rectal temperature.)   ___ ___ _____
   • Probe covers   ___ ___ _____
   • Toilet tissue (rectal temperature)   ___ ___ _____
   • Water-soluble lubricant (rectal temperature)   ___ ___ _____
   • Gloves   ___ ___ _____
   • Towel (axillary temperature)   ___ ___ _____
5. Plugged the probe into the thermometer, if using an electronic thermometer.   ___ ___ _____
6. Decontaminated your hands.   ___ ___ _____
7. Identified the person. Checked the identification (ID) bracelet against the assignment sheet. Also called the person by name.   ___ ___ _____

Procedure

8. Provided for privacy. Positioned the person for an oral, rectal, axillary, or tympanic membrane temperature.   ___ ___ _____
9. Put on the gloves if contact with blood, body fluid, secretion, or excretion was likely.   ___ ___ _____
10. Inserted the probe into the probe cover.   ___ ___ _____
11. For an *oral temperature:*
    a. Asked the person to open the mouth and raise the tongue.   ___ ___ _____
    b. Placed the covered probe at the base of the tongue and to one side.   ___ ___ _____
    c. Asked the person to lower the tongue and close the mouth.   ___ ___ _____
12. For a *rectal temperature:*
    a. Placed some lubricant on a tissue.   ___ ___ _____
    b. Lubricated the end of the covered probe.   ___ ___ _____
    c. Exposed the anal area.   ___ ___ _____
    d. Raised the upper buttock.   ___ ___ _____
    e. Inserted the probe ½ inch into the rectum.   ___ ___ _____
    f. Held the probe in place.   ___ ___ _____

Date of Satisfactory Completion _____   Instructor's Initials _____

Procedure—cont'd	S	U	Comments

13. For *axillary temperature*:
    a. Helped the person remove an arm from the gown. Did not expose the person. ___ ___ _____
    b. Dried the axilla with a towel. ___ ___ _____
    c. Placed the covered probe in the axilla. ___ ___ _____
    d. Placed the person's arm over the chest. ___ ___ _____
    e. Held the probe in place. ___ ___ _____
14. For a *tympanic membrane temperature*:
    a. Asked the person to turn his or her head so the ear was in front of you. ___ ___ _____
    b. Pulled up and back on the ear to straighten the ear canal. ___ ___ _____
    c. Inserted the covered probe gently. ___ ___ _____
15. Started the thermometer. ___ ___ _____
16. Held the probe in place until you heard a tone or saw a flashing or steady light. ___ ___ _____
17. Read the temperature on the display. ___ ___ _____
18. Removed the probe. Pressed the eject button to discard the cover. ___ ___ _____
19. For a *temporal artery temperature*:
    a. Asked the person to turn his or her face toward you. ___ ___ _____
    b. Placed the device near the center of the forehead. Pressed the button. ___ ___ _____
    c. While the button was depressed, slid the device across the forehead and over the temporal artery, ending in front of the ear. (If the person had perspiration on the forehead, continued to slid the device to the back of the ear.) Followed manufacturer instructions. ___ ___ _____
20. Noted the person's name and temperature on your note pad or assignment sheet. Noted the temperature site. ___ ___ _____
21. Returned the probe to the holder. ___ ___ _____
22. Helped the person put the gown back on (axillary temperature). For a rectal temperature:
    a. Wiped the anal area with toilet tissue to remove lubricant. ___ ___ _____
    b. Covered the person. ___ ___ _____
    c. Disposed of used toilet tissue. ___ ___ _____
    d. Removed the gloves. Practiced hand hygiene. ___ ___ _____

Post-Procedure
23. Provided for comfort. ___ ___ _____
24. Placed the call light within reach. ___ ___ _____
25. Unscreened the person. ___ ___ _____
26. Completed a safety check of the room. ___ ___ _____
27. Returned the thermometer to the charging unit. ___ ___ _____
28. Decontaminated your hands. ___ ___ _____
29. Reported and recorded the temperature. Noted the temperature site when reporting and recording. A rectal temperature was noted with an "R" after the value. An axillary temperature was noted with an "Ax" after the value. Reported an abnormal temperature at once. ___ ___ _____

Date of Satisfactory Completion _____   Instructor's Initials _____

NNAAP™ Skill   **CD-ROM**   **VIDEO CLIP**   **VIDEO**   ## Taking a Radial Pulse

Name: _____   Date: _____

	S	U	Comments
Quality of Life			
Remembered to:			
• Knock before entering the person's room	____	____	_____
• Address the person by name	____	____	_____
• Introduce yourself by name and title	____	____	_____
• Explain the procedure to the person before beginning and during the procedure	____	____	_____
• Protect the person's rights during the procedure	____	____	_____
• Handle the person gently during the procedure	____	____	_____

Pre-Procedure

	S	U	Comments
1. Followed *Delegation Guidelines: Taking Pulses.* Saw *Promoting Safety and Comfort: Taking Pulses.*	____	____	_____
	____	____	_____
2. Practiced hand hygiene.	____	____	_____
3. Identified the person. Checked the identification (ID) bracelet against the assignment sheet. Called the person by name.	____	____	_____
4. Provided for privacy.	____	____	_____

Procedure

	S	U	Comments
5. Had the person sit or lie down.	____	____	_____
6. Located the radial pulse on the thumb side of the person's wrist. Used your first 2 or 3 middle fingers.	____	____	_____
7. Noted if the pulse was strong or weak, regular or irregular.	____	____	_____
8. Counted the pulse for 30 seconds. Multiplied the number of beats by 2. Or counted the pulse for 1 minute if:			
a. Directed by the nurse and care plan.	____	____	_____
b. Required by center policy.	____	____	_____
c. The pulse was irregular.	____	____	_____
d. Required for your state competency test.	____	____	_____
9. Noted the person's name and pulse on your note pad or assignment sheet. Noted the strength of the pulse. Noted if it was regular or irregular.	____	____	_____

Post-Procedure

	S	U	Comments
10. Provided for comfort.	____	____	_____
11. Placed the call light within reach.	____	____	_____
12. Unscreened the person.	____	____	_____
13. Completed a safety check of the room.	____	____	_____
14. Decontaminated your hands.	____	____	_____
15. Reported and recorded the pulse rate and your observations. Reported an abnormal pulse at once.	____	____	_____

Date of Satisfactory Completion _____   Instructor's Initials _____

VIDEO CLIP **VIDEO** ## Taking an Apical Pulse

Name: _____   Date: _____

	S	U	Comments

Quality of Life
Remembered to:
- Knock before entering the person's room
- Address the person by name
- Introduce yourself by name and title
- Explain the procedure to the person before beginning and during the procedure
- Protect the person's rights during the procedure
- Handle the person gently during the procedure

Pre-Procedure
1. Followed *Delegation Guidelines: Taking Pulses.* Saw *Promoting Safety and Comfort: Using a Stethoscope.*
2. Practiced hand hygiene.
3. Collected a stethoscope and antiseptic wipes.
4. Decontaminated your hands.
5. Identified the person. Checked the identification (ID) bracelet against the assignment sheet. Also called the person by name.
6. Provided for privacy.

Procedure
7. Cleaned the earpieces and diaphragm with the wipes.
8. Had the person sit or lie down.
9. Exposed the nipple area of the left chest. Exposed a woman's breasts to the extent necessary.
10. Warmed the diaphragm in your palm.
11. Placed the earpieces in your ears.
12. Found the apical pulse. Placed the diaphragm 2 to 3 inches to the left of the breastbone and below the left nipple.
13. Counted the pulse for 1 minute. Noted if the pulse was regular or irregular.
14. Covered the person. Removed the earpieces.
15. Noted the person's name and pulse on your note pad or assignment sheet. Noted if the pulse was regular or irregular.

Post-Procedure
16. Provided for comfort.
17. Placed the call light within reach.
18. Unscreened the person.
19. Completed a safety check of the room.
20. Cleaned the earpieces and diaphragm with the wipes.
21. Returned the stethoscope to its proper place.
22. Decontaminated your hands.
23. Reported and recorded your observations. Reported the pulse rate with *Ap* for apical. Reported an abnormal pulse rate at once.

Date of Satisfactory Completion _____   Instructor's Initials _____

Taking an Apical-Radial Pulse

Name: _____   Date: _____

Quality of Life	S	U	Comments
Remembered to:			
• Knock before entering the person's room	____	____	_____
• Address the person by name	____	____	_____
• Introduce yourself by name and title	____	____	_____
• Explain the procedure to the person before beginning and during the procedure	____	____	_____
• Protect the person's rights during the procedure	____	____	_____
• Handle the person gently during the procedure	____	____	_____

Pre-Procedure

	S	U	Comments
1. Followed *Delegation Guidelines:* *Taking Pulses.* Saw *Promoting Safety and Comfort:*	____	____	_____
a. *Using a Stethoscope.*	____	____	_____
b. *Taking Pulses.*	____	____	_____
2. Asked a co-worker to help you.	____	____	_____
3. Practiced hand hygiene.	____	____	_____
4. Collected a stethoscope and antiseptic wipes.	____	____	_____
5. Decontaminated your hands.	____	____	_____
6. Identified the person. Checked the identification (ID) bracelet against the assignment sheet. Also called the person by name.	____	____	_____
7. Provided for privacy.	____	____	_____

Procedure

	S	U	Comments
8. Cleaned the earpieces and diaphragm with the wipes.	____	____	_____
9. Had the person sit or lie down.	____	____	_____
10. Exposed the nipple area of the left chest. Exposed a woman's breasts to the extent necessary.	____	____	_____
11. Warmed the diaphragm in your palm.	____	____	_____
12. Placed the earpieces in your ears.	____	____	_____
13. Found the apical pulse. The co-worker found the radial pulse.	____	____	_____
14. Gave the signal to begin counting.	____	____	_____
15. Counted the pulse for 1 minute.	____	____	_____
16. Gave the signal to stop counting.	____	____	_____
17. Covered the person. Removed the stethoscope earpieces.	____	____	_____
18. Noted the person's name and apical and radial pulses on your note pad or assignment sheet. Subtracted the radial pulse from the apical pulse for the pulse deficit. Noted if the pulses were regular or irregular.	____	____	_____

Post-Procedure

	S	U	Comments
19. Provided for comfort.	____	____	_____
20. Placed the call light within reach.	____	____	_____
21. Unscreened the person.	____	____	_____
22. Completed a safety check of the room.	____	____	_____
23. Cleaned the earpieces and diaphragm with the wipes.	____	____	_____

Date of Satisfactory Completion _____   Instructor's Initials _____

Post-Procedure—cont'd	**S**	**U**	**Comments**
24. Returned the stethoscope to its proper place.	____	____	_____
25. Decontaminated your hands.	____	____	_____
26. Reported and recorded your observations. (Reported an abnormal pulse at once.) Included:			
a. The apical and radial pulse rates	____	____	_____
b. The pulse deficit	____	____	_____

Date of Satisfactory Completion _____   Instructor's Initials _____

NNAAP™ Skill   CD-ROM   VIDEO CLIP   VIDEO   **Counting Respirations**

Name: _____   Date: _____

Procedure	S	U	Comments
1. Followed *Delegation Guidelines: Respirations.*	____	____	_____
2. Kept your fingers or stethoscope over the pulse site.	____	____	_____
3. Did not tell the person you were counting respirations.	____	____	_____
4. Began counting when the chest rose. Counted each rise and fall of the chest as 1 respiration.	____	____	_____
5. Noted the following:			
a. If respirations were regular	____	____	_____
b. If both sides of the chest rose equally	____	____	_____
c. The depth of the respirations	____	____	_____
d. If the person had any pain or difficulty breathing	____	____	_____
e. An abnormal respiratory pattern	____	____	_____
6. Counted respirations for 30 seconds. Multiplied the number by 2. Counted respirations for 1 minute if:			
a. Directed by the nurse and care plan.	____	____	_____
b. Required by center policy.	____	____	_____
c. Respirations were abnormal or irregular.	____	____	_____
d. Required for the state competency test.	____	____	_____
7. Noted the person's name, respiratory rate, and any other observations on your note pad or assignment sheet.	____	____	_____

Post-Procedure

	S	U	Comments
8. Provided for comfort.	____	____	_____
9. Placed the call light within reach.	____	____	_____
10. Unscreened the person.	____	____	_____
11. Completed a safety check of the room.	____	____	_____
12. Decontaminated your hands.	____	____	_____
13. Reported and recorded the respiratory rate and your observations. Reported abnormal respirations at once.	____	____	_____

Date of Satisfactory Completion _____   Instructor's Initials _____

NNAAP™ Skill   CD-ROM   VIDEO CLIP   VIDEO   **Measuring Blood Pressure**

Name: _____   Date: _____

	S	U	Comments

Quality of Life
Remembered to:
- Knock before entering the person's room
- Address the person by name
- Introduce yourself by name and title
- Explain the procedure to the person before beginning and during the procedure
- Protect the person's rights during the procedure
- Handle the person gently during the procedure

Pre-Procedure
1. Followed *Delegation Guidelines: Measuring Blood Pressure.*
   Saw *Promoting Safety and Comfort:*
   a. *Using a Stethoscope.*
   b. *Equipment.*
2. Practiced hand hygiene.
3. Collected the following:
   - Sphygmomanometer
   - Stethoscope
   - Antiseptic wipes
4. Decontaminated your hands.
5. Identified the person. Checked the identification (ID) bracelet against the assignment sheet. Also called the person by name.
6. Provided for privacy.

Procedure
7. Wiped the earpieces and diaphragm with the wipes. Warmed the diaphragm in your palm.
8. Had the person sit or lie down.
9. Positioned the person's arm level with the heart. The palm was up.
10. Stood no more than 3 feet away from the manometer. The aneroid type was directly in front of you or mounted on the wall.
11. Exposed the upper arm.
12. Squeezed the cuff to expel any remaining air. Closed the valve on the bulb.
13. Found the brachial artery at the inner aspect of the elbow (on the little finger side of the arm). Used your fingertips.
14. Located the arrow on the cuff. Placed the arrow on the cuff over the brachial artery. Wrapped the cuff around the upper arm at least 1 inch above the elbow. It was even and snug.
15. Placed the stethoscope earpieces in your ears.
16. Found the radial or brachial pulse.
17. *Method 1:*
    a. Inflated the cuff until you could no longer feel the pulse. Noted this point.
    b. Inflated the cuff 30 mm Hg beyond the point where you last felt the pulse.

Date of Satisfactory Completion _____   Instructor's Initials _____

Procedure—cont'd	S	U	Comments

Procedure—cont'd

18. *Method 2:*
    a. Inflated the cuff until you longer felt felt the pulse. Noted this point.
    b. Inflated the cuff 30 mm Hg beyond the point where you last felt the pulse.
    c. Deflated the cuff slowly. Noted the point where you felt the pulse.
    d. Waited 30 seconds.
    e. Inflated the cuff 30 mm Hg beyond the point where you felt the pulse return.
19. Placed the diaphragm of the stethoscope over the brachial artery. Did not place it under the cuff.
20. Deflated the cuff at an even rate of 2 to 4 millimeters per second. Turned the valve counter-clockwise to deflate the cuff.
21. Noted the point where you heard the first sound. This was the systolic reading. It was near the point where the radial pulse disappeared.
22. Continued to deflate the cuff. Noted the point where the sound disappeared. This was the diastolic reading.
23. Deflated the cuff completely. Removed it from the person's arm. Removed the stethoscope earpieces from your ears.
24. Noted the person's name and blood pressure on your note pad or assignment sheet.
25. Returned the cuff to the case or the wall holder.

Post-Procedure

26. Provided for comfort.
27. Placed the call light within reach.
28. Unscreened the person.
29. Completed a safety check of the room.
30. Cleaned the earpieces and diaphragm with the wipes.
31. Returned the equipment to its proper place.
32. Decontaminated your hands.
33. Reported and recorded the blood pressure. Reported an abnormal blood pressure at once.

Date of Satisfactory Completion _____ Instructor's Initials _____

NNAAP™ Skill   CD-ROM   VIDEO CLIP   VIDEO   **Measuring Weight and Height**

Name: _____   Date: _____

	S	U	Comments
Quality of Life			
Remembered to:			
• Knock before entering the person's room	___	___	_____
• Address the person by name	___	___	_____
• Introduce yourself by name and title	___	___	_____
• Explain the procedure to the person before beginning and during the procedure	___	___	_____
• Protect the person's rights during the procedure	___	___	_____
• Handle the person gently during the procedure	___	___	_____

Pre-Procedure

	S	U	Comments
1. Followed *Delegation Guidelines: Weight and Height.* Saw *Promoting Safety and Comfort: Weight and Height.*	___	___	_____
2. Asked the person to void.	___	___	_____
3. Practiced hand hygiene.	___	___	_____
4. Brought the scale and paper towels (for standing scale) to the person's room or transported the person by wheelchair to the wheelchair platform scale.	___	___	_____
5. Decontaminated your hands.			
6. Identified the person. Checked the identification (ID) bracelet against the assignment sheet. Also called the person by name.	___	___	_____
7. Provided for privacy.			

Procedure

	S	U	Comments
8. Placed the paper towels on the scale platform.	___	___	_____
9. Raised the height rod.	___	___	_____
10. Moved the weights to zero (0). The pointer was in the middle.	___	___	_____
11. Had the person remove the robe and footwear. Assisted as needed.	___	___	_____
12. Helped the person stand on the scale. The person stood in the center of the scale. Arms were at the sides.	___	___	_____
13. Moved the weights until the balance pointer was in the middle.	___	___	_____
14. If using a wheelchair scale, pushed the person sitting in the wheelchair onto the scale. Noted the weight. Safely moved the person in the wheelchair off the platform. Subtracted the weight of the wheelchair from the total weight. That was the value recorded.	___	___	_____
15. Noted the weight on your note pad or assignment sheet.	___	___	_____
16. Asked the person to stand very straight.	___	___	_____
17. Lowered the height rod until it rested on the person's head.	___	___	_____
18. Noted the height on your note pad or assignment sheet.	___	___	_____
19. Raised the height rod. Helped the person step off of the scale.	___	___	_____
20. Helped the person put on a robe and non-skid footwear if he or she was to be up. Or helped the person back to bed.	___	___	_____
21. Lowered the height rod. Adjusted the weights to zero (0) if this was center policy.	___	___	_____

Date of Satisfactory Completion _____   Instructor's Initials _____

Post-Procedure	S	U	Comments
22. Provided for comfort.	___	___	_____
23. Placed the call light within reach.	___	___	_____
24. Raised or lowered bed rails. Followed the care plan.	___	___	_____
25. Unscreened the person.	___	___	_____
26. Completed a safety check of the room.	___	___	_____
27. Discarded the paper towels.	___	___	_____
28. Returned the scale to its proper place.	___	___	_____
29. Decontaminated your hands.	___	___	_____
30. Reported and recorded the measurements.	___	___	_____

Date of Satisfactory Completion _____ Instructor's Initials _____

Measuring Height—The Person is in Bed

Name: _____   Date: _____

Quality of Life	S	U	Comments
Remembered to:			
• Knock before entering the person's room	___	___	_____
• Address the person by name	___	___	_____
• Introduce yourself by name and title	___	___	_____
• Explain the procedure to the person before beginning and during the procedure	___	___	_____
• Protect the person's rights during the procedure	___	___	_____
• Handle the person gently during the procedure	___	___	_____

Pre-Procedure

1. Followed *Delegation Guidelines: Weight and Height.*
   Saw *Promoting Safety and Comfort: Weight and Height.*
2. Practiced hand hygiene.
3. Asked a co-worker to help you.
4. Collected a measuring tape and ruler.
5. Decontaminated your hands.
6. Identified the person. Checked the identification (ID) bracelet against the assignment sheet. Also called the person by name.
7. Provided for privacy.
8. Raised the bed for body mechanics. Bed rails were up if used.

Procedure

9. Lowered the bed rails (if up).
10. Positioned the person supine if the position was allowed.
11. Had your co-worker hold the end of the measuring tape at the person's heel.
12. Pulled the measuring tape along the person's body. Pulled until it extended past the head.
13. Placed the ruler flat across the top of the person's head. It extended from the person's head to the measuring tape. Made sure the ruler was level.
14. Noted the height on your note pad or assignment sheet.

Post-Procedure

15. Provided for comfort.
16. Placed the call light within reach.
17. Lowered the bed to its lowest position.
18. Raised or lowered bed rails. Followed the care plan.
19. Completed a safety check of the room.
20. Returned equipment to its proper place.
21. Decontaminated your hands.
22. Reported and recorded the height.

Date of Satisfactory Completion _____   Instructor's Initials _____

Preparing the Person for an Examination

Name: _____   Date: _____

Quality of Life	S	U	Comments
Remembered to:			
• Knock before entering the person's room	___	___	_____
• Address the person by name	___	___	_____
• Introduce yourself by name and title	___	___	_____
• Explain the procedure to the person before beginning and during the procedure	___	___	_____
• Protect the person's rights during the procedure	___	___	_____
• Handle the person gently during the procedure	___	___	_____

Pre-Procedure

	S	U	Comments
1. Followed *Delegation Guidelines: Preparing the Person.*	___	___	_____
Saw *Promoting Safety and Comfort: Preparing the Person.*	___	___	_____
2. Practiced hand hygiene.	___	___	_____
3. Collected the following:			
• Flashlight	___	___	_____
• Sphygmomanometer	___	___	_____
• Stethoscope	___	___	_____
• Thermometer	___	___	_____
• Tongue depressors (blades)	___	___	_____
• Laryngeal mirror	___	___	_____
• Ophthalmoscope	___	___	_____
• Otoscope	___	___	_____
• Nasal speculum	___	___	_____
• Percussion (reflex) hammer	___	___	_____
• Tuning fork	___	___	_____
• Tape measure	___	___	_____
• Gloves	___	___	_____
• Water-soluble lubricant	___	___	_____
• Vaginal speculum	___	___	_____
• Cotton-tipped applicators	___	___	_____
• Specimen containers and labels	___	___	_____
• Disposable bag	___	___	_____
• Kidney basin	___	___	_____
• Towel	___	___	_____
• Bath blanket	___	___	_____
• Tissues	___	___	_____
• Drape (sheet, bath blanket, drawsheet, or paper drape)	___	___	_____
• Paper towels	___	___	_____
• Cotton balls	___	___	_____
• Waterproof pad	___	___	_____
• Eye chart (Snellen chart)	___	___	_____
• Slides	___	___	_____
• Gown	___	___	_____
• Alcohol wipes	___	___	_____
• Wastebasket	___	___	_____
• Container for soiled instruments	___	___	_____
• Marking pencils or pens	___	___	_____
4. Decontaminated your hands.	___	___	_____

Date of Satisfactory Completion _____   Instructor's Initials _____

	S	U	Comments
Pre-Procedure—cont'd			
5. Identified the person. Checked the identification (ID) bracelet against the assignment sheet. Also called the person by name.	_____	_____	_____
6. Provided for privacy.	_____	_____	_____
Procedure			
7. Had the person put on the gown. Told the person to remove all clothes. Assisted as needed.	_____	_____	_____
8. Asked the person to void. Collected a urine specimen if needed. Provided for privacy.	_____	_____	_____
9. Transported the person to the exam room. (This was not done for an exam in the person's room).	_____	_____	_____
10. Measured weight and height. Recorded the measurements on the exam form.	_____	_____	_____
11. Helped the person onto the exam table. Provided a step stool if necessary. (Omitted this step for an exam in the person's room.)	_____	_____	_____
12. Raised the far bed rail (if used). Raised the bed to its highest level. (This step was not done if an exam table was used.)	_____	_____	_____
13. Measured vital signs. Recorded them on the exam form.	_____	_____	_____
14. Positioned the person as directed.	_____	_____	_____
15. Draped the person.	_____	_____	_____
16. Placed a waterproof pad under the buttocks.	_____	_____	_____
17. Raised the bed rail near you (if used).	_____	_____	_____
18. Provided adequate lighting.	_____	_____	_____
19. Put the call light on for the examiner. Did not leave the person alone.	_____	_____	_____
Post-Procedure			
20. Assisted the examiner as needed.	_____	_____	_____
21. Processed specimens according to directions (if any).	_____	_____	_____
22. Performed hand hygiene.	_____	_____	_____
23. Assisted the person off the exam table or, if in bed, helped the person to a comfortable position.	_____	_____	_____
24. After the person left the exam room, cleaned the area and put away all equipment and supplies.	_____	_____	_____
25. Completed a safety check of the room.	_____	_____	_____

Date of Satisfactory Completion _____ Instructor's Initials _____

Collecting a Random Urine Specimen

Name: _____   Date: _____

Quality of Life	S	U	Comments
Remembered to:			
• Knock before entering the person's room	___	___	_____
• Address the person by name	___	___	_____
• Introduce yourself by name and title	___	___	_____
• Explain the procedure to the person before beginning and during the procedure	___	___	_____
• Protect the person's rights during the procedure	___	___	_____
• Handle the person gently during the procedure	___	___	_____

Pre-Procedure

	S	U	Comments
1. Followed *Delegation Guidelines: Urine Specimens.* Saw *Promoting Safety and Comfort: Urine Specimens.*	___	___	_____
2. Practiced hand hygiene.	___	___	_____
3. Collected the following before going to the person's room:			
• Laboratory requisition slip	___	___	_____
• Specimen container and lid	___	___	_____
• Specimen label	___	___	_____
• Plastic bag(s)	___	___	_____
• BIOHAZARD label (if needed)	___	___	_____
• Gloves	___	___	_____
4. Arranged collected items in the person's bathroom.	___	___	_____
5. Decontaminated your hands.	___	___	_____
6. Identified the person. Checked the identification (ID) bracelet against the assignment sheet. Also called the person by name.	___	___	_____
7. Labeled the container in the person's presence.	___	___	_____
8. Put on gloves.	___	___	_____
9. Collected the following:			
• Voiding receptacle—bedpan and cover, urinal, commode, or specimen pan			
• Graduate to measure output	___	___	_____
10. Provided for privacy.	___	___	_____

Procedure

	S	U	Comments
11. Asked the person to void into the receptacle. Reminded the person to put toilet tissue in the wastebasket or toilet. Toilet tissue was not put in the bedpan or specimen pan.	___	___	_____
12. Took the receptacle to the bathroom.	___	___	_____
13. Poured about 120 mL (milliliters) (4 oz [ounces]) into the specimen container.	___	___	_____
14. Placed the lid on the specimen container. Put the container in the plastic bag. Did not let the container touch the outside of the bag. Some facilities require double-bagging of the specimen. Applied a BIOHAZARD symbol according to center policy.	___	___	_____
15. Measured urine intake and output (I&O) if ordered. Included the amount in the specimen container.	___	___	_____
16. Emptied, cleaned, and disinfected equipment. Returned equipment to its proper place.	___	___	_____

Date of Satisfactory Completion _____   Instructor's Initials _____

Procedure—cont'd   S   U   Comments

17. Removed the gloves and practiced hand hygiene.   _____ _____ _____
    Put on clean gloves.

18. Assisted with hand washing.   _____ _____ _____

19. Removed the gloves. Practiced hand hygiene.   _____ _____ _____

Post-Procedure

20. Provided for comfort.   _____ _____ _____

21. Placed the call light within reach.   _____ _____ _____

22. Raised or lowered bed rails. Followed the care plan. _____ _____ _____

23. Unscreened the person.   _____ _____ _____

24. Completed a safety check of the room.   _____ _____ _____

25. Decontaminated your hands.   _____ _____ _____

26. Took the specimen and the requisition slip to the   _____ _____ _____
    storage area. Followed center policy. Wore gloves.

27. Reported and recorded your observations.   _____ _____ _____

Date of Satisfactory Completion _____   Instructor's Initials _____

VIDEO CLIP VIDEO ### Collecting a Midstream Specimen

Name: _____ Date: _____

	S	U	Comments
Quality of Life Remembered to:			
• Knock before entering the person's room	____	____	_____
• Address the person by name	____	____	_____
• Introduce yourself by name and title	____	____	_____
• Explain the procedure to the person before beginning and during the procedure	____	____	_____
• Protect the person's rights during the procedure	____	____	_____
• Handle the person gently during the procedure	____	____	_____
Pre-Procedure			
1. Followed *Delegation Guidelines: Urine Specimens.*	____	____	_____
Saw *Promoting Safety and Comfort: Urine Specimens.*	____	____	_____
2. Practiced hand hygiene.	____	____	_____
3. Collected the following:			
• Laboratory requisition slip	____	____	_____
• Midstream specimen kit—includes specimen container, label, and towelettes; may include sterile gloves	____	____	_____
• Plastic bag(s)	____	____	_____
• Sterile gloves (if not part of kit)	____	____	_____
• BIOHAZARD label (if needed)			
4. Arranged your work area.	____	____	_____
5. Decontaminated your hands.	____	____	_____
6. Identified the person. Checked the identification (ID) bracelet against the assignment sheet. Also called the person by name.	____	____	_____
7. Put on disposable gloves.	____	____	_____
8. Collected the following:			
• Voiding receptacle—bedpan and cover, urinal, commode, or specimen pan if needed	____	____	_____
• Supplies for perineal care	____	____	_____
• Graduate to measure output	____	____	_____
• Paper towel	____	____	_____
9. Provided for privacy.	____	____	_____
Procedure			
10. Provided perineal care. (Wore gloves for this step. Decontaminated your hands after removing gloves.)	____	____	_____
11. Opened the sterile kit.	____	____	_____
12. Put on the sterile gloves.	____	____	_____
13. Opened the packet of towelettes inside the kit.	____	____	_____
14. Opened the sterile specimen container. Did not touch the inside of the container or the lid. Sat the lid down so the inside was up.	____	____	_____
15. *For a female*—cleaned the perineal area with the towelettes.			
a. Spread the labia with your thumb and index finger. Used your non-dominant hand. (This hand was then contaminated and did not touch anything sterile.)	____	____	_____
b. Cleaned the urethral area from front to back. Used a clean towellette for each stroke.	____	____	_____
c. Kept the labia separated to collect the urine specimen.	____	____	_____

Date of Satisfactory Completion _____ Instructor's Initials _____

Procedure—cont'd	S	U	Comments

16. *For a male*—cleaned the penis with towelettes.
   a. Held the penis with your non-dominant hand. (This hand was then contaminated and did not touch anything sterile.)
   b. Cleaned the penis starting at the meatus. Cleaned in a circular motion. Started at the center and worked outward.
   c. Kept holding the penis until the specimen was collected.
17. Asked the person to void into the receptacle.
18. Passed the specimen container into the stream of urine. (If female, kept the labia separated.)
19. Collected about 30 to 60 mL (1 to 2 oz) of urine.
20. Removed the specimen container before the person stopped voiding.
21. Released the labia or penis. Allowed the person to finish voiding into the receptacle.
22. Put the lid on the specimen container. Touched only the outside of the container and lid. Wiped the outside of the container. Sat the container on a paper towel.
23. Provided toilet tissue after the person was done voiding.
24. Took the receptacle to the bathroom.
25. Measured urine if intake and output (I&O) was ordered. Included the amount in the specimen container.
26. Emptied, cleaned, and disinfected equipment. Returned equipment to its proper place.
27. Removed the gloves and practiced hand hygiene. Put on clean disposable gloves.
28. Labeled the specimen container in the person's presence. Placed the container in the plastic bag. Did not let the container touch the outside of the bag. (Double-bagged the specimen if required by facility.) Applied a *BIOHAZARD* label according to center policy.
29. Assisted with hand washing.
30. Removed the gloves. Practiced hand hygiene.

Post-Procedure
31. Provided for comfort.
32. Placed the call light within reach.
33. Raised or lowered bed rails. Followed the care plan.
34. Unscreened the person.
35. Completed a safety check of the room.
36. Decontaminated your hands.
37. Took the specimen and the requisition slip to the storage area. Followed center policy. Wore gloves.
38. Reported and recorded your observations.

Date of Satisfactory Completion _____   Instructor's Initials _____

VIDEO CLIP VIDEO **Collecting a 24-Hour Urine Specimen**

Name: _____ Date: _____

	S	U	Comments
Quality of Life			
Remembered to:			
• Knock before entering the person's room	___	___	_____
• Address the person by name	___	___	_____
• Introduce yourself by name and title	___	___	_____
• Explain the procedure to the person before beginning and during the procedure	___	___	_____
• Protect the person's rights during the procedure	___	___	_____
• Handle the person gently during the procedure	___	___	_____
Pre-Procedure			
1. Followed *Delegation Guidelines:* *Urine Specimens.* Saw *Promoting Safety and Comfort:*	___	___	_____
a. *Urine Specimens.*	___	___	_____
b. *The 24-Hour Urine Specimen.*	___	___	_____
2. Practiced hand hygiene.	___	___	_____
3. Collected the following:			
• Laboratory requisition slip	___	___	_____
• Urine container for a 24-hour collection	___	___	_____
• Specimen label	___	___	_____
• Preservative if needed	___	___	_____
• Bucket with ice if needed	___	___	_____
• Two 24-HOUR URINE labels	___	___	_____
• Funnel	___	___	_____
• BIOHAZARD label	___	___	_____
4. Arranged collected items in the person's bathroom.	___	___	_____
5. Placed one 24-HOUR URINE label in the bathroom. Placed the other near the bed.	___	___	_____
6. Decontaminated your hands.	___	___	_____
7. Identified the person. Checked the identification (ID) bracelet against the assignment sheet. Also called the person by name.	___	___	_____
8. Labeled the urine container in the person's presence. Applied the BIOHAZARD label.	___	___	_____
9. Put on gloves.	___	___	_____
10. Collected the following:			
• Voiding receptacle—bedpan and cover, urinal, commode, or specimen pan	___	___	_____
• Gloves	___	___	_____
• Graduate for output	___	___	_____
11. Provided for privacy.	___	___	_____
Procedure			
12. Asked the person to void. Provided a voiding receptacle.	___	___	_____
13. Measured and discarded the urine. Noted the time. This started the 24-hour collection period.	___	___	_____
14. Marked the time on the collection container.	___	___	_____
15. Emptied, cleaned, and disinfected equipment. Returned equipment to its proper place.	___	___	_____
16. Removed the gloves and practiced hand hygiene. Put on clean gloves.	___	___	_____
17. Assisted with hand washing.	___	___	_____

Date of Satisfactory Completion _____ Instructor's Initials _____

Procedure—cont'd	S	U	Comments
18. Removed the gloves. Practiced hand hygiene.	___	___	___
19. Marked the time the test began and the time it will end on the room and bathroom labels.	___	___	___
20. Reminded the person to:			
a. Use the voiding receptacle when voiding during the next 24 hours.	___	___	___
b. Not have a bowel movement (BM) when voiding.	___	___	___
c. Put toilet tissue in the toilet or wastebasket.	___	___	___
d. Put on the call light after voiding.	___	___	___
21. Returned to the room when the person signaled for you. Knocked before entering the room.	___	___	___
22. Did the following after every voiding:			
a. Decontaminated your hands. Put on gloves.	___	___	___
b. Measured urine if intake and output (I&O) was ordered.	___	___	___
c. Poured urine into the container using the funnel. Did not spill any urine. Re-started the test if you spilled or discarded the urine.	___	___	___
d. Emptied, cleaned, and disinfected equipment. Returned equipment to its proper place.	___	___	___
e. Removed the gloves and practiced hand hygiene. Put on clean gloves.	___	___	___
f. Assisted with hand washing.	___	___	___
g. Removed the gloves. Practiced hand hygiene.	___	___	___
23. Asked the person to void at the end of the 24-hour period. Did the following:			
a. Decontaminated your hands. Put on gloves.	___	___	___
b. Measured urine if I&O was ordered.	___	___	___
c. Poured urine into the container using the funnel. Did not spill any urine. Restarted the test if you spilled or discarded the urine.	___	___	___
d. Emptied, cleaned, and disinfected equipment. Returned equipment to its proper place.	___	___	___
e. Removed the gloves and practiced hand hygiene. Put on clean gloves.	___	___	___
f. Assisted with hand washing.	___	___	___
g. Removed the gloves. Practiced hand hygiene.	___	___	___
Post-Procedure			
24. Provided for comfort.	___	___	___
25. Placed the call light within reach.	___	___	___
26. Raised or lowered bed rails. Followed the care plan.	___	___	___
27. Put on gloves.			
28. Removed the labels from the room and bathroom.	___	___	___
29. Cleaned and returned equipment to its proper place. Discarded disposable items.	___	___	___
30. Removed the gloves. Practiced hand hygiene.	___	___	___
31. Unscreened the person.	___	___	___
32. Completed a safety check of the room.	___	___	___
33. Took the specimen and the requisition slip to the storage area. Wore gloves.	___	___	___
34. Reported and recorded your observations.	___	___	___

Date of Satisfactory Completion _____   Instructor's Initials _____

Testing Urine with Reagent Strips

Name: _____ Date: _____

	S	U	Comments
Quality of Life			
Remembered to:			
• Knock before entering the person's room	___	___	___
• Address the person by name	___	___	___
• Introduce yourself by name and title	___	___	___
• Explain the procedure to the person before beginning and during the procedure	___	___	___
• Protect the person's rights during the procedure	___	___	___
• Handle the person gently during the procedure	___	___	___

Pre-Procedure

	S	U	Comments
1. Followed *Delegation Guidelines: Testing Urine.* Saw *Promoting Safety and Comfort:*			
a. *Testing Urine.*	___	___	___
b. *Using Reagent Strips.*	___	___	___
2. Practiced hand hygiene.	___	___	___
3. Collected gloves and the reagent strips ordered.	___	___	___
4. Decontaminated your hands.	___	___	___
5. Identified the person. Checked the identification (ID) bracelet against the assignment sheet. Also called the person by name.	___	___	___
6. Put on gloves.	___	___	___
7. Collected equipment for the urine specimen.	___	___	___
8. Provided for privacy.	___	___	___

Procedure

	S	U	Comments
9. Collected the urine specimen.	___	___	___
10. Removed the strip from the bottle. Put the cap on the bottle at once. It was on tight.	___	___	___
11. Dipped the test strip areas into the urine.	___	___	___
12. Removed the strip after the correct amount of time. Saw the manufacturer instructions.	___	___	___
13. Tapped the strip gently against the container. This removed excess urine.	___	___	___
14. Waited the required amount of time. Saw the manufacturer instructions.	___	___	___
15. Compared the strip with the color chart on the bottle. Read the results.	___	___	___
16. Discarded disposable items and the specimen.	___	___	___
17. Emptied, cleaned, and disinfected equipment. Returned equipment to its proper place.	___	___	___
18. Removed the gloves. Practiced hand hygiene.	___	___	___

Post-Procedure

	S	U	Comments
19. Provided for comfort.	___	___	___
20. Placed the call light within reach.	___	___	___
21. Raised or lowered bed rails. Followed the care plan.	___	___	___
22. Unscreened the person.	___	___	___
23. Completed a safety check of the room.	___	___	___
24. Decontaminated your hands.	___	___	___
25. Reported and recorded the results and any other observations.	___	___	___

Date of Satisfactory Completion _____ Instructor's Initials _____

Straining Urine

Name: _____   Date: _____

Quality of Life	S	U	Comments

Remembered to:
- Knock before entering the person's room
- Address the person by name
- Introduce yourself by name and title
- Explain the procedure to the person before beginning and during the procedure
- Protect the person's rights during the procedure
- Handle the person gently during the procedure

Pre-Procedure
1. Followed *Delegation Guidelines: Testing Urine.* Saw *Promoting Safety and Comfort: Testing Urine.*
2. Practiced hand hygiene.
3. Collected the following before going to the person's room:
   - Laboratory requisition slip
   - Gauze or strainer
   - Specimen container
   - Specimen label
   - Two STRAIN ALL URINE labels
   - Plastic bag
   - BIOHAZARD label if needed
   - Gloves
4. Arranged collected items in the person's bathroom.
5. Placed one STRAIN ALL URINE label in the bathroom. Placed the other near the bed.
6. Decontaminated your hands.
7. Identified the person. Checked the identification (ID) bracelet against the assignment sheet. Also called the person by name.
8. Labeled the specimen container in the person's presence.
9. Put on gloves.
10. Collected the following:
    - Voiding receptacle—bedpan and cover, urinal, commode, or specimen pan
    - Graduate
    - Gloves
11. Provided for privacy.

Procedure
12. Asked the person to use the voiding receptacle for urinating. Asked the person to put on the call light after voiding.
13. Removed the gloves. Practiced hand hygiene.
14. Returned to the room when the person signaled for you. Knocked before entering the room.
15. Decontaminated your hands. Put on gloves.
16. Placed the gauze or strainer into the graduate.
17. Poured urine into the graduate. Urine passed through the gauze or strainer.

Date of Satisfactory Completion _____   Instructor's Initials _____

Procedure—cont'd	S	U	Comments
18. Placed the gauze or strainer in the specimen container if any crystals, stones, or particles appeared.	___	___	_____
19. Placed the specimen container in the plastic bag. Did not let the container touch the outside of the bag. Applied a *BIOHAZARD* symbol according to center policy.	___	___	_____
20. Measured urine if intake and output (I&O) was ordered.	___	___	_____
21. Emptied, cleaned, and disinfected equipment. Returned equipment to its proper place.	___	___	_____
22. Removed the gloves and practiced hand hygiene. Put on gloves.	___	___	_____
23. Assisted with hand washing.	___	___	_____
24. Removed the gloves. Practiced hand hygiene.	___	___	_____

Post-Procedure

	S	U	Comments
25. Provided for comfort.	___	___	_____
26. Placed the call light within reach.	___	___	_____
27. Raised or lowered bed rails. Followed the care plan.	___	___	_____
28. Unscreened the person.	___	___	_____
29. Completed a safety check of the room.	___	___	_____
30. Decontaminated your hands.	___	___	_____
31. Took the specimen container and requisition slip to the laboratory or storage area. Wore gloves.	___	___	_____
32. Reported and recorded your observations.	___	___	_____

Date of Satisfactory Completion _____ Instructor's Initials _____

VIDEO **Collecting a Stool Specimen**

Name: _____   Date: _____

	S	U	Comments
Quality of Life			
Remembered to:			
• Knock before entering the person's room	___	___	_____
• Address the person by name	___	___	_____
• Introduce yourself by name and title	___	___	_____
• Explain the procedure to the person before beginning and during the procedure	___	___	_____
• Protect the person's rights during the procedure	___	___	_____
• Handle the person gently during the procedure	___	___	_____

Pre-Procedure

1. Followed *Delegation Guidelines:*
   Stool Specimens.
   Saw *Promoting Safety and Comfort:*
   Stool Specimens.
2. Practiced hand hygiene.
3. Collected the following before going to the person's room:
   • Laboratory requisition slip
   • Specimen pan for the toilet
   • Specimen container and lid
   • Specimen label
   • Tongue blade
   • Disposable bag
   • Plastic bag(s)
   • BIOHAZARD label (if needed)
   • Gloves
4. Arranged collected items in the person's bathroom.
5. Decontaminated your hands.
6. Identified the person. Checked the identification (ID) bracelet against the assignment sheet. Also called the person by name.
7. Labeled the specimen container in the person's presence.
8. Put on gloves.
9. Collected the following:
   • Receptacle for voiding—bedpan and cover, urinal, commode, or specimen pan
   • Toilet tissue
10. Provided for privacy.

Procedure

11. Asked the person to void. Provided the receptacle for voiding if the person did not use the bathroom. Emptied, cleaned, and disinfected the device. Returned it to its proper place.
12. Put the specimen pan on the toilet if the person used the bathroom. Placed it at the back of the toilet. Or provided a bedpan or commode.
13. Asked the person not to put toilet tissue into the bedpan, commode, or specimen pan. Provided a bag for toilet tissue.
14. Placed the call light and toilet tissue within reach. Raised or lowered bed rails. Followed the care plan.

Date of Satisfactory Completion _____   Instructor's Initials _____

Procedure—cont'd	S	U	Comments
15. Removed the gloves. Decontaminated your hands. Left the room.			
16. Returned when the person signaled. Or checked on the person every 5 minutes. Knocked before entering.			
17. Decontaminated your hands. Put on clean gloves.			
18. Lowered the bed rail near you if up.			
19. Removed the bedpan (if used). Noted the color, amount, consistency, and odor of stools.			
20. Provided perineal care if needed.			
21. Collected the specimen:			
a. Used a tongue blade to take about 2 tablespoons of stool to the specimen container. Took the sample from the middle of a formed stool.			
b. Included pus, mucus, or blood present in the stool.			
c. Took stool from 2 different places in the bowel movement (BM) if required by center policy.			
d. Put the lid on the specimen container.			
e. Placed the container in the plastic bag. Did not let the container touch the outside of the bag. (Double-bagged if required by facility.) Applied a *BIOHAZARD* symbol according to center policy.			
22. Wrapped the tongue blade in toilet tissue. Discarded it in the disposable bag.			
23. Emptied, cleaned, and disinfected equipment. Returned equipment to its proper place.			
24. Removed the gloves and practiced hand hygiene. Put on clean gloves.			
25. Assisted with hand washing.			
26. Removed the gloves. Practiced hand hygiene.			
Post-Procedure			
27. Provided for comfort.			
28. Placed the call light within reach.			
29. Raised or lowered bed rails. Followed the care plan.			
30. Unscreened the person.			
31. Completed a safety check of the room.			
32. Took the specimen and requisition slip to the storage area. Followed center policy. Wore gloves.			
33. Reported and recorded your observations.			

Date of Satisfactory Completion _____   Instructor's Initials _____

VIDEO CLIP **VIDEO** **Testing a Stool Specimen for Blood**

Name: _____   Date: _____

	S	U	Comments

Quality of Life
Remembered to:
- Knock before entering the person's room
- Address the person by name
- Introduce yourself by name and title
- Explain the procedure to the person before beginning and during the procedure
- Protect the person's rights during the procedure
- Handle the person gently during the procedure

Pre-Procedure
1. Followed *Delegation Guidelines:*
   Testing Stools for Blood.
   Saw *Promoting Safety and Comfort*
   a. *Stool Specimens.*
   b. *Testing Stool for Blood.*
2. Practiced hand hygiene.
3. Collected the following before going to the person's room:
   - Occult blood test kit
   - Tongue blades (if needed)
   - Gloves
4. Arranged collected items in the person's bathroom.
5. Decontaminated your hands.
6. Identified the person. Checked the identification (ID) bracelet against the assignment sheet. Also called the person by name.
7. Put on gloves.
8. Collected the following:
   - Equipment for collecting a stool specimen
   - Paper towels
9. Provided for privacy.

Procedure
10. Collected a stool specimen.
11. Practiced hand hygiene. Put on clean gloves.
12. Opened the test kit.
13. Used a tongue blade to obtain a small amount of stool.
14. Applied a thin smear of stool on *box A* on the test paper.
15. Used another tongue blade to obtain stool from another part of the specimen.
16. Applied a thin smear of stool on *box B* on the test paper.
17. Closed the packet.
18. Turned the test packet to the other side. Opened the flap. Applied developer (from the kit) to *boxes A and B*. Followed the manufacturer instructions.
19. Waited 10 to 60 seconds as required by the manufacturer instructions.
20. Noted the color changes on the assignment sheet.
21. Disposed of test packet.
22. Wrapped the tongue blades in toilet tissue. Then discarded them.
23. Emptied, cleaned, and disinfected equipment. Returned equipment to its proper place.
24. Removed the gloves. Practiced hand hygiene.

Date of Satisfactory Completion _____   Instructor's Initials _____

Post-Procedure	S	U	Comments
25. Provided for comfort.	____	____	_____
26. Placed the call light within reach.	____	____	_____
27. Raised or lowered bed rails. Followed the care plan.	____	____	_____
28. Completed a safety check of the room.	____	____	_____
29. Decontaminated your hands.	____	____	_____
30. Reported and recorded the test results and other observations.	____	____	_____

VIDEO CLIP **VIDEO** ## Collecting a Sputum Specimen

Name: _____   Date: _____

	S	U	Comments

Quality of Life

Remembered to:

- Knock before entering the person's room
- Address the person by name
- Introduce yourself by name and title
- Explain the procedure to the person before beginning and during the procedure
- Protect the person's rights during the procedure
- Handle the person gently during the procedure

Pre-Procedure

1. Followed *Delegation Guidelines:*
   Sputum Specimens.
   Saw *Promoting Safety and Comfort:*
   Sputum Specimens.
2. Practiced hand hygiene.
3. Collected the following before going to the person's room:
   - Laboratory requisition slip
   - Sputum specimen container and lid
   - Specimen label
   - Plastic bag(s)
   - *BIOHAZARD* label (if needed)
4. Arranged collected items in the person's bathroom.
5. Decontaminated your hands.
6. Identified the person. Checked the identification (ID) bracelet against the assignment sheet. Also called the person by name.
7. Labeled the specimen container in the person's presence.
8. Collected gloves and tissues.
9. Provided for privacy. If able, the person used the bathroom for this procedure.

Procedure

10. Put on gloves.
11. Asked the person to rinse the mouth out with clear water. Did not have them use mouthwash.
12. Had the person hold the container. Only touched the outside.
13. Asked the person to cover the mouth and nose with tissues when coughing. Followed center policy for used tissues.
14. Asked the person to take 2 or 3 deep breaths and cough up sputum.
15. Had the person expectorate directly into the container. Sputum did not touch the outside of the container.
16. Collected 1 to 2 tablespoons of sputum unless told to collect more.
17. Put the lid on the container.
18. Placed the container in the plastic bag. Did not let the container touch the outside of the bag. (Double-bagged, if required by facility.) Applied a *BIOHAZARD* symbol according to center policy.
19. Removed gloves and decontaminated your hands. Put on clean gloves.
20. Assisted with hand washing.
21. Removed the gloves. Decontaminated your hands.

Date of Satisfactory Completion _____   Instructor's Initials _____

Post-Procedure	**S**	**U**	**Comments**
22. Provided for comfort.	———	———	———————
23. Placed the call light within reach.	———	———	———————
24. Raised or lowered bed rails. Followed the care plan.	———	———	———————
25. Unscreened the person.	———	———	———————
26. Completed a safety check of the room.	———	———	———————
27. Decontaminated your hands.	———	———	———————
28. Delivered the specimen and requisition slip to the storage area. Followed center policy. Wore gloves.	———	———	———————
29. Reported and recorded your observations.	———	———	———————

Date of Satisfactory Completion _____   Instructor's Initials _____

VIDEO CLIP **VIDEO** **Measuring Blood Glucose**

Name: _____   Date: _____

	S	U	Comments
Quality of Life			
Remembered to:			
• Knock before entering the person's room	___	___	_____
• Address the person by name	___	___	_____
• Introduce yourself by name and title	___	___	_____
• Explain the procedure to the person before beginning and during the procedure	___	___	_____
• Protect the person's rights during the procedure	___	___	_____
• Handle the person gently during the procedure	___	___	_____

Pre-Procedure

1. Followed *Delegation Guidelines: Blood Glucose Testing.* Saw *Promoting Safety and Comfort: Blood Glucose Testing.*
2. Practiced hand hygiene.
3. Collected the following:
   • Sterile lancet
   • Antiseptic wipes
   • Gloves
   • Cotton balls
   • Glucose meter
   • Reagent strips (Used correct strips for the meter. Checked expiration date.)
   • Paper towels
   • Warm washcloth
4. Read the manufacturer instructions for lancet and glucose meter.
5. Arranged your work area.
6. Identified the person. Checked the identification (ID) bracelet against the assignment sheet. Also called the person by name.
7. Provided privacy.
8. Raised the bed for body mechanics. Far bed rail was up if used.

Procedure

9. Helped the person to a comfortable position.
10. Put on gloves.
11. Prepared the supplies:
    a. Opened the antiseptic wipes.
    b. Removed a reagent strip from the bottle. Placed it on the paper towel. Placed the cap securely on the bottle.
    c. Prepared the lancet.
    d. Turned on the glucose meter.
    e. Followed the prompts. Entered username and person's ID number, if required. Scanned the bar code on the bottle of reagent strips if needed.
    f. Inserted a reagent strip into the glucose meter.
12. Performed a skin puncture to obtain a drop of blood:
    a. Inspected the person's finger. Selected a puncture site.
    b. Warmed the finger. Rubbed it gently or applied a warm washcloth.

Date of Satisfactory Completion _____   Instructor's Initials _____

Procedure—cont'd	S	U	Comments
c. Massaged the hand and finger toward the puncture site. Lowered the finger below the person's waist. These actions increased blood flow to the site.	___	___	___
d. Held the finger with thumb and forefinger. Used your non-dominant hand. Held the finger until large drop of blood formed.	___	___	___
e. Cleaned the site with antiseptic wipe. *Did not touch the site after cleaning.*	___	___	___
f. Allowed the site to dry.	___	___	___
g. Picked up the sterile lancet.	___	___	___
h. Placed the lancet against the puncture site.	___	___	___
i. Pushed the button on the lancet to puncture the skin. (Followed the manufacturer instructions.)	___	___	___
j. Wiped away the first blood drop. Used a cotton ball.	___	___	___
k. Applied gentle pressure below the puncture site.	___	___	___
l. Allowed a large drop of blood to form.	___	___	___
13. Collected and tested the specimen. Followed the manufacturer instructions and center policy for glucose meter use.			
a. Held the test area of the reagent strip close to the drop of blood.	___	___	___
b. Lightly touched the reagent strip to the drop of blood. Did not smear the blood. The meter tested the sample when enough blood was applied.	___	___	___
c. Applied pressure to the puncture site until the bleeding stopped. Used a cotton ball. Allowed person, if able, to apply pressure to the site.	___	___	___
d. Read the results on the display. Noted the results on your note pad or assignment sheet. Told person the results.	___	___	___
e. Turned off the glucose meter.	___	___	___
14. Discarded the lancet in the sharps container.	___	___	___
15. Discarded the cotton balls following center policy.	___	___	___
16. Removed and discarded gloves. Decontaminated your hands.	___	___	___
Post-Procedure			
17. Provided for comfort.	___	___	___
18. Placed the call light within reach.	___	___	___
19. Lowered the bed to its lowest position.	___	___	___
20. Raised or lowered bed rails. Followed the care plan.	___	___	___
21. Unscreened the person.	___	___	___
22. Discarded used supplies.	___	___	___
23. Completed a safety check of the room.	___	___	___
24. Followed center policy for soiled linens.	___	___	___
25. Decontaminated your hands.	___	___	___
26. Reported and recorded your observations.	___	___	___

Date of Satisfactory Completion _____   Instructor's Initials _____

Preparing The Person's Room

Name: _____   Date: _____

Procedure	S	U	Comments
1. Followed *Delegation Guidelines: Admitting, Transferring, and Discharging Residents.*	___	___	_____
2. Practiced hand hygiene.			
3. Collected the following:			
• Admission kit—wash basin, soap, toothpaste, toothbrush, water pitcher and cup, and so on	___	___	_____
• Bedpan (and urinal if for a man)	___	___	_____
• Admission form	___	___	_____
• Thermometer	___	___	_____
• Sphygmomanometer	___	___	_____
• Stethoscope	___	___	_____
• Gown or pajamas (if needed)	___	___	_____
• Towels and washcloth	___	___	_____
• IV (intravenous) pole (if needed)	___	___	_____
• Other items requested by the nurse	___	___	_____
4. Placed the following on the over-bed table:			
• Thermometer	___	___	_____
• Sphygmomanometer	___	___	_____
• Stethoscope	___	___	_____
• Admission form	___	___	_____
5. Placed the water pitcher and cup on the bedside stand or over-bed table.	___	___	_____
6. Placed the following in the bedside stand:			
• Admission kit	___	___	_____
• Bedpan and urinal	___	___	_____
• Gown or pajamas	___	___	_____
• Towels and washcloth	___	___	_____
7. *If the person arrived by stretcher:*			
a. Made a surgical bed.	___	___	_____
b. Raised the bed to its highest level.	___	___	_____
8. *If the person was ambulatory or arrived by wheelchair:*			
a. Left the bed closed.	___	___	_____
b. Lowered the bed to its lowest position.	___	___	_____
9. Attached the call light to the bed linens.	___	___	_____
10. Decontaminated your hands.	___	___	_____

Date of Satisfactory Completion _____   Instructor's Initials _____

Admitting the Person

Name: _____   Date: _____

Quality of Life	S	U	Comments

Remembered to:

- Knock before entering the person's room
- Address the person by name
- Introduce yourself by name and title
- Explain the procedure to the person before beginning and during the procedure
- Protect the person's rights during the procedure
- Handle the person gently during the procedure

Pre-Procedure

1. Followed *Delegation Guidelines:*
   Admitting, Transferring, and Discharging Residents.
   Saw *Promoting Safety and Comfort:*
   Admitting, Transferring, and Discharging Residents.
2. Practiced hand hygiene.
3. Prepared the room.

Procedure

4. Checked the person's name on the admission form.
5. Greeted the person by name. Asked if he or she preferred a certain name.
6. Introduced yourself to the person and others present. Gave your name and title. Explained that you assist the nurse in giving care.
7. Introduced the roommate.
8. Provided for privacy. Asked family or friends to leave the room. Told them how much time you needed and directed them to the waiting area. Allowed a family member or friend to stay if the person preferred.
9. Allowed the person to stay dressed if his or her condition permitted. Or helped the person change into a gown or pajamas.
10. Provided for comfort. The person was in bed or in a chair as directed by the nurse.
11. Assisted the nurse with assessments:
    a. Measured vital signs.
    b. Measured weight and height.
    c. Collected information for the admission form as requested by the nurse.
12. Completed a clothing and personal belongings list.
13. Helped the person put away clothes and personal items. Put them in the closet, drawers, and bedside stand. (The family may have wanted to help with this step.)
14. Explained ordered activity limits.
15. Oriented the person to the area:
    a. Gave names of the nurses and nursing assistants.
    b. Identified items in the bedside stand. Explained the purpose of each.
    c. Explained how to use the over-bed table.
    d. Showed how to use the call light.

Date of Satisfactory Completion _____   Instructor's Initials _____

Procedure—cont'd	S	U	Comments
e. Showed how to use the bed, TV, and light controls.	___	___	_____
f. Explained how to make phone calls. Placed the phone within reach.	___	___	_____
g. Showed the person the bathroom. Also showed how to use the call light in the bathroom.	___	___	_____
h. Explained visiting hours and policies.	___	___	_____
i. Explained where to find the nurses' station, lounge, chapel, dining room, and other areas.	___	___	_____
j. Identified staff—housekeeping, dietary, physical therapy, and others. Also identified students in the agency.	___	___	_____
k. Explained when meals and snacks are served.	___	___	_____
16. Filled the water pitcher and cup if oral fluids were allowed.	___	___	_____
17. Placed the call light within reach.	___	___	_____
18. Placed other controls and needed items within reach.	___	___	_____
19. Provided a denture container if needed. Labeled it with the person's name, room, and bed number.	___	___	_____
20. Labeled the person's property and personal care items with his or her name (if not completed by the family).	___	___	_____

Post-Procedure

	S	U	Comments
21. Provided for comfort.	___	___	_____
22. Lowered the bed to its lowest position.	___	___	_____
23. Raised or lowered bed rails. Followed the care plan.	___	___	_____
24. Completed a safety check of the room.	___	___	_____
25. Decontaminated your hands.	___	___	_____
26. Reported and recorded your observations.	___	___	_____

Date of Satisfactory Completion _____   Instructor's Initials _____

Moving the Person to a New Room

Name: _____   Date: _____

	S	U	Comments
Quality of Life			
Remembered to:			
• Knock before entering the person's room	___	___	_____
• Address the person by name	___	___	_____
• Introduce yourself by name and title	___	___	_____
• Explain the procedure to the person before beginning and during the procedure	___	___	_____
• Protect the person's rights during the procedure	___	___	_____
• Handle the person gently during the procedure	___	___	_____
Pre-Procedure			
1. Followed *Delegation Guidelines: Admitting, Transferring, and Discharging Residents.* Saw *Promoting Safety and Comfort: Admitting, Transferring, and Discharging Residents.*	___	___	_____
2. Asked a co-worker to help you.	___	___	_____
3. Practiced hand hygiene.	___	___	_____
4. Collected the following:			
• Wheelchair or stretcher	___	___	_____
• Utility cart	___	___	_____
• Bath blanket	___	___	_____
5. Decontaminated your hands.	___	___	_____
6. Identified the person. Checked the identification (ID) bracelet against the assignment sheet. Also called the person by name.	___	___	_____
7. Provided for privacy.	___	___	_____
Procedure			
8. Collected the person's belongings and and care equipment. Placed them on the cart.	___	___	_____
9. Transferred the person to a wheelchair or a stretcher. Covered the person with a bath blanket.	___	___	_____
10. Transported the person to the new room. Your co-worker brought the cart.	___	___	_____
11. Helped transfer the person to the bed or chair. Helped position the person.	___	___	_____
12. Helped arrange the person's belongings and equipment.	___	___	_____
13. Reported the following to the receiving nurse:			
a. How the person tolerated the transfer	___	___	_____
b. Any observations made during the transfer	___	___	_____
c. That the nurse will bring the medical record, care plan, Kardex, and medications	___	___	_____
Post-Procedure			
14. Returned the wheelchair or stretcher and the cart to the storage area.	___	___	_____
15. Decontaminated your hands.	___	___	_____
16. Reported and recorded the following:			
• The time of the transfer	___	___	_____
• Who helped you with the transfer	___	___	_____
• Where the person was taken	___	___	_____

Date of Satisfactory Completion _____   Instructor's Initials _____

Post-Procedure—cont'd	S	U	Comments
• How the person was transferred (bed, wheelchair, or stretcher)	___	___	___
• How the person tolerated the transfer	___	___	___
• Who received the person	___	___	___
• Any other observations	___	___	___
17. Stripped the bed and cleaned the unit. Decontaminated your hands and put on gloves for this step. (The housekeeping staff may do this step.)	___	___	___
18. Removed the gloves. Decontaminated your hands.	___	___	___
19. Followed center policy for dirty linens.	___	___	___
20. Made a closed bed.	___	___	___
21. Decontaminated your hands.	___	___	___

Date of Satisfactory Completion _____   Instructor's Initials _____

Transferring or Discharging the Person

Name: _____   Date: _____

	S	U	Comments
Quality of Life			
Remembered to:			
• Knock before entering the person's room	___	___	_____
• Address the person by name	___	___	_____
• Introduce yourself by name and title	___	___	_____
• Explain the procedure to the person before beginning and during the procedure	___	___	_____
• Protect the person's rights during the procedure	___	___	_____
• Handle the person gently during the procedure	___	___	_____

Pre-Procedure

1. Followed *Delegation Guidelines:*
   Admitting, Transferring, and Discharging Residents.
   Saw *Promoting Safety and Comfort:*
   Admitting, Transferring, and Discharging Residents.   ___ ___ _____
2. Asked a co-worker to help you.   ___ ___ _____
3. Practiced hand hygiene.   ___ ___ _____
4. Identified the person. Checked the identification (ID)
   bracelet against the assignment sheet.
   Also called the person by name.   ___ ___ _____
5. Provided for privacy.   ___ ___ _____

Procedure

6. Helped the person dress as needed.   ___ ___ _____
7. Helped the person pack. Checked all drawers and
   closets. Checked the bathroom. Made sure all items
   were collected.   ___ ___ _____
8. Checked off the clothing and personal belongings list.
   Made sure the person had eyeglasses, hearing aids,
   and dentures. Gave the list to the nurse.   ___ ___ _____
9. Told the nurse that the person was ready for the
   final visit. The nurse:
   a. Gave prescriptions written by the doctor.   ___ ___ _____
   b. Provided discharge instructions.   ___ ___ _____
   c. Got valuables from the safe.   ___ ___ _____
   d. Had the person sign the clothing and personal
      belongings list.   ___ ___ _____
10. *If the person left by wheelchair:*
    a. Got a wheelchair and a utility cart for the person's
       items. Asked a co-worker to help you.   ___ ___ _____
    b. Helped the person into the wheelchair.   ___ ___ _____
    c. Took the person to the exit area.   ___ ___ _____
    d. Locked the wheelchair wheels.   ___ ___ _____
    e. Helped the person out of the wheelchair and into
       the car.   ___ ___ _____
    f. Helped put the person's items into the car.   ___ ___ _____
11. *If the person left by ambulance:*
    a. Raised the bed rails.   ___ ___ _____
    b. Raised the bed to its highest level.   ___ ___ _____
    c. Placed the call light within reach.   ___ ___ _____
    d. Waited for the ambulance attendants.   ___ ___ _____

Date of Satisfactory Completion _____   Instructor's Initials _____

Post-Procedure	S	U	Comments
12. Returned the wheelchair and cart to the storage area.	___	___	___
13. Decontaminated your hands.	___	___	___
14. Reported and recorded the following:			
• The time of the discharge	___	___	___
• Who helped you with the procedure	___	___	___
• How the person was transported	___	___	___
• Who was with the person	___	___	___
• The person's destination	___	___	___
• Any other observations	___	___	___
15. Stripped the bed and cleaned the unit. Decontaminated your hands and put on gloves for this step. (The housekeeping staff may do this step.)	___	___	___
16. Removed the gloves. Decontaminated your hands.	___	___	___
17. Followed center policy for dirty linens.	___	___	___
18. Made a closed bed.	___	___	___
19. Decontaminated your hands.	___	___	___

Date of Satisfactory Completion _____ Instructor's Initials _____

NNAAP™ Skill **CD-ROM** **VIDEO CLIP** **VIDEO** **Applying Compression Stockings**

Name: _____   Date: _____

Quality of Life	S	U	Comments
• Knock before entering the person's room	___	___	_____
• Address the person by name	___	___	_____
• Introduce yourself by name and title	___	___	_____
• Explain the procedure to the person before beginning and during the procedure	___	___	_____
• Protect the person's rights during the procedure	___	___	_____
• Handle the person gently during the procedure	___	___	_____

Pre-Procedure

	S	U	Comments
1. Followed *Delegation Guidelines: Compression Stockings.* Saw *Promoting Safety and Comfort: Compression Stockings.*	___	___	_____
2. Practiced hand hygiene.	___	___	_____
3. Obtained compression stockings in the correct size and length. (Checked if nurse measured the leg.)	___	___	_____
4. Identified the person. Checked the identification (ID) bracelet against the assignment sheet. Also called the person by name.	___	___	_____
5. Provided for privacy.	___	___	_____
6. Raised the bed for body mechanics. Bed rails were up if used.	___	___	_____

Procedure

	S	U	Comments
7. Lowered the bed rail near you.	___	___	_____
8. Positioned the person supine.	___	___	_____
9. Exposed the legs. Fan-folded top linens toward the thighs.	___	___	_____
10. Turned the stocking inside out down to the heel.	___	___	_____
11. Slipped the foot of the stocking over the toes, foot, and heel. Made sure the stocking heel was properly positioned on the person's heel.	___	___	_____
12. Grasped the stocking top. Pulled the stocking up the leg. It turned right side out as it was pulled up. The stocking was even and snug.	___	___	_____
13. Removed twists, creases, or wrinkles.	___	___	_____
14. Repeated for the other leg:			
a. Turned the stocking inside out down to the heel.	___	___	_____
b. Slipped the foot of the stocking over the toes, foot, and heel. Made sure the stocking heel was properly positioned on the person's heel.	___	___	_____
c. Grasped the stocking top. Pulled the stocking up the leg. It turned right side out as it was pulled up. The stocking was even and snug.	___	___	_____
d. Removed twists, creases, or wrinkles.	___	___	_____

Post-Procedure

	S	U	Comments
15. Covered the person.	___	___	_____
16. Provided for comfort.	___	___	_____
17. Placed the call light within reach.	___	___	_____
18. Lowered the bed to its lowest position.	___	___	_____
19. Raised or lowered bed rails. Followed the care plan.	___	___	_____
20. Unscreened the person.	___	___	_____
21. Completed a safety check of the room.	___	___	_____
22. Decontaminated your hands.	___	___	_____
23. Reported and recorded your observations.	___	___	_____

Date of Satisfactory Completion _____   Instructor's Initials _____

Applying Elastic Bandages

Name: _____   Date: _____

	S	U	Comments
Quality of Life			
Remembered to:			
• Knock before entering the person's room	___	___	_____
• Address the person by name	___	___	_____
• Introduce yourself by name and title	___	___	_____
• Explain the procedure to the person before beginning and during the procedure	___	___	_____
• Protect the person's rights during the procedure	___	___	_____
• Handle the person gently during the procedure	___	___	_____
Pre-Procedure			
1. Followed *Delegation Guidelines: Elastic Bandages.* Saw *Promoting Safety and Comfort: Elastic Bandages.*	___	___	_____
2. Practiced hand hygiene.	___	___	_____
3. Collected the following:			
• Elastic bandage as directed by the nurse	___	___	_____
• Tape or clips (unless the bandage had Velcro)	___	___	_____
4. Identified the person. Checked the identification (ID) bracelet against the assignment sheet. Also called the person by name.	___	___	_____
5. Provided for privacy.	___	___	_____
6. Raised the bed for body mechanics. Bed rails were up if used.	___	___	_____
Procedure			
7. Lowered the bed rail near you.	___	___	_____
8. Helped the person to a comfortable position. Exposed the part to be bandaged.	___	___	_____
9. Made sure the area was clean and dry.	___	___	_____
10. Held the bandage so the roll was up. The loose end was on the bottom.	___	___	_____
11. Applied the bandage to the smallest part of the wrist, foot, ankle, or knee.	___	___	_____
12. Made two circular turns around the part.	___	___	_____
13. Made over-lapping spiral turns in an upward direction. Each turn overlapped about ½ to ⅔ of the previous turn. Each over-lap was equal.	___	___	_____
14. Applied the bandage smoothly with firm, even pressure. It was not tight.	___	___	_____
15. Ended the bandage with two circular turns.	___	___	_____
16. Secured the bandage in place with Velcro, tape, or clips. The clips were not under any body part.	___	___	_____
17. Checked the fingers or toes for coldness or cyanosis (bluish color). Asked about pain, itching, numbness, or tingling. Removed the bandage if any were noted. Reported your observations.	___	___	_____
Post-Procedure			
18. Provided for comfort.	___	___	_____
19. Placed the call light within reach.	___	___	_____
20. Lowered the bed to its lowest position.	___	___	_____

Date of Satisfactory Completion _____   Instructor's Initials _____

Post-Procedure—cont'd	S	U	Comments
21. Raised or lowered bed rails. Followed the care plan.	————	————	————————————
22. Unscreened the person.	————	————	————————————
23. Completed a safety check of the room.	————	————	————————————
24. Decontaminated your hands.	————	————	————————————
25. Reported and recorded your observations.	————	————	————————————

Date of Satisfactory Completion ——————————————— Instructor's Initials ————————————————

VIDEO CLIP   VIDEO   ## Applying a Dry, Non-Sterile Dressing

Name: _____   Date: _____

	S	U	Comments

Quality of Life
Remembered to:
- Knock before entering the person's room
- Address the person by name
- Introduce yourself by name and title
- Explain the procedure to the person before beginning and during the procedure
- Protect the person's rights during the procedure
- Handle the person gently during the procedure

Pre-Procedure
1. Followed *Delegation Guidelines:*
   Applying Dressings.
   Saw *Promoting Safety and Comfort:*
   Applying Dressings.
2. Practiced hand hygiene.
3. Collected the following:
   - Gloves
   - Personal protective equipment (PPE) as needed
   - Tape
   - Dressings as directed by the nurse
   - Saline solution as directed by the nurse
   - Cleansing solution as directed by the nurse
   - Adhesive remover
   - Dressing set with scissors and forceps
   - Plastic bag
   - Bath blanket
4. Decontaminated your hands.
5. Identified the person. Checked the identification (ID) bracelet against the assignment sheet. Also called the person by name.
6. Provided for privacy.
7. Arranged your work area. You did not have to reach over or turn your back on the work area.
8. Raised the bed for body mechanics.
   Bed rails were up if used.

Procedure
9. Lowered the bed rail near you if up.
10. Helped the person to a comfortable position.
11. Covered the person with a bath blanket.
    Fan-folded top linens to the foot of the bed.
12. Exposed the affected body part.
13. Made a cuff on the plastic bag. Placed it within reach.
14. Decontaminated your hands.
15. Put on needed PPE. Put on gloves.
16. Removed tape. Held the skin down.
    Gently pulled the tape toward the wound.
17. Removed any adhesive from the skin. Wet a 4 × 4 gauze dressing with adhesive remover. Cleaned away from the wound.

Date of Satisfactory Completion _____   Instructor's Initials _____

Procedure—cont'd	S	U	Comments
18. Removed gauze dressings. Started with the top dressing and removed each layer. Kept the soiled side of each dressing away from the person's sight. Put dressings in the plastic bag. They did not touch the outside of the bag.	———	———	———————
19. Removed the dressing over the wound very gently. Moistened the dressing with saline, if it stuck to the wound.	———	———	———————
20. Observed the wound, drain site, and wound drainage.	———	———	———————
21. Removed the gloves and put them in a plastic bag. Decontaminated your hands.	———	———	———————
22. Opened new dressings.	———	———	———————
23. Cut the length of tape needed.	———	———	———————
24. Put on clean gloves.	———	———	———————
25. Cleaned the wound with saline as directed by the nurse.	———	———	———————
26. Applied dressings as directed by the nurse.	———	———	———————
27. Secured the dressings in place with tape.	———	———	———————
28. Removed the gloves. Put them in the bag.	———	———	———————
29. Removed and discarded PPE.	———	———	———————
30. Decontaminated your hands.	———	———	———————
31. Covered the person. Removed the bath blanket.	———	———	———————
Post-Procedure			
32. Provided for comfort.	———	———	———————
33. Placed the call light within reach.	———	———	———————
34. Lowered the bed to its lowest position.	———	———	———————
35. Raised or lowered bed rails. Followed the care plan.	———	———	———————
36. Returned equipment and supplies to the proper place. Left extra dressings and tape in the room.	———	———	———————
37. Discarded used supplies in the bag. Tied the bag closed. Discarded the bag following center policy. (Wore gloves for this step.)	———	———	———————
38. Cleaned your work area. Followed the Bloodborne Pathogen Standard.	———	———	———————
39. Unscreened the person.	———	———	———————
40. Completed a safety check of the room.	———	———	———————
41. Decontaminated your hands.	———	———	———————
42. Reported and recorded your observations.	———	———	———————

Date of Satisfactory Completion —————————   Instructor's Initials —————————

VIDEO CLIP   VIDEO   **Applying Warm and Cold Applications**

Name: _____   Date: _____

	S	U	Comments
Quality of Life			
Remembered to:			
• Knock before entering the person's room	___	___	_____
• Address the person by name	___	___	_____
• Introduce yourself by name and title	___	___	_____
• Explain the procedure to the person before beginning and during the procedure	___	___	_____
• Protect the person's rights during the procedure	___	___	_____
• Handle the person gently during the procedure	___	___	_____
Pre-Procedure			
1. Followed *Delegation Guidelines: Applying Warm and Cold.*	___	___	_____
Saw *Promoting Safety and Comfort: Applying Warm and Cold.*	___	___	_____
2. Practiced hand hygiene.	___	___	_____
3. Collected the following:			
a. For a *warm compress:*			
• Basin	___	___	_____
• Bath thermometer	___	___	_____
• Small towel, washcloth, or gauze squares	___	___	_____
• Plastic wrap or aquathermia pad	___	___	_____
• Ties, tape, or rolled gauze	___	___	_____
• Bath towel	___	___	_____
• Waterproof pad	___	___	_____
b. For a *warm soak:*			
• Water basin or arm or foot bath	___	___	_____
• Bath thermometer	___	___	_____
• Waterproof pad	___	___	_____
• Bath blanket	___	___	_____
• Towel	___	___	_____
c. For a *sitz bath:*			
• Disposable sitz bath	___	___	_____
• Bath thermometer	___	___	_____
• Two bath blankets, bath towels, and a clean gown	___	___	_____
d. For a *warm or cold pack:*			
• Commercial pack	___	___	_____
• Pack cover	___	___	_____
• Ties, tape, or rolled gauze (if needed)	___	___	_____
• Waterproof pad	___	___	_____
e. For an *aquathermia pad:*			
• Aquathermia pad and heating unit	___	___	_____
• Distilled water	___	___	_____
• Flannel cover or other cover as directed by the nurse	___	___	_____
• Ties, tape, or rolled gauze	___	___	_____
f. For an *ice bag, ice collar, ice glove, or dry cold pack:*			
• Ice bag, collar, glove, or cold pack	___	___	_____
• Crushed ice (except for cold pack)	___	___	_____
• Flannel cover or other cover as directed by the nurse	___	___	_____
• Paper towels	___	___	_____

Date of Satisfactory Completion _____   Instructor's Initials _____

	S	U	Comments
Pre-Procedure—cont'd			
g. For a *cold compress:*			
• Large basin with ice	____	____	_____
• Small basin with cold water	____	____	_____
• Gauze squares, washcloths, or small towels	____	____	_____
• Waterproof pad	____	____	_____
4. Identified the person. Checked the identification (ID) bracelet against the assignment sheet. Also called the person by name.	____	____	_____
5. Provided for privacy.	____	____	_____
Procedure			
6. Positioned the person for the procedure.	____	____	_____
7. Placed the waterproof pad (if needed) under the body part.	____	____	_____
8. For a *warm compress:*			
a. Filled the basin ½ to ⅔ full with warm water as directed by the nurse. Measured water temperature.	____	____	_____
b. Placed the compress in the water.	____	____	_____
c. Wrung out the compress.	____	____	_____
d. Applied the compress over the area. Noted the time.	____	____	_____
e. Covered the compress quickly. Used one of the following as directed by the nurse:			
1. Applied plastic wrap and then a bath towel. Secured the towel in place with ties, tape, or rolled gauze.	____		_____
2. Applied an aquathermia pad.	____		_____
9. For a *warm soak:*			
a. Filled a container ½ full with warm water as directed by the nurse. Measured water temperature.	____	____	_____
b. Placed the body part into the water. Padded the edge of the container with a towel. Noted the time.	____	____	_____
c. Covered the person with a bath blanket for warmth.	____	____	_____
10. For a *sitz bath:*			
a. Placed the disposable sitz bath on the toilet seat.	____	____	_____
b. Filled the sitz bath ⅔ full with water as directed by the nurse. Measured water temperature.	____	____	_____
c. Secured the gown above the waist.	____	____	_____
d. Helped the person sit on the sitz bath. Noted the time.	____	____	_____
e. Provided for warmth. Placed a bath blanket around the shoulders. Placed another over the legs.	____	____	_____
f. Stayed with the person if he or she was weak or unsteady.	____	____	_____
11. For a *warm or cold pack:*			
a. Squeezed, kneaded, or struck the pack as directed by the manufacturer.	____	____	_____
b. Placed the pack in the cover.	____	____	_____
c. Applied the pack. Noted the time.	____	____	_____
d. Secured the pack in place with ties, tape, or rolled gauze. Some packs are secured with Velcro straps.	____	____	_____
12. For an *aquathermia pad:*			
a. Filled the heating unit to the fill line with distilled water.	____	____	_____
b. Removed the bubbles. Placed the pad and tubing below the heating unit. Tilted the heating unit from side to side.	____	____	_____

Date of Satisfactory Completion _____ Instructor's Initials _____

	S	U	Comments

Pre-Procedure—cont'd

   c. Set the temperature as the nurse directed (usually 105°F [40.5°C]). Removed the key. _____ _____ _____

   d. Placed the pad in the cover. _____ _____ _____

   e. Plugged in the unit. Allowed water to warm to the desired temperature. _____ _____ _____

   f. Set the heating unit on the bedside stand. Kept the pad and connecting hoses level with the unit. Hoses did not have kinks. _____ _____ _____

   g. Applied the pad to the body part. Noted the time. _____ _____ _____

   h. Secured the pad in place with ties, tape, or rolled gauze. Did not use pins. _____ _____ _____

13. For an _ice bag, collar, or glove:_

   a. Filled the device with water. Put in the stopper. Turned the device upside down and checked for leaks. _____ _____ _____

   b. Emptied the device. _____ _____ _____

   c. Filled the device ½ to ⅔ full with crushed ice or ice chips. _____ _____ _____

   d. Removed excess air. Bent, twisted, or squeezed the device. Or pressed it against a firm surface. _____ _____ _____

   e. Placed the cap or stopper on securely. _____ _____ _____

   f. Dried the device with paper towels. _____ _____ _____

   g. Placed the device in the cover. _____ _____ _____

   h. Applied the device. Noted the time. _____ _____ _____

   i. Secured the device in place with ties, tape, or rolled gauze. _____ _____ _____

14. For a _cold compress:_

   a. Placed the small basin with cold water into the large basin with ice. _____ _____ _____

   b. Placed the compress into the cold water. _____ _____ _____

   c. Wrung out the compress. _____ _____ _____

   d. Applied the compress to the part. Noted the time. _____ _____ _____

15. Placed the call light within reach. Unscreened the person. _____ _____ _____

16. Raised or lowered bed rails. Followed the care plan. _____ _____ _____

17. Checked the person every 5 minutes. Checked for signs and symptoms of complications. Removed the application if complications occurred. Told the nurse at once. _____ _____ _____

18. Checked the application every 5 minutes. Changed the application if cooling (warm applications) or warming (cold applications) occurred. _____ _____ _____

19. Removed the application at the specified time. Warm and cold applications are usually left on for 15 to 20 minutes. (If bed rails were up, lowered the near one for this step.) _____ _____ _____

Post-Procedure

20. Provided for comfort. _____ _____ _____

21. Placed the call light within reach. _____ _____ _____

22. Raised or lowered bed rails. Followed the care plan. _____ _____ _____

23. Unscreened the person. _____ _____ _____

24. Cleaned and returned re-usable items to the proper place. Followed center policy for soiled linens. Wore gloves. _____ _____ _____

25. Completed a safety check of the room. _____ _____ _____

26. Removed and discarded the gloves. Decontaminated your hands. _____ _____ _____

27. Reported and recorded your observations. _____ _____ _____

Date of Satisfactory Completion _____   Instructor's Initials _____

Caring for Eyeglasses

Name: _____   Date: _____

Quality of Life	S	U	Comments
Remembered to:			
• Knock before entering the person's room	_____	_____	_____
• Address the person by name	_____	_____	_____
• Introduce yourself by name and title	_____	_____	_____
• Explain the procedure to the person before beginning and during the procedure	_____	_____	_____
• Protect the person's rights during the procedure	_____	_____	_____
• Handle the person gently during the procedure	_____	_____	_____

Pre-Procedure

	S	U	Comments
1. Followed *Delegation Guidelines: Eyeglasses.*	_____	_____	_____
Saw *Promoting Safety and Comfort: Eyeglasses.*	_____	_____	_____
2. Practiced hand hygiene.	_____	_____	_____
3. Collected the following:			
• Eyeglass case	_____	_____	_____
• Cleaning solution or warm water	_____	_____	_____
• Disposable lens cloth or cotton cloth	_____	_____	_____

Procedure

	S	U	Comments
	_____	_____	_____
4. Removed the eyeglasses:			
a. Held the frames in front of the ears.	_____	_____	_____
b. Lifted the frames from the ears. Brought the eyeglasses down away from the face.	_____	_____	_____
5. Cleaned the lenses with cleaning solution or warm water. Cleaned in a circular motion. Dried the lenses with the cloth.			
6. *If the person did not wear the glasses:*			
a. Opened the eyeglass case.	_____	_____	_____
b. Folded the glasses. Put them in the case. Did not touch the clean lenses.	_____	_____	_____
c. Placed the eyeglass case in the top drawer of the bedside stand.	_____	_____	_____
7. *If the person wore the eyeglasses:*			
a. Unfolded the eyeglasses.	_____	_____	_____
b. Held the frames at each side. Placed them over the ears.	_____	_____	_____
c. Adjusted the eyeglasses so the nosepiece rested on the nose.	_____	_____	_____
d. Returned the eyeglass case to the top drawer in the bedside stand.	_____	_____	_____

Post-Procedure

	S	U	Comments
8. Provided for comfort.	_____	_____	_____
9. Placed the call light within reach.	_____	_____	_____
10. Returned the cleaning solution to its proper place.	_____	_____	_____
11. Discarded the disposable cloth.	_____	_____	_____
12. Completed a safety check of the room.	_____	_____	_____
13. Decontaminated your hands.	_____	_____	_____
14. Reported and recorded your observations.	_____	_____	_____

Date of Satisfactory Completion _____   Instructor's Initials _____

Adult CPR—One Rescuer

Name: _____   Date: _____

Procedure	S	U	Comments

1. Made sure the scene was safe. _____ _____ _____
2. Took 5 to 10 seconds to check for a response and breathing:
   a. Checked if the person was responding. Tapped or _____ _____ _____
      gently shook the person, called the person by name,
      and shouted: "Are you okay?"
   b. Checked for no breathing or no normal breathing (gasping). _____ _____ _____
3. Called for help. Activated the Emergency Medical _____ _____ _____
   Services (EMS) system or center's emergency
   response system if the person was not responding
   and not breathing or not breathing normally (gasping).
4. Got or asked someone to bring an automated _____ _____ _____
   external defibrillator (AED) if available.
5. Positioned the person supine on a hard, flat surface. _____ _____ _____
   Logrolled the person so there was no twisting of
   the spine. Placed the arms alongside the body.
6. Checked for a carotid pulse. This took 5 to 10 seconds. _____ _____ _____
   Started chest compressions if you did not feel a pulse.
7. Exposed the person's chest. _____ _____ _____
8. Gave chest compressions at a rate of 100 per minute. _____ _____ _____
   Pushed hard and fast. Established a regular rhythm.
   Counted out loud. Pressed down at least 2 inches.
   Allowed the chest to recoil between compressions.
   Gave 30 chest compressions.
9. Opened the airway. Used the head tilt–chin lift method. _____ _____ _____
10. Gave 2 breaths. Each breath took only 1 second. _____ _____ _____
    Each breath made the chest rise. (If the first breath
    did not make the chest rise, tried opening the airway
    again. Used the head tilt–chin lift method.)
11. Continued the cycle of 30 compressions followed by _____ _____ _____
    2 breaths. Limited interruptions in compressions to
    less than 10 seconds. Continued cycles until the
    AED arrived. Or continued until help arrived or
    the person began to move. If movement occurred,
    placed the person in the recovery position.

Date of Satisfactory Completion _____   Instructor's Initials _____

Adult CPR—Two Rescuers

Name: _____   Date: _____

Procedure	S	U	Comments
1. Made sure the scene was safe.	____	____	_____
2. *Rescuer 1:* Took 5 to 10 seconds to check for a response and breathing:			
a. Checked if the person was responding. Tapped or gently shook the person. Called the person by name. Shouted: "Are you okay?"	____	____	_____
b. Checked for no breathing or no normal breathing (gasping).	____	____	_____
3. *Rescuer 2:*			
a. Activated the Emergency Medical Services (EMS) system or center's emergency response system if the person was not responding and not breathing or not breathing normally (gasping).	____	____	_____
b. Got an automated external defibrillator (AED), if one was available.	____	____	_____
4. *Rescuer 1:* Positioned the person supine on a hard, flat surface. Logrolled the person so there was no twisting of the spine. Placed the arms alongside the body.	____	____	_____
5. When the second rescuer returned, 2-person CPR began.			
a. *Rescuer 1:* Gave chest compressions at a rate of 100 per minute. Pushed hard and fast. Established a regular rhythm. Counted out loud. Pressed down at least 2 inches. Allowed the chest to recoil between compressions. Gave 30 chest compressions. Paused to allow the other rescuer to give 2 breaths.	____	____	_____
b. *Rescuer 2:*			
1. Opened the airway. Used the head tilt–chin lift method.	____	____	_____
2. Gave 2 breaths every 30 compressions. Each breath took only 1 second and made the chest rise. (If the first breath did not make the chest rise, tried opening the airway again. Used the head tilt–chin lift method.	____	____	_____
c. Continued cycles of 30 compressions and 2 breaths.	____	____	_____
d. Changed position every 2 minutes (after about 5 cycles of 30 compressions and 2 breaths). The switch took no more than 5 seconds.	____	____	_____
e. Continued until the AED arrived. Or continued until help took over or the person began to move. If movement occurred, placed the person in the recovery position.	____	____	_____

Date of Satisfactory Completion _____   Instructor's Initials _____

Adult CPR with AED—Two Rescuers

Name: _____   Date: _____

Procedure	S	U	Comments

Procedure

1. Made sure the scene was safe.
2. *Rescuer 1:* Took 5 to 10 seconds to check for a response and breathing. Tapped or gently shook the person. Called the person by name, if known. Shouted: "Are you okay?"
3. *Rescuer 2:*
   a. Activated the Emergency Medical Services (EMS) system or the center's emergency response system if the person was not responding and not breathing or not breathing normally (gasping).
   b. Got an automated external defibrillator (AED) if one was available.
4. *Rescuer 1:*
   a. Positioned the person supine on a hard, flat surface. Logrolled the person so there was no twisting of the spine. Placed the arms alongside the body.
   b. Checked for a carotid pulse. This took 5 to 10 seconds. Started chest compressions if you did not feel a pulse.
   c. Exposed the person's chest.
   d. Gave chest compressions at a rate of 100 per minute. Pushed hard and fast. Established a regular rhythm. Counted out loud. Pressed down at least 2 inches. Allowed the chest to recoil between compressions. Gave 30 chest compressions.
   e. Opened the airway. Used the head tilt–chin lift method.
   f. Gave 2 breaths. Each breath took only 1 second. Each breath made the chest rise. (If the first breath did not make the chest rise, tried opening the airway again. Used the head tilt–chin lift method.)
   g. Continued the cycle of 30 compressions followed by 2 breaths. Limited interruptions in compressions to less than 10 seconds.
5. *Rescuer 2:*
   a. Opened the case with the AED.
   b. Turned on the AED.
   c. Applied adult electrode pads to the person's chest. Followed the instructions and diagram provided with the AED.
   d. Attached the connecting cables to the AED.
   e. Cleared away from the person. Made sure no one was touching the person.
   f. Allowed the AED to analyze the person's heart rhythm.
   g. Made sure everyone was clear of the person if the AED advised a "shock." Loudly instructed others not to touch the person. Said: "I am clear, you are clear, everyone is clear!" Looked to make sure no one was touching the person.
   h. Pressed the "shock" button when the AED advised a "shock."

Date of Satisfactory Completion _____   Instructor's Initials _____

Procedure—cont'd	S	U	Comments

6. *Rescuers 1 and 2:*

   a. Performed 2-person CPR:

      1. Began with compressions. One rescuer gave chest compressions at a rate of at least 100 per minute. Pushed hard and fast. Established a regular rhythm. Counted out loud. Allowed the chest to recoil between compressions. Gave 30 chest compressions. Paused to allow the other rescuer to give 2 breaths.

7. Repeated the following after 2 minutes of cardiopulmonary respiration (CPR) (5 cycles of 30 compressions and 2 breaths). Then changed positions and continued CPR beginning with compressions.

   a. Cleared away from the person. Made sure no one was touching the person.

   b. Allowed the AED to analyze the person's heart rhythm.

   c. Made sure everyone was clear of the person if the AED advised a "shock." Loudly instructed others not to touch the person. Said: "I am clear, you are clear, everyone is clear!" Looked to make sure no one was touching the person.

   d. Pressed the "shock" button when the AED advised a "shock."

8. Continued until help took over or the person began to move. If movement occurred, placed the person in the recovery position.

Date of Satisfactory Completion _____   Instructor's Initials _____

Assisting with Post-Mortem Care

Name: _____   Date: _____

	S	U	Comments

Pre-Procedure

1. Followed *Delegation Guidelines:*
   Care of the Body After Death.
   Saw *Promoting Safety and Comfort:*
   Care of the Body After Death.
2. Practiced hand hygiene.
3. Collected the following:
   - Post-mortem kit (shroud or body bag, gown, identification [ID] tags, gauze squares, safety pins)
   - Bed protectors
   - Wash basin
   - Bath towel and washcloths
   - Denture cup
   - Tape
   - Dressings
   - Gloves
   - Cotton balls
   - Valuables envelope
4. Provided for privacy.
5. Raised the bed for body mechanics.
6. Made sure the bed was flat.

Procedure

7. Put on gloves.
8. Positioned the body supine. Arms and legs were straight. A pillow was under the head and shoulders. Or raised the head of the bed 15 to 20 degrees, if center policy.
9. Closed the eyes. Gently pulled the eyelids over the eyes. Applied moist cotton balls gently over the eyelids if the eyes did not stay closed.
10. Inserted dentures if it is center policy to do so. If not, placed them in a labeled denture cup.
11. Closed the mouth. If necessary, placed a rolled towel under the chin to keep the mouth closed.
12. Followed center policy for jewelry. Removed all jewelry, except for wedding rings if this is center policy. Listed the jewelry that you removed. Placed the jewelry and the list in a valuables envelope.
13. Placed cotton balls over the rings. Taped them in place.
14. Removed drainage containers.
15. Removed tubes and catheters. Used the gauze squares as needed. (Omitted this step if autopsy will be performed.)
16. Bathed soiled areas with plain water. Dried thoroughly.
17. Placed a bed protector under the buttocks.
18. Removed soiled dressings. Replaced them with clean ones.
19. Put a clean gown on the body. Positioned the body supine. Arms and legs were straight. A pillow was under the head and shoulders. Or the head of the bed was raised 15 to 20 degrees if center policy.
20. Brushed and combed the hair if necessary.

Date of Satisfactory Completion _____   Instructor's Initials _____

Procedure—cont'd	S	U	Comments
21. Covered the body to the shoulders with a sheet if the family was to view the body.	___	___	_____
22. Gathered the person's belongings. Put them in a bag labeled with the person's name. Made sure you included eyeglasses, hearing aids, and other valuables.	___	___	_____
23. Removed supplies, equipment, and linens. Straightened the room. Provided soft lighting.	___	___	_____
24. Removed the gloves. Decontaminated your hands.	___	___	_____
25. Let the family view the body. Provided for privacy. Returned to the room after they left.	___	___	_____
26. Decontaminated your hands. Put on gloves.	___	___	_____
27. Filled out the ID tags. Tied one to the ankle or to the right big toe.	___	___	_____
28. Placed the body in the body bag or covered it with a sheet. Or applied the shroud.			
a. Positioned the shroud under the body.	___	___	_____
b. Brought the top down over the head.	___	___	_____
c. Folded the bottom up over the feet.	___	___	_____
d. Folded the sides over the body.	___	___	_____
e. Pinned or taped the shroud in place.	___	___	_____
29. Attached the second ID tag to the shroud, sheet, or body bag.	___	___	_____
30. Left the denture cup with the body.	___	___	_____
31. Pulled the privacy curtain around the bed. Or closed the door.	___	___	_____
Post-Procedure			
32. Removed the gloves. Decontaminated your hands.	___	___	_____
33. Stripped the unit after the body had been removed. Wore gloves.	___	___	_____
34. Removed the gloves. Decontaminated your hands.	___	___	_____
35. Reported the following:			
• The time the body was taken by the funeral director	___	___	_____
• What was done with jewelry, other valuables, and personal items	___	___	_____
• What was done with dentures	___	___	_____

Date of Satisfactory Completion _____ Instructor's Initials _____

COMPETENCY EVALUATION REVIEW

PREPARING FOR THE COMPETENCY EVALUATION

After completing your state's training program, you need to pass the competency evaluation. The purpose of the competency evaluation is to make sure you can do your job safely. This section will help you prepare for the test.

COMPETENCY EVALUATION

The competency evaluation has a written test and a skills test. The number of questions varies with each state. Each question has four possible answers. Although some questions may appear to have more than one possible answer, there is only one best answer. You will have about 1 minute to read and answer each question. Some questions take less time to read and answer. Other questions take longer. You should have enough time to take the test without feeling rushed.

The content of the written test varies depending on your state. Content may include:

- Activities of Daily Living—hygiene, dressing and grooming, nutrition and hydration, elimination, rest/sleep/comfort
- Basic Nursing Skills—infection control, safety/emergency, therapeutic/technical procedures (e.g., vital signs, bedmaking), data collection and reporting
- Restorative Skills—prevention, self-care/independence
- Emotional and Mental Health Needs
- Spiritual and Cultural Needs
- The Person's Rights
- Legal and Ethical Behavior
- Being a Member of the Health Care Team
- Communication

The written test is given as a paper and pencil test in most states. Some test sites may use computers. You do not need computer experience to take the test on the computer. If you have difficulty reading English, you may request to take an oral test. Talk with your instructor or employer about details for computer testing or oral testing.

The skills test involves performing five nursing skills you learned in your training program. These skills are chosen randomly. You do not select the skills. You are allowed about 30 minutes to do the skills. See p. 491 for more information about the skills test.

TAKING THE COMPETENCY EVALUATION

To register for the test, you need to complete an application. Your instructor or employer tells you when and where the tests are given. There is a fee for the evaluation. If you work in a nursing center, the employer may pay this fee. If you pay the fee, you may need to purchase a money order or certified check. Make sure your name is on the money order or certified check. Cash and personal checks may not be accepted.

Plan to arrive at the test site about 15 to 30 minutes before the evaluation begins. Most centers do not admit you if you are late. Know the exact location of the test site and room. Actually drive or take transportation to the test site a few days or a week before the test. Making a "dry run" lets you know how much time you need to travel, park, and get to the test site. It will also help decrease your anxiety level on the test day.

To be admitted to the test, you need two pieces of identification (ID). The first form of ID is a government-issued document such as a driver's license or passport. It must have a current photo and your signature. The name on the ID must be the same as the name on your application form. If your name has changed and you have not been able to have the name changed on your identification documents, ask your instructor or employer what to do. The second form of ID must include your name and signature. Examples include a library card, hunting license, or credit card.

Take several sharpened Number 2 pencils to the test. For the skills test you will need a watch with a second hand. You may need a person to play the role of the patient or resident. Ask your instructor or employer how this is done in your state.

Taking the written test and skills test may take several hours. You may want to bring snacks or lunch and a beverage to the testing site. Eating and drinking are not allowed during the test. However, you may be told where you can eat while waiting for the test.

You cannot bring textbooks, study notes, or other materials into the testing room. The only exception may be a language translation dictionary that you show to the proctor (a person who monitors the test) before the test begins. Cell phones, pagers, calculators, or other electronic devices are not permitted during testing. Children and pets are not allowed in the testing areas.

STUDYING FOR THE COMPETENCY EVALUATION

You began to prepare for the written and skills test during your training program. You learned the basic nursing content and skills needed to provide safe, quality care. The following suggestions can help you study for the competency evaluation:

- Begin to study at least 2 to 3 weeks before the test. Plan to study for 1 to 2 hours each day.
- Decide on a specific time to study. Choose a study time that is best for you. This may be early in the morning before others are awake. It may be in the evening after others go to sleep. Try to choose a time when you are mentally alert.
- Choose a specific area to study in. This area should be quiet, well lit, and comfortable. You should have enough room to write and to spread out your books, notes, and other study aids—such as a CD or DVD. The area does not need to be noise-free. The testing site is not absolutely quiet. You want to concentrate and not be distracted by the noise around you.
- Collect everything you need before settling down to study. This includes your textbook, notes, paper, highlighters, pens or pencils, CD, and DVD.
- Take short breaks when you need them. Take a break when your mind begins to wander or if you feel sleepy.
- Develop a study plan. Write your plan down so you can refer to it. Study one content area before going on to the next. For example, study personal hygiene before going on to vital signs. Do not jump from one subject to another.
- Use a variety of ways to study:
  - Use index cards to help you review abbreviations and terminology. Put the abbreviation or term on the front of the card and place the meaning on the back. Take the cards with you and review them whenever you have a break or are waiting.
  - Tape key points. You can listen to the tape while cooking or riding in the car.
  - Study groups are another way to prepare for a test. Group members can quiz each other.
- To remember what you are learning, try these ideas:
  - Relax when you study. When relaxed, you learn information quickly and recall it with greater ease.
  - Repeat what you are learning. Say it out loud. This helps you remember the idea.
  - Make the information you are learning meaningful. Think about how the information will help you be a good nursing assistant.
  - Write down what you are learning. Writing helps you remember information. Prepare study sheets.
  - Be positive about what you are learning. You remember what you find interesting.

- Suggestions for studying if you have children:
  - When you first come home from work or school, spend time with your children. Then plan study time.
  - Select educational programs on TV that your children can watch as you study. Or get a CD-ROM from the library.
  - When you take your study breaks, spend time with your children.
  - Ask other adults to take care of the children while you study.
- Take the two 75-question practice tests in this section. Each question has the correct answer and the reason why an answer is correct or incorrect. If you practice taking tests, you are more likely to pass them. Take the practice tests under conditions similar to the real test. Work within time limits.
- If your state has a practice test and a candidate handbook, study the content. Some states have practice tests on-line.

MANAGING ANXIETY

Almost everyone dreads taking tests. It is common and normal to experience anxiety before taking a test. If used wisely, anxiety can actually help you do well. When you are anxious, that means you are concerned. You may be concerned about how prepared you are to take the test. Or you may be concerned about how you will feel about yourself if you do not pass the test. Being concerned usually results in some action. To overcome anxiety before the test:

- Study and prepare for the test. That helps increase your confidence as you recall or clarify what you have learned. Anxiety decreases as confidence increases. When you think you know the information, keep studying. This reinforces your learning.
- Develop a positive mental attitude. You can pass this test. You took tests in your training program and passed them. Praise yourself. Talk to yourself in a positive way. If a negative thought enters your mind, stop it at once. Challenge the mental thought and tell yourself you will pass the test.
- Visualize success. Think about how wonderful you will feel when you are notified that you have passed the test.
- Perform breathing exercises. Breathe slowly and deeply.
- Perform regular exercise. Exercise helps you stay physically fit. It also helps keep you calm.
- Good nourishment helps you think clearly. Eat a nourishing meal before the test. Do not skip breakfast. Vitamin C helps fight short-term stress. Protein and calcium help overcome the effects of long-term stress. Complex carbohydrates (pasta, nuts, yogurt) can help

settle your nerves. Eat familiar foods the day before and the day of the test. Do not eat foods that could cause stomach or intestinal upset.

- Maintain a normal routine the day before the test.
- Get a good night's sleep before the test. Go to bed early enough so you do not oversleep or are too tired to get up. Set your alarm clock properly. You may want to set two alarm clocks.
- Do not "cram" the evening before or the day of the test. Last-minute cramming increases your anxiety. Do something relaxing with family and friends.
- Avoid drinking large amounts of coffee, colas, water, or other beverages. You do not want to be uncomfortable with a full bladder when you take the test.
- Wear comfortable clothes. Dress in layers so that you are prepared for a cold or warm room.
- If you are a woman, remember that worry and anxiety can affect your menstrual cycle. Wear a panty liner, sanitary napkin, or tampon if you think your period may start. This eliminates worry about soiling your clothing during the test.
- Allow plenty of time for travel, traffic, and parking.
- Arrive early enough to use the restroom before the test begins.
- Do not talk about the test with others. Their panic or anxiety may affect your self-confidence.

TAKING THE TEST

Follow these guidelines for taking the test:

- Listen carefully and follow the instructions given by the proctor (person administering the test).
- When you receive the test, make certain you have all the test pages.
- Read and follow all directions carefully.
- You are not allowed to ask questions about the content of the test questions.
- Do deep-breathing and muscle-relaxation exercises as needed.
- Cheating of any kind is not allowed. If the proctor sees you giving or receiving any type of assistance, your test booklet is taken and you must leave the testing site.
- If using a computer answer sheet, completely fill in the bubble.
- If you make a mistake, erase the wrong answer completely. Do not make any stray marks on the paper. Not erasing completely or leaving stray marks could cause the computer to misread your answer.
- Do not worry or get anxious if people finish the test before you do. Persons who finish a test early do not necessarily score better than those who finish later.
- You cannot take any evaluation materials or notes out of the testing room.

ANSWERING MULTIPLE-CHOICE QUESTIONS

Pace yourself during the test. First, answer all the questions that you know. Then go back and answer skipped questions. Sometimes you will remember the answer later. Or another test question may give you a clue to the one you skipped. Spending too much time on a question can cost you valuable time later. To help you answer the questions or statements:

- Always read the questions or statements carefully. Do not scan or glance at questions. Scanning or glancing can cause you to miss important key words. Read each word of the question.
- Before reading the answers, decide what the answer is in your own words. Then read all four answers to the question. Select the one best answer.
- Do not read into a question. Take the question as it is asked. Do not add your own thoughts and ideas to the question. Do not assume or suppose "what if." Just respond to the information provided.
- Trust your common sense. If unsure of an answer, select your first choice. Do not change your answer unless you are absolutely sure of the correct answer. Your first reaction is usually correct.
- Look for key words in every question. Sometimes key words are in italics, highlighted, or underlined. Common key words are: *always, never, first, except, best, not, correct, incorrect, true,* or *false.*
- Know which words can make a statement correct (e.g., *may, can, usually, most, at least, sometimes*). The word "except" can make a question a false statement.
- Be careful of answers with these key words or phrases: *always, never, every, only, all, none, at all times,* or *at no time.* These words and phrases do not allow for exceptions. In nursing, exceptions are generally present. However, sometimes answers containing these words are correct. For example, which of the following is correct and which are incorrect?
  a. Always use a turning sheet.
  b. Never shake linens.
  c. Soap is used for all baths.
  d. The call light must always be attached to the bed.
  The correct answer is b. Incorrect answers are a, c, and d.
- Omit answers that are obviously wrong. Then choose the best of the remaining answers.
- Go back to the questions you skipped. Answer all questions by eliminating or narrowing your choices. Always mark an answer even if you are not sure.
- Review the test a second time for completeness and accuracy before turning it in.

- Make sure you have answered each question. Also check that you have given only one answer for each question.
- Remember, the test is not designed to trick or confuse you. The written competency evaluation tests what you know, not what you do not know. You know more than you are asked.

ON-LINE TESTING

The test may be given by computer at the test site. Ask your instructor what computer skills you will need. You usually do not need keyboard or typing skills. You will use a computer mouse to select answers. Also, you will usually receive instruction before the test begins. This will let you practice using the computer before starting the test.

NOTE: This review covers selected chapters based on Competency Evaluation requirements.

CHAPTER 1 THE NURSING ASSISTANT WORKING IN LONG-TERM CARE

- Provide medical, nursing, dietary, recreational, rehabilitative, social services. Housekeeping and laundry services are also provided.
- Residents are older or disabled.
- Some residents are recovering from illness, injury, or surgery.
- Some residents return home when well enough. Some residents need nursing care until death.
- Long-term care centers include board and care homes (group homes), assisted living residences, skilled nursing facilities (SNFs), hospices, Alzheimer's or dementia care units, and rehabilitation and subacute care units.

THE NURSING TEAM

- Provides quality care to people.
- Care is coordinated by a registered nurse (RN).

Nursing Assistants

- Report to the nurse supervising their work.
- Provide basic nursing care under the supervision of a licensed nurse.
- Need formal training and must pass a competency test.

THE INTERDISCIPLINARY HEALTH CARE TEAM (HEALTH TEAM)

- Involves many health care workers whose skills and knowledge focus on total care.
- Works together to provide coordinated care to meet each person's needs.
- Follows the direction of the RN leading the team.

MEETING STANDARDS

Survey Process

- Surveys are done to see if agencies meet standards for licensure, certification, and accreditation.
  - A license is issued by the state. A center must have a license to operate and provide care.
  - Certification is required to receive Medicare and Medicaid funds.
  - Accreditation is voluntary. It signals quality and excellence.

Your Role

- Provide quality care.
- Protect the person's rights.
- Provide for the person's and your own safety.
- Help keep the center clean and safe.
- Conduct yourself in a professional manner.
- Have good work ethics.
- Follow center policies and procedures.
- Answer questions honestly and completely.

FEDERAL AND STATE LAWS

Nurse Practice Acts

- Each state has a nurse practice act. It regulates nursing practice in that state
- A state's nurse practice act is used to decide what nursing assistants can do. Some nurse practice acts also regulate nursing assistant roles, functions, education, and certification requirements. Some states have separate laws for nursing assistants.
- Nursing assistants must be able to function with skill and safety. They can have their certification, license, or registration denied, revoked, or suspended. The National Council of State Boards of Nursing (NCSBN) lists these reasons for doing so:
  - Substance abuse or dependency.
  - Abandoning, abusing, or neglecting a resident.
  - Fraud or deceit. Examples include:
    - Filing false personal information
    - Providing false information when applying for initial certification or re-instatement.
  - Violating professional boundaries.
  - Giving unsafe care.
  - Performing acts beyond the nursing assistant role.
  - Misappropriation (stealing, theft) or mis-using property.
  - Obtaining money or property from a resident. Fraud, falsely representing oneself, and through force are examples.
  - Having been convicted of a crime. Examples include murder, assault, kidnapping, rape or sexual assault, sexual crimes involving children, criminal mistreatment of children or a vulnerable adult, drug trafficking, embezzlement, theft, and arson.

- Failing to conform to the standards of nursing assistants.
- Putting patients and residents at risk for harm.
- Violating resident's privacy.
- Failing to maintain the confidentiality of resident information.

THE OMNIBUS BUDGET RECONCILIATION ACT OF 1987 (OBRA)

- The purpose of OBRA, a federal law, is to improve the quality of life of nursing center residents.
- OBRA sets minimum training and competency evaluation requirements for nursing assistants. Each state must have a nursing assistant training and competency evaluation program (NATCEP). A nursing assistant must successfully complete a NATCEP to work in a nursing center, hospital, or home care agency receiving Medicare funds.
- OBRA requires at least 75 hours of instruction. Some states have more hours. Sixteen hours of supervised training in a laboratory or clinical setting are required.
- OBRA requires a nursing assistant registry in each state. It is an official record that lists persons who have successfully completed the NATCEP.
- Re-training and a new competency evaluation program are required for nursing assistants who have not worked for 24 months.
- Each state's NATCEP must meet OBRA requirements.

ROLES, RESPONSIBILITIES, AND STANDARDS

- OBRA, state laws, and legal and advisory opinions direct what you can do.
- Rules for you to follow:
  - You are an assistant to the nurse.
  - A nurse assigns and supervises your work.
  - You report observations about the person's physical and mental status to the nurse. Report changes in the person's condition or behavior at once.
  - The nurse decides what should be done for a person. You do not make these decisions.
  - Review directions and the care plan with the nurse before going to the person.
  - Perform no nursing task that you are not trained to do.
  - Perform no nursing task that you are not comfortable doing without a nurse's supervision.
  - Perform only the nursing tasks that your state and job description allow.
- Role limits for nursing assistants:
  - Never give medications.

- Never insert tubes or objects into body openings. Do not remove tubes from the body.
- Never take oral or telephone orders from doctors.
- Never perform procedures that require sterile technique.
- Never tell the person or family the person's diagnosis or treatment plans.
- Never diagnose or prescribe treatments or medications for anyone.
- Never supervise others, including other nursing assistants.
- Never ignore an order or request to do something. This includes nursing tasks that you can do, those you cannot do, and those that are beyond your legal limits.
- Review Box 1-5, Nursing Assistant Standards, in the textbook.
- Always obtain a written job description when you apply for a job. Do not take a job that requires you to:
  - Act beyond the legal limits of your role.
  - Function beyond your training limits.
  - Perform acts that are against your morals or religion.

DELEGATION

- RNs can delegate tasks to you. In some states, licensed practical nurses/licensed vocational nurses (LPNs/LVNs) can delegate tasks to you.
- Nursing assistants cannot delegate. You cannot delegate any task to other nursing assistants or to any other worker.
- Delegation decisions must protect the person's health and safety. The delegating nurse is legally responsible for his or her actions and the actions of others who performed the delegated tasks.
- If you perform a task that places the person at risk, you may face serious legal problems.
- *The Five Rights of Delegation*
  - The right task. Does your state allow you to perform the task? Were you trained to do the task? Do you have experience performing the task? Is the task in your job description?
  - The right circumstances. Do you have experience performing the task given the person's condition and needs? Do you understand the purposes of the task for the person? Can you perform the task safely under the current circumstances? Do you have the equipment and supplies to safely complete the task? Do you know how to use the equipment and supplies?
  - The right person. Are you comfortable performing the task? Do you have concerns about performing the task?

- The right directions and communication. Did the nurse give clear directions and instructions? Did you review the task with the nurse? Do you understand what the nurse expects?
- The right supervision. Is a nurse available to answer questions? Is a nurse available if the person's condition changes or if problems occur?

Your Role in Delegation

- When you agree to perform a task, you are responsible for your own actions. You must complete the task safely. Report to the nurse what you did and the observations you made.
- You should refuse to perform a task when:
  - The task is beyond the legal limits of your role.
  - The task is not in your job description.
  - You were not prepared to perform the task.
  - The task could harm the person.
  - The person's condition has changed.
  - You do not know how to use the supplies or equipment.
  - Directions are not ethical or legal.
  - Directions are against center policies.
  - Directions are unclear or incomplete.
  - A nurse is not available for supervision.
- Never ignore an order or request to do something. Tell the nurse about your concerns.

CHAPTER 1 REVIEW QUESTIONS

Circle the BEST answer.

1. Nursing assistants do all the following *except*
   a. Provide quality care
   b. Follow agency policies and procedures
   c. Conduct themselves in an unprofessional manner
   d. Help keep the agency clean and safe
2. Nursing assistants report to
   a. Other nursing assistants
   b. Licensed nurses
   c. The administrator
   d. The medical director
3. The interdisciplinary health care team does all the following *except*
   a. Involves many health care workers
   b. Follows the direction of the physician
   c. Works together to provide coordinated care
   d. Follows the direction of the RN
4. Nursing assistants perform nursing tasks delegated to them by an RN or LPN/LVN.
   a. True
   b. False
5. A resident asks you about his or her medical condition. You
   a. Tell the nurse about the resident's request
   b. Tell the resident what is in his or her medical record

   c. Ignore the question
   d. Tell another nursing assistant about the resident's request
6. You answer the telephone. The doctor starts to give you an order. You
   a. Take the order from the doctor
   b. Politely give your name and title, ask the doctor to wait for the nurse, and promptly find the nurse
   c. Politely ask the doctor to call back later
   d. Ask the doctor if the nurse may call him back
7. You can have your certification revoked for all the following *except*
   a. Substance abuse or dependency
   b. Abandoning a patient or resident
   c. Performing acts beyond the nursing assistant role
   d. Giving safe care
8. When should you refuse a task?
   a. The task is not in your job description.
   b. The task is within the legal limits of your role.
   c. The directions for the task are clear.
   d. A nurse is available for questions and supervision.
9. A nurse delegates a task that you did not learn in your training. The task is in your job description. What is your appropriate response to the nurse?
   a. "I cannot do that task."
   b. "I did not learn that task in my training. Can you show me how to do it?"
   c. "I will ask the other nursing assistant to watch me do the task."
   d. "I will ask the other nursing assistant to do the task for me."
10. You are busy with a new resident. It is time for another resident's bath. You may delegate the bath to another nursing assistant.
    a. True
    b. False

Answers to these questions are on p. 505.

CHAPTER 2 RESIDENT RIGHTS, ETHICS, AND LAWS

- Centers must protect and promote resident rights. Residents must be free to exercise their rights without interference. If residents are not able to exercise their rights, legal representatives do so for them.

The Omnibus Budget Reconciliation Act of 1987 (OBRA)

- OBRA is a federal law.
- OBRA requires that nursing centers provide care in a manner and in a setting that maintains or improves each person's quality of life, health, and safety.

- OBRA requires nursing assistant training and competency evaluation.
- Resident rights are a major part of OBRA.

Information
- The right to information includes:
  - Access to medical records, incident reports, contracts, and financial records.
  - Information about his or her health condition.
  - Information about his or her doctor, including name, specialty, and contact information.
- Report any request for information to the nurse.

Refusing Treatment
- The person has the right to refuse treatment or to take part in research.
- A person who does not give consent or refuses treatment cannot be treated against his or her wishes.
- The center must find out what the person is refusing and why.
- Advance directives are part of the right to refuse treatment.
- Report any treatment refusal to the nurse.

Privacy and Confidentiality
- Residents have the right to:
  - Personal privacy. The person's body is not exposed unnecessarily. Only staff directly involved in care and treatments are present. The person must give consent for others to be present. A person has the right to use the bathroom in private. Privacy is maintained for all personal care measures.
  - Visit with others in private—in areas where others cannot see or hear them. This includes phone calls.
  - Send and receive mail without others interfering. No one can open mail the person sends or receives without his or her consent. Mail is given to the person within 24 hours of delivery to the center.
- Information about the person's care, treatment, and condition is kept confidential. So are medical and financial records. Consent is needed to release information to other agencies or persons.

Personal Choice
- Residents have the right to make their own choices. They can:
  - Choose their own doctor.
  - Take part in planning and deciding their care and treatment.
  - Choose activities, schedules, and care based on their preferences.
  - Choose when to get up and go to bed, what to wear, what to eat, and how to spend their time.
  - Choose friends and visitors inside and outside the center.

Grievances
- Residents have the right to voice concerns, ask questions, and complain about treatment or care.
- The center must promptly try to correct the matter.
- No one can punish the person in any way for voicing the grievance.

Work
- The person is not required to work or perform services for the center.
- The person has the right to work or perform services if he or she wants to.
- Residents volunteer or are paid for their services.

Taking Part in Resident and Family Groups
- The resident has the right to:
  - Form and take part in resident and family groups.
  - Take part in social, cultural, religious, and community events. The resident has the right to help in getting to and from events of his or her choice.

Care and Security of Personal Items
- The resident has the right to:
  - Keep and use personal items, such as clothing and some furnishings.
  - Have his or her property treated with care and respect. Items are labeled with the person's name.
- Protect yourself and the center from being accused of stealing a person's property. Do not go through a person's closet, drawers, purse, or other space without the person's knowledge and consent. If you have to inspect closets and drawers, follow center policy for reporting and recording the inspection.

Freedom From Abuse, Mistreatment, and Neglect
- Residents have the right to be free from:
  - Verbal, sexual, physical, or mental abuse.
  - Involuntary seclusion—separating a person from others against his or her will, confining a person to a certain area, keeping the person away from his or her room without consent.
- No one can abuse, neglect, or mistreat a resident. This includes center staff, volunteers, staff from other agencies or groups, other residents, family members, visitors, and legal representatives.

Freedom From Restraint
- Residents have the right not to have body movements restricted by restraints or medications.
- Restraints are used only if required to treat the person's medical symptoms if necessary to protect the person or others from harm. If a restraint is required, a doctor's order is needed.

Quality of Life

- Residents must be cared for in a manner that promotes dignity and self-esteem. Physical, psychological, and mental well-being must be promoted. Review Box 2-2, OBRA-Required Actions That Promote Dignity and Privacy, in your textbook.
- Centers must provide activity programs that promote physical, intellectual, social, spiritual, and emotional well-being. Many centers provide religious services for spiritual health. You assist residents to and from activity programs. You may need to help them with activities.
- Residents have a right to a safe, clean, comfortable, and home-like setting. The center must provide a setting and services that meet the person's needs and preferences. The setting and staff must promote the person's independence, dignity, and well-being.

OMBUDSMAN PROGRAM

- The Older Americans Act requires an ombudsman program in every state.
- Ombudsmen are employed by a state agency. They are not nursing center employees.
- **Ombudsmen** protect the health, safety, welfare, and rights of residents. They also may investigate and resolve complaints, provide support to resident and family groups, and help the center manage difficult problems.
- Because a family or resident may share a concern with you, you must know the state and center policies and procedures for contacting an ombudsman.

ETHICAL ASPECTS

- Ethics is the knowledge of what is right conduct and wrong conduct. It also deals with choices or judgments about what should or should not be done. An ethical person does not cause a person harm.
- Ethical behavior involves not being prejudiced or biased. To be prejudiced or biased means to make judgments and have views before knowing the facts. You should not judge a person by your values and standards. Also, do not avoid persons whose standards and values differ from your own.
- Ethical problems involve making choices. You must decide what is the right thing to do.

Boundaries

- **Professional boundaries** separate helpful behaviors from behaviors that are not helpful.
- A **boundary violation** is an act or behavior that meets your needs, not the person's. The act or behavior is unethical. Boundary violations include

abuse, keeping secrets with a person, or giving a lot of personal information about yourself to another. Review Box 2-3, Code of Conduct for Nursing Assistants, in the textbook.

- **Professional sexual misconduct** is an act, behavior, or comment that is sexual in nature. It is sexual misconduct even if the person consents or makes the first move.
- To maintain professional boundaries, review Box 2-4, Rules for Maintaining Professional Boundaries. Be alert to **boundary signs** (acts, behaviors, or thoughts that warn of a boundary crossing or violation).

LEGAL ASPECTS

- **Negligence** is an unintentional wrong. The negligent person did not act in a reasonable and careful manner. As a result, harm was caused to the person or property of another. The person did not mean to cause harm.
- **Malpractice** is negligence by a professional person.
- You are legally responsible (liable) for your own actions. The nurse is liable as your supervisor.
- **Defamation** is injuring a person's name and reputation by making false statements to a third person. **Libel** is making false statements in print, writing, or through pictures or drawings. **Slander** is making false statements orally. Never make false statements about a patient, resident, co-worker, or any other person.
- **False imprisonment** is the unlawful restraint or restriction of a person's freedom of movement. It involves threatening to restrain a person, restraining a person, and preventing a person from leaving the center.
- **Invasion of privacy** is violating a person's right not to have his or her name, photo, or private affairs exposed or made public without giving consent. Review Box 2-6, Protecting the Right to Privacy, in the textbook.
- The Health Insurance Portability and Accountability Act (HIPAA) protects the privacy and security of a person's health information. **Protected health information** refers to identifying information and information about the person's health care. Direct any questions about the person or the person's care to the nurse.
- **Fraud** is saying or doing something to trick, fool, or deceive a person. The act is fraud if it does or could cause harm to a person or the person's property.
- **Assault** is intentionally attempting or threatening to touch a person's body without the person's consent. The person fears bodily harm. **Battery** is touching a person's body without his or her consent. Protect yourself from being accused of assault and battery. Explain to the person what is to be done and get the person's consent.

Informed Consent

- A person has the right to decide what will be done to his or her body and who can touch his or her body. Consent is informed when the person clearly understands all aspects of treatment.
- Persons who cannot give consent are persons who are under the legal age or are mentally incompetent. Unconscious, sedated, or confused persons also do not give consent. Informed consent is given by a responsible party—wife, husband, daughter, son, legal representative.
- You are never responsible for obtaining written consent.

Reporting Abuse

- **Abuse** is
  - The willful infliction of injury, unreasonable confinement, intimidation, or punishment that results in physical harm, pain, or mental anguish. Intimidation means to make afraid with threats of force or violence.
  - Depriving the person (or the person's caregiver) of the goods or services needed to attain or maintain well-being.
- Abuse also includes involuntary seclusion.
- **Vulnerable adults** are persons 18 years old or older who have disabilities or conditions that make them at risk to be wounded, attacked, or damaged. They have problems caring for or protecting themselves due to:
  - A mental, emotional, physical, or developmental disability
  - Brain damage
  - Changes from aging
  - All residents are vulnerable. Older persons and children are at risk for abuse.
- **Elder abuse** is any knowing, intentional, or negligent act by a person to an older adult. It may include physical abuse, neglect, verbal abuse, involuntary seclusion, financial exploitation, emotional abuse, sexual abuse, or abandonment. Review Box 2-7, Signs of Elder Abuse, in the textbook.
- If you suspect a person is being abused, report your observations to the nurse.

CHAPTER 2 REVIEW QUESTIONS
Circle the BEST answer.

1. Residents have all the following rights *except*
   a. Refusing a treatment
   b. Making a telephone call in private
   c. Choosing activities to attend
   d. Being punished for voicing a grievance
2. OBRA does not require nursing assistant training and competency evaluation.
   a. True
   b. False
3. The person has a right to take part in planning and deciding their care and treatment.
   a. True
   b. False
4. The person is required to work for the center.
   a. True
   b. False
5. A resident offers you a gift certificate for being kind to her. You should
   a. Say "thank you" and accept the gift
   b. Accept the gift and give it to charity
   c. Thank the resident for thinking of you, then explain it is against policy for you to accept the gift
   d. Accept the gift and give it to your daughter
6. To protect a person's privacy, you should do the following *except*
   a. Keep all information about the person confidential
   b. Discuss the person's treatment or diagnosis with the nurse supervising your work
   c. Open the person's mail
   d. Allow the person to visit with others in private
7. What should you do if you suspect an older person is being abused?
   a. Report the situation to the health department.
   b. Notify the nurse and discuss the observations with him or her.
   c. Notify the doctor about the suspected abuse.
   d. Ask the family why they are abusing the person.
8. A resident needs help going to the bathroom. You do not answer her call light promptly. She gets up without help, falls, and breaks a leg. This is an example of
   a. Negligence
   b. Defamation
   c. False imprisonment
   d. Slander
9. Examples of defamation include all the following *except*
   a. Implying or suggesting that a person uses drugs
   b. Saying that a person is insane or mentally ill
   c. Implying that a person steals money from staff
   d. Burning a resident with water that is too hot
10. Which statement about ethics is *false?*
    a. An ethical person does not judge others by his or her values and standards.
    b. An ethical person avoids persons whose standards and values differ from his or her own.
    c. An ethical person is not prejudiced or biased.
    d. An ethical person does not cause harm to another person.
11. Examples of false imprisonment include all of the following *except*
    a. Threatening to restrain a resident
    b. Restraining a resident without a doctor's order
    c. Treating the resident with respect
    d. Preventing a resident from leaving the agency

12. To protect yourself from being accused of assault and battery, you should explain to the resident what you plan to do before touching him or her and get consent.
   a. True
   b. False

Answers to these questions are on p. 505.

CHAPTER 3 WORK ETHICS
HEALTH, HYGIENE, AND APPEARANCE

- To give safe and effective care, you must be physically and mentally healthy. You need a balanced diet, sleep and rest, good body mechanics, and exercise on a regular basis.
- Personal hygiene needs careful attention. Bathe daily, use deodorant or antiperspirant, and brush your teeth often. Shampoo often. Keep fingernails clean, short, and neatly shaped.
- Review Box 3-1, Practices for a Professional Appearance, in your textbook.

TEAMWORK

- Practice good work ethics—work when scheduled, be cheerful and friendly, perform delegated tasks, be kind to others, be available to help others.
- Be ready to work when your shift starts. Arrive on your nursing unit a few minutes early. Stay the entire shift. When it is time to leave, report off duty to the nurse.
- A good attitude is needed. Review Box 3-2, Qualities and Traits for Good Work Ethics, in your textbook.
- Gossiping is unprofessional and hurtful. To avoid being a part of **gossip**:
  - Remove yourself from a group or situation in which gossip is occurring.
  - Do not make or repeat any comment that can hurt another person.
  - Do not make or repeat any comment that you do not know to be true.
  - Do not talk about residents, family members, visitors, co-workers, or the center at home or in social settings.
- **Confidentiality** means trusting others with personal and private information. The person's information is shared only among health team members involved in his or her care. Agency and co-worker information also is confidential.
- Your speech and language must be professional:
  - Do not swear or use foul, vulgar, or abusive language.
  - Do not use slang.
  - Speak softly, gently, and clearly.
  - Do not shout or yell.
  - Do not fight or argue with a resident, family member, visitor, or co-worker.

- A courtesy is a polite, considerate, or helpful comment or act.
  - Address others by Miss, Mrs., Ms., Mr., or Doctor. Use a first name only if the person asks you to do so.
  - Say "please" and "thank you." Say "I'm sorry" when you make a mistake or hurt someone.
  - Let residents, families, and visitors enter elevators first.
  - Be thoughtful—compliment others, give praise.
  - Wish the person and family well when they leave the center.
  - Hold doors open for others.
  - Help others willingly when asked.
  - Do not take credit for another person's deeds. Give the person credit for the action.
- Keep personal matters out of the workplace:
  - Make personal phone calls during meals and breaks.
  - Do not let family and friends visit you on the unit.
  - Do not use the agency's computers and other equipment for personal use.
  - Do not take agency supplies for personal use.
  - Do not discuss personal problems at work.
  - Control your emotions.
  - Do not borrow money from or lend money to co-workers.
  - Do not sell things or engage in fund-raising at work.
  - Do not have cell phones or personal pagers on while at work.
- Leave for and return from breaks and meals on time. Tell the nurse when you leave and return to the unit.

MANAGING STRESS

- These guidelines can help you reduce or cope with stress:
  - Exercise regularly.
  - Get enough sleep or rest.
  - Eat healthy.
  - Plan personal and quiet time for yourself.
  - Use common sense about what you can do.
  - Do one thing at a time.
  - Do not judge yourself harshly.
  - Give yourself praise.
  - Have a sense of humor.
  - Talk to the nurse if your work or a person is causing too much stress.

HARASSMENT

- **Harassment** means to trouble, torment, offend, or worry a person by one's behavior or comments. Harassment can be sexual. Or it can involve age, race, ethnic background, religion, or disability. You must respect others. Do not offend others by your gestures, remarks, or use of touch. Do not offend others with jokes, photos, or other pictures.

CHAPTER 3 REVIEW QUESTIONS
Circle the BEST answer.

1. You believe you have good work ethics. This means you do the following *except*
   a. Work when scheduled
   b. Act cheerful and friendly
   c. Refuse to help others
   d. Perform tasks assigned by the nurse
2. A nursing assistant is gossiping about a co-worker. You should
   a. Stay with the group and listen to what is being said
   b. Repeat the comment to your family
   c. Remove yourself from the group in which gossip is occurring
   d. Repeat the comment to another co-worker
3. You want to maintain confidentiality about others. You do the following *except*
   a. Share information about a resident with a nurse who is on another unit
   b. Avoid talking about a resident in the elevator, hallway, or dining area
   c. Avoid talking about co-workers and residents when others are present
   d. Avoid eavesdropping
4. When you are at work, you should do which of the following?
   a. Swear and use foul language.
   b. Use slang.
   c. Argue with a visitor.
   d. Speak clearly and softly.
5. To give safe and effective care, you do all of the following *except*
   a. Eat a balanced diet
   b. Get enough sleep and rest
   c. Exercise on a regular basis
   d. Drink too much alcohol
6. While at work, you should do all of the following *except*
   a. Be courteous to others
   b. Make personal phone calls
   c. Admit when you are wrong or make mistakes
   d. Respect others

Answers to these questions are on p. 505.

CHAPTER 4 COMMUNICATING WITH THE HEALTH TEAM
COMMUNICATION

- For good communication:
  - Use words that mean the same thing to you and the receiver of the message.
  - Use familiar words.
  - Be brief and concise.
  - Give information in a logical and orderly manner.
  - Give facts and be specific.

THE MEDICAL RECORD

- The **medical record** is a way for the health team to share information about the person. It is a legal document.
- If you know a person in the agency but you do not give care to that person, you have no right to review the person's chart. To do so is an invasion of privacy.
- A person or legal representative may ask you for the chart. Report the request to the nurse.
- Follow your agency's policies about recording in the medical record.

RESIDENT CARE CONFERENCES

- The registered nurse (RN) may conduct a care conference to share information and ideas about the person's care. The RN, nursing assistants, and other health team members take part in the conference. The person has the right to take part in care planning conferences. Sometimes the family is involved. The person may refuse actions suggested by the health team.

REPORTING AND RECORDING

- The health team communicates by reporting and recording.

Reporting

- You report care and observations to the nurse. Follow these rules:
  - Be prompt, thorough, and accurate.
  - Give the person's name and room and bed numbers.
  - Give the time your observations were made or the care was given.
  - Report only what you observed or did yourself.
  - Give reports as often as the person's condition requires or when the nurse asks you to.
  - Report any changes from normal or changes in the person's condition at once.
  - Use your written notes to give a specific, concise, and clear report.

Recording

- Rules for recording are:
  - Always use ink. Use the color required by the center.
  - Include the date and time for every recording.
  - Make sure writing is readable and neat.
  - Use only center-approved abbreviations.
  - Use correct spelling, grammar, and punctuation.
  - Do not use ditto marks.
  - Never erase or use correction fluid. Follow the center's procedure for correcting errors.
  - Sign all entries with your name and title as required by center policy.
  - Do not skip lines.
  - Make sure each form is stamped with the person's name and other identifying information.

- Record only what you observed and did yourself.
- Never chart a procedure, treatment, or care measure until after it is completed.
- Be accurate, concise, and factual. Do not record judgments or interpretations.
- Record in a logical and sequential manner.
- Be descriptive. Avoid terms with more than one meaning.
- Use the person's exact words whenever possible. Use quotation marks to show that the statement is a direct quote.
- Chart any changes from normal or changes in the person's condition. Also chart that you informed the nurse (include the nurse's name), what you told the nurse, and the time you made the report.
- Do not omit information.
- Record safety measures. Example: Reminding a person not to get out of bed.
- Review the 24-hour clock, Figure 4-9, in your textbook.

MEDICAL TERMINOLOGY AND ABBREVIATIONS

- Medical terminology and abbreviations are used in health care. Someone may use a word or phrase that you do not understand. If so, ask the nurse to explain its meaning.
- Review Box 4-3, Medical Terminology, in the textbook.
- Use only the abbreviations accepted by the center. If you are not sure that an abbreviation is acceptable, write the term out in full. See the inside of the back cover of the textbook for common abbreviations.

COMPUTERS AND OTHER ELECTRONIC DEVICES

- Computers contain vast amounts of information about a person. Therefore, the right to privacy must be protected. If allowed access, you must follow the agency's policies. Review Box 4-5, Using the Center's Computer and Other Electronic Devices, in your textbook.

PHONE COMMUNICATIONS

- Guidelines for answering phones:
  - Answer the call after the first ring if possible.
  - Do not answer the phone in a rushed or hasty manner.
  - Give a courteous greeting. Identify the nursing unit and your name and title.
  - When taking a message, write down the caller's name, phone number, date and time, and message.
  - Repeat the message and phone number back to the caller.
  - Ask the caller to "Please hold" if necessary.
  - Do not lay the phone down or cover the receiver with your hand when not speaking to the caller. The caller may hear confidential information.
  - Return to a caller on hold within 30 seconds.
  - Do not give confidential information to any caller.
  - Transfer a call if appropriate. Tell the caller you are going to transfer the call. Give the name and phone number in case the call gets disconnected.
  - End the conversation politely.
  - Give the message to the appropriate person.

DEALING WITH CONFLICT

- These guidelines can help you deal with conflict:
  - Ask your supervisor for some time to talk privately about the problem.
  - Approach the person with whom you have the conflict. Ask to talk privately. Be polite and professional.
  - Agree on a time and place to talk.
  - Talk in a private setting. No one should hear you or the other person.
  - Explain the problem and what is bothering you. Give facts and specific behaviors. Focus on the problem. Do not focus on the person.
  - Listen to the person. Do not interrupt.
  - Identify ways to solve the problem. Offer your thoughts. Ask for the co-worker's ideas.
  - Set a date and time to review the matter.
  - Thank the person for meeting with you.
  - Carry out the solution.
  - Review the matter as scheduled.

CHAPTER 4 REVIEW QUESTIONS
Circle the BEST answer.

1. For good communication, you should do the following *except*
   a. Use words with more than one meaning
   b. Use words familiar to the person or family
   c. Give facts in a brief and concise manner
   d. Give information in a logical and orderly manner
2. When you record in a person's chart, you do the following *except*
   a. Record what you observed and did
   b. Record the person's response to the treatment or procedure
   c. Use abbreviations that are not on the accepted list for the center
   d. Record the time the observation was made or the treatment performed
3. When reporting care and observations to the nurse, you do all of the following *except*
   a. Give the person's name and room and bed numbers
   b. Report only what you observed or did yourself
   c. Report any changes from normal or changes in the person's condition at once
   d. Report any changes from normal or changes in the person's condition at the end of the shift

Answers to these questions are on p. 505.

CHAPTER 5 ASSISTING WITH THE NURSING PROCESS

- The **nursing process** is the method nurses use to plan and deliver nursing care.
- You play a key role by making observations as you care and talk with the person.
- **Observation** is using the senses of sight, hearing, touch, and smell to collect information. Box 5-1, Basic Observations, in your textbook lists the basic observations you need to make and report to the nurse. Examples are:
  - Can the person give his or her name, the time, and location when asked?
  - Can the person move the arms and legs?
  - Is the skin pale or flushed?
  - Is there drainage from the eyes? What color is the drainage?
  - Does the person like the food served?
  - Can the person bathe without help?
- Observations you need to report to the nurse at once are:
  - A change in the person's ability to respond
  - A change in the person's mobility
  - Complaints of sudden, severe pain
  - A sore or reddened area on the person's skin
  - Complaints of a sudden change in vision
  - Complaints of pain or difficulty breathing
  - Abnormal respirations
  - Complaints or signs of difficulty swallowing
  - Vomiting
  - Bleeding
  - Vital signs outside their normal ranges
- **Objective data (signs)** are seen, heard, felt, or smelled by an observer. For example, you can feel a pulse.
- **Subjective data (symptoms)** are things a person tells you about that you cannot observe through your senses. For example, you cannot see the person's nausea.
- The nurse communicates delegated tasks to you. This is the purpose of an assignment sheet. An assignment sheet tells you about each person's care, what measures and tasks need to be done, and which nursing unit tasks to do. Talk to the nurse about any unclear assignment.

CHAPTER 5 REVIEW QUESTIONS
Circle the BEST answer.

1. Which statement about observations is *false?*
   a. You make observations as you care and talk with people.
   b. Observation uses the senses of smell, sight, touch, and hearing.
   c. A reddened area on the person's skin is reported to the nurse at once.
   d. You report observations to the doctor.

2. Objective data include all of the following *except*
   a. The person has pain in his abdomen
   b. The person's pulse is 76
   c. The person's urine is dark amber
   d. The person's breath has an odor

Answers to these questions are on p. 505.

CHAPTER 6 UNDERSTANDING THE RESIDENT
CARING FOR THE PERSON

- The whole person needs to be considered when you provide care—physical, social, psychological, and spiritual parts. These parts are woven together and cannot be separated.
- Follow these rules to address persons with dignity and respect:
  - Call persons by their titles—Mrs. Dennison, Mr. Smith, Miss Turner, or Dr. Gonzalez.
  - Do not call persons by their first names unless they ask you to.
  - Do not call persons by any other name unless they ask you to.
  - Do not call persons Grandma, Papa, Sweetheart, Honey, or other name.

BASIC NEEDS

- A **need** is something necessary or desired for maintaining life and mental well-being.
- According to Maslow, basic needs must be met for a person to survive and function:
  - *Physiological or physical needs*—are required for life. They are oxygen, food, water, elimination, rest, and shelter.
  - *Safety and security needs*—relate to feeling safe from harm, danger, and fear.
  - *Love and belonging needs*—relate to love, closeness, affection, and meaningful relationships with others. Family, friends, and the health team can meet love and belonging needs.
  - *Self-esteem needs*—relate to thinking well of oneself and to seeing oneself as useful and having value. People often lack self-esteem when ill, injured, older, or disabled.
  - *The need for self-actualization*—involves learning, understanding, and creating to the limit of a person's capacity. Rarely, if ever, is it totally met.

CULTURE AND RELIGION

- **Culture** refers to the characteristics of a group of people. People come from many cultures, races, and nationalities. Family practices, food choices, hygiene habits, clothing styles, and language are part of their culture. The person's culture also influences health beliefs and practices.

- **Religion** relates to spiritual beliefs, needs, and practices. A person's religion influences health and illness practices. Many may want to pray and observe religious practices. Assist residents to attend religious services as needed. If a person wants to see a spiritual leader or adviser, tell the nurse. Provide privacy during the visit.
- A person may not follow all the beliefs and practices of his or her culture or religion. Some people do not practice a religion.
- Respect and accept the person's culture and religion. Learn about practices and beliefs different from your own. Do not judge a person by your standards.

BEHAVIOR ISSUES

- Many people do not adjust well to illness, injury, and disability. They have some of the following behaviors:
  - *Anger*. Anger may be communicated verbally and nonverbally. Verbal outbursts, shouting, and rapid speech are common. Some people are silent. Others are uncooperative and may refuse to answer questions. Nonverbal signs include rapid movements, pacing, clenched fists, and a red face. Glaring and getting close to you when speaking are other signs. Violent behaviors can occur.
  - *Demanding behavior*. Nothing seems to please the person. The person is critical of others.
  - *Self-centered behavior*. The person cares only about his or her own needs. The needs of others are ignored. The person becomes impatient if needs are not met.
  - *Aggressive behavior*. The person may swear, bite, hit, pinch, scratch, or kick. Protect the person, others, and yourself from harm.
  - *Withdrawal*. The person has little or no contact with family, friends, and staff. Some people are generally not social and prefer to be alone.
  - *Inappropriate sexual behavior*. Some people make inappropriate sexual remarks or touch others in the wrong way. These behaviors may be on purpose. Or they are caused by disease, confusion, dementia, or medication side effects.
- You cannot avoid persons with unpleasant behaviors or who lose control. Review Box 6-1, Dealing With Behavior Issues, in your textbook.

COMMUNICATING WITH THE PERSON

- For effective communication between you and the person, you must:
  - Follow the rules of communication in Chapter 4.
  - Understand and respect the patient or resident as a person.
  - View the person as a physical, psychological, social, and spiritual human being.
  - Appreciate the person's problems and frustrations.
  - Respect the person's rights.

- Respect the person's religion and culture.
- Give the person time to understand the information that you give.
- Repeat information as often as needed.
- Ask questions to see if the person understood you.
- Be patient. People with memory problems may ask the same question many times.
- Include the person in conversations when others are present.

Verbal Communication

- When talking with a person, follow these rules:
  - Face the person.
  - Position yourself at the person's eye level.
  - Control the loudness and tone of your voice.
  - Speak clearly, slowly, and distinctly.
  - Do not use slang or vulgar words.
  - Repeat information as needed.
  - Ask one question at a time and wait for an answer.
  - Do not shout, whisper, or mumble.
  - Be kind, courteous, and friendly.
- Use written words if the person cannot speak or hear but can read. Keep written messages brief and concise. Use a black felt pen on white paper, and print in large letters.
- Some persons cannot speak or read. Ask questions that have "yes" and "no" answers. A picture board may be helpful.

Nonverbal Communication

- Messages are sent with gestures, facial expressions, posture, body movements, touch, and smell. Nonverbal messages more accurately reflect a person's feelings than words do. A person may say one thing but act another way. Watch the person's eyes, hand movements, gestures, posture, and other actions.
- Touch conveys comfort, caring, love, affection, interest, trust, concern, and reassurance. Touch should be gentle. Touch means different things to different people. Some people do not like to be touched.
- People send messages through their **body language**—facial expressions, gestures, posture, hand and body movements, gait, eye contact, and appearance. Your body language should show interest, enthusiasm, caring, and respect for the person. Often you need to control your body language. Control reactions to odors from body fluids, secretions, or excretions.

Communication Methods

- *Listening* means to focus on verbal and nonverbal communication. You use sight, hearing, touch, and smell. To be a good listener:
  - Face the person.
  - Have good eye contact with the person.
  - Lean toward the person. Do not sit back with your arms crossed.

- Respond to the person. Nod your head and ask questions.
  - Avoid communication barriers.
- *Paraphrasing* is restating the person's message in your own words.
- *Direct questions* focus on certain information. You ask the person something you need to know.
- *Open-ended questions* lead or invite the person to share thoughts, feelings, or ideas. The person chooses what to talk about.
- *Clarifying* lets you make sure that you understand the message. You can ask the person to repeat the message, say you do not understand, or restate the message.
- *Focusing* deals with a certain topic. It is useful when a person wanders in thought.
- *Silence* is a very powerful way to communicate. Silence on your part shows caring and respect for the person's situation and feelings.

Communication Barriers
- *Language.* You and the person must use and understand the same language.
- *Cultural differences.* A person from another country may attach different meanings to verbal and nonverbal communication from what you intended.
- *Changing the subject.* Avoid changing the subject whenever possible.
- *Giving your opinions.* Opinions involve judging values, behavior, or feelings. Let others express feelings and concerns. Do not make judgments or jump to conclusions.
- *Talking a lot when others are silent.* Talking too much is usually because of nervousness and discomfort with silence.
- *Failure to listen.* Do not pretend to listen. It shows lack of caring and interest. You may miss complaints of pain, discomfort, or other symptoms that you must report to the nurse.
- *Pat answers.* "Don't worry." "Everything will be okay." These make the person feel that you do not care about his or her concerns, feelings, and fears.
- *Illness and disability.* Speech, hearing, vision, cognitive function, and body movements may be affected. Verbal and nonverbal communication are affected.
- *Age.* Values and communication styles vary among age-groups.

PERSONS WITH SPECIAL NEEDS
- Common courtesies and manners apply to any person with a disability. Review Box 6-2, Disability Etiquette, in the textbook.
- The person who is comatose is unconscious and cannot respond to others. Often the person can feel touch and pain. Assume that the person hears and understands you. Use touch and give care gently. Practice these measures:

- Knock before entering the person's room.
- Tell the person your name, the time, and the place every time you enter the room.
- Give care on the same schedule every day.
- Explain what you are going to do.
- Tell the person when you are finishing care.
- Use touch to communicate care, concern, and comfort.
- Tell the person what time you will be back to check on him or her.
- Tell the person when you are leaving the room.

FAMILY AND FRIENDS
- If you need to give care when visitors are there, protect the person's right to privacy. Politely ask the visitors to leave the room when you give care. A partner or family member may help you if the patient or resident consents.
- Treat family and visitors with courtesy and respect.
- Do not discuss the person's condition with family and friends. Refer questions to the nurse. A visitor may upset or tire a person. Report your observations to the nurse.

CHAPTER 6 REVIEW QUESTIONS
Circle the BEST answer.
1. While caring for a person, you need to
   a. Consider only the person's physical and social needs
   b. Consider the person's physical, social, psychological, and spiritual needs
   c. Consider only the person's cultural needs
   d. Ignore the person's spiritual needs
2. When referring to residents, you should
   a. Refer to them by their room number
   b. Call them "Honey"
   c. Call them by their first name
   d. Call them by their name and title
3. Based on Maslow's theory of basic needs, which person's needs must be met first?
   a. The person who wants to talk about her granddaughter's wedding
   b. The person who is uncomfortable in the dining room
   c. The person who wants mail opened
   d. The person who asks for more water
4. Which statement about culture is *false*?
   a. A person's culture influences health beliefs and practices.
   b. You must respect a person's culture.
   c. You should ignore the person's culture while you give his or her care.
   d. You should learn about another person's culture that is different from yours.

5. Which statement about religion and spiritual beliefs is *false*?
   a. A person's religion influences health and illness practices.
   b. You should assist a person to attend services in the nursing center.
   c. Many people find comfort and strength from religion during illness.
   d. A person must follow all beliefs of his or her religion.

6. A person is angry and is shouting at you. You should do the following *except*
   a. Stay calm and professional
   b. Yell so the person will listen to you
   c. Listen to what the person is saying
   d. Report the person's behavior to the nurse

7. A person tries to scratch and kick you. You should
   a. Protect yourself from harm
   b. Argue with the person
   c. Become angry with the person
   d. Refuse to care for the person

8. When speaking with another person, you do all of the following *except*
   a. Position yourself at the person's eye level
   b. Speak slowly, clearly, and distinctly
   c. Shout, mumble, and whisper
   d. Ask one question at a time

9. Which statement about listening is *false*?
   a. You use sight, hearing, touch, and smell when you listen.
   b. You observe nonverbal cues.
   c. You have good eye contact with the person.
   d. You sit back with your arms crossed.

10. Which statement about silence is *false*?
    a. Silence is a powerful way to communicate.
    b. Silence gives people time to think.
    c. You should talk a lot when the other person is silent.
    d. Silence helps when the person is upset and needs to gain control.

11. A person speaks a foreign language. You should do the following *except*
    a. Keep messages short and simple
    b. Use gestures and pictures
    c. Shout or speak loudly
    d. Repeat the message in other words

12. When caring for a person who is comatose, you do the following *except*
    a. Tell the person your name when you enter the room
    b. Explain what you are doing
    c. Use touch to communicate care and comfort
    d. Make jokes about how sick the person is

13. A person is in a wheelchair. You should do all of the following *except*
    a. Lean on a person's wheelchair
    b. Sit or squat to talk to a person in a wheelchair or chair
    c. Think about obstacles before giving directions to a person in a wheelchair
    d. Extend the same courtesies to the person as you would to anyone else

14. A person's daughter is visiting and you need to provide care to the person. You
    a. Expose the person's body in front of the visitor
    b. Politely ask the visitor to leave the room
    c. Decide to not provide the care at all
    d. Discuss the person's condition with the visitor

Answers to these questions are on p. 505.

CHAPTER 8 THE OLDER PERSON
GROWTH AND DEVELOPMENT

- Aging is normal. It is not a disease. Normal changes occur in body structure and function. Psychological and social changes also occur.
- **Growth** refers to the physical changes that are measured and that occur in a steady and orderly manner.
- **Development** relates to changes in mental, emotional, and social function.
- Growth and development occur in a sequence, order, and pattern. Review Box 8-1, Stages of Growth and Development, in your textbook.

SOCIAL CHANGES

- Physical reminders of growing old affect self-esteem and may threaten self-image, feelings of self-worth, and independence.
- People cope with aging in their own way. How they cope depends on their health status, life experiences, finances, education, and social support systems.
- *Retirement.* Many people enjoy retirement. Others are in poor health and have medical bills that can make retirement hard.
- *Reduced income.* Retirement usually means reduced income. The retired person still has expenses. Reduced income may force life-style changes. One example is the person avoids health care or needed drugs.
- *Social relationshoips.* Social relationships change throughout life. Family time helps prevent loneliness, as do hobbies, religious and community events, and new friends.
- *Children as caregivers.* Some older persons feel more secure when their children care for them. Others feel unwanted and useless. Some lose dignity and self-respect. Tensions may occur among the child, parent, and other household members.
- *Death of a partner.* When death occurs, the person loses a lover, friend, companion, and confidant. Grief may be great. The person's life will likely change.

PHYSICAL CHANGES

- Body processes slow down. Energy level and body efficiency decline.

- *The integumentary system.* The skin loses its elasticity, strength, and fatty tissue layer. Wrinkles appear. Dry skin and itching occur. The skin is fragile and easily injured. The person is more sensitive to cold. Nails become thick and tough. Feet may have poor circulation. White or gray hair is common. Hair thins. Facial hair may occur in women. Hair is drier. The risk of skin cancer increases.
- *The musculoskeletal system.* Muscle and bone strength are lost. Bones become brittle and break easily. Vertebrae shorten. Joints become stiff and painful. Mobility decreases. There is a gradual loss of height.
- *The nervous system.* Confusion, dizziness, and fatigue may occur. Responses are slower. The risk for falls increases. Forgetfulness increases. Memory is shorter. Events from long ago are remembered better than recent ones. Older persons have a harder time falling asleep. Sleep periods are shorter. Older persons wake often during the night and have less deep sleep. Less sleep is needed. They may rest or nap during the day. They may go to bed early and get up early.
- *The senses.* Hearing and vision losses occur. Taste and smell dull. Touch and sensitivy to pain, pressure, hot, and cold are reduced.
- *The circulatory system.* The heart muscle weakens. Arteries narrow and are less elastic. Poor circulation occurs in many body parts.
- *The respiratory system.* Respiratory muscles weaken. Lung tissue becomes less elastic. Difficult, labored, or painful breathing may occur with activity. The person may lack strength to cough and clear the airway of secretions. Respiratory infections and diseases may develop.
- *The digestive system.* Less saliva is produced. The person may have difficulty swallowing (dysphagia). Indigestion may occur. Loss of teeth and ill-fitting dentures cause chewing problems and digestion problems. Flatulence and constipation can occur. Fewer calories are needed as energy and activity levels decline. More fluids are needed.
- *The urinary system.* Urine is more concentrated. Bladder muscles weaken. Bladder size decreases. Urinary frequency or urgency may occur. Many older persons have to urinate at night. Urinary incontinence may occur. In men, The prostate gland enlarges. This may cause difficulty urinating or frequent urination.
- *The reproductive system.* In men, testosterone decreases. An erection takes longer. Orgasm is less forceful. Women experience menopause. Female hormones of estrogen and progesterone decrease. The uterus, vagina, and genitalia shrink (atrophy). Vaginal walls thin. Ther is vaginal dryness. Arousal takes longer. Orgasm is less intense.

Needing Nursing Center Care
- The person needing nursing center care may suffer some or all of these losses:
  - Loss of identity as a productive member of a family and community

  - Loss of possessions—home, household items, car, and so on
  - Loss of independence
  - Loss of real-world experiences—shopping, traveling, cooking, driving, hobbies
  - Loss of health and mobility
- The person may feel useless, powerless, and hopeless. The health team helps the person cope with loss and improve quality of life. Treat the person with dignity and respect. Also practice good communication skills. Follow the care plan.

CHAPTER 8 REVIEW QUESTIONS
Circle the Best answer.

1. Which is a developmental task of late adulthood?
   a. Accepting changes in appearance
   b. Adjusting to decreased strength
   c. Developing a satisfactory sex life
   d. Performing self-care
2. Which statement is *false*?
   a. Physical changes occur with aging.
   b. Energy level and body efficiency decline with age.
   c. Some people age faster than others.
   d. Normal aging means loss of health.
3. As a person ages, the integumentary system changes. Which statement is *false*?
   a. Dry skin and itching occur.
   b. Nails become thick and tough.
   c. The person is less sensitive to cold.
   d. Skin is injured more easily.
4. Which statement is *false* about the musculo-skeletal system and aging?
   a. Strength decreases.
   b. Vertebrae shorten.
   c. Mobility increases.
   d. Bone mass decreases.
5. Which statement about the nervous system and aging is *false*?
   a. Reflexes slow.
   b. Memory may be shorter.
   c. Sleep patterns change.
   d. Forgetfulness decreases.
6. Which statement about the digestive system and aging is *false*?
   a. Appetite decreases.
   b. Less saliva is produced.
   c. Flatulence and constipation may decrease.
   d. Teeth may be lost.
7. Which statement about the urinary system and aging is *false*?
   a. Urine becomes more concentrated.
   b. Urinary frequency may occur.
   c. Urinary urgency may occur.
   d. Bladder muscles become stronger.

Answers to these questions are on p. 505.

CHAPTER 10 SAFETY
ACCIDENT RISK FACTORS

- *Age.* Older persons are at risk for falls and other injuries.
- *Awareness of surroundings.* People need to know their surroundings to protect themselves from injury.
- *Agitated and aggressive behaviors.* Pain, confusion, fear, and decreased awareness of surroundings can cause these behaviors.
- *Impaired vision.* Persons can fall or trip over items. Some have problems reading labels on containers.
- *Impaired hearing.* Persons have problems hearing explanations and instructions. They may not hear warning signals or fire alarms. They do not know to move to safety.
- *Impaired smell and touch.* Illness and aging affect smell and touch.
- *Impaired mobility.* Some diseases and injuries affect mobility. A person may be aware of danger but is unable to move to safety.
- *Medications.* Medications have side effects. Report behavior changes and the person's complaints.

IDENTIFYING THE PERSON

- You must give the right care to the right person. To identify the person:
  - Compare identifying information on the assignment sheet or treatment card with that on the identification (ID) bracelet.
  - Call the person by name when checking the ID bracelet. Just calling the person by name is not enough to identify him or her. Confused, disoriented, drowsy, hard-of-hearing, or distracted persons may answer to any name.
  - Some nursing centers have photo ID systems. Use this system safely.
  - Alert and oriented persons may choose not to wear ID bracelets. Follow center policy and the care plan to identify the person.

PREVENTING BURNS

- Smoking, spilled hot liquids, very hot water, and electrical devices are common causes of burns. See p. 130 in your textbook for safety measures to prevent burns.

PREVENTING POISONING

- Medications and household products are common poisons. Poisoning in adults may result from carelessness, confusion, or poor vision when reading labels. To prevent poisoning:
  - Make sure patients and residents cannot reach hazardous materials.
  - Follow agency policy for storing personal care items.

PREVENTING SUFFOCATION

- **Suffocation** is when breathing stops from the lack of oxygen. Death occurs if the person does not start breathing.
- To prevent suffocation, review Box 10-3, Safety Measures to Prevent Suffocation.

Choking

- Choking or foreign-body airway obstruction (FBAO) occurs when a foreign body obstructs the airway. Air cannot pass through the air passages to the lungs. The body does not get enough oxygen. This can lead to cardiac arrest.
- Choking often occurs during eating. A large, poorly chewed piece of meat is the most common cause. Other common causes include laughing and talking while eating.
- With *mild airway obstruction*, some air moves in and out of the lungs. The person is conscious. Usually the person can speak. Often forceful coughing can remove the object.
- With *severe airway obstruction*, the conscious person clutches at the throat—the "universal sign of choking." The person has difficulty breathing. Some persons cannot breathe, speak, or cough. The person appears pale and cyanotic. Air does not move in and out of the lungs. If the obstruction is not removed, the person will die. Severe airway obstruction is an emergency.
- Use abdominal thrusts to relieve FBAO. Chest thrusts are used for very obese persons and pregnant women.
- Call for help when a person has an obstructed airway. Report and record what happened, what you did, and the person's response.

PREVENTING EQUIPMENT ACCIDENTS

- All equipment is unsafe if broken, not used correctly, or not working properly. Inspect all equipment before use. Review Box 10-4, Safety Measures to Prevent Equipment Accidents, in the textbook.

WHEELCHAIR AND STRETCHER SAFETY

- Review Box 10-5, Wheelchair and Stretcher Safety, in the textbook.

HANDLING HAZARDOUS SUBSTANCES

- A hazardous substance is any chemical in the workplace that can cause harm. Hazardous substances include oxygen, mercury, disinfectants, and cleaning agents.
- Hazardous substance containers must have a warning label. If a label is removed or damaged, do not use the substance. Take the container to the nurse. Do not leave the container unattended.

- Check the Material Safety Data Sheet (MSDS) before using a hazardous substance, cleaning up a leak or spill, or disposing of the substance. Tell the nurse about a leak or spill right away. Do not leave a leak or spill unattended.

FIRE SAFETY

- Faulty electrical equipment and wiring, over-loaded electrical circuits, and smoking are major causes of fires.
- Safety measures are needed where oxygen is used and stored:
  - NO SMOKING signs are placed on the door and near the person's bed.
  - The person and visitors are reminded not to smoke in the room.
  - Smoking materials are removed from the room.
  - Electrical items are turned off before being unplugged.
  - Wool blankets and fabrics that cause static electricity are not used.
  - The person wears a cotton gown or pajamas.
  - Electrical items are in good working order.
  - Lit candles and other open flames are not allowed.
  - Materials that ignite easily are removed from the room.
- Review Box 10-7, Fire Prevention Measures, in the textbook.
- Know your center's policies and procedures for fire emergencies. Know where to find fire alarms, fire extinguishers, and emergency exits. Remember the word RACE:
  - R—*rescue*. Rescue persons in immediate danger. Move them to a safe place.
  - A—*alarm*. Sound the nearest fire alarm. Notify the telephone operator.
  - C—*confine*. Close doors and windows. Turn off oxygen or electrical items.
  - E—*extinguish*. Use a fire extinguisher on a small fire.
- Remember the word PASS for using a fire extinguisher:
  - P—*pull* the safety pin.
  - A—*aim* low. Aim at the base of the fire.
  - S—*squeeze* the lever. This starts the stream of water.
  - S—*sweep* back and forth. Sweep side to side at the base of the fire.
- Do not use elevators during a fire.

DISASTERS

- A **disaster** is a sudden catastrophic event. The agency has procedures for disasters that could occur in your area. Follow them to keep patients, residents, visitors, staff, and yourself safe.

WORKPLACE VIOLENCE

- **Workplace violence** consists of violent acts (including assault or threat of assault) directed toward persons at work or while on duty. Review Box 10-8, Measures to Prevent or Control Workplace Violence, in the textbook.

CHAPTER 10 REVIEW QUESTIONS
Circle the BEST answer.

1. You see a water spill in the hallway. What will you do?
   a. Ask housekeeping to wipe up the spill right away.
   b. Wipe up the spill right away.
   c. Report the spill to the nurse.
   d. Ask the resident to walk around the spill.
2. An electrical outlet in a person's room does not work. What will you do?
   a. Tell the administrator about the problem.
   b. Tell another nursing assistant about the problem.
   c. Try to repair the electrical outlet.
   d. Follow the center's policy for reporting the problem.
3. Accident risk factors include all of the following *except*
   a. Walking without difficulty
   b. Hearing problems
   c. Dulled sense of smell
   d. Poor vision
4. To prevent a person from being burned, you should do the following *except*
   a. Supervise the smoking of persons who are confused
   b. Turn cold water on first; turn hot water off first
   c. Do not let the person sleep with a heating pad
   d. Allow smoking in bed
5. To prevent suffocation, you should do all of the following *except*
   a. Make sure dentures fit properly
   b. Check the care plan for swallowing problems before serving food or liquids
   c. Leave a person alone in a bathtub or shower
   d. Position the person in bed properly
6. Which statement about mild airway obstruction is *false?*
   a. Some air moves in and out of the lungs.
   b. The person is conscious.
   c. Usually the person cannot speak.
   d. Forceful coughing will often remove the object.
7. The "universal sign of choking" is
   a. Clutching at the chest
   b. Clutching at the throat
   c. Not being able to talk
   d. Not being able to breathe

8. Which statement about wheelchair safety is *false*?
   a. Lock the wheels before transferring a resident to or from a wheelchair.
   b. The person's feet should rest on the footplate when you are pushing the wheelchair.
   c. Let the footplates fall back onto a person's legs.
   d. Check for flat or loose tires.
9. Which of the following is *not* a safety measure with oxygen?
   a. NO SMOKING signs are placed on the resident's door and near the bed.
   b. Lit candles and other open flames are permitted in the room.
   c. Electrical items are turned off before being unplugged.
   d. The person wears a cotton gown or pajamas.
10. You have discovered a fire in the nursing center. You should do the following *except*
   a. Rescue persons in immediate danger
   b. Sound the nearest fire alarm
   c. Open doors and windows and keep oxygen on
   d. Use a fire extinguisher on a small fire that has not spread to a larger area
11. When using a fire extinguisher, you do all of the following *except*
   a. Pull the safety pin on the fire extinguisher
   b. Aim at the top of the flames
   c. Squeeze the lever to start the stream
   d. Sweep the stream back and forth

Answers to these questions are on p. 505.

CHAPTER 11 PREVENTING FALLS
- Falls are a leading cause of injuries and deaths among older persons. A history of falls increases the risk of falling again.
- Most falls occur in resident rooms and bathrooms. Most occur between 1800 (6:00 PM) and 2100 (9:00 PM). Falls are more likely during shift changes.
- Causes for falls are poor lighting, cluttered floors, needing to use the bathroom, and out-of-place furniture. So are wet and slippery floors, bathtubs, and showers. Review Box 11-1, Factors Increasing the Risk of Falls, in the textbook.
- Agencies have fall prevention programs. Review Box 11-2, Safety Measures to Prevent Falls, in the textbook. The person's care plan also lists measures specific for the person.

BED RAILS
- A **bed rail** (*side rail*) is a device that serves as a guard or barrier along the side of the bed.
- The nurse and care plan tell you when to raise bed rails. They are needed by persons who are unconscious or sedated with medications. Some confused and disoriented people need them. If a person needs bed rails, keep them up at all times except when giving bedside nursing care.

- Bed rails present hazards. The person can fall when trying to get out of bed. Or the person can get caught, trapped, entangled, or strangled.
- Bed rails are considered restraints if the person cannot get out of bed or lower them without help.
- Bed rails cannot be used unless they are needed to treat a person's medical symptoms. The person or legal representative must give consent for raised bed rails. The need for bed rails is carefully noted in the person's medical record and the care plan. If a person uses bed rails, check the person often. Record when you checked the person and your observations.
- To prevent falls:
  - Never leave the person alone when the bed is raised.
  - Always lower the bed to its lowest position when you are done giving care.
  - If a person does not use bed rails and you need to raise the bed, ask a co-worker to stand on the far side of the bed to protect the person from falling.
  - If you raise the bed to give care, always raise the far bed rail if you are working alone.
  - Be sure the person who uses raised bed rails has access to items on the bedside stand and over-bed table. The call light, water pitcher and cup, tissues, phone, and TV and light controls should be within the person's reach.

HAND RAILS AND GRAB BARS
- Hand rails give support to persons who are weak or unsteady when walking.
- Grab bars provide support for sitting down or getting up from a toilet. They also are used for getting in and out of the shower or tub.

WHEEL LOCKS
- Bed wheels are locked at all times except when moving the bed.
- Wheelchair and stretcher wheels are locked when transferring a person.

TRANSFER/GAIT BELTS
- Use a **transfer belt (gait belt)** to support a person who is unsteady or disabled. Always follow the manufacturer instructions. Apply the belt over clothing and under the breasts. The belt buckle is never positioned over the person's spine. Tighten the belt so it is snug. You should be able to slide your open, flat hand under the belt. Tuck the excess strap under the belt. Remove the belt after the procedure.
- Check with the nurse and care plan before using a transfer/gait belt if the person has:
  - A colostomy, ileostomy, gastrostomy, or urostomy
  - A gastric tube

- Chronic obstructive pulmonary disease
- An abdominal wound, incision, or drainage tube
- A chest wound, incision, or drainage tube
- Monitoring equipment
- A hernia
- Other conditions or care equipment involving the chest or abdomen

THE FALLING PERSON

- If a person starts to fall, do not try to prevent the fall. You could injure yourself and the person. Ease the person to the floor and protect the person's head. Do not let the person get up before the nurse checks for injuries. An incident report is completed after all falls.

CHAPTER 11 REVIEW QUESTIONS

Circle the BEST answer.

1. Most falls occur in
   a. Resident rooms and bathrooms
   b. Dining rooms
   c. Hallways
   d. Activity rooms
2. Which statement about falls is *false?*
   a. Poor lighting, cluttered floors, and throw rugs may cause falls.
   b. Improper shoes and needing to use the bathroom may cause falls.
   c. Most falls occur between 6:00 PM and 9:00 PM.
   d. Falls are less likely to occur during shift changes.
3. You note the following after a person got dressed. Which is unsafe?
   a. Non-skid footwear is worn.
   b. Pant cuffs are dragging on the floor.
   c. Clothing fits properly.
   d. The belt is fastened.
4. Which statement about bed rails is *false?*
   a. The nurse and care plan tell you when to raise bed rails.
   b. Bed rails are considered restraints.
   c. You may leave a person alone when the bed is raised and the bed rails are down.
   d. Bed rails can present hazards because people try to climb over them.
5. Which statement about transfer/gait belts is *false?*
   a. To use the belt safely, follow the manufacturer instructions.
   b. Always apply the belt over clothing.
   c. Tighten the belt so it is very snug and breathing is impaired.
   d. Place the belt buckle off center so it is not over the spine.

6. A person becomes faint in the hallway and begins to fall. You should do the following *except*
   a. Ease the person to the floor
   b. Protect the person's head
   c. Let the person get up before the nurse checks him or her
   d. Help the nurse complete the incident report

Answers to these questions are on p. 505.

CHAPTER 12 RESTRAINT ALTERNATIVES AND SAFE RESTRAINT USE

- The Centers for Medicare and Medicaid Services (CMS) has rules for using restraints. These rules protect the person's rights and safety.
- Restraints may be used only to treat a medical symptom or for the immediate physical safety of the person or others. Restraints may be used only when less restrictive measures fail to protect the person or others. They must be discontinued at the earliest possible time.
- A **physical restraint** is any manual method or physical or mechanical device, material, or equipment attached to or near the person's body that he or she cannot remove easily and that restricts freedom of movement or normal access to one's body.
- A **chemical restraint** is a medication that is used for discipline or convenience and not required to treat medical symptoms. The medication or dosage is not a standard treatment for the person's condition.
- Federal, state, and accrediting agencies have guidelines about restraint use. They do not forbid restraint use. They require considering or trying all other appropriate alternatives first.

RESTRAINT ALTERNATIVES

- Knowing and treating the cause of harmful behaviors can prevent restraint use. There are many alternatives to restraints, such as answering the call light promptly. For other alternatives see Box 12-2, Alternatives to Restraint Use, in the textbook.

SAFE RESTRAINT USE

- Restraints are used only when necessary to treat a person's medical symptoms—physical, emotional, or behavioral problems. Sometimes restraints are needed to protect the person or others.

Physical and Chemical Restraints

- *Physical restraints* are applied to the chest, waist, elbows, wrists, hands, or ankles. They confine the person to a bed or chair. Or they prevent movement of a body part.
- Some furniture or barriers prevent free movement:
  - Geriatric chairs or chairs with attached trays
  - Any chair placed so close to the wall that the person cannot move

- Bed rails
- Sheets tucked in so tightly that they restrict movement
- Wheelchair locks if the person cannot release them
- Medications or medication dosages are *chemical restraints* if they:
  - Control behavior or restrict movement
  - Are not standard treatment for the person's condition

Complications of Restraint Use

- Restraints can cause many complications. Injuries occur as the person tries to get free of the restraint. Injuries also occur from using the wrong restraint, applying it wrong, or keeping it on too long. Cuts, bruises, and fractures are common. The most serious risk is death from strangulation. Review Box 12-1, Risks of Restraint Use, in the textbook.
- Restraints may also affect a person's dignity and self-esteem. Depression, anger, and agitation are common. So are embarrassment, humiliation, and mistrust.

Legal Aspects

- *Restraints must protect the person.* A restraint is used only when it is the best safety measure for the person.
- *A doctor's order is required.* The doctor gives the reason for the restraint, what body part to restrain, what to use, and how long to use it.
- *The least restrictive method is used.* It allows the greatest amount of movement or body access possible.
- *Restraints are used only after other measures fail to protect the person.* Box 12-2 lists alternatives to restraint use.
- *Unnecessary restraint is false imprisonment.* If you apply an unneeded restraint, you could face false imprisonment charges.
- *Consent is required.* The person must understand the reason for the restraint. If the person cannot give consent, his or her legal representative must give consent before a restraint can be used. The doctor or nurse provides the necessary information and obtains the consent. However, using restraints cannot be refused if used as a last resort because the person's behavior causes an immediate threat to self or others.

Safety Guidelines

- Review Box 12-3, Safety Measures for Using Restraints, in the textbook.
- *Observe for increased confusion and agitation.* Restraints can increase confusion and agitation. Restrained persons need repeated explanations and reassurance. Spending time with them has a calming effect.
- *Protect the person's quality of life.* Restraints are used for as short a time as possible. You must meet the person's physical, emotional, and social needs.
- *Follow the manufacturer instructions.* The restraint must be snug and firm but not tight. You could be negligent if you do not apply or secure a restraint properly.

- *Apply restraints with enough help to protect the person and staff from injury.*
- *Observe the person at least every 15 minutes or more often as noted in the care plan.* Injuries and deaths can result from improper restraint use and poor observation.
- *Remove or release the restraint, reposition the person, and meet basic needs at least every 2 hours or as often as noted in the care plan.* This includes food, fluid, comfort, safety, hygiene, and elimination needs and giving skin care. Perform range-of-motion exercises or help the person walk.

Reporting and Recording

- Report and record the following:
  - Type of restraint applied.
  - Body part or parts restrained.
  - Reason for the restraint.
  - Safety measures taken.
  - Time you applied the restraint.
  - Time you removed or released the restraint.
  - Care given when restraint was removed.
  - Person's vital signs.
  - Skin color and condition.
  - Condition of the limbs.
  - Pulse felt in the restrained part.
  - Changes in the person's behavior.
  - Complaints of discomfort; a tight restraint; difficulty breathing; or pain, numbness, or tingling in the restrained part. Report these complaints to the nurse at once.

CHAPTER 12 REVIEW QUESTIONS
Circle the BEST answer.

1. A geriatric chair or a bed rail may be considered a restraint if free movement is restricted.
   a. True
   b. False
2. Which statement about the use of restraints is *false?*
   a. A person may be embarrassed and humiliated when restraints are on.
   b. A person may experience depression and agitation when restraints are on.
   c. Restraints can be used for staff convenience.
   d. Restraints can cause serious injury and death.
3. Restraints can increase a person's confusion and agitation.
   a. True
   b. False
4. The person with a restraint should be observed at least every
   a. 15 minutes
   b. 30 minutes
   c. Hour
   d. 2 hours

5. Restraints need to be removed at least every
   a. Hour
   b. 2 hours
   c. 3 hours
   d. 4 hours
6. You should record all the following *except*
   a. The type of restraint used
   b. The consent for the restraint
   c. The time you removed the restraint
   d. The care you gave when the restraint was removed

Answers to these questions are on p. 505.

CHAPTER 13 PREVENTING INFECTION
MICROORGANISMS

- A **microorganism (microbe)** is a small *(micro)* living plant or animal *(organism)*.
- Some microbes are harmful and can cause infections **(pathogens)**. Others do not usually cause infection **(non-pathogens)**.

Multidrug-Resistant Organisms

- *Multidrug-resistant organisms (MDROs)* can resist the effects of antibiotics. Such organisms are able to change their structures to survive in the presence of antibiotics. The infections they cause are harder to treat.
- MDROs are caused by doctors prescribing antibiotics when they are not needed (over-prescribing). Not taking antibiotics for the prescribed length of time is also a cause.
- Two common types of MDROs are resistant to many antibiotics:
  - *Methicillin-resistant* Staphylococcus aureus *(MRSA)*
  - *Vancomycin-resistant* Enterococcus *(VRE)*

INFECTION

- An **infection** is a disease state resulting from the invasion and growth of microbes in the body.
- Review Box 13-1, Signs and Symptoms of Infection, in the textbook.

Healthcare-Associated Infection

- A **healthcare-associated infection (HAI)** is an infection that develops in a person cared for in any setting where health care is given. Hospitals, nursing centers, clinics, and home care settings are examples. HAIs also are called *nosocomial infections.*
- The health team must prevent the spread of HAIs by:
  - Medical asepsis. This includes hand hygiene.
  - Surgical asepsis.
  - Standard Precautions and Transmission-Based Precautions.
  - The Bloodborne Pathogen Standard.

Infection in Older Persons

- Older persons may not show the normal signs and symptoms of infection. The person may have only a slight fever or no fever at all. Redness and swelling may be very slight. The person may not complain of pain. Confusion and delirium may occur.
- Infections can become life-threatening before the older person has obvious signs and symptoms. Be alert to minor changes in the person's behavior or condition. Review Box 13-1, Signs and Symptoms of Infection, in the textbook. Report any concerns to the nurse at once.

MEDICAL ASEPSIS

- **Asepsis** is being free of disease-producing microbes.
- **Medical asepsis (clean technique)** refers to the practices used to:
  - Remove or destroy pathogens.
  - Prevent pathogens from spreading from one person or place to another person or place.

Common Aseptic Practices

- To prevent the spread of microbes, wash your hands:
  - After urinating or having a bowel movement.
  - After changing tampons or sanitary pads.
  - After contact with your own or another person's blood, body fluids, secretions, or excretions. This includes saliva, vomitus, urine, feces, vaginal discharge, mucus, semen, wound drainage, pus, and respiratory secretions.
  - After coughing, sneezing, or blowing your nose.
  - Before and after handling, preparing, or eating food.
  - After smoking a cigarette, cigar, or pipe.
- Also do the following:
  - Provide all persons with their own linens and personal care items.
  - Cover your nose and mouth when coughing, sneezing, or blowing your nose.
  - Bathe, wash hair, and brush your teeth regularly.
  - Wash fruits and raw vegetables before eating or serving them.
  - Wash cooking and eating utensils with soap and water after use.

Hand Hygiene

- *Hand hygiene is the easiest and most important way to prevent the spread of infection.* Practice hand hygiene before and after giving care. Review Box 13-2, Rules of Hand Hygiene, in the textbook.

Supplies and Equipment

- Most health care equipment is disposable. Bedpans, urinals, wash basins, water pitchers, and drinking cups are multi-use items. Do not "borrow" them for another person.
- Non-disposable items are cleaned and then disinfected. Then they are sterilized.

Other Aseptic Measures
- Review Box 13-3, Aseptic Measures, in the textbook.

ISOLATION PRECAUTIONS
- Isolation precautions prevent the spread of **communicable diseases (contagious diseases).** They are diseases caused by pathogens that spread easily.
- The CDC's isolation precautions guideline has two tiers of precautions:
  - Standard Precautions
  - Transmission-Based Precautions

Standard Precautions
- Standard Precautions reduce the risk of spreading pathogens and known and unknown infections. Standard Precautions are used for all persons whenever care is given. They prevent the spread of infection from:
  - Blood.
  - All body fluids, secretions, and excretions even if blood is not visible. Sweat is not known to spread infections.
  - Non-intact skin (skin with open breaks).
  - Mucous membranes.
- Review Box 13-4, Standard Precautions, in the textbook.

Transmission-Based Precautions
- Some infections require Transmission-Based Precautions. Review Box 13-5, Transmission-Based Precautions, in the textbook.
- Agency policies may differ from those in the book. The rules in Box 13-6, Rules for Isolation Precautions, in the textbook are a guide for giving safe care.

Protective Measures
- Isolation precautions involve wearing personal protective equipment (PPE)—gloves, a gown, a mask, and goggles or a face shield.
- Removing linens, trash, and equipment from the room may require double-bagging.
- Follow agency procedures when collecting specimens and transporting persons.
- Wear gloves whenever contact with blood, body fluids, secretions, excretions, mucous membranes, and non-intact skin is likely. Wearing gloves is the most common protective measure used with Standard Precautions and Transmission-Based Precautions. Remember the following when using gloves:
  - The outside of gloves is contaminated.
  - Gloves are easier to put on when your hands are dry.
  - Do not tear gloves when putting them on.
  - You need a new pair for every person.
  - Remove and discard torn, cut, or punctured gloves at once. Practice hand hygiene. Then put on a new pair.
  - Wear gloves once. Discard them after use.
  - Put on clean gloves just before touching mucous membranes or non-intact skin.
  - Put on new gloves whenever gloves become contaminated with blood, body fluids, secretions, or excretions. A task may require more than one pair of gloves.
  - Change gloves if interacting with the person involves touching portable computer keyboards or other mobile equipment that is transported from room to room.
  - Put on gloves last when worn with other PPE.
  - Change gloves whenever moving from a contaminated body site to a clean body site.
  - Make sure gloves cover your wrists. If you wear a gown, gloves cover the cuffs.
  - Remove gloves so the inside part is on the outside. The inside is clean.
  - Decontaminate your hands after removing gloves.
- Latex allergies are common and can cause skin rashes. Asthma and shock are more serious problems. Report skin rashes and breathing problems at once. If you or a resident has a latex allergy, wear latex-free gloves.
- Gowns must completely cover your neck to your knees. The gown front and sleeves are considered contaminated. A wet gown is contaminated. Gowns are used once. When removing a gown, roll it away from you. Keep it inside out.
- Masks are disposable. A wet or moist mask is contaminated. When removing a mask, touch only the ties or elastic bands. The front of the mask is contaminated.
- The outside of goggles or a face shield is contaminated. Use the device's ties, headband, or ear-pieces to remove the device.
- Contaminated items, linens, and trash are bagged to remove them from the person's room. Leak-proof plastic bags are used. They have the BIOHAZARD symbol. Double-bagging is not needed unless the outside of the bag is soiled.

Meeting Basic Needs
- Love, belonging, and self-esteem needs are often unmet when Transmission-Based Precautions are used. Visitors and staff often avoid the person. The person may feel lonely, unwanted, and rejected. He or she may feel dirty and undesirable. The person may feel ashamed and guilty for having a contagious disease. You can help meet the person's needs.

BLOODBORNE PATHOGEN STANDARD
- The health team is at risk for exposure to the human immunodeficiency virus (HIV) and the hepatitis B virus (HBV). HIV and HBV are bloodborne pathogens found in the blood.

- The Bloodborne Pathogen Standard is intended to protect you from exposure.
- Staff at risk for exposure to HIV and HBV receive free training.
- *Hepatitis B vaccination.* You can receive the hepatitis B vaccination within 10 working days of being hired. The agency pays for it. If you refuse the vaccination, you must sign a statement. You can have the vaccination at a later date.

Engineering and Work Practice Controls

- *Engineering controls* reduce employee exposure in the workplace. There are special containers for contaminated sharps (needles, broken glass) and specimens. These containers are puncture-resistant, leak-proof, and color-coded in red. They have the BIOHAZARD symbol.
- *Work practice controls* reduce exposure risk. All tasks involving blood or other potentially infectious materials (OPIM) are done in ways to limit splatters, splashes, and sprays. Other controls include:
  - Do not eat, drink, smoke, apply cosmetics or lip balm, or handle contact lenses in areas of occupational exposure.
  - Do not store food or drinks where blood or OPIM are kept.
  - Practice hand hygiene after removing gloves.
  - Wash hands as soon as possible after skin contact with blood or OPIM.
  - Never recap, bend, or remove needles by hand.
  - Never shear or break contaminated needles.
  - Discard contaminated needles and sharp instruments (razors) in containers that are closable, puncture-resistant, and leak-proof.

Personal Protective Equipment (PPE)

- This includes gloves, goggles, face shields, masks, laboratory coats, gowns, shoe covers, and surgical caps. For safe handling and use of PPE:
  - Remove PPE before leaving the work area.
  - Remove PPE when a garment becomes contaminated.
  - Place used PPE in marked areas or containers when being stored, washed, decontaminated, or discarded.
  - Wear gloves when you expect contact with blood or OPIM.
  - Wear gloves when handling or touching contaminated items or surfaces.
  - Replace worn, punctured, or contaminated gloves.
  - Never wash or decontaminate disposable gloves for re-use.
  - Discard utility gloves that show signs of cracking, peeling, tearing, or puncturing. Utility gloves are decontaminated for re-use if the process will not ruin them.

Equipment

- Contaminated equipment is cleaned and decontaminated. Decontaminate work surfaces with a proper disinfectant:
  - Upon completing tasks
  - At once when there is obvious contamination
  - After any spill of blood or OPIM
  - At the end of the work shift when surfaces become contaminated

Laundry

- The Occupational and Safety Health Administration (OSHA) requires these measures for contaminated laundry:
  - Handle it as little as possible.
  - Wear gloves or other needed PPE.
  - Bag contaminated laundry where it is used.
  - Mark laundry bags or containers with the BIOHAZARD symbol for laundry sent off-site.
  - Place wet, contaminated laundry in leak-proof containers before transport. The containers are color-coded in red or have the BIOHAZARD symbol.

Exposure Incidents

- Report exposure incidents at once. Medical evaluation, follow-up, and required tests are free. Your blood is tested for HIV and HBV. Confidentiality is important.

CHAPTER 13 REVIEW QUESTIONS
Circle the BEST answer.

1. A healthcare-associated infection (nosocomial infection) is
   a. An infection free of disease-producing microbes
   b. An infection that develops in a person cared for in any setting where health care is given
   c. An infection acquired by health care workers
   d. An infection acquired only by older persons
2. Which statement about hand hygiene is *false*?
   a. Hand hygiene is the easiest way to prevent the spread of infection.
   b. Hand hygiene is the most important way to prevent the spread of infection.
   c. Hand hygiene is practiced before and after giving care to a person.
   d. If hands are visibly soiled, hand hygiene can be done with an alcohol-based hand rub.
3. When washing your hands, you should do all of the following *except*
   a. Stand away from the sink so your clothes do not touch the sink
   b. Keep your hands lower than your elbows
   c. Wash your hands for at least 15 seconds
   d. Dry your arms from the forearms to the fingertips

4. Which statement about wearing gloves is *false*?
   a. The insides of gloves are contaminated.
   b. You need a new pair of gloves for each person you care for.
   c. Change gloves when moving from a contaminated body site to a clean body site.
   d. Gloves need to cover your wrists.
5. Which statement is *false*?
   a. Gowns must cover you from your neck to your waist.
   b. A moist mask is contaminated.
   c. The outside of goggles is contaminated.
   d. You should wash your hands after removing a gown, mask, or goggles.
6. Which statement about PPE is *false*?
   a. Remove PPE when a garment becomes contaminated.
   b. Wear gloves when handling or touching contaminated items or surfaces.
   c. Wash or decontaminate disposable gloves for re-use.
   d. Remove PPE before leaving the work area.

Answers to these questions are on p. 505.

CHAPTER 14 BODY MECHANICS AND SAFE RESIDENT HANDLING, POSITIONING, AND TRANSFERS
PRINCIPLES OF BODY MECHANICS

- Your strongest and largest muscles are in the shoulders, upper arms, hips, and thighs. Use these muscles to lift and move persons and heavy objects.
- For good body mechanics:
  - Bend your knees and squat to lift a heavy object. Do not bend from your waist.
  - Hold items close to your body and base of support.
- Review Box 14-1, Rules for Body Mechanics, in your textbook.

ERGONOMICS

- **Ergonomics** is the science of designing a job to fit the worker. The task, work station, equipment, and tools are changed to help reduce stress on the worker's body. The goal is to prevent injury and disorders of the muscles, tendons, ligaments, joints, cartilage, and nervous system.
- Early signs and symptoms of injury include pain, limited joint movement, or soft tissue swelling. Always report a work-related injury as soon as possible. Early attention can help prevent the problem from becoming worse.

POSITIONING THE PERSON

- The person must be properly positioned at all times. Regular position changes and good alignment promote comfort and well-being. Breathing is

easier. Circulation is promoted. Pressure ulcers and contractures are prevented.
- Whether in bed or in a chair, the person is repositioned at least every 2 hours. To safely position a person:
  - Use good body mechanics.
  - Ask a co-worker to help you if needed.
  - Explain the procedure to the person.
  - Be gentle when moving the person.
  - Provide for privacy.
  - Use pillows as directed by the nurse for support and alignment.
  - Provide for comfort after positioning.
  - Place the call light within reach after positioning.
  - Complete a safety check before leaving the room.
  - Use pillows and positioning devices to support body parts and keep the person in good alignment.
- **Fowler's position** is a semi-sitting position. The head of the bed is raised between 45 and 60 degrees. The knees may be slightly elevated.
- The **supine position (dorsal recumbent position)** is the back-lying position.
- A person in the **prone position** lies on the abdomen with the head turned to one side.
- A person in the **lateral position (side-lying position)** lies on one side or the other.
- The **Sims' position (semi-prone side position)** is a left side-lying position.
- Persons who sit in chairs must hold their upper bodies and heads erect. For good alignment:
  - The person's back and buttocks are against the back of the chair.
  - Feet are flat on the floor or wheelchair footplates. Never leave feet unsupported.
  - Backs of the knees and calves are slightly away from the edge of the seat.

PREVENTING WORK-RELATED INJURIES

- To prevent work-related injuries:
  - Wear shoes that provide good traction.
  - Use assist equipment and devices whenever possible.
  - Get help from other staff.
  - Plan and prepare for the task. Know what equipment you will need and on what side of the bed to place the chair or wheelchair.
  - Schedule harder tasks early in your shift.
  - Tell the resident what he or she can do to help. Give clear, simple instructions.
  - Do not hold or grab the person under the arms.
- For additional guidelines, review Box 14-2, Preventing Work-Related Injuries, in the textbook.

PROTECTING THE SKIN

- Protect the person's skin from friction and shearing. Both cause infection and pressure ulcers. To reduce friction and shearing:

- Roll the person.
- Use a lift sheet (turning sheet).
- Use a turning pad, slide board, slide sheet, or large incontinence product.

MOVING PERSONS IN BED

- Before moving a person in bed, you need to know from the nurse and care plan:
  - What procedure to use
  - How many workers are needed to move the person safely
  - Position limits and restrictions
  - How far you can lower the head of the bed
  - Any limits in the person's ability to move or be repositioned
  - What equipment is needed—trapeze, lift sheet, slide sheet, mechanical lift
  - How to position the person
  - If the person uses bed rails
  - What observations to report and record:
    - Who helped you with the procedure
    - How much help the person needed
    - How the person tolerated the procedure
    - How you positioned the person
    - Complaints of pain or discomfort
  - When to report observations
  - What specific concerns to report at once

Moving the Person Up in Bed

- You can sometimes move light-weight adults up in bed alone if they can assist and use a trapeze. Two or more staff members are needed to move heavy, weak, and very old persons up in bed. Always protect the person and yourself from injury.
- Assist devices are used to reduce shearing and friction. Such assist devices include a drawsheet (lift sheet), flat sheet folded in half, turning pad, slide sheet, and large incontinence product.

TURNING PERSONS

- Turning persons onto their sides helps prevent complications from bedrest. Certain procedures and care measures also require the side-lying position. After the person is turned, position him or her in good alignment. Use pillows as directed to support the person in the side-lying position.
- **Logrolling** is turning the person as a unit, in alignment, with one motion. The spine is kept straight.

SITTING ON THE SIDE OF THE BED (DANGLING)

- Many older persons become dizzy or faint when getting out of bed too fast. They need to sit on the side of the bed before walking or transferring. Some persons

increase activity in stages—bedrest, to sitting on the side of the bed, to sitting in a chair, to walking.
- While dangling, the person coughs and deep breathes. He or she moves the legs back and forth in circles to stimulate circulation. Provide for warmth during dangling.
- Observations to report and record:
  - Pulse and respiratory rates
  - Pale or bluish skin color (cyanosis)
  - Complaints of light-headedness, dizziness, or difficulty breathing
  - How well the activity was tolerated
  - The length of time the person dangled
  - The amount of help needed
  - Other observations and complaints

TRANSFERRING PERSONS

- The rules of body mechanics apply during transfers.
- Arrange the room so there is enough space for a safe transfer. Correct placement of the chair, wheelchair, or other device also is needed for a safe transfer.
- Have the person wear non-skid footwear for transfers.
- Lock the wheels of the bed, wheelchair, stretcher, or other assist device.
- After the transfer, position the person in good alignment.
- Transfer belts (gait belts) are used to support persons during transfers and reposition persons in chairs and wheelchairs.

Bed to Chair or Wheelchair Transfers

- Safety is important for transfers. In transferring, the strong side moves first. Help the person out of bed on his or her strong side. Help the person from the wheelchair to the bed on his or her strong side.
- The person must not put his or her arms around your neck.

Mechanical Lifts

- Persons who cannot help themselves are transferred with mechanical lifts. So are persons who are too heavy for the staff to transfer.
- Before using a mechanical lift, you must be trained in its use. The sling, straps, hooks, and chains must be in good repair. The person's weight must not exceed the lift's capacity. At least two staff members are needed. Always follow the manufacturer instructions for using the lift.
- Falling from the lift is a common fear. To promote the person's mental comfort, always explain the procedure before you begin. Also show the person how the lift works.

CHAPTER 14 REVIEW QUESTIONS
Circle the BEST answer.

1. To lift and move residents and heavy objects you should
   a. Use the muscles in your lower arms
   b. Use the muscles in your legs
   c. Use the muscles in your shoulders, upper arms, hips, and thighs
   d. Use the muscles in your abdomen

2. For good body mechanics, you should do all of the following *except*
   a. Bend your knees and squat to lift a heavy object
   b. Bend from your waist to lift a heavy object
   c. Hold items close to your body and base of support
   d. Bend your legs; do not bend your back

3. Which statement is *false*?
   a. A person must be properly positioned at all times.
   b. Regular position changes and good alignment promote comfort and well-being.
   c. Regular position changes and good alignment promote pressure ulcers and contractures.
   d. When a person is in good alignment, breathing is easier and circulation is promoted.

4. In Fowler's position
   a. The head of the bed is flat
   b. The head of the bed is raised to 90 degrees
   c. The head of the bed is raised between 45 and 60 degrees
   d. The head of the bed is raised between 30 and 35 degrees

5. Friction and shearing are reduced by doing all of the following *except*
   a. Rolling the person
   b. Using a lift sheet or turning pad
   c. Using a pillow
   d. Using a slide board or slide sheet

6. After a person is turned, you must position him or her in good alignment.
   a. True
   b. False

7. Which statement about dangling is *false*?
   a. Many older persons become dizzy or faint when they first dangle.
   b. The person should cough and deep breathe while dangling.
   c. The person moves his or her legs before dangling.
   d. You should cover the person's shoulders with a robe or blanket while dangling.

8. You are transferring a person from the bed to a wheelchair. Which statement is *false*?
   a. The person should wear non-skid footwear.
   b. The person may put his or her arm around your neck.
   c. You should use a gait/transfer belt.
   d. You should lock the wheelchair wheels.

9. A person has a weak left side and a strong right side. In transferring the person from the bed to the wheelchair, his or her strong (right) side moves first.
   a. True
   b. False

10. Before using a mechanical lift, you do all of the following *except*
    a. Check the sling, straps, and chains to ensure good repair
    b. Check the person's weight to be sure it does not exceed the lift's capacity
    c. Follow the manufacturer instructions for using the lift
    d. Operate the lift without a co-worker

Answers to these questions are on p. 505.

CHAPTER 15 THE RESIDENT'S UNIT
- A resident unit is the personal space, furniture, and equipment provided for the person by the nursing center. Resident units are as personal and home-like as possible.

Comfort
- Age, illness, and activity are factors that affect comfort.
- Temperature, ventilation, noise, odors, and lighting are factors that are controlled to meet the person's needs.

Temperature and Ventilation
- Older persons, and those who are ill, may need higher temperatures for comfort.
- To protect older and ill persons from cool areas and drafts:
  - Keep room temperatures warm.
  - Make sure they wear the correct clothing.
  - Offer lap robes to cover the legs.
  - Provide enough blankets for warmth.
  - Cover them with bath blankets when giving care.
  - Move them from drafty areas.

Odors
- To reduce odors in nursing centers:
  - Empty, clean, and disinfect bedpans, urinals, commodes, and kidney basins promptly.
  - Check to make sure toilets are flushed.
  - Check incontinent people often.
  - Clean persons who are wet or soiled from urine, feces, or wound drainage.
  - Change wet or soiled linens and clothing promptly.
  - Keep laundry containers closed.
  - Follow agency policy for wet or soiled linens and clothing.

- Dispose of incontinence and ostomy products promptly.
- Provide good hygiene to prevent body and breath odors.
- Use room deodorizers as needed.
- If you smoke, practice hand washing after handling smoking materials and before giving care. Give careful attention to your uniform, hair, and breath because of smoke odors.

Noise
- To decrease noise:
  - Control your voice.
  - Handle equipment carefully.
  - Keep equipment in good working order.
  - Answer phones, call lights, and intercoms promptly.

Lighting
- Adjust lighting to meet the person's needs. Glares, shadows, and dull lighting can cause falls, headaches, and eyestrain. A bright room is cheerful. Dim light is better for relaxing and rest. Persons with poor vision need bright light. Always keep light controls within the person's reach.

ROOM FURNITURE AND EQUIPMENT
- Rooms are furnished and equipped to meet basic needs.

The Bed
- Beds are raised to give care. They are positioned at the lowest level when not giving care.
- Bed wheels are locked at all times except when moving the bed.
- Use bed rails as the nurse and care plan direct.
- Basic bed positions:
  - *Flat*—the usual sleeping position.
  - *Fowler's position*—a semi-sitting position. The head of the bed is raised between 45 and 60 degrees.
  - *High-Fowler's position*—a semi-sitting position. The head of the bed is raised between 60 and 90 degrees.
  - *Semi-Fowler's position*—the head of the bed is raised 30 degrees. Some agencies define semi-Fowler's position as when the head of the bed is raised 30 degrees and the knee portion is raised 15 degrees. Know the definition used by your agency.
  - *Trendelenburg's position*—the head of the bed is lowered and the foot of the bed is raised. A doctor orders the position.
  - *Reverse Trendelenburg's position*—the head of the bed is raised and the foot of the bed is lowered. A doctor orders the position.

Bed Safety
- *Entrapment* means the person can get caught, trapped, or entangled in spaces created by bed rails, the mattress, the bed frame, or the head-board

and foot-board. Serious injuries and deaths have occurred from entrapment. If a person is at risk for entrapment, report your concerns to the nurse at once. If a person is caught, trapped, or entangled, try to release the person. Call for the nurse at once.

The Over-bed Table
- Only clean and sterile items are placed on the over-bed table. Never place bedpans, urinals, or soiled linens on the over-bed table or on top of the bedside stand.
- Clean the table and bedside stand after using them as a work surface.

Privacy Curtains
- Always pull the curtain completely around the bed before giving care. Privacy curtains do not block sound or conversations.

The Call System
- The call light must always be kept within the person's reach—in the room, bathroom, and shower or tub room. You must:
  - Place the call light on the person's strong side.
  - Remind the person to signal when help is needed.
  - Answer call lights promptly.
  - Answer bathroom and shower or tub room call lights at once.
- Persons with limited hand mobility may need special communication measures.
- Be careful when using the intercom. Remember confidentiality. Persons nearby can hear what you and the person say.

Closet and Drawer Space
- The person must have free access to the closet and its contents. You must have the person's permission to open or search closets or drawers.
- Agency staff can inspect a person's closet or drawers if hoarding is suspected. The person is informed of the inspection and is present when it takes place. Have a co-worker present when you inspect a person's closet.

General Rules
- Keep the person's room clean, neat, safe, and comfortable. Follow the rules in Box 15-1, Maintaining the Person's Unit, and Box 15-2, OBRA and CMS Requirements for Resident Rooms.

CHAPTER 15 REVIEW QUESTIONS
Circle the BEST answer.
1. Serious injuries and death have occurred from entrapment.
   a. True
   b. False

2. You should never place bedpans, urinals, or soiled linens on the over-bed table.
   a. True
   b. False
3. You should clean the bedside stand if you use it for a work surface.
   a. True
   b. False
4. The following protect a person from drafts *except*
   a. Wearing enough clothing
   b. Lap robes
   c. Using a sheet when giving care
   d. Providing blankets
5. To reduce odors, you do all of the following *except*
   a. Empty bedpans and commodes promptly
   b. Keep laundry containers open
   c. Check to make sure toilets are flushed
   d. Clean persons who are wet or soiled from urine or feces
6. Which statement about the call light is *false?*
   a. The call light must always be within the person's reach.
   b. Place the call light on the person's strong side.
   c. You have to answer the call lights only for residents assigned to you.
   d. Answer call lights promptly.
7. You suspect a person is hoarding food in her closet. Before you inspect the closet, what do you do?
   a. Tell another nursing assistant what you suspect
   b. Inspect the closet without telling the resident
   c. Tell the family
   d. Ask the resident if you can inspect the closet

Answers to these questions are on p. 505.

CHAPTER 16   BEDMAKING

- Clean, dry, and wrinkle-free linens promote comfort. Skin breakdown and pressure ulcers are prevented.
- To keep beds neat and clean:
  - Straighten linens whenever loose or wrinkled and at bedtime.
  - Check for and remove food and crumbs after meals.
  - Check linens for dentures, eyeglasses, hearing aids, sharp objects, and other items.
  - Change linens whenever they become wet, soiled, or damp.
  - Follow Standard Precautions and the Bloodborne Pathogen Standard.

TYPES OF BEDS

- Beds are made in these ways:
  - A closed bed is not used until bedtime. Or the bed is ready for a new resident. Top linens are not folded back.
  - An open bed is in use. Top linens are fan-folded back so the person can get into bed. A closed bed becomes an open bed by fan-folding back the top linens.
  - An occupied bed is made with the person in it.
  - A surgical bed is made to transfer a person from a stretcher. This bed is also made for persons who arrive by ambulance.

LINENS

- When handling linens and making beds:
  - Practice medical asepsis.
  - Always hold linens away from your body and uniform. Your uniform is considered dirty.
  - Never shake linens.
  - Place clean linens on a clean surface.
  - Never put clean or dirty linens on the floor.
- Collect enough linens. Do not bring unneeded linens into the person's room. Once in the room, extra linens are considered contaminated. They cannot be used for another person.
- Roll each piece of dirty linen away from you. The side that touched the person is inside the roll and away from you.

Making Beds

- When making beds, safety and medical asepsis are important. Use good body mechanics. Follow the rules for safe resident handling, moving, and transfers. Practice hand hygiene before handling clean linens and after handling dirty linens. To save time and energy, make beds with a co-worker.
- Review Box 16-1, Rules for Bedmaking, in the textbook.

The Occupied Bed

- You make an occupied bed when the person stays in bed. Keep the person in good alignment. Follow restrictions or limits in the person's movement or position. Explain each procedure step to the person before it is done. This is important even if the person cannot respond to you.

CHAPTER 16 REVIEW QUESTIONS
Circle the BEST answer.

1. Once in the person's room, extra linens are considered contaminated. They can be used for another person.
   a. True
   b. False
2. Roll each piece of dirty linen away from you. The side that touched the person is inside the roll.
   a. True
   b. False

3. Wear gloves when removing linens from the person's bed.
   a. True
   b. False
4. To keep beds neat and clean, do the following *except*
   a. Straighten linens whenever loose or wrinkled
   b. Check for and remove food and crumbs after meals
   c. Check linens for dentures, eyeglasses, and hearing aids
   d. Change linens monthly
5. Which statement is *false?*
   a. Practice medical asepsis when handling linens.
   b. Always hold linens away from your body and uniform.
   c. Shake linens to remove crumbs.
   d. Put dirty linens in the dirty laundry bin.

Answers to these questions are on p. 505.

CHAPTER 17 HYGIENE

- Besides cleansing, good hygiene prevents body and breath odors. It is relaxing and increases circulation.
- Culture and personal choice affect hygiene.

DAILY CARE

- Most people have hygiene routines and habits. Hygiene measures are often done before and after meals and at bedtime. You assist with hygiene whenever it is needed. Protect the person's right to privacy and to personal choice.

ORAL HYGIENE

- Oral hygiene keeps the mouth and teeth clean. It prevents mouth odors and infections, increases comfort, and makes food taste better. Mouth care also reduces the risk for cavities and periodontal disease.
- Assist with oral hygiene after sleep, after meals, and at bedtime. Follow the care plan.
- Follow Standard Precautions and the Bloodborne Pathogen Standard.
- Report and record:
  - Dry, cracked, swollen, or blistered lips
  - Mouth or breath odor
  - Redness, swelling, irritation, sores, or white patches in the mouth or on the tongue
  - Bleeding, swelling, or redness of the gums
  - Loose teeth
  - Rough, sharp, or chipped areas on dentures

Brushing and Flossing Teeth
- Flossing removes plaque and tartar from the teeth as well as food from between the teeth. Flossing is usually done after brushing. If done once a day, bedtime is the best time to floss.

- Some persons need help gathering and setting up equipment for oral hygiene. You may have to perform oral care for persons who are weak, cannot move their arms, or are too confused to brush their teeth.

Mouth Care for the Unconscious Person
- Unconscious persons have dry mouths and crusting on the tongue and mucous membranes. Oral hygiene keeps the mouth clean and moist. It also helps prevent infection.
- Use sponge swabs to apply the cleaning agent. To prevent cracking of the lips, apply a lubricant to the lips. Check the care plan.
- To prevent aspiration by the unconscious person:
  - Position the person on one side with the head turned well to the side.
  - Use only a small amount of fluid to clean the mouth.
  - Do not insert dentures. Dentures are not worn when the person is unconscious.
- When giving oral hygiene, keep the person's mouth open with a padded tongue blade.
- Mouth care is given at least every 2 hours. Follow the nurse's direction and the care plan.

Denture Care
- Mouth care is given and dentures are cleaned as often as natural teeth. Dentures are usually removed at bedtime. Remind people not to wrap dentures in tissues or napkins.
- Dentures are slippery when wet. Hold them firmly. During cleaning, hold them over a basin of water lined with a towel. Use a cleaning agent and follow the manufacturer instructions.
- Hot water causes dentures to lose their shape. If dentures are not worn after cleaning, store them in a container with cool water or a denture soaking solution.
- Label the denture cup with the person's name, room number, and bed number. Report lost or damaged dentures to the nurse at once. Losing or damaging dentures is negligent conduct.
- Many people do not like being seen without their dentures. Privacy is important. If you clean dentures, return them to the person as quickly as possible.
- Persons with partial dentures have some natural teeth. They need to brush and floss the natural teeth.

BATHING

- Bathing cleans the skin. The mucous membranes of the genital and anal areas are cleaned as well. A bath is refreshing and relaxing. Circulation is stimulated and body parts are exercised. You have time to talk to the person. You also can make observations.
- Review Box 17-1, Rules for Bathing, in the textbook.

- Soap dries the skin. Therefore, older persons usually need a complete bath or shower twice a week. Partial baths are taken on the other days. Some bathe daily but not with soap. Thorough rinsing is needed when using soap. Lotions and oils keep the skin soft.
- Water temperature for complete bed baths and partial bed baths is between 110°F and 115°F. Older persons have fragile skin and need lower water temperatures. Measure water temperature according to agency policy.
- Report and record:
  - The color of the skin, lips, nail beds, and sclera
  - The location and description of rashes
  - Dry skin
  - Bruises or open areas
  - Pale or reddened areas, especially over bony parts
  - Drainage or bleeding from wounds or body openings
  - Swelling of the feet and legs
  - Corns or calluses on the feet
  - Skin temperature
  - Complaints of pain or discomfort
- Use caution when applying powders. Do not use powders near persons with respiratory disorders. Do not sprinkle or shake powder onto the person. To safely apply powder:
  - Turn away from the person.
  - Sprinkle a small amount onto your hands or a cloth.
  - Apply the powder in a thin layer.
  - Make sure powder does not get on the floor. Powder is slippery and can cause falls.

The Complete Bed Bath

- The complete bed bath involves washing the person's entire body in bed. Wash around the person's eyes with water. Do not use soap. Gently wipe from the inner to the outer aspect of the eye. Use a clean part of the washcloth for each stroke. Ask the person if you should use soap to wash the face. Let the person wash the genital area if he or she is able.
- Give a back massage after the bath. Apply deodorant or antiperspirant, lotion, and powder as requested. Comb and brush the hair. Empty and clean the wash basin.

The Partial Bath

- The partial bath involves bathing the face, hands, axillae (underarms), back, buttocks, and perineal area. You assist the person as needed. Most need help washing the back.

Tub Baths and Showers

- Falls, burns, and chilling from water are risks. Review Box 17-2, Safety Measures for Tub Baths and Showers, in the textbook.
- A tub bath can cause a person to feel faint, weak, or tired. The person may need a transfer bench, a tub with a side entry door, a wheelchair or stretcher lift, or a mechanical lift to get in and out of the tub.
- Some people can use a regular shower. Have the person use the grab bars for support during the shower. Use a bath mat if the shower does not have non-skid surfaces. Never let weak or unsteady persons stand in the shower. They may need to use shower chairs, shower stalls or cabinets, or shower trolleys. Some shower rooms have two or more stations. Protect the person's privacy. Properly screen and cover the person.
- Water temperature for tub baths and showers is usually 105°F. Report and record dizziness and light-headedness.

THE BACK MASSAGE

- The back massage relaxes muscles and stimulates circulation.
- Massages are given after the bath and with evening care. You also can give back massages at other times, such as after re-positioning a person.
- Observe the skin for breaks, bruises, reddened areas, and other signs of skin breakdown.
- Lotion reduces friction during the massage. It is warmed before applying.
- Use firm strokes. Keep your hands in contact with the person's skin.
- After the massage, apply some lotion to the elbows, knees, and heels.
- Back massages are dangerous for persons with certain heart diseases, back injuries, back surgeries, skin diseases, and some lung disorders. Check with the nurse and the care plan before giving back massages to persons with these conditions.
- Do not massage reddened bony areas. Reddened areas signal skin breakdown and pressure ulcers. Massage can lead to more tissue damage.
- Wear gloves if the person's skin is not intact. Always follow Standard Precautions and the Bloodborne Pathogen Standard.
- Report and record skin breakdown, redness, and bruising.

PERINEAL CARE

- Perineal care involves cleaning the genital and anal areas. It is done daily during the bath and whenever the area is soiled with urine or feces. The person does perineal care if able.
- Perineal and perineum are not common terms. Most people understand privates, private parts, crotch, genitals, or the area between the legs. Use terms the person understands.
- Standard Precautions, medical asepsis, and the Bloodborne Pathogen Standard are followed.

- Work from the cleanest area to the dirtiest—commonly called cleaning from "front to back." On a woman, clean from the urethra (cleanest) to the anal (dirtiest) area. On a male, start at the meatus of the urethra and work outward.
- Use warm water. Use washcloths, towelettes, cotton balls, or swabs according to center policy. Rinse thoroughly. Pat dry. Water temperature is usually 105°F to 109°F.
- Report and record:
  - Bleeding, redness, swelling, irritation
  - Complaints of pain or burning
  - Signs of urinary or fecal incontinence
  - Signs of skin breakdown
  - Discharge from the vagina or urinary tract
  - Odors

CHAPTER 17 REVIEW QUESTIONS
Circle the BEST answer.

1. Oral hygiene does all of the following *except*
   a. Keeps the mouth and teeth clean
   b. Prevents mouth odors and infections
   c. Decreases comfort
   d. Makes food taste better
2. When giving oral hygiene, you should report and record all of the following *except*
   a. Dry, cracked, swollen, or blistered lips
   b. Redness, sores, or white patches in the mouth
   c. Bleeding, swelling, or redness of the gums
   d. The number of fillings a person has
3. A person is unconscious. When you do mouth care, you do all of the following *except*
   a. Use only a small amount of fluid to clean the mouth
   b. Use your fingers to keep the mouth open
   c. Explain what you are doing
   d. Give mouth care at least every 2 hours
4. Which statement about dentures is *false*?
   a. Dentures are slippery when wet.
   b. During cleaning, hold dentures over a basin of water lined with a towel.
   c. Store dentures in cool water.
   d. Remind people to wrap their dentures in tissues or napkins.
5. Bathing does all of the following *except*
   a. Cleanses the skin
   b. Stimulates circulation
   c. Makes a person tense
   d. Permits you to observe the person's skin
6. The water temperature for a complete bed bath is
   a. 102°F to 108°F
   b. 110°F to 115°F
   c. 115°F to 120°F
   d. 120°F to 125°F

7. Which statement is *false*?
   a. Use powder near persons with respiratory disorders.
   b. Before applying powder, check with the nurse and the care plan.
   c. Before applying powder, sprinkle a small amount of powder onto your hands.
   d. Apply powder in a thin layer.
8. When washing a person's eyes, you should do all of the following *except*
   a. Use only water
   b. Gently wipe from the inner to the outer aspect of the eye
   c. Gently wipe from the outer to the inner aspect of the eye
   d. Use a clean part of the washcloth for each stroke
9. Which statement is *false*?
   a. A back massage relaxes and stimulates circulation.
   b. Massages are given after the bath and with evening care.
   c. You can observe the person's skin before beginning the massage.
   d. You should use cold lotion for the massage.
10. When giving female perineal care, you should work from the urethra to the anal area.
    a. True
    b. False
11. When giving male perineal care, start at the meatus and work outward.
    a. True
    b. False

Answers to these questions are on p. 505.

CHAPTER 18 GROOMING
- Hair care, shaving, and nail and foot care prevent infection and promote comfort. They also affect love, belonging, and self-esteem needs.

HAIR CARE
- You assist patients and residents with brushing and combing hair and with shampooing according to the care plan. The nursing process reflects the person's culture, personal choice, skin and scalp condition, health history, and self-care ability.

Brushing and Combing Hair
- Brushing and combing prevent tangled, matted hair.
- When brushing and combing hair, start at the scalp and brush or comb to the hair ends.
- Never cut hair for any reason. Tell the nurse if you think the person's hair needs to be cut.
- Special measures are needed for curly, coarse, and dry hair. Check the care plan.

- When giving hair care, place a towel across the person's back and shoulders to protect garments from falling hair. If the person is in bed, give hair care before changing the linens and pillowcase.

Shampooing

- Shampooing frequency depends on the person's needs and preferences. Usually, shampooing is done weekly on the person's bath or shower day.
- Hair is dried and styled as quickly as possible after the shampoo.
- During shampooing, report and record:
  - Scalp sores
  - Flaking
  - Itching
  - Presence of nits or lice
  - Patches of hair loss
  - Very dry or very oily hair
  - Matted or tangled hair
  - How the person tolerated the procedure
- Keep shampoo away from and out of eyes. Have the person hold a washcloth over the eyes.
- Wear gloves if the person has scalp sores.
- Follow Standard Precautions and the Bloodborne Pathogen Standard.

SHAVING

- Review Box 18-1, Rules for Shaving, in your textbook.

Caring for Mustaches and Beards

- Wash and comb mustaches and beards daily and as needed. Ask the person how to groom his mustache or beard.
- Never trim a mustache or beard without the person's consent.

Shaving Legs and Underarms

- Many women shave their legs and underarms. This practice varies among cultures. Legs and underarms are shaved after bathing when the skin is soft.

NAIL AND FOOT CARE

- Nail and foot care prevent infection, injury, and odors.
- Nails are easier to trim and clean right after soaking or bathing.
- Use nail clippers to cut fingernails. Never use scissors. Use extreme caution to prevent damage to nearby tissues.
- Follow Standard Precautions and the Bloodborne Pathogen Standard.
- Report and record:
  - Reddened, irritated, or calloused areas
  - Breaks in the skin

- Corns on top of and between the toes
- Very thick nails
- Loose nails
- You do not cut or trim toenails if a person has diabetes or poor circulation to the legs and feet or takes medications that affect blood clotting. Also, do not cut or trim toenails if the person has very thick nails or ingrown toenails. The nurse or podiatrist cuts toenails and provides foot care for these persons.
- When doing foot care, check between the toes for cracks and sores. If left untreated, a serious infection could occur.
- The feet of persons with decreased sensation or circulatory problems may easily burn because they do not feel hot temperatures.
- After soaking, apply lotion to the feet. Because the lotion can cause slippery feet, help the person put on non-skid footwear before you transfer the person or let the person walk.

CHANGING CLOTHING AND HOSPITAL GOWNS

- Garments are changed after the bath and whenever wet or soiled.
- When changing clothing:
  - Provide for privacy.
  - Encourage the person to do as much as possible.
  - Let the person choose what to wear. Make sure the right undergarments are chosen.
  - Remove clothing from the strong or "good" (unaffected) side first.
  - Put clothing on the weak (affected) side first.
  - Support the arm or leg when removing or putting on a garment.

CHAPTER 18 REVIEW QUESTIONS
Circle the BEST answer.

1. Hair care, shaving, and nail and foot care prevent infection and promote comfort.
   a. True
   b. False
2. If a person's hair is matted, you may cut the hair.
   a. True
   b. False
3. When giving hair care, place a towel across the person's back and shoulders to protect garments from falling hair.
   a. True
   b. False
4. You should wear gloves when shampooing a person who has scalp sores.
   a. True
   b. False

5. A person takes an anticoagulant. Therefore, he shaves with a blade razor.
   a. True
   b. False
6. You should wear gloves when shaving a person.
   a. True
   b. False
7. Never trim a mustache or beard without the person's consent.
   a. True
   b. False
8. Mustaches and beards need daily care.
   a. True
   b. False
9. A person has diabetes. You can cut his or her toenails.
   a. True
   b. False
10. Fingernails are cut with
    a. Scissors
    b. Nail clippers
    c. An emery board
    d. A nail file
11. Which statement is *false*?
    a. Provide privacy when a person is changing clothes.
    b. Most residents wear street clothes during the day.
    c. Let the person choose what to wear.
    d. You may tear a person's clothing.

Answers to these questions are on p. 505.

CHAPTER 19 NUTRITION AND FLUIDS

- Food and water are necessary for life. A poor diet and poor eating habits:
  - Increase the risk for infection
  - Cause healing problems
  - Affect physical and mental function, increasing the risk for accidents and injuries

BASIC NUTRITION

- **Nutrition** is the process involved in the ingestion, digestion, absorption, and use of foods and fluids by the body. Good nutrition is needed for growth, healing, and body functions.
- A *nutrient* is a substance that is ingested, digested, absorbed, and used by the body.

Nutrients

- A well-balanced diet ensures an adequate intake of essential nutrients.
- *Protein*—is needed for tissue growth and repair. Sources include meat, fish, poultry, eggs, milk and milk products, cereals, beans, peas, and nuts.
- *Carbohydrates*—provide energy and fiber for bowel elimination. They are found in fruits, vegetables, breads, cereals, and sugar.

- *Fats*—provide energy, add flavor to food, and help the body use certain vitamins. Sources include meats, lard, butter, shortening, oils, milk, cheese, egg yolks, and nuts.
- *Vitamins*—are needed for certain body functions. The body stores vitamins A, D, E, and K. Vitamin C and the B complex vitamins must be ingested daily.
- *Minerals*—are needed for bone and tooth formation, nerve and muscle function, fluid balance, and other body processes.
- *Water*—is needed for all body processes.

FACTORS AFFECTING EATING AND NUTRITION

- *Age.* Many changes occur in the digestive system with aging.
- *Culture.* Culture influences dietary practices, food choices, and food preparation.
- *Religion.* Selecting, preparing, and eating food often involve religious practices. A person may follow all, some, or none of the dietary practices of his or her faith.
- *Appetite.* Illness, medications, anxiety, pain, and depression can cause loss of appetite. Unpleasant sights, thoughts, and smells are other causes.
- *Personal choice.* Food likes and dislikes are influenced by foods served in the home. Usually, food likes expand with age and social experiences.
- *Body reactions.* People usually avoid foods that cause allergic reactions. They also avoid foods that cause nausea, vomiting, diarrhea, indigestion, gas, or headaches.
- *Illness.* Appetite usually decreases during illness and recovery from injuries. However, nutritional needs are increased.
- *Disability.* Disease or injury can affect the hands, wrists, and arms. Adaptive equipment lets the person eat independently.

OBRA DIETARY REQUIREMENTS

- OBRA has requirements for food served in nursing centers:
  - Each person's nutritional and dietary needs are met.
  - The person's diet is well-balanced. It is nourishing and tastes good. Food is well-seasoned.
  - Food is appetizing. It has an appealing aroma and is attractive.
  - Hot food is served hot. Cold food is served cold.
  - Food is served promptly.
  - Food is prepared to meet each person's needs. Some people need food cut, ground, or chopped. Others have special diets ordered by the doctor.
  - Other foods are offered if the person refused the food served. Substituted food must have a similar nutritional value to the first foods served.

- Each person receives at least 3 meals a day. A bedtime snack is offered.
- The center provides needed adaptive equipment and utensils.

SPECIAL DIETS

The Sodium-Controlled Diet

- A sodium-controlled diet decreases the amount of sodium in the body. The diet involves:
  - Omitting high-sodium foods. Review Box 19-4, High-Sodium Foods, in the textbook.
  - Not adding salt when eating.
  - Limiting the amount of salt used in cooking.

Diabetes Meal Planning

- Diabetes meal planning is for people with diabetes. It involves the person's food preferences and calories needed. It also involves eating meals and snacks at regular times.
- Serve the person's meals and snacks on time to maintain a certain blood sugar level.
- Always check the tray to see what was eaten. Tell the nurse what the person did and did not eat. If not all the food was eaten, between-meal nourishment is needed. The nurse tells you what to give. Tell the nurse about changes in the person's eating habits.

The Dysphagia Diet

- **Dysphagia** means difficulty swallowing. Food thickness is changed to meet the person's needs. Review Box 19-5, Dysphagia Diet, in the textbook.
- You may need to feed a person with dysphagia. To promote the person's comfort:
  - Know the signs and symptoms of dysphagia. Review Box 19-6 in the textbook.
  - Feed the person according to the care plan and swallow guide.
  - Follow aspiration precautions. Review Box 19-7 in the textbook.
  - Report changes in how the person eats.
  - Report choking, coughing, or difficulty breathing during or after meals. Also report abnormal breathing or respiratory sounds. Report these observations at once.

FLUID BALANCE

- Fluid balance is needed for health. The amount of fluid taken in (**input**) and the amount of fluid lost (**output**) must be equal. If fluid intake exceeds fluid output, body tissues swell with water (**edema**).
- **Dehydration** is a decrease in the amount of water in body tissues. Fluid output exceeds intake. Common causes are poor fluid intake, vomiting, diarrhea, bleeding, excess sweating, and increased urine production.

Normal Fluid Requirements

- An adult needs 1500 mL of water daily to survive. About 2000 to 2500 mL of fluid per day is needed for normal fluid balance. Water requirements increase with hot weather, exercise, fever, illness, and excess fluid loss.
- Older persons may have a decreased sense of thirst. Their bodies need water, but they may not feel thirsty. Offer fluids according to the care plan.

Special Fluid Orders

- The doctor may order the amount of fluid a person can have in 24 hours. Intake and output (I&O) records are kept.
- *Encourage fluids.* The person drinks an increased amount of fluid.
- *Restrict fluids.* Fluids are limited to a certain amount.
- *Nothing by mouth (NPO).* The person cannot eat or drink.
- *Thickened liquids.* All liquids are thickened, including water.

INTAKE AND OUTPUT

- All fluids taken by mouth are measured and recorded—water, milk, and so forth. So are foods that melt at room temperature—ice cream, sherbet, pudding, gelatin, and Popsicles.
- Output includes urine, vomitus, diarrhea, and wound drainage.

Measuring Intake and Output

- To measure intake and output, you need to know:
  - 1 ounce (oz) equals 30 mL.
  - A pint is about 500 mL.
  - A quart is about 1000 mL.
  - The serving sizes of bowls, dishes, cups, pitchers, glasses, and other containers.
- An I&O record is kept at the bedside. Record I&O measurements in the correct column. Amounts are totaled at the end of the shift. The totals are recorded in the person's chart.
- The urinal, commode, bedpan, or specimen pan is used for voiding. Remind the person not to void in the toilet. Also remind the person not to put toilet tissue into the receptacle.

MEETING FOOD AND FLUID NEEDS

Preparing for Meals

- Preparing residents for meals promotes their comfort:
  - Assist with elimination needs.
  - Provide oral hygiene. Make sure dentures are in place.
  - Make sure eyeglasses and hearing aids are in place.

- Make sure incontinent persons are clean and dry.
- Position the person in a comfortable position.
- Assist with hand washing.

Serving Meal Trays
- Food is served in containers that keep foods at the correct temperature. Hot food is kept hot. Cold food is kept cold.
- Prompt serving keeps food at the correct temperature.

Feeding the Person
- Serve food and fluid in the order the person prefers. Offer fluids during the meal.
- Use teaspoons to feed the person.
- Persons who need to be fed are often angry, humiliated, and embarrassed. Some are depressed or refuse to eat. Let them do as much as possible. If strong enough, let them hold milk or juice glasses. Never let them hold hot drinks.
- Tell the visually impaired person what is on the tray. Describe what you are offering. For persons who feed themselves, use the numbers on the clock for the location of foods.
- Many people pray before eating. Allow time and privacy for prayer.
- Meals provide social contact with others. Engage the person in pleasant conversations. Also, sit facing the person.
- Report and record:
  - The amount and kind of food eaten
  - Complaints of nausea or dysphagia
  - Signs and symptoms of dysphagia
  - Signs and symptoms of aspiration
- The person will eat better if not rushed.
- Wipe the person's hands, face, and mouth as needed during the meal.

Between-Meal Snacks
- Many special diets involve between-meal snacks. These snacks are served upon arrival on the nursing unit. Follow the same considerations and procedures for serving meal trays and feeding persons.

Calorie Counts
- Calorie records are kept for some people. On a flow sheet, note what the person ate and how much. A nurse or dietitian converts these portions into calories.

Providing Drinking Water
- Patients and residents need fresh drinking water. Follow the agency's procedure for providing fresh water.
- Water glasses and pitchers can spread microbes. To prevent the spread of microbes:
  - Label the water pitcher with the person's name and room and bed numbers.
  - Do not touch the rim or inside of the water glass, cup, or pitcher.

- Do not let the ice scoop touch the rim or inside of the water glass, cup, or pitcher.
- Place the ice scoop in the holder or on a towel, not in the ice container or dispenser.
- Make sure the person's water pitcher and cup are clean and free of cracks and chips.

CHAPTER 19 REVIEW QUESTIONS
Circle the BEST answer.
1. A person is on a sodium-controlled diet. Which statement is *true?*
   a. High-sodium foods are allowed.
   b. Salt is added at the table.
   c. Pretzels and potato chips are a good snack.
   d. The amount of salt used in cooking is limited.
2. A person is a diabetic. You should do all of the following *except*
   a. Serve his meals and snacks late
   b. Always check his tray to see what he ate
   c. Tell the nurse what he ate and did not eat
   d. Provide a between-meal snack as the nurse directs
3. A person has dysphagia. You should do all of the following *except*
   a. Report choking and coughing during a meal at once
   b. Report difficulty in breathing during a meal at the end of the shift
   c. Report changes in how the person eats
   d. Follow aspiration precautions
4. Older persons have a decreased sense of thirst.
   a. True
   b. False
5. When feeding a person, you do all of the following *except*
   a. Use a teaspoon to feed the person
   b. Offer fluids during the meal
   c. Let the person do as much as possible
   d. Stand so you can feed 2 people at once
6. A person is visually impaired. You do all of the following *except*
   a. Tell the person what is on the tray
   b. Use the numbers on a clock to tell the person the location of food
   c. If feeding the person, describe what you are offering
   d. Let the person guess what is served
7. A person is on intake and output. He just ate ice cream. This is recorded as intake.
   a. True
   b. False
8. A person drank a pint of milk at lunch. You know he drank
   a. 250 mL of milk
   b. 350 mL of milk
   c. 500 mL of milk
   d. 750 mL of milk

9. The soup bowl holds 6 ounces. A person ate all of the soup. You record his intake as
   a. 50 mL
   b. 120 mL
   c. 180 mL
   d. 200 mL

Answers to these questions are on p. 505.

CHAPTER 21 URINARY ELIMINATION
NORMAL URINATION

- Healthy adults produce about 1500mL of urine a day.
- The frequency of urination is affected by amount of fluid intake, habits, availability of toilet facilities, activity, work, and illness. People usually void at bedtime, after sleep, and before meals. Some people void every 2 to 3 hours. The need to void at night disturbs sleep. Review Box 22-1, Rules for Normal Urination, in the textbook.
- Observe urine for color, clarity, odor, amount, and particles. Normal urine is pale yellow, straw-colored, or amber. It is clear with no particles. A faint odor is normal.
- Some foods and drugs affect urine color. Ask the nurse to observe urine that looks or smells abnormal.
- Report the following urinary problems:
  - **Dysuria**—painful or difficult urination
  - **Hematuria**—blood in the urine
  - **Nocturia**—frequent urination at night
  - **Oliguria**—scant amount of urine; less than 500mL in 24 hours
  - **Polyuria**—abnormally large amounts of urine
  - **Urinary frequency**—voiding at frequent intervals
  - **Urinary incontinence**—the loss of bladder control
  - **Urinary urgency**—the need ot void at once

Bedpans

- Follow Standard Precautions and the Bloodborne Pathogen Standard when handling bedpans, urinals, commodes, and their contents.
- Thoroughly clean and disinfect bedpans, urinals, and commodes after use.

Urinals

- Some men need support when standing to use the urinal.
- You may have to place and hold the urinal for some men. This may embarrass both the person and you. Act in a professional manner at all times.
- Remind men to hang urinals on bed rails and to signal after using them.

URINARY INCONTINENCE

- Urinary incontinence is the loss of bladder control.
- If urinary incontinence is a new problem, tell the nurse at once.

- Incontinence is embarrassing. Garments are wet, and odors develop. Skin irritation, infection, and pressure ulcers are risks. The person's pride, dignity, and self-esteem are affected. Social isolation, loss of independence, and depression are common.
- Good skin care and dry garments and linens are essential. Promoting normal urinary elimination prevents incontinenced in some people. Other people may need bladder training.
- Review Box 21-2, Nursing Measures for Person with Urinary Inconcontinenc, in the textbook.
- Caring for persons with incontinence is stressful. Remember, the person does not choose to be incontinent. If you find yourself short-tempered and impatient, talk to the nurse at once. Kindness, empathy, understanding, and patience are needed.

CATHETERS

- An indwelling catheter (retention or Foley cather) drains urine constantly into a drainage bag.
- The catheter must not pull at the insertion site. Hold the catheter securely during catheter care. Then properly secure the catheter. Also make sure the tubing is not under the person. Besides obstructing urine flow, lying on the tubing is uncomfortable. It can also cause skin breakdown.
- Follow Standard Precautions and the Bloodborne Pathogen Standard. Review Box 21-3, Caring for Persons With Indwelling catheters, in the textbook.
- Report and record:
  - Complaints of pain, burning, irritation, or the need to void
  - Crusting, abnormal drainage, or secretions
  - The color, clarity, and odor of urine
  - Particles in the urine
  - Urine leaking at the insertion site
  - Drainage system leaks

Drainage Systems

- A closed drainage system is used for indwelling catheters. The drainage bag hangs from the bed frame, chair, or wheelchair. It must not touch the floor. The bag is always kept lower than the person's bladder. Do not hang the drainage bag on a bed rail.
- If the drainage system is disconnected accidentally, tell the nurse at once. Do not touch the ends of the catheter or tubing. Do the following:
  - Practice hand hygiene. Put on gloves.
  - Wipe the end of the tube with an antiseptic wipe.
  - Wipe the end of the catheter with another antiseptic wipe.
  - Do not put the ends down. Do not touch the ends after you clean them.
  - Connect the tubing to the catheter.
  - Discard the wipes into a biohazard bag.
  - Remove the gloves. Practice hand hygiene.
- Check with the nurse and care plan about when to empty and measure the urine in the drainage bag.

Follow Standard Precautions and the Bloodborne Pathogen Standard.
- A leg bag is a drainage system that attaches to the thigh or calf. Empty and measure a leg bag when it is half full.
- Report and record:
  - The amount of urine measured
  - The color, clarity, and odor of urine
  - Particles in the urine
  - Complaints of pain, burning, irritation, or the need to urinate
  - Drainage system leaks

Condom Catheters
- Condom catheters are often used for incontinent men. They are also called external catheters, Texas catheters, and urinary sheaths.
- These catheters are changed daily after perineal care.
- To apply a condom catheter, follow the manufacturer's instructions. Thoroughly wash and dry the penis before applying the catheter.
- Some condom catheters are self-adhering. Other catheters are secured in place with elastic tape in a spiral manner. Never use adhesive tape to secure catheters. It does not expand. Blood flow to the penis is cut off, injuring the penis.
- When removing or applying a condom catheter, report and record the following observations to the nurse at once.
  - Reddened or open areas on the penis
  - Swelling of the penis
  - Color, clarity, and odor of urine
  - Particles in the urine
  - Blood in the urine
  - Cloudy urine

BLADDER TRAINING
- Bladder training helps some persons with urinary incontinence. Control of urination is the goal. Bladder control promotes comfort and quality of life. It also increases self-esteem. You assist with bladder training as directed by the nurse and the care plan.

CHAPTER 21 REVIEW QUESTIONS
Circle the BEST answer.
1. Which statement is false?
   a. Normal urine is yellow, straw-colored, or amber.
   b. Urine with a strong odor is normal.
   c. A person normally voids 1500mL a day.
   d. Observe urine for color, clarity, odor, amount, and particles.
2. Which observation does not need to be reported o the nurse promptly?
   a. Complaints of urgency
   b. Burning on urination
   c. Painful or difficult urination
   d. Clear amber urine

3. Which statement is false?
   a. Incontinence is embarrassing.
   b. Caring for persons with incontinence may be stressful.
   c. Incontinence is a personal choice.
   d. Be kind and patient to persons who are incontinent.
4. A person with a catheter complains of pain. You should notify the nurse at once.
   a. True
   b. False
5. Which statement is false?
   a. The urinary drainage system should hang from the bed frame or chair.
   b. The urinary drainage system should hang on a bed rail.
   c. The urinary drainage system must be off the floor.
   d. The urine drainage system must be kept lower than the person's bladder.
6. Which statement is false?
   a. Condom catheters are changed daily.
   b. Follow the manufacturer's instructions when applying a condom catheter.
   c. Use adhesive tape to secure a condom catheter in place.
   d. Report and record open or reddened areas on the penis at once.
7. The goal of bladder training is to
   a. Allow the person to use the toilet
   b. Keep the catheter
   c. Gain control of urination
   d. Decrease self-esteem
Answers to these questions are on p. 505.

CHAPTER 22 BOWEL ELIMINATION
NORMAL BOWEL ELIMINATION
Observations
- Stools are normally brown, soft, formed, moist, and shaped like the rectum. They have a normal odor caused by bacterial action in the intestines. Certain food and drugs cause odors.
- Carefully observe stools before disposing of them. Observe and report the color, amount, consistency, odor, and shape of stools. Also, observe and report the presence of blood or mucus, frequency of defecation, and any complaints of pain or discomfort.

FACTORS AFFECTING BOWEL ELIMINATION
- *Privacy.* Bowel elimination is a private act.
- Habits. Many people have a bowel movement after breakfast. Some read. Defecation is easier when a person is relaxed.

- *Diet—high-fiber foods.* Fiber helps prevent constipation.
- *Diet—other foods.* Some foods cause constipation. Other foods cause frequent stools or diarrhea.
- *Fluids.* Drinking 6 to 8 glasses of water daily promotes normal bowel elimination. Warm fluids—coffee, tea, hot cider, warm water—increase peristalsis.
- *Activity.* Exercise and activity maintain muscle tone and stimulate peristalsis.
- *Drugs.* Drugs can prevent constipation or control diarrhea. Some have diarrhea or constipation as side effects.
- *Disability.* Some people cannot control bowel movements. A bowel training program is needed.
- *Aging.* Older persons are at risk for constipation. Some older persons lose bowel control and have fecal incontinence.
- To provide comfort and safety during bowel elimination, review Box 22-1, Safety and Comfort During Bowel Elimination, in the textbook. Follow Standard Precautions and the Bloodborne Pathogen Standard.

COMMON PROBLEMS

- Common problems include constipation, fecal impaction, diarrhea, fecal incontinence, and flatulence.

Constipation

- **Constipation** is the passage of a hard, dry stool.
- Common causes of constipation are a low fiber diet and ignoring the urge to defecate. Other causes include decreased fluid intake, inactivity, drugs, aging, and certain diseases.
- Dietary changes, fluids, and activity prevent or relieve constipation. So do drugs and enemas.

Fecal Impaction

- A **fecal impaction** is the prolonged retention and buildup of feces in the rectum.
- Fecal impaction results if constipation is not relieved. The person cannot defecate. Liquid feces pass around the hardened fecal mass in the rectum. The liquid feces seep from the anus.
- Abdominal discomfort, abdominal distention, nausea, cramping, and rectal pain are common. Older persons have poor appetite or confusion. Some persons have a fever. Report these signs and symptoms to the nurse.

Diarrhea

- Diarrhea is the frequent passage of liquid stools.
- The need to have a bowel movement is urgent. Some people cannot get to a bathroom in time. Abdominal cramping, nausea, and vomiting may occur.
- Assist with elimination needs promptly, dispose of stools promptly, and give good skin care. Liquid stools irritate the skin. So does frequent wiping with toilet paper. Skin breakdown and pressure ulcers are risks.

- Follow Standard Precautions and the Bloodborne Pathogen Stnadard when in contact with stools.
- Report signs of diarrhea at once. Ask the nurse to observe the stool.

Fecal Incontinence

- Fecal incontinence is the inability to control the passage of feces and gas through the anus.
- Fecal incontinence affects the person emotionally. Frustration, embarrassment, anger, and humiliation are common. The person may need:
  - Bowel training
  - Help with elimination after meals and every 2 to 3 hours
  - Incontinence products to keep garments and linens clean
  - Good skin care

Flatulence

- **Flatulence** is the excessive formation of gas or air in the stomach and intestines.
- Causes include swallowing air while eating and drinking and bacterial action in the intestines. Other causes may be gas-forming foods, constipation, bowel and abdominal surgeries, and drugs that decrease peristalsis.
- If flatus is not expelled, the intestines distend (swell or enlarge from the pressure of gases). Abdominal cramping or pain, shortness of breath, and a swollen abdomen occur. "Bloating" is a common complaint. Exercise, walking, moving in bed, and the left side-lying position often produce flatus. Enemas and drugs may be ordered.

BOWEL TRAINING

- Bowel training has two goals:
  - To gain control of bowel movements.
  - To develop a regular pattern of elimination. Fecal impactions, constipation, and fecal incontinence are prevented.
  - Factors that promote elimination are part of the care plan and bowel training program.

ENEMAS

- An **enema** is the introduction of fluid into the rectum and lower colon.
- Doctors order enemas:
  - To remove feces
  - To relieve constipation, fecal impaction, or flatulence
  - To clean the bowel of feces before certain surgeries and diagnostic procedures

Reviw Box 22-2, Safety and Comfort Measures for Giving Enemas, in the textbook.

The Person with an Ostomy

- Sometimes part of the intestines is removed surgically. An **ostomy** is sometimes necessary. An ostomy is a surgically created opening. The opening is called a **stoma**. The person wears a pouch over the stoma to collect stools and flatus.

- Stools irritate the skin. Skin care prevents skin breakdown around the stoma. It prevents stools from having contact with the skin. The skin barrier is part of the pouch or a separate device.
- The pouch has an adhesive backing that is applied to the skin. Some pouches are secured to ostomy belts.
- The pouch is changed every 3 to 7 days and when it leaks. Frequent pouch changes can damage the skin.
- Many pouches have a drain at the bottom that closes with a clip, clamp, or wire closure. The drain is opened to empty the pouch. The drain is wiped with toilet tissue before it is closed.

CHAPTER 22 REVIEW QUESTIONS

Circle the BEST answer.

1. Which statement is *false*?
   a. Lack of privacy can prevent defecation.
   b. Low-fiber foods promote defecation.
   c. Drinking 6 to 8 glasses of water daily promotes normal bowel elimination.
   d. Exercise stimulates peristalsis.
2. Which of the following does *not* prevent constipation?
   a. A high-fiber diet
   b. Increased fluid intake
   c. Exercise
   d. Ignoring the urge to defecate
3. A person has fecal incontinence. You should do all of the following *except*
   a. Be patient
   b. Help with elimination after meals
   c. Provide good skin care
   d. Scold the person for being incontinent
4. The preferred position for an enema is the
   a. Sims' position or the left side-lying position
   b. Prone position
   c. Supine position
   d. Trendelenburg's position

Answers to these questions are on p. 505.

CHAPTER 23 EXERCISE AND ACTIVITY

BEDREST

- The doctor may order bedrest to treat a health problem.

Complications of Bedrest

- Pressure ulcers, constipation, and fecal impactions can result. Urinary tract infections and renal calculi (kidney stones) can occur. So can blood clots and pneumonia.

- The musculo-skeletal system is affected by lack of exercise and activity. These complications must be prevented to maintain normal movement:
  - A **contracture** is the lack of joint mobility caused by abnormal shortening of a muscle. Common sites are the fingers, wrists, elbows, toes, ankles, knees, and hips. The person is permanently deformed and disabled.
  - **Atrophy** is the decrease in size or the wasting away of tissue. Tissues shrink in size.
- **Orthostatic hypotension (postural hypotension)** is abnormally low blood pressure when the person suddenly stands up. The person is dizzy and weak and has spots before the eyes. Fainting can occur. To prevent orthostatic hypotension, have the person change slowly from a lying or sitting position to a standing position.

Positioning

- Supportive devices are often used to support and maintain the person in a certain position:
  - *Bed-boards*—are placed under the mattress to prevent the mattress from sagging.
  - *Foot-boards*—are placed at the foot of mattresses to prevent plantar flexion that can lead to footdrop.
  - *Trochanter rolls*—prevent the hips and legs from turning outward (external rotation).
  - *Hip abduction wedges*—keep the hips abducted.
  - *Hand rolls or hand grips*—prevent contractures of the thumb, fingers, and wrist.
  - *Splints*—keep the elbows, wrists, thumbs, fingers, ankles, and knees in normal position.
  - *Bed cradles*—keep the weight of top linens off the feet and toes.

RANGE-OF-MOTION EXERCISES

- **Range-of-motion (ROM)** exercises involve moving the joints through their complete range of motion. They are usually done at least 2 times a day.
- *Active ROM*—exercises are done by the person.
- *Passive ROM*—someone moves the joints through their range of motion.
- *Active-assistive ROM*—the person does the exercises with some help.
- Review Box 23-2, Joint Movements, in the textbook.
- Range-of-motion exercises can cause injury if not done properly. Practice these rules:
  - Exercise only the joints the nurse tells you to exercise.
  - Expose only the body part being exercised.
  - Use good body mechanics.
  - Support the part being exercised.
  - Move the joint slowly, smoothly, and gently.
  - Do not force a joint beyond its present range of motion.
  - Do not force a joint to the point of pain.

- Ask the person if he or she has pain or discomfort.
- Perform ROM exercises to the neck only if allowed by center policy.

AMBULATION

- **Ambulation** is the act of walking.
- Follow the care plan when helping a person walk. Use a gait (transfer) belt if the person is weak or unsteady. The person uses hand rails along the wall. Always check the person for orthostatic hypotension.
- When you help the person walk, walk to the side and slightly behind the person on the person's weak side. Encourage the person to use the hand rail on his or her strong side.

Walking Aids

- A cane is held on the strong side of the body. The cane tip is about 6 to 10 inches to the side of the foot. It is about 6 to 10 inches in front of the foot on the strong side. The grip is level with the hip. To walk:
  - Step A: The cane is moved forward 6 to 10 inches.
  - Step B: The weak leg (opposite the cane) is moved forward even with the cane.
  - Step C: The strong leg is moved forward and ahead of the cane and the weak leg.
- A walker gives more support than a cane. Wheeled walkers are common. They have wheels on the front legs and rubber tips on the back legs. The person pushes the walker about 6 to 8 inches in front of his or her feet.
- Braces support weak body parts, prevent or correct deformities, or prevent joint movement. A brace is applied over the ankle, knee, or back. Skin and bony points under braces are kept clean and dry. Report redness or signs of skin breakdown at once. Also report complaints of pain or discomfort.

CHAPTER 23 REVIEW QUESTIONS
Circle the BEST answer.

1. To prevent orthostatic hypotension, you should
   a. Move a person from the lying position to the sitting position quickly
   b. Move a person from the sitting position to the standing position quickly
   c. Move a person from the lying or sitting position to a standing position slowly
   d. Keep the person in bed
2. Exercise helps prevent contractures and muscle atrophy.
   a. True
   b. False
3. When performing ROM exercises, you should force a joint to the point of pain.
   a. True
   b. False
4. A person's left leg is weaker than his right. The person holds the cane on his right side.
   a. True
   b. False

Answers to these questions are on p. 505.

CHAPTER 24 COMFORT, REST, AND SLEEP

- Comfort is a state of well-being. Many factors affect comfort.

ASSISTING WITH PAIN RELIEF

- **Pain or discomfort** means to ache, hurt, or be sore. Pain is subjective. You cannot see, hear, touch, or smell pain or discomfort. You must rely on what the person says.
- Report the person's complaints of pain and your observations to the nurse.
- Review Box 24-3, Nursing Measures to Promote Comfort and Relieve Pain, in the textbook.

Factors Affecting Pain

- *Past experience.* The severity of pain, its cause, how long it lasted, and if relief occurred all affect the person's current response to pain.
- *Anxiety.* Pain and anxiety are related. Pain can cause anxiety. Anxiety increases how much pain the person feels. Reducing anxiety helps lessen pain.
- *Rest and sleep.* Pain seems worse when a person is tired or restless.
- *Attention.* The more a person thinks about pain, the worse it seems.
- *Personal and family duties.* Often pain is ignored when there are children to care for. Some deny pain if a serious illness is feared.
- *The value or meaning of pain.* To some people, pain is a weakness. For some persons, pain means avoiding daily routines and people. Some people like doting and pampering by others. The person values pain and wants such attention.
- *Support from others.* Dealing with pain is often easier when family and friends offer comfort and support. Just being nearby helps. Facing pain alone is hard for persons.
- *Culture.* Culture affects pain responses. Non–English-speaking persons may have problems describing pain.
- *Illness.* Some diseases cause decreased pain sensations.
- *Age.* Older persons may have decreased pain sensations. They may not feel pain or it may not feel severe. The person is at risk for undetected disease or injury. Chronic pain may mask new pain.
- *Persons with dementia.* Persons with dementia may not be able to complain of pain. Changes in usual behavior may signal pain. Loss of appetite also signals pain. Report any changes in a person's usual behavior to the nurse.

Signs and Symptoms

- You cannot see, hear, touch, or smell the person's pain. Rely on what the person tells you. Promptly report any information you collect about pain. Use the person's exact words when reporting and recording pain. The nurse needs the following information:
  - *Location*. Where is the pain?
  - *Onset and duration*. When did the pain start? How long has it lasted?
  - *Intensity*. Ask the person to rate the pain. Use a pain scale.
  - *Description*. Ask the person to describe the pain.
  - *Factors causing pain*. Ask when the pain started and what the person was doing.
  - *Factors affecting pain*. Ask what makes the pain better and what makes it worse.
  - *Vital signs*. Increases often occur with acute pain. They may be normal with chronic pain.
  - *Other signs and symptoms*. Dizziness, nausea, vomiting, weakness, numbness, and tingling.
- Review Box 24-2, Signs and Symptoms of Pain, in the textbook.

PROMOTING SLEEP

- Sleep is a basic need. Tissue healing and repair occur during sleep. Sleep lowers stress, tension, and anxiety. It refreshes and renews the person. The person regains energy and mental alertness. The person thinks and functions better after sleep.

Factors Affecting Sleep

- *Illness*. Illness increases the need for sleep.
- *Nutrition*. Sleep needs increase with weight gain. Foods with caffeine prevent sleep.
- *Exercise*. People tire after exercise. Being tired helps people sleep well. Exercise before bedtime interferes with sleep. Exercise is avoided 2 hours before bedtime.
- *Environment*. People adjust to their usual sleep settings.
- *Medications and other substances*. Sleeping pills promote sleep. Medications for anxiety, depression, and pain may cause the person to sleep.
- *Emotional problems*. Fear, worry, depression, and anxiety affect sleep.

Sleep Disorders

- **Insomnia** is a chronic condition in which the person cannot sleep or stay asleep all night.
- **Sleep deprivation** means that the amount and quality of sleep are decreased. Sleep is interrupted.
- **Sleepwalking** is when the person leaves the bed and walks about. If a person is sleepwalking, protect the person from injury. Guide sleepwalkers back to bed. They startle easily. Awaken them gently.

Promoting Sleep

- To promote sleep, allow a flexible bedtime, provide a comfortable room temperature, and have the person void before going to bed. Review Box 24-6, Nursing Measures to Promote Sleep, in the textbook for other measures.

CHAPTER 24 REVIEW QUESTIONS
Circle the BEST answer.

1. A person complains of pain. You will do all of the following *except*
   a. Ask where the pain is
   b. Ask when the pain started
   c. Ask what the intensity of the pain is on a scale of 1 to 10
   d. Ask what he or she is complaining about
2. Persons with dementia may not complain of pain. Which of the following might be a signal of pain for a person with dementia?
   a. Illness
   b. Mental alertness
   c. Loss of appetite
   d. Forgetfulness
3. You can promote rest for a person by doing all of the following *except*
   a. Ask the person if he or she would like coffee or tea
   b. Place the call light within reach
   c. Provide a quiet setting
   d. Follow the person's routines and rituals before rest
4. To promote sleep for a person, you should do all of the following *except*
   a. Follow the person's wishes
   b. Follow the care plan
   c. Follow the person's rituals and routines before bedtime
   d. Tell the person when to go to bed

Answers to these questions are on p. 505.

CHAPTER 25 OXYGEN NEEDS AND RESPIRATORY THERAPIES
ALTERED RESPIRATORY FUNCTION

- Hypoxia means that cells do not have enough oxygen.
- Restlessness, dizziness, and disorientation are signs of hypoxia.
- Review Box 25-1, Signs and Symptoms of Hypoxia, in the textbook. Report signs and symptoms of hypoxia to the nurse at once. Hypoxia is life-threatening.

Abnormal Respirations

- Adults normally have 12 to 20 respirations per minute. They are quiet, effortless, and regular. Both sides of the chest rise and fall equally. Report these observations at once:
  - **Tachypnea**—rapid breathing. Respirations are 20 or more per minute.
  - **Bradypnea**—slow breathing. Respirations are fewer than 12 per minute.
  - **Apnea**—lack or absence of breathing.
  - **Hypoventilation**—respirations are slow, shallow, and sometimes irregular.
  - **Hyperventilation**—respirations are rapid and deeper than normal.
  - **Dyspnea**—difficult, labored, or painful breathing.
  - **Cheyne-Stokes respirations**—respirations gradually increase in rate and depth. Then they become shallow and slow. Breathing may stop for 10 to 20 seconds.
  - **Orthopnea**—breathing deeply and comfortably only when sitting.
  - **Kussmaul respirations**—very deep and rapid respirations.

PROMOTING OXYGENATION

Positioning

- Breathing is usually easier in semi-Fowler's and Fowler's positions. Persons with difficulty breathing often prefer the **orthopneic position** (sitting up and leaning over a table to breathe).

Deep Breathing and Coughing

- Deep breathing moves air into most parts of the lungs. Coughing removes mucus. Deep breathing and coughing are usually done every 2 hours while the person is awake.

Oxygen Devices

- A nasal cannula allows eating and drinking. Tight prongs can irritate the nose. Pressure on the ears and cheekbones is possible.
- A simple face mask covers the nose and mouth. Talking and eating are hard to do with a mask. Listen carefully. Moisture can build up under the mask. Keep the face clean and dry. Masks are removed for eating. Usually oxygen is given by cannula during meals.

Oxygen Flow Rates

- When giving care and checking the person, always check the flow rate. Tell the nurse at once if it is too high or too low. A nurse or respiratory therapist will adjust the flow rate.

Oxygen Safety

- You do not give oxygen. You assist the nurse in providing safe care.
- Always check the oxygen level when you are with or near persons using oxygen systems that contain a limited amount of oxygen. Oxygen tanks and liquid oxygen systems are examples. Report a low oxygen level to the nurse at once.
- Follow the rules for fire and the use of oxygen in Chapter 10.
- Never remove the oxygen device.
- Make sure the oxygen device is secure but not tight.
- Check for signs of irritation from the oxygen device—behind the ears, under the nose, around the face, and cheekbones.
- Keep the face clean and dry when a mask is used.
- Never shut off the oxygen flow.
- Do not adjust the flow rate unless allowed by your state and agency.
- Tell the nurse at once if the flow rate is too high or too low.
- Tell the nurse at once if the humidifier is not bubbling.
- Secure tubing to the person's garment. Follow agency policy.
- Make sure there are no kinks in the tubing.
- Make sure the person does not lie on any part of the tubing.
- Report signs of hypoxia, respiratory distress, or abnormal breathing to the nurse at once.
- Give oral hygiene as directed. Follow the care plan.
- Make sure the oxygen device is clean and free of mucus.

CHAPTER 25 REVIEW QUESTIONS

Circle the BEST answer.

1. Which statement is *false*?
   a. Restlessness, dizziness, and disorientation are signs of hypoxia.
   b. Hypoxia is life-threatening.
   c. Report signs and symptoms of hypoxia at the end of the shift.
   d. Anything that affects respiratory function can cause hypoxia.
2. Adults normally have
   a. 8 to 10 respirations per minute
   b. 12 to 20 respirations per minute
   c. 10 to 12 respirations per minute
   d. 20 to 24 respirations per minute
3. Dyspnea is
   a. Difficult, labored, or painful breathing
   b. Slow breathing with fewer than 12 respirations per minute
   c. Rapid breathing with 24 or more respirations per minute
   d. Lack or absence of breathing

4. Which statement about positioning is *false?*
   a. Breathing is usually easier in semi-Fowler's or Fowler's position.
   b. Persons with difficulty breathing often prefer the orthopneic position.
   c. Position changes are needed at least every 4 hours.
   d. Follow the person's care plan for positioning preferences.
5. A person has a nasal cannula. Which statement is *false?*
   a. You will leave the nasal cannula on while the person is eating.
   b. You will watch the nose area for irritation.
   c. You will watch the ears and cheekbones for skin breakdown.
   d. You will take the nasal cannula off while the person is eating.

Answers to these questions are on p. 505.

CHAPTER 26 MEASURING VITAL SIGNS
VITAL SIGNS
- Accuracy is essential when you measure, record, and report vital signs. If unsure of your measurements, promptly ask the nurse to take them again.
- Report the following at once:
  - Any vital sign that is changed from a prior measurement
  - Vital signs above or below the normal range

BODY TEMPERATURE
- Thermometers are used to measure temperature. It is measured using the Fahrenheit (F) and centigrade or Celsius (C) scales.
- Temperature sites are the mouth, rectum, axilla (underarm), tympanic membrane (ear), and temporal artery (forehead).
- Review Box 26-1, Temperature Sites, in the textbook.
- Normal ranges for body temperatures vary by site:
  - Oral: 97.6°F to 99.6°F
  - Rectal: 98.6°F to 100.6°F
  - Axillary: 96.6°F to 98.6°F

- Tympanic membrane: 98.6°F
- Temporal artery: 99.6°F
- Older persons have lower body temperatures than younger persons.

Taking Temperatures
- *The oral site.* The thermometer remains in place 2 to 3 minutes or as required by center policy.
- *The rectal site.* Lubricate the bulb end of the rectal thermometer. Insert the thermometer ½ inch into the rectum. Hold the thermometer in place for 2 minutes or as required by center policy. Privacy is important.
- *The axillary site.* The axilla must be dry. The thermometer stays in place for 5 to 10 minutes or as required by center policy.

Electronic Thermometers
- Tympanic membrane thermometers are gently inserted into the ear. The temperature is measured in 1 to 3 seconds. These thermometers are not used if there is ear drainage.
- Temporal artery thermometers measure body temperature at the temporal artery in the forehead. These thermometers measure body temperature in 3 to 4 seconds. Follow the manufacturer instructions for using, cleaning, and storing the device.

PULSE
Pulse Rate
- The adult pulse rate is between 60 and 100 beats per minute. Report these abnormal rates to the nurse at once:
  - *Tachycardia*—the heart rate is more than 100 beats per minute.
  - *Bradycardia*—the heart rate is less than 60 beats per minute.

Rhythm and Force of the Pulse
- The rhythm of the pulse should be regular. Report and record an irregular pulse rhythm.
- Report and record if the pulse force is strong, full, bounding, weak, thready, or feeble.

Taking Pulses
- The radial pulse is used for routine vital signs. Do not use your thumb to take a pulse. Count the pulse for 30 seconds and multiply by 2 if the agency policy permits. If the pulse is irregular, count it for 1 minute. Report and record if the pulse is regular or irregular.
- The apical pulse is on the left side of the chest slightly below the nipple. Count the apical pulse for 1 minute.

RESPIRATIONS
- The healthy adult has 12 to 20 respirations per minute. Respirations are normally quiet, effortless, and regular. Both sides of the chest rise and fall equally.
- Count respirations when the person is at rest. Count respirations right after taking a pulse.
- Count respirations for 30 seconds and multiply the number by 2 if the agency policy permits. If an abnormal pattern is noted, count the respirations for 1 minute.
- Report and record:
  - The respiratory rate
  - Equality and depth of respirations
  - If the respirations were regular or irregular
  - If the person has pain or difficulty breathing
  - Any respiratory noises
  - An abnormal respiratory pattern

BLOOD PRESSURE
Normal and Abnormal Blood Pressures
- Blood pressure has normal ranges:
  - *Systolic pressure* (upper number)—less than 120 mm Hg
  - *Diastolic pressure* (lower number)—less than 80 mm Hg
- **Hypertension**—blood pressure measurements that remain above a systolic pressure of 140 mm Hg or a diastolic pressure of 90 mm Hg. Report any systolic measurement above 120 mm Hg. Also report a diastolic pressure above 80 mm Hg.
- **Hypotension**—when the systolic blood pressure is below 90 mm Hg and the diastolic pressure is below 60 mm Hg. Report a systolic pressure below 90 mm Hg. Also report a diastolic pressure below 60 mm Hg.
- Review Box 26-3, Guidelines for Measuring Blood Pressure, in your textbook.

WEIGHT AND HEIGHT
- When weighing a person, follow the manufacturer instructions and center procedures for using the scales. Follow these guidelines when measuring weight and height:

- The person wears only a gown or pajamas. No footwear is worn.
- The person voids before being weighed.
- Weigh the person at the same time of day. Before breakfast is the best time.
- Use the same scale for daily, weekly, and monthly weights.
- Balance the scale at zero before weighing the person.

CHAPTER 26 REVIEW QUESTIONS
Circle the BEST answer.
1. Which statement about taking a rectal temperature is *false*?
   a. The bulb end of the thermometer needs to be lubricated.
   b. The thermometer is held in place for 5 minutes.
   c. Privacy is important.
   d. The normal range is 98.6°F to 100.6°F.
2. Which pulse rate should you report at once?
   a. A pulse rate of 52 beats per minute
   b. A pulse rate of 60 beats per minute
   c. A pulse rate of 76 beats per minute
   d. A pulse rate of 100 beats per minute
3. Which statement is *false*?
   a. An irregular pulse is counted for 1 minute.
   b. You may use your thumb to take a radial pulse rate.
   c. The radial pulse is usually used to count a pulse rate.
   d. Tachycardia is a fast pulse rate.
4. Which blood pressure should you report?
   a. 120/80 mm Hg
   b. 88/62 mm Hg
   c. 110/70 mm Hg
   d. 92/68 mm Hg
5. The person must wear footwear when being measured for weight and height.
   a. True
   b. False

Answers to these questions are on p. 505.

CHAPTER 30 WOUND CARE
- A **wound** is a break in the skin or mucous membrane.
- The wound is a portal of entry for microbes. Infection is a major threat. Wound care involves preventing infection and further injury to the wound and nearby tissues.

SKIN TEARS
- A **skin tear** is a break or rip in the skin.
- Skin tears are caused by friction, shearing, pulling, or pressure on the skin. Bumping a hand, arm, or leg on

any hard surface can cause a skin tear. Beds, bed rails, chairs, wheelchair footplates, and tables are dangers. So is holding the person's arm or leg too tight.
- Skin tears are painful. They are portals of entry for microbes. Wound complications can develop. Tell the nurse at once if you cause or find a skin tear.
- Review Box 30-2, Measures to Prevent Skin Tears, in the textbook.

VASCULAR ULCERS
- *Vascular ulcers* are open sores on the lower legs or feet. They are caused by decreased blood flow through the arteries or veins.
- Review Box 30-3, Measures to Prevent Vascular Ulcers, in the textbook.
- *Venous ulcers (stasis ulcers)* are open sores on the lower legs or feet. They are caused by poor blood flow through the veins. The heels and inner aspect of the ankles are common sites for venous ulcers.
- *Arterial ulcers* are open wounds on the lower legs or feet caused by poor arterial blood flow. They are found between the toes, on top of the toes, and on the outer side of the ankle.
- A *diabetic foot ulcer* is an open wound on the foot caused by complications from diabetes. When nerves are affected, the person can lose sensation in a foot or leg. The person may not feel pain, heat, or cold. Therefore, the person may not feel a cut, blister, burn, or other trauma to the foot. Infection and a large sore can develop. When blood flow to the foot decreases, tissues and cells do not get needed oxygen and nutrients. A sore does not heal properly. Tissue death (gangrene) can occur.

Prevention and Treatment
- Check the person's feet and legs every day. Report any sign of a problem to the nurse at once. Follow the care plan to prevent and treat circulatory ulcers.

Elastic Stockings
- Elastic stockings also are called anti-embolism or anti-embolic (AE) stockings. They also are called TED hose.
- The person usually has two pairs of stockings. One pair is washed; the other pair is worn.
- Stockings should not have twists, creases, or wrinkles after you apply them.
- Stockings are applied before the person gets out of bed.

WARM AND COLD APPLICATIONS
Warm Applications
- Heat relieves pain, relaxes muscles, promotes healing, reduces tissue swelling, and decreases joint stiffness.

Complications
- High temperatures can cause burns. Report pain, excessive redness, and blisters at once. Also observe for pale skin.
- Metal implants pose risks. Pacemakers and joint replacements are made of metal. Do not apply heat to an implant area.

Cold Applications
- Cold applications reduce pain, prevent swelling, and decrease circulation and bleeding.

Complications
- Complications include pain, burns, blisters, and poor circulation. Burns and blisters occur from intense cold. They also occur when dry cold is in direct contact with the skin.

Applying Warm and Cold
- Protect the person from injury during warm and cold applications. Review Box 30-8, Rules for Applying Warm and Cold, in the textbook.

CHAPTER 30 REVIEW QUESTIONS
Circle the BEST answer.

1. All of the following can cause a skin tear *except*
   a. Friction and shearing
   b. Holding a person's arm or leg too tight
   c. Rings, watches, and bracelets
   d. Trimmed, short nails
2. A person is diabetic. Which statement is *false?*
   a. The person may not feel pain in her feet.
   b. The person may not feel heat or cold in her feet.
   c. You need to check her feet weekly for foot problems.
   d. The person is at risk for diabetic foot ulcers.
3. Which statement about elastic stockings is *false?*
   a. Elastic stockings are also called anti-embolic stockings.
   b. Elastic stockings should be wrinkle-free after being applied.
   c. A person usually has two pairs of elastic stockings.
   d. Elastic stockings are applied after a person gets out of bed.
4. Complications from a warm application include all of the following *except*
   a. Excessive redness
   b. Blisters
   c. Pale skin
   d. Cyanotic (bluish) nail beds
5. When applying warm or cold, you should do all of the following *except*
   a. Ask the nurse what the temperature of the application should be

b. Cover dry warm or cold applications before applying them

c. Observe the skin every 2 hours

d. Know how long to leave the application in place

Answers to these questions are on p. 505.

CHAPTER 31 PRESSURE ULCERS

- A **pressure ulcer** is a localized injury to the skin and/or underlying tissue. Pressure ulcers usually occur over a bony prominence—the back of the head, shoulder blades, elbows, hips, spine, sacrum, knees, ankles, heels, and toes.
- *Decubitus ulcer, bed sore,* and *pressure sore* are other terms for pressure ulcer.
- Pressure, shearing, and friction are common causes of skin breakdown and pressure ulcers. Risk factors include breaks in the skin, poor circulation to an area, moisture, dry skin, and irritation by urine and feces.

Persons at Risk

- Persons at risk for pressure ulcers are those who:
  - Are confined to a bed or chair
  - Need some or total help in moving
  - Are agitated or have involuntary muscle movements
  - Have loss of bowel or bladder control
  - Are exposed to moisture
  - Have poor nutrition
  - Have poor fluid balance
  - Have lowered mental awareness
  - Have problems sensing pain or pressure
  - Have circulatory problems
  - Are older
  - Are obese or very thin

Pressure Ulcer Stages

- In persons with light skin, a reddened bony area is the first sign of a pressure ulcer. In persons with dark skin, a bony area may appear red, blue, or purple. The area may feel warm or cool. The person may complain of pain, burning, tingling, or itching in the area.
- Figure 31-4 in the textbook shows the stages of pressure ulcers.
- Box 31-2 in the textbook describes pressure ulcer stages.

Prevention and Treatment

- Preventing pressure ulcers is much easier than trying to heal them. Review Box 31-3, Measures to Prevent Pressure Ulcers, in the textbook.
- The person at risk for pressure ulcers may be placed on a foam, air, alternating air, gel, or water mattress.
- Protective devices are often used to prevent and treat pressure ulcers and skin breakdown. Protective devices include:
  - Bed cradle
  - Heel and elbow protectors
  - Heel and foot elevators
  - Gel or fluid-filled pads and cushions
  - Eggcrate-type pads
  - Special beds
  - Other equipment—pillows, trochanter rolls, and foot-boards

CHAPTER 31 REVIEW QUESTIONS
Circle the BEST answer.

1. You may expect to find a pressure ulcer at all of the following sites *except*
   a. Back of the head
   b. Ears
   c. Top of the thigh
   d. Toes
2. Which of the following is not a protective device used to prevent and treat pressure ulcers?
   a. Heel elevator
   b. Bed cradle
   c. Drawsheet
   d. Elbow protector
3. In obese people, pressure ulcers can occur between abdominal folds.
   a. True
   b. False
4. Pressure ulcers never occur over a bony prominence.
   a. True
   b. False

Answers to these questions are on p. 505.

CHAPTER 32 HEARING, SPEECH, AND VISION PROBLEMS
HEARING LOSS

- Hearing loss is not being able to hear the range of sounds associated with normal hearing. Deafness is the most severe form of hearing loss.
- Obvious signs and symptoms of hearing loss include:
  - Speaking too loudly
  - Leaning forward to hear
  - Turning and cupping the better ear toward the speaker
  - Answering questions or responding inappropriately
  - Asking for words to be repeated
  - Asking others to speak louder or to speak more slowly and clearly
  - Having trouble hearing over the phone
  - Finding it hard to follow conversations when two or more people are talking
  - Turning up the TV, radio, or music volume so loud that others complain

- Persons with hearing loss may wear hearing aids or lip-read (speech-read). They watch facial expressions, gestures, and body language. Some people learn American Sign Language (ASL). Others may have hearing assistance dogs.
- Review Box 32-1, Measures to Promote Hearing, in the textbook.
- Hearing aids are battery-operated. If they do not seem to work properly:
  - Check if the hearing aid is on. It has an on and off switch.
  - Check the battery position.
  - Insert a new battery if needed.
  - Clean the hearing aid. Follow the nurse's direction and the manufacturer instructions.
- Hearing aids are turned off when not in use. The battery is removed.
- Handle and care for hearing aids properly. If lost or damaged, report it to the nurse at once.

EYE DISORDERS

- *Glaucoma.* Glaucoma results when fluid builds up in the eye and causes pressure on the optic nerve. The optic nerve is damaged. Vision loss with eventual blindness occurs. Medications and surgery can control glaucoma and prevent further damage to the optic nerve. Prior damage cannot be reversed.
- *Cataract.* Cataract is a clouding of the lens in the eye. Signs and symptoms include cloudy, blurry, or dimmed vision. Persons may also be sensitive to light and glares or see halos around lights. Poor vision at night and double vision in one eye are other symptoms. Surgery is the only treatment. Review the list of post-operative care measures on p. XXX in the textbook.

Impaired Vision and Blindness
- Birth defects, accidents, and eye diseases are among the many causes of impaired vision and blindness. They also are complications of some diseases.
- Review Box 32-4, Caring for Blind and Visually Impaired Persons, in the textbook.

Corrective Lenses
- Clean eyeglasses daily and as needed.
- Protect eyeglasses from loss or damage. When not worn, put them in their case.
- Contact lenses are cleaned, removed, and stored according to the manufacturer instructions.

CHAPTER 32 REVIEW QUESTIONS
Circle the BEST answer.

1. A person is hard-of-hearing. You do all of the following *except*
   a. Face the person when speaking
   b. Speak clearly, distinctly, and slowly
   c. Use facial expressions and gestures to give clues
   d. Use long sentences
2. A person has taken his hearing aid out for the evening. You do all of the following *except*
   a. Make sure the hearing aid is turned off
   b. Keep the battery in the hearing aid
   c. Place the hearing aid in a safe place
   d. Handle the hearing aid carefully
3. A person is blind. You do all of the following *except*
   a. Identify yourself when you enter her room
   b. Describe people, places, and things thoroughly
   c. Rearrange her furniture without telling her
   d. Encourage her to do as much for herself as possible
4. Fluid buildup in the eye that causes pressure on the optic nerve is
   a. Cataract
   b. Cerumen
   c. Glaucoma
   d. Tinnitus

Answers to these questions are on p. 506.

CHAPTER 33 CANCER, IMMUNE SYSTEM, AND SKIN DISORDERS
CANCER
- Cancer is the second leading cause of death in the United States.
- Review Box 33-1, Some Signs and Symptoms of Cancer, in the textbook.
- Surgery, radiation therapy, and chemotherapy are the most common treatments.
- Persons with cancer have many needs. They include:
  - Pain relief or control
  - Rest and exercise
  - Fluids and nutrition
  - Preventing skin breakdown
  - Preventing bowel problems (constipation, diarrhea)
  - Dealing with treatment side effects
  - Psychological and social needs
  - Spiritual needs
  - Sexual needs
- Anger, fear, and depression are common. Some surgeries are disfiguring. The person may feel unwhole, unattractive, or unclean. The person and family need support.
- Talk to the person. Do not avoid the person because you are uncomfortable. Use touch and listening to show that you care.
- Spiritual needs are important. A spiritual leader may provide comfort.

IMMUNE SYSTEM DISORDERS
- The immune system protects the body from microbes, cancer cells, and other harmful substances. It defends against threats inside and outside the body.

Acquired Immunodeficiency Syndrome

- Acquired immunodeficiency syndrome (AIDS) is caused by a virus. The virus is spread through body fluids—blood, semen, vaginal secretions, and breast milk. The human immunodeficiency virus (HIV) is not spread by saliva, tears, sweat, sneezing, coughing, insects, or casual contact.
- Persons with AIDS are at risk for pneumonia, tuberculosis, Kaposi's sarcoma (a cancer), and nervous system damage.
- To protect yourself and others from the virus, follow Standard Precautions and the Bloodborne Pathogen Standard.
- Review Box 33-3, Caring for the Person With AIDS, in the textbook.
- Older persons also get AIDS. They get and spread HIV through sexual contact and intravenous (IV) drug use. Aging and some diseases can mask the signs and symptoms of AIDS. Older persons are less likely to be tested for HIV/AIDS.

CHAPTER 33 REVIEW QUESTIONS
Circle the BEST answer.

1. A person with cancer may need all the following *except*
   a. Pain relief or control
   b. Avoidance from you
   c. Fluids and nutrition
   d. Psychological support
2. Which statement about HIV is *false?*
   a. HIV is spread through body fluids.
   b. Standard Precautions and the Bloodborne Pathogen Standard are followed.
   c. Older persons cannot get and spread HIV.
   d. Older persons are less likely to be tested for HIV/AIDS.
3. The immune system defends against threats inside and outside the body.
   a. True
   b. False

Answers to these questions are on p. 506.

CHAPTER 34 NERVOUS SYSTEM AND MUSCULO-SKELETAL DISORDERS
NERVOUS SYSTEM DISORDERS

Stroke
- Stroke is also called a brain attack or cerebro-vascular accident (CVA). It is the third leading cause of death in the United States. Review Box 34-1, Warning Signs of Stroke, in the textbook.
- The effects of stroke include:
  - Loss of face, hand, arm, leg, or body control
  - **Hemiplegia**—paralysis on one side of the body
  - Changing emotions (crying easily or mood swings, sometimes for no reason)

- Difficulty swallowing (dysphagia)
- Aphasia or slowed or slurred speech
- Changes in sight, touch, movement, and thought
- Impaired memory
- Urinary frequency, urgency, or incontinence
- Loss of bowel control or constipation
- Depression and frustration
- The health team helps the person regain the highest possible level of function. Review Box 34-2, Care of the Person With a Stroke, in the textbook.

Aphasia
- **Aphasia** is the total or partial loss of the ability to use or understand language.
- *Expressive aphasia* relates to difficulty expressing or sending out thoughts. Thinking is clear. The person knows what to say but has difficulty or cannot speak the words.
- *Receptive aphasia* relates to difficulty understanding language. The person has trouble understanding what is said or read. People and common objects are not recognized.

Parkinson's Disease
- Parkinson's disease is a slow, progressive disorder with no cure. Persons over the age of 50 are at risk. Signs and symptoms become worse over time. They include:
  - *Tremors*—often start in one finger and spread to the whole arm. Pill-rolling movements—rubbing the thumb and index finger—may occur. The person may have trembling in the hands, arms, legs, jaw, and face.
  - *Rigid, stiff muscles*—in the arms, legs, neck, and trunk.
  - *Slow movements*—the person has a slow, shuffling gait.
  - *Stooped posture and impaired balance*—it is hard to walk. Falls are a risk.
  - *Mask-like expression*—the person cannot blink and smile. A fixed stare is common.
- Other signs and symptoms that develop over time include swallowing and chewing problems, constipation, and bladder problems. Sleep problems, depression, and emotional changes (fear, insecurity) can occur. So can memory loss and slow thinking. The person may have slurred, monotone, and soft speech. Some people talk too fast or repeat what they say.
- Medications are ordered to treat and control the disease. Exercise and physical therapy improve strength, posture, balance, and mobility. Therapy is needed for speech and swallowing problems. The person may need help with eating and self-care. Safety measures are needed to prevent falls and injury.

Multiple Sclerosis
- Multiple sclerosis (MS) is a chronic disease. The myelin (which covers nerve fibers) in the brain and spinal cord is destroyed. Nerve impulses are not sent

to and from the brain in a normal manner. Functions are impaired or lost. There is no cure.

- Symptoms usually start between the ages of 20 and 40. Signs and symptoms depend on the damaged area. They may include vision problems, muscle weakness in the arms and legs, balance problems that affect standing and walking. Tingling, prickling, or numb sensations may occur. Also, partial or complete paralysis and pain may occur.
- Persons with MS are kept active as long as possible and as independent as possible. Skin care, hygiene, and range-of-motion (ROM) exercises are important. So are turning, positioning, and deep breathing and coughing. Bowel and bladder elimination is promoted. Injuries and complications from bedrest are prevented.

Spinal Cord Injury

- Spinal cord injuries can permanently damage the nervous system. Common causes are stab or gunshot wounds, motor vehicle crashes, falls, and sports injuries.
- The higher the level of injury, the more functions are lost:
  - Lumbar injuries—sensory and muscle function in the legs is lost. The person has **paraplegia**—paralysis in legs and lower trunk.
  - Thoracic injuries—sensory and muscle function below the chest is lost. The person has paraplegia.
  - Cervical injuries—sensory and muscle function of the arms, legs, and trunk is lost. Paralysis in the arms, legs, and trunk is called **quadriplegia** or **tetraplegia.**
- Review Box 34-3, Care of Persons With Paralysis, in the textbook.

MUSCULO-SKELETAL DISORDERS

Arthritis

- Arthritis means joint inflammation.
- *Osteoarthritis (degenerative joint disease).* The fingers, spine (neck and lower back), and weight-bearing joints (hips, knees, and feet) are often affected. Treatment involves pain relief, heat applications, exercise, rest and joint care, weight control, and a healthy life-style. Falls are prevented. Help is given with activities of daily living (ADL) as needed. Toilet seat risers are helpful when hips and knees are affected. So are chairs with higher seats and armrests. Some people need joint replacement surgery.
- *Rheumatoid arthritis.* Rheumatoid arthritis (RA) causes joint pain, swelling, stiffness, and loss of function. Joints are tender, warm, and swollen. Fatigue and fever are common. The person does not feel well. The person's care plan may include rest balanced with exercise, proper positioning, joint care, weight control, measures to reduce stress, and measures to prevent falls. Medications are ordered for pain relief and to reduce inflammation. Heat and cold applications may be ordered. Some persons

need joint replacement surgery. Emotional support is needed. Persons with RA need to stay as active as possible. Give encouragement and praise. Listen when the person needs to talk.

CHAPTER 34 REVIEW QUESTIONS
Circle the BEST answer.

1. The person had a stroke. Care includes all of the following *except*
   a. Place the call light on the person's strong side
   b. Re-position the person every 2 hours
   c. Perform ROM exercises as ordered
   d. Place objects on the affected side
2. The person with hemiplegia
   a. Is paralyzed on one side of the body
   b. Has both arms paralyzed
   c. Has both legs paralyzed
   d. Has all extremities paralyzed
3. The person with multiple sclerosis should be kept active as long as possible.
   a. True
   b. False
4. The person has paralysis in the legs and lower trunk. This is called
   a. Quadriplegia
   b. Paraplegia
   c. Hemiplegia
   d. Tetraplegia
5. Fever is a common symptom of osteoarthritis.
   a. True
   b. False

Answers to these questions are on p. 506.

CHAPTER 35 CARDIOVASCULAR AND RESPIRATORY DISORDERS
CARDIOVASCULAR DISORDERS

Angina

- Angina is chest pain. It is from reduced blood flow to part of the heart muscle. Chest pain is described as tightness, pressure, squeezing, or burning in the chest. Pain can occur in the shoulders, arms, neck, jaw, or back. The person may be pale, feel faint, and perspire. Dyspnea is common. Nausea, fatigue, and weakness may occur. Some persons complain of "gas" or indigestion.
- Rest often relieves symptoms in 3 to 15 minutes. Chest pain lasting longer than a few minutes and not relieved by rest and nitroglycerin may signal heart attack. The person needs emergency care.

Myocardial Infarction

- Myocardial infarction (MI) also is called *heart attack, acute myocardial infarction (AMI)*, and *acute coronary syndrome (ACS).*

- Blood flow to the heart muscle is suddenly blocked. Part of the heart muscle dies. MI is an emergency. Sudden cardiac death (*sudden cardiac arrest*) can occur.
- Review Box 35-2, Signs and Symptoms of Myocardial Infarction, in the textbook.

Heart Failure

- Heart failure or congestive heart failure (CHF) occurs when the heart is weakened and cannot pump normally. Blood backs up. Tissue congestion occurs.
- Medications are given to strengthen the heart. They also reduce the amount of fluid in the body. A sodium-controlled diet is ordered. Oxygen is given. Semi-Fowler's position is preferred for breathing. Intake and output (I&O), daily weight, elastic stockings, and range-of-motion exercises are part of the care plan.

RESPIRATORY DISORDERS

Chronic Obstructive Pulmonary Disease

- Two disorders are grouped under chronic obstructive pulmonary disease (COPD). They are chronic bronchitis and emphysema. These disorders obstruct airflow. Lung function is gradually lost.
- *Chronic bronchitis.* Bronchitis means inflammation of the bronchi. Chronic bronchitis occurs after repeated episodes of bronchitis. Smoking is the major cause. Smoker's cough in the morning is often the first symptom of chronic bronchitis. Over time, the cough becomes more frequent. The person has difficulty breathing and tires easily. The person must stop smoking. Oxygen therapy and breathing exercises are often ordered. If a respiratory tract infection occurs, the person needs prompt treatment.
- *Emphysema.* In emphysema, the alveoli enlarge and become less elastic. They do not expand and shrink normally when breathing in and out. Air becomes trapped when exhaling. Smoking is the most common cause. The person has shortness of breath and a cough. Sputum may contain pus. Fatigue is common. The person works hard to breathe in and out. Breathing is easier when the person sits upright and slightly forward. The person must stop smoking. Respiratory therapy, breathing exercises, oxygen, and medication therapy are ordered.

Asthma

- In asthma, the airway becomes inflamed and narrow. Extra mucus is produced. Dyspnea results. Wheezing and coughing are common. So are pain and tightening in the chest. Asthma usually is triggered by allergies. Other triggers include air pollutants and irritants, smoking and second-hand smoke, respiratory tract infections, exertion, and cold air. Asthma is treated with medications. Severe attacks may require emergency care.

Pneumonia

- Pneumonia is an inflammation and infection of lung tissue. Bacteria, viruses, and other microbes are causes.
- High fever, chills, painful cough, chest pain on breathing, and rapid pulse occur. Shortness of breath and rapid breathing also occur. Cyanosis may be present. Sputum is thick and white, green, yellow, or rust-colored. Other signs and symptoms are nausea, vomiting, headache, tiredness, and muscle aches.
- Medications are ordered for infection and pain. Fluid intake is increased. Intravenous therapy and oxygen may be needed. Semi-Fowler's position eases breathing. Rest is important. Standard Precautions are followed. Isolation precautions are used depending on the cause.

Tuberculosis

- Tuberculosis (TB) is a bacterial infection in the lungs. TB is spread by airborne droplets with coughing, sneezing, speaking, singing, or laughing. Those who have close, frequent contact with an infected person are at risk. TB is more likely to occur in close, crowded areas. Age, poor nutrition, and human immunodeficiency virus (HIV) infection are other risk factors.
- Signs and symptoms are tiredness, loss of appetite, weight loss, fever, and night sweats. Cough and sputum production increase over time. Sputum may contain blood. Chest pain occurs.
- Medications for TB are given. Standard Precautions and isolation precautions are needed. The person must cover the mouth and nose with tissues when sneezing, coughing, or producing sputum. Tissues are flushed down the toilet, placed in a BIOHAZARD bag, or placed in a paper bag and burned. Hand washing after contact with sputum is essential.

CHAPTER 35 REVIEW QUESTIONS
Circle the BEST answer.

1. Which statement about angina is *false?*
   a. Angina is chest pain.
   b. The person may be pale and perspire.
   c. Rest often relieves the symptoms.
   d. You do not report angina to the nurse.
2. A person has heart failure. You do all of the following *except*
   a. Measure intake and output
   b. Measure weight daily
   c. Promote a diet that is high in salt
   d. Restrict fluids as ordered
3. Which position is usually best for the person with pneumonia?
   a. Semi-Fowler's
   b. Prone
   c. Supine
   d. Trendelenburg's

4. A bacterial infection in the lungs is
   a. Asthma
   b. Bronchitis
   c. Tuberculosis
   d. Emphysema

Answers to these questions are on p. 506.

CHAPTER 36 DIGESTIVE AND ENDOCRINE DISORDERS
DIGESTIVE DISORDERS
Vomiting
- These measures are needed:
  - Follow Standard Precautions and the Bloodborne Pathogen Standard.
  - Turn the person's head well to one side. This prevents aspiration.
  - Place a kidney basin under the person's chin.
  - Move vomitus away from the person.
  - Provide oral hygiene.
  - Observe vomitus for color, odor, and undigested food. If it looks like coffee grounds, it contains undigested blood. This signals bleeding. Report your observations.
  - Measure, report, and record the amount of vomitus. Also record the amount on the intake and output (I&O) record.
  - Save a specimen for laboratory study.
  - Dispose of vomitus after the nurse observes it.
  - Eliminate odors.
  - Provide for comfort.

Hepatitis
- Hepatitis is an inflammation of the liver. It can be mild or cause death. Signs and symptoms are listed in Box 36-2 in the textbook. Some people do not have symptoms.
- Protect yourself and others. Follow Standard Precautions and the Bloodborne Pathogen Standard. Isolation precautions are ordered as necessary. Assist the person with hygiene and hand washing as needed.

THE ENDOCRINE SYSTEM
Diabetes
- In this disorder the body cannot produce or use insulin properly. Insulin is needed for glucose to move from the blood into the cells. Sugar builds up in the blood. Cells do not have enough sugar for energy and cannot function.
- Diabetes must be controlled to prevent complications. Complications include blindness, renal failure, nerve damage, and damage to the gums and teeth. Heart and blood vessel diseases are other problems. They can lead to stroke, heart attack, and slow healing. Foot and leg wounds and ulcers are very serious.

- Good foot care is needed. Corns, blisters, calluses, and other foot problems can lead to an infection and amputation.
- Blood glucose is monitored for:
  - *Hypoglycemia*—low sugar in the blood.
  - *Hyperglycemia*—high sugar in the blood.
- Review Table 36-1 in the textbook for the causes, signs, and symptoms of hypoglycemia and hyperglycemia. Both can lead to death if not corrected. You must call for the nurse at once.

CHAPTER 36 REVIEW QUESTIONS
Circle the BEST answer.
1. A person is vomiting. You should do all of the following *except*
   a. Follow Standard Precautions and the Bloodborne Pathogen Standard
   b. Keep the person supine
   c. Provide oral hygiene
   d. Observe vomitus for color, odor, and undigested food
2. A person with diabetes is trembling, sweating, and feels faint. You
   a. Tell the nurse immediately
   b. Tell the nurse at the end of the shift
   c. Tell another nursing assistant
   d. Ignore the symptoms
3. All of the following are signs and symptoms of hepatitis except
   a. Itching
   b. Diarrhea
   c. Skin rash
   d. Increased appetite

Answers to these questions are on p. 506.

CHAPER 37 URINARY AND REPRODUCTIVE DISORDERS
URINARY SYSTEM DISORDERS
Urinary Tract Infections (UTIs)
- UTIs are common. Catheters, poor perineal hygiene, immobility, and poor fluid intake are common causes.

Prostate Enlargement
- The prostate grows larger as a man grows older. This is called benign prostatic hyperplasia (BPH). The enlarged prostate presses against the urethra. This obstructs urine flow through the urethra. Bladder function is gradually lost. Most men in their 60s and older have some symptoms of BPH.

REPRODUCTIVE DISORDERS
Sexually Transmitted Diseases
- A sexually transmitted disease (STD) is spread by oral, vaginal, or anal sex. Some people do not have

signs and symptoms or are not aware of an infection. Others know but do not seek treatment because of embarrassment. Standard Precautions and the Bloodborne Pathogen Standard are followed.

CHAPTER 37 REVIEW QUESTIONS
Circle the BEST answer.

1. Which statement is *false*?
   a. Older persons are at high risk for urinary tract infections.
   b. Skin irritation and infection can occur if urine leaks onto the skin.
   c. Benign prostatic hypertrophy may cause urinary problems in women.
   d. Some people may not be aware of having a sexually transmitted disease.
2. An STD is spread by oral, vaginal, or anal sex.
   a. True
   b. False
3. A person with an STD always has signs and symptoms.
   a. True
   b. False

Answers to these questions are on p. 506.

CHAPTER 38 MENTAL HEALTH DISORDERS
- The whole person has physical, social, psychological, and spiritual parts. Each part affects the other.
- **Mental health** means the person copes with and adjusts to every-day stresses in ways accepted by society.
- **Mental illness** is a disturbance in the ability to cope with or adjust to stress. Behavior and function are impaired. Mental disorder, emotional illness, and psychiatric disorder also mean mental illness.

ANXIETY DISORDERS
- **Anxiety** is a vague, uneasy feeling in response to stress. The person may not know why or the cause. The person senses danger or harm—real or imagined. Some anxiety is normal. Review Box 38-1, Signs and Symptoms of Anxiety, in the textbook.
- Coping and defense mechanisms are used to relieve anxiety. Review Box 38-2, Defense Mechanisms, in the textbook.
- Some common anxiety disorders include panic disorder, phobias, obsessive-compulsive disorder, and post-traumatic stress disorder.
- *Panic disorder*. **Panic** is an intense and sudden feeling of fear, anxiety, terror, or dread. Onset is sudden with no obvious reason. The person cannot function. Signs and symptoms of anxiety are severe.
- *Phobias*. **Phobia** means an intense fear. The person has an intense fear of an object, situation, or activity that has little or no actual danger. The person avoids what is feared. When faced with the fear, the person has high anxiety and cannot function.
- *Obsessive-compulsive disorder (OCD)*. An **obsession** is a recurrent, unwanted thought, idea, or image. **Compulsion** is repeating an act over and over again. The act may not make sense, but the person has much anxiety if the act is not done. Some persons with OCD also have depression, eating disorders, substance abuse, and other anxiety disorders.
- *Post-traumatic stress disorder (PTSD)*. PTSD occurs after a terrifying ordeal. The ordeal involved physical harm or the threat of physical harm. Review Box 38-3, Signs and Symptoms of Post-Traumatic Stress Disorder, in the textbook. Flashbacks are common. A **flashback** is reliving the trauma in thoughts during the day and in nightmares during sleep. During a flashback, the person may lose touch with reality. He or she may believe that the trauma is happening all over again. Signs and symptoms usually develop about 3 months after the harmful event. Or they may emerge years later. PTSD can develop at any age.

SCHIZOPHRENIA
- *Schizophrenia* means split mind. It is a severe, chronic, disabling brain disorder that involves:
  - **Psychosis**—a state of severe mental impairment. The person does not view the real or unreal correctly.
  - **Delusion**—a false belief.
  - **Hallucination**—seeing, hearing, smelling, or feeling something that is not real.
  - **Paranoia**—a disorder of the mind. The person has false beliefs (delusions). He or she is suspicious about a person or situation.
  - **Delusion of grandeur**—an exaggerated belief about one's importance, wealth, power, or talents.
  - **Delusion of persecution**—the false belief that one is being mistreated, abused, or harassed.
- The person with schizophrenia has problems relating to others. He or she may be paranoid. The person may have difficulty organizing thoughts. Responses are inappropriate. Communication is disturbed. The person may withdraw. Some people regress to an earlier time or condition. Some persons with schizophrenia attempt suicide.

MOOD DISORDERS
- Mood disorders involve feelings, emotions, and moods.

Bipolar Disorder
- The person with bipolar disorder has severe extremes in mood, energy, and ability to function. There are emotional lows (depression) and emotional highs (mania). This disorder is also called manic-depressive illness. This disorder must be managed

throughout life. Review Box 38-4, Signs and Symptoms of Bipolar Disorder, in the textbook. Bipolar disorder can damage relationships and affect school or work performance. Some people are suicidal.

Major Depression
- Depression involves the body, mood, and thoughts. Symptoms affect work, study, sleep, eating, and other activities. The person is very sad.
- Depression is common in older persons. They have many losses—death of family and friends, loss of health, loss of body functions, loss of independence. Loneliness and the side effects of some medications also are causes. Review Box 38-5, Signs and Symptoms of Depression in Older Persons, in the textbook. Depression in older persons is often overlooked or a wrong diagnosis is made.

SUBSTANCE ABUSE AND ADDICTION

Alcoholism
- Alcohol affects alertness, judgment, coordination, and reaction time. Over time, heavy drinking damages the brain, central nervous system, liver, heart, kidneys, and stomach. It causes changes in the heart and blood vessels. It also can cause forgetfulness and confusion. Alcoholism is a chronic disease. There is no cure. However, alcoholism can be treated. Counseling and medications are used to help the person stop drinking. The person must avoid all alcohol to avoid a relapse.
- Alcohol effects vary with age. Even small amounts can make older persons feel "high." Older persons are at risk for falls, vehicle crashes, and other injuries from drinking. Mixing alcohol with some medications can be harmful or fatal. Alcohol also makes some health problems worse.

SUICIDE
- **Suicide** means to kill oneself.
- People think about suicide when they feel hopeless or when they cannot see solutions to their problems. Suicide is most often linked to depression, alcohol or substance abuse, or stressful events. Review Box 38-6, Risk Factors for Suicide, in the textbook.
- If a person mentions or talks about suicide, take the person seriously. Call for the nurse at once. Do not leave the person alone.

CARE AND TREATMENT
- Treatment of mental health disorders involves having the person explore his or her thoughts and feelings. This is done through psychotherapy and behavior,

group, occupational, art, and family therapies. Often medications are ordered.
- The care plan reflects the person's needs. The physical, safety and security, and emotional needs of the person must be met.
- Communication is important. Be alert to nonverbal communication.

CHAPTER 38 REVIEW QUESTIONS
Circle the BEST answer.

1. A person may not know why anxiety occurs.
   a. True
   b. False
2. Panic is an intense and sudden feeling of fear, anxiety, terror, or dread.
   a. True
   b. False
3. A person with an obsessive-compulsive disorder has a ritual that is repeated over and over again.
   a. True
   b. False
4. A person talks about suicide. You must do all of the following *except*
   a. Call the nurse at once
   b. Stay with the person
   c. Leave the person alone
   d. Take the person seriously
5. Which statement about depression in older persons is *false*?
   a. Depression is often overlooked in older persons.
   b. Depression rarely occurs in older persons.
   c. Loneliness may be a cause of depression in older persons.
   d. Side effects of some medications may cause depression in older persons.
6. Which statement is *false*?
   a. Communication is important when caring for a person with a mental health disorder.
   b. You should be alert to nonverbal communication when caring for a person with a mental health disorder.
   c. The care plan reflects the needs of the person.
   d. The focus is only on the person's emotional needs.

Answers to these questions are on p. 506.

CHAPTER 39 CONFUSION AND DEMENTIA
- Changes in the brain and nervous system occur with aging. Review Box 39-1, Changes in the Nervous System From Aging, in the textbook.
- Changes in the brain can affect **cognitive function**—memory, thinking, reasoning, ability to understand, judgment, and behavior.

CONFUSION

- Confusion has many causes. Diseases, infections, hearing and vision loss, brain injury, and medication side effects are some causes.
- When caring for the confused person:
  - Follow the person's care plan.
  - Provide for safety.
  - Face the person and speak clearly.
  - Call the person by name every time you are in contact with him or her.
  - State your name. Show your name tag.
  - Give the date and time each morning. Repeat as needed during the day and evening.
  - Explain what you are going to do and why.
  - Give clear, simple directions and answers to questions.
  - Ask clear, simple questions. Give the person time to respond.
  - Keep calendars and clocks with large numbers in the person's room.
  - Have the person wear eyeglasses and hearing aids as needed.
  - Use touch to communicate.
  - Place familiar objects and pictures within the person's view.
  - Provide newspapers, magazines, TV, and radio. Read to the person if appropriate.
  - Discuss current events with the person.
  - Maintain the day-night cycle.
  - Provide a calm, relaxed, and peaceful setting.
  - Follow the person's routine.
  - Break tasks into small steps when helping the person.
  - Do not rearrange furniture or the person's belongings.
  - Encourage the person to take part in self-care.
  - Be consistent.

DEMENTIA

- **Dementia** is the loss of cognitive function that interferes with routine personal, social, and occupational activities.
- Dementia is not a normal part of aging. Most older people do not have dementia.
- Some early warning signs include problems with dressing, cooking, and driving as well as getting lost in familiar places and misplacing items.
- Alzheimer's disease is the most common type of permanent dementia.

ALZHEIMER'S DISEASE

- Alzheimer's disease (AD) is a brain disease. Memory, thinking, reasoning, judgment, language, behavior, mood, and personality are affected.

Signs of AD

- The classic sign of AD is gradual loss of short-term memory. Warning signs include:
  - Asking the same questions over and over again.
  - Repeating the same story—word for word, again and again.
  - Forgetting activities that were once done regularly with ease.
  - Losing the ability to pay bills or balance a checkbook.
  - Getting lost in familiar places. Or misplacing household objects.
  - Neglecting to bathe or wearing the same clothes over and over again. Meanwhile, the person insists that a bath was taken or that clothes were changed.
  - Relying on someone else to make decisions or answer questions that he or she would have handled.
- Review Box 39-5, Signs of Alzheimer's Disease, in the textbook for other signs of AD.

Behaviors

- The following behaviors are common with AD:
  - *Wandering*. Persons with AD are not oriented to person, place, and time. They may wander away from home and not find their way back. The person cannot tell what is safe or dangerous.
  - *Sundowning*. With sundowning, signs, symptoms, and behaviors of AD increase during hours of darkness. As daylight ends, confusion, restlessness, anxiety, agitation, and other symptoms increase.
  - *Hallucinations*. The person with AD may see, hear, or feel things that are not real.
  - *Delusions*. People with AD may think they are some other person. A person may believe that the caregiver is someone else.
  - *Catastrophic reactions*. The person reacts as if there is a disaster or tragedy.
  - *Agitation and restlessness*. The person may pace, hit, or yell.
  - *Aggression and combativeness*. These behaviors include hitting, pinching, grabbing, biting, or swearing.
  - *Screaming*. Persons with AD may scream to communicate.
  - *Abnormal sexual behaviors*. Sexual behaviors may involve the wrong person, the wrong time, and the wrong place. Persons with AD cannot control behavior.
  - *Repetitive behaviors*. Persons with AD repeat the same motions over and over again.

CARE OF PERSONS WITH AD AND OTHER DEMENTIAS

- People with AD do not choose to be forgetful, incontinent, agitated, or rude. Nor do they choose to have other behaviors, signs, and symptoms of the disease. The disease causes the behaviors.
- Safety, hygiene, nutrition and fluids, elimination, and activity needs must be met. So must comfort and sleep needs. Review Box 39-9, Care of Persons With AD and Other Dementias, in the textbook.
- The person can have other health problems and injuries. However, the person may not recognize pain, fever, constipation, incontinence, or other signs and symptoms. Carefully observe the person. Report any change in the person's usual behavior to the nurse.
- Infection is a risk. Provide good skin care, oral hygiene, and perineal care after bowel and bladder elimination.
- Supervised activities meet the person's needs and cognitive abilities.
- Impaired communication is a common problem. Avoid giving orders, wanting the truth, and correcting the person's errors.
- Always look for dangers in the person's room and in the hallways, lounges, dining areas, and other areas on the nursing unit. Remove the danger if you can.
- Every staff member must be alert to persons who wander. Such persons are allowed to wander in safe areas.

The Family

- The family may have physical, emotional, social, and financial stresses. The family often feels hopeless. No matter what is done, the person only gets worse. Anger and resentment may result. Guilt feelings are common.
- The family is an important part of the health team. They may help plan the person's care. For many persons, family members provide comfort. The family also needs support and understanding from the health team.

CHAPTER 39 REVIEW QUESTIONS

Circle the BEST answer.

1. Cognitive function involves all of the following *except*
   a. Memory and thinking
   b. Reasoning and understanding
   c. Personality and mood
   d. Judgment and behavior
2. When caring for a confused person, you do all of the following *except*
   a. Provide for safety
   b. Maintain the day-night schedule
   c. Keep calendars and clocks in the person's room
   d. Ask difficult-to-understand questions and give complex directions

3. Which statement about dementia is *false*?
   a. Dementia is a normal part of aging.
   b. The person may have changes in personality.
   c. Alzheimer's disease is the most common type of dementia.
   d. The person may have changes in behavior.
4. When caring for persons with AD, you do all of the following *except*
   a. Provide good skin care
   b. Talk to them in a calm voice
   c. Observe them closely for unusual behavior
   d. Allow personal choice in wandering

Answers to these questions are on p. 506.

CHAPTER 41 REHABILITATION AND RESTORATIVE NURSING CARE

- A **disability** is any lost, absent, or impaired physical or mental function.
- **Rehabilitation** is the process of restoring the person to his or her highest possible level of physical, psychological, social, and economic function. The focus is on improving abilities. This promotes function at the highest level of independence.

REHABILITATION AND THE WHOLE PERSON

- Rehabilitation takes longer in older persons. Changes from aging affect healing, mobility, vision, hearing, and other functions. Chronic health problems can slow recovery.

Physical Aspects

- Rehabilitation starts when the person first seeks health care. Complications, such as contractures and pressure ulcers, are prevented.
- *Self-care.* Self-care for activities of daily living (ADL) is a major goal. Self-help devices are often needed.
- *Elimination.* Bowel or bladder training may be needed. Fecal impaction, constipation, and fecal incontinence are prevented.
- *Mobility.* The person may need crutches, a walker, a cane, a brace, or a wheelchair.
- *Nutrition.* The person may need a dysphagia diet or enteral nutrition.
- *Communication.* Speech therapy and communication devices may be helpful.

Psychological and Social Aspects

- A disability can affect function and appearance. Self-esteem and relationships may suffer. The person may feel unwhole, useless, unattractive, unclean, or undesirable. The person may deny the disability. The person may expect therapy to correct the problem. He or she may be depressed, angry, and hostile.
- Successful rehabilitation depends on the person's attitude. The person must accept his or her limits and

be motivated. The focus is on abilities and strengths. Despair and frustration are common. Progress may be slow. Old fears and emotions may recur.
- Remind persons of their progress. They need help accepting disabilities and limits. Give support, reassurance, and encouragement. Spiritual support helps some people. Psychological and social needs are part of the care plan.

THE REHABILITATION TEAM

- Rehabilitation is a team effort. The person is the key member. The health team and family help the person set goals and plan care. All help the person regain function and independence.

Your Role

- Every part of your job focuses on promoting the person's independence. Preventing decline in function also is a goal. Review Box 41-2, Assisting With Rehabilitation and Restorative Care, in the textbook.

Quality of Life

- To promote quality of life:
  - *Protect the right to privacy.* The person re-learns old skills or practices new skills in private. Others do not need to see mistakes, falls, spills, clumsiness, anger, or tears.
  - *Encourage personal choice.* This gives the person control.
  - *Protect the right to be free from abuse and mistreatment.* Sometimes improvement is not seen for weeks. Repeated explanations and demonstrations may have little or no results. You and other staff and family may become upset and short-tempered. However, no one can shout, scream, or yell at the person. Nor can they call the person names or hit or strike the person. Unkind remarks are not allowed. Report signs of abuse or mistreatment.
  - *Learn to deal with your anger and frustration.* The person does not choose loss of function. If the process upsets you, discuss your feelings with the nurse.

- *Encourage activities.* Provide support and reassurance to the person with the disability. Remind the person that others with disabilities can give support and understanding.
- *Provide a safe setting.* The setting must meet the person's needs. The over-bed table, bedside stand, and call light are moved to the person's strong side.
- *Show patience, understanding, and sensitivity.* The person may be upset and discouraged. Give support, encouragement, and praise when needed. Stress the person's abilities and strengths. Do not give pity or sympathy.

CHAPTER 41 REVIEW QUESTIONS
Circle the BEST answer.
1. Successful rehabilitation depends on the person's attitude.
   a. True
   b. False
2. A person with a disability may be depressed, angry, and hostile.
   a. True
   b. False
3. A person needs rehabilitation. You should do all of the following *except*
   a. Let the person re-learn old skills in private
   b. Let the person practice new skills in private
   c. Encourage the person to make choices
   d. Shout at the person
4. You saw a family member hit and scream at a person. You need to report your observations to the nurse.
   a. True
   b. False
5. A person has a weak left arm. You will
   a. Place the call light on his left side
   b. Place the call light on his right side
   c. Give him sympathy
   d. Give him pity

Answers to these questions are on p. 506.

PRACTICE EXAMINATION 1

This test contains 75 questions. For each question, circle the BEST answer.

1. A nurse asks you to give a person his medication when he is done in the bathroom. Your response to the nurse is
   A. "I will give the medication for you."
   B. "I will ask the other nursing assistant to give the medication."
   C. "I am sorry but I cannot give that medication. I will let you know when he is out of the bathroom."
   D. "I refuse to give that medication."

2. An ethical person
   A. Does not judge others
   B. Avoids persons whose standards and values are different from his or hers
   C. Is prejudiced and biased
   D. Causes harm to another person

3. You smell alcohol on the breath of a co-worker. You
   A. Ignore the situation
   B. Tell the co-worker to get counseling
   C. Take a break and drink some alcohol, too
   D. Tell the nurse at once

4. A person's call light goes unanswered. He gets out of bed and falls. His leg is broken. This is
   A. Neglect
   B. Emotional abuse
   C. Physical abuse
   D. Malpractice

5. Your mom asks you about a person on your unit. How should you respond?
   A. "She is walking better now that she is receiving physical therapy."
   B. "I'm sorry but I cannot talk about her. It is unprofessional and violates her privacy and confidentiality."
   C. "Don't tell anyone I told you but she is getting worse."
   D. "She has been very sad recently and needs visitors."

6. You are going off duty. The nursing assistant coming on duty is on the unit with you. A person puts her call light on. Your response is
   A. "I'm ready to go. I will let you answer that light."
   B. "I've been here all day so I am not answering that light."
   C. "No one helped me answer lights when I came on duty."
   D. "I will answer that light so you can get organized for the shift."

7. When recording in the medical record, you
   A. Write in pencil
   B. Spell words incorrectly
   C. Use only center-approved abbreviations
   D. Record what your co-worker did

8. You are answering the phone in the nurses' station. You
   A. Answer in a rushed manner
   B. Give a courteous greeting
   C. End the conversation and hang up without saying good-bye
   D. Give confidential information about a resident to the caller

9. A person who was admitted to the nursing center yesterday does not feel safe. You
   A. Are rude as you care for the person
   B. Ignore the person's requests for information
   C. Show the person around the nursing center
   D. Act rushed as you care for the person

10. A person is angry and is shouting at you. You should
    A. Yell back at the person
    B. Stay calm and professional
    C. Put the person in a room away from others
    D. Call the family

11. When speaking with another person, you
    A. Use medical terms that may not be familiar to the person
    B. Mumble your words as you talk
    C. Ask several questions at a time
    D. Speak clearly and distinctly

12. To use a transfer or gait belt safely, you should
    A. Ignore the manufacturer instructions
    B. Leave the excess strap dangling
    C. Apply the belt over bare skin
    D. Apply the belt under the breasts

13. When you are listening to a person, you
    A. Look around the room
    B. Sit with your arms crossed
    C. Act rushed and not interested in what the person is saying
    D. Have good eye contact with the person

14. When caring for a person who is comatose, you
    A. Make jokes about how sick the person is
    B. Care for the person without talking to him or her
    C. Explain what you are doing to him or her
    D. Discuss your problems with the other nursing assistant in the room with you

15. You need to give care to a person when a visitor is present. You
    A. Politely ask the visitor to leave the room
    B. Do the care in the presence of the visitor
    C. Expose the person's body in front of the visitor
    D. Rudely tell the visitor where to wait while you care for the person

16. A person tells you he wants to talk with a minister. You
    A. Ignore the request
    B. Tell the nurse
    C. Ask what the person wants to discuss with the minister
    D. Tell the person there is no need to talk with a minister

17. When you care for a person who has a restraint, you
    A. Observe the person every 15 minutes
    B. Remove the restraint and reposition the person every 4 hours
    C. Apply the restraint tightly
    D. Apply the restraint incorrectly

18. As a person ages
    A. The skin becomes less dry
    B. Muscle strength increases
    C. Reflexes are faster
    D. Bladder muscles weaken

19. A person you are caring for touches your buttocks several times. You
    A. Tell the person you like being touched
    B. Ask the person not to touch you again
    C. Tell the person's daughter
    D. Tell the person's girlfriend

20. You are transporting a person in a wheelchair. You
    A. Pull the chair backward
    B. Let the person's feet touch the floor
    C. Push the chair forward
    D. Rest the footplates on the person's leg

21. You cannot read the person's name on the identification (ID) bracelet. You
    A. Tell the nurse so a new bracelet can be made
    B. Ignore the fact that you cannot read the name
    C. Ask another nursing assistant to identify the person
    D. Tell the family the person needs a new ID bracelet

22. The universal sign of choking is
    A. Holding your breath
    B. Clutching at the throat
    C. Having difficulty breathing
    D. Coughing

23. A person is on a diabetic diet. You
    A. Serve the person's meals late
    B. Let the person eat whenever he or she is hungry
    C. Sometimes check the tray to see what was eaten
    D. Tell the nurse about changes in the person's eating habits

24. With mild airway obstruction
    A. The person is usually unconscious
    B. The person cannot speak
    C. Forceful coughing often does not remove the object
    D. Forceful coughing often can remove the object

25. To relieve severe airway obstruction in a conscious adult, you do
    A. Abdominal thrusts
    B. Back thrusts
    C. Chest compressions
    D. A finger sweep

26. Faulty electrical equipment
    A. Can be used in a nursing center
    B. Should be given to the nurse
    C. Should be taken home by you for repair
    D. Should be used only with alert persons

27. A warning label has been removed from a hazardous substance container. You
    A. May use the substance if you know what is in the container
    B. Leave the container where it is
    C. Take the container to the nurse and explain the problem
    D. Tell another nursing assistant about the missing label

28. A person's beliefs and values are different from your views. What should you do?
    A. Refuse to care for the person.
    B. Delegate care to another nursing assistant.
    C. Tell the nurse about your concerns.
    D. Tell the person how you feel.

29. You find a person smoking in the nursing center. You should
    A. Ignore the situation
    B. Tell the person to leave
    C. Tell another nursing assistant
    D. Ask the person to put the cigarette out and show him or her where smoking is permitted

30. During a fire, the first thing you do is
    A. Rescue persons in immediate danger
    B. Sound the nearest fire alarm
    C. Close doors and windows to confine the fire
    D. Extinguish the fire

31. A person with Alzheimer's disease has increased restlessness and confusion as daylight ends. You
    A. Try to reason with the person
    B. Ask the person to tell you what is bothering him or her
    C. Provide a calm, quiet setting late in the day
    D. Complete his or her treatments and activities late in the day

32. To prevent suffocation, you should
    A. Make sure dentures fit loosely
    B. Cut food into large pieces
    C. Make sure the person can chew and swallow the food served
    D. Ignore loose teeth or dentures

33. When using a wheelchair, you should
    A. Lock both wheels before you transfer a person to and from the wheelchair
    B. Lock only one wheel before you transfer a person to and from the wheelchair
    C. Let the person's feet touch the floor when the chair is moving
    D. Let the person stand on the footplates

34. A person begins to fall while you are walking him or her. You should
    A. Try to prevent the fall
    B. Ease the person to the floor
    C. Yell at the person for falling
    D. Tell the nurse at the end of the shift

35. A person has a restraint on. You know that
    A. Restraints are used for staff convenience
    B. Death from strangulation is a risk factor when using a restraint
    C. Restraints may be used to punish a person
    D. A written nurse's order is required for a restraint

36. Before feeding a person, you
    A. Tell the other nursing assistant
    B. Go to the restroom
    C. Wash your hands
    D. Tell the nurse

37. When wearing gloves, you remember to
    A. Wear them several times before discarding them
    B. Wear the same ones from room to room
    C. Wear gloves with a tear or puncture
    D. Change gloves when they become contaminated with urine

38. When washing your hands, you
    A. Use hot water
    B. Let your uniform touch the sink
    C. Keep your watch at your wrist
    D. Keep your hands and forearms lower than your elbows

39. You need to move a box from the floor to the counter in the utility room. You
    A. Bend from your waist to pick up the box
    B. Hold the box away from your body as you pick it up
    C. Bend your knees and squat to lift the box
    D. Stand with your feet close together as you pick up the box

40. The nurse asks you to place a person in Fowler's position. You
    A. Put the bed flat
    B. Raise the head of the bed between 45 and 60 degrees
    C. Raise the head of the bed between 80 and 90 degrees
    D. Raise the head of the bed 15 degrees

41. You accidentally scratch a person. This is
    A. Neglect
    B. Negligence
    C. Malpractice
    D. Physical abuse

42. You positioned a person in a chair. For good body alignment, you
    A. Have the person's back and buttocks against the back of the chair
    B. Leave the person's feet unsupported
    C. Have the backs of the person's knees touch the edge of the chair
    D. Have the person sit on the edge of the chair

43. You need to transfer a person with a weak left leg from the bed to the wheelchair. You
    A. Get the person out of bed on the left side
    B. Get the person out of bed on the right side
    C. Keep the person in bed
    D. Ask the person which side moves first

44. A person tries to scratch and kick you. You should
    A. Protect yourself from harm
    B. Argue with the person
    C. Become angry with the person
    D. Ignore the person

45. When moving a person up in bed
    A. Window coverings may be left open so people can look in
    B. Body parts may be exposed
    C. Ask the person to help
    D. Ask the person to lie still

46. For comfort, most older persons prefer
    A. Rooms that are cold
    B. Restrooms that smell of urine
    C. Loud talking and laughter in the nurses' station
    D. Lighting that meets their needs

47. Call lights are
    A. Placed on the person's strong side
    B. Answered when time permits
    C. Kept on the bedside table
    D. Kept on the person's weak side

48. A nurse asks you to inspect a person's closet. You
    A. Tell the nurse you cannot do this
    B. Inspect the closet when the person is in the dining room
    C. Ask the person if you can inspect his or her closet
    D. Tell the nurse to inspect the closet

49. When changing bed linens, you
    A. Hold the linens close to your uniform
    B. Shake the sheet when putting it on the bed
    C. Take only needed linens into the person's room
    D. Put dirty linens on the floor
50. To use a fire extinguisher, you
    A. Keep the safety pin in the extinguisher
    B. Direct the hose or nozzle at the top of the fire
    C. Squeeze the lever to start the stream
    D. Sweep the stream at the top of the fire
51. When doing mouth care for an unconscious person, you
    A. Do not need to wear gloves
    B. Give mouth care at least every 2 hours
    C. Place the person in a supine position
    D. Keep the mouth open with your fingers
52. A person is angry because he did not get to the activity room on time because a co-worker did not come to work. How should you respond to him?
    A. "It's not my fault. A co-worker called off today and we are short-staffed."
    B. "I'm sorry you were late for activities. I will try to plan better."
    C. "I am doing the best I can."
    D. "I'm just too busy."
53. You are asked to clean a person's dentures. You
    A. Use hot water
    B. Hold the dentures firmly and line the basin with a towel
    C. Wrap the dentures in tissues after cleaning
    D. Store the dentures in a denture cup with the person's room number on it
54. When bathing a person, you notice a rash that was not there before. You
    A. Do nothing
    B. Tell the person
    C. Tell the nurse and record it in the medical record
    D. Tell the person's daughter
55. When washing a person's eyes, you
    A. Use soap
    B. Clean the eye near you first
    C. Wipe from the inner aspect to the outer aspect of the eye
    D. Wipe from the outer aspect to the inner aspect of the eye
56. When giving a back massage, you
    A. Use cold lotion
    B. Use light strokes
    C. Massage reddened bony areas
    D. Look for bruises and breaks in the skin
57. You need to give perineal care to a female. You
    A. Separate the labia and clean downward from front to back
    B. Separate the labia and clean upward from back to front
    C. Wear gloves only if there is drainage
    D. Only use water
58. When giving a person a tub bath or shower, you
    A. Do not give the person a call light
    B. Turn the hot water on first, then the cold water
    C. Stay within hearing distance if the person can be left alone
    D. Direct water toward the person while adjusting the water temperature
59. A person is on an anticoagulant. You
    A. Use a safety razor
    B. Use an electric razor
    C. Let him grow a beard
    D. Let him choose which type of razor to use
60. A person with a weak left arm wants to remove his or her sweater. You
    A. Let the person do it without any assistance
    B. Help the person remove the sweater from his or her right arm first
    C. Help the person remove the sweater from his or her left arm first
    D. Tell the person to keep the sweater on
61. When talking with a person, you should call the person
    A. "Honey"
    B. By his or her first name
    C. By his or her title—Mr. or Mrs. or Miss
    D. "Grandpa" or "Grandma"
62. A person has an indwelling catheter. You
    A. Let the person lie on the tubing
    B. Disconnect the catheter from the drainage tubing every 8 hours
    C. Secure the catheter to the lower leg
    D. Measure and record the amount of urine in the drainage bag
63. A person needs to eat a diet that contains carbohydrates. Carbohydrates
    A. Are needed for tissue repair and growth
    B. Provide energy and fiber for bowel elimination
    C. Add flavor to food and help the body use certain vitamins
    D. Are needed for nerve and muscle function
64. You are taking a rectal temperature with a thermometer. You
    A. Insert the thermometer before lubricating it
    B. Leave the privacy curtain open
    C. Leave the thermometer in place for 10 minutes
    D. Hold the thermometer in place

65. A person has a blood pressure (BP) of 86/58 mm Hg. You
    A. Report the BP to the nurse at once
    B. Record the BP but do not tell the nurse
    C. Ask the unit secretary to tell the nurse
    D. Retake the BP in 30 minutes before telling the nurse
66. On which person would you take an oral temperature?
    A. An unconscious person
    B. A person receiving oxygen
    C. A person who breathes through his or her mouth
    D. A conscious person
67. When caring for a person who is blind or visually impaired, you
    A. Offer the person your arm and have the person walk a half step behind you
    B. Do as much for the person as possible
    C. Shout at the person when talking with him or her
    D. Touch the person before indicating your presence
68. You are caring for a person with dementia. You
    A. Misplace the person's clothes
    B. Choose the activities the person attends
    C. Send personal items home
    D. Let the family make choices if the person cannot
69. When caring for a person with a disability, you
    A. Can shout or scream at the person
    B. Can hit or strike the person
    C. Can call the person names
    D. Discuss your anger with the nurse
70. While bathing a person, you
    A. Keep doors and windows open
    B. Wash from the dirtiest areas to the cleanest areas
    C. Encourage the person to help as much as possible
    D. Rub the skin dry

71. When a person is dying
    A. Assume that the person can hear you
    B. Oral care is done every 5 hours
    C. Skin care is done weekly
    D. Re-position the person every 3 hours
72. A person is on intake and output. You
    A. Measure only liquids such as water and juice
    B. Measure ice cream and gelatin as part of intake
    C. Measure intravenous (IV) fluids
    D. Measure tube feedings
73. A person has been on bedrest. You need to have the person walk. What will you do first?
    A. Help the person move quickly.
    B. Have the person dangle before getting out of bed.
    C. Have the person sit in a chair.
    D. Walk with the person as soon as he or she gets out of bed.
74. Your ring accidentally causes a skin tear on an elderly person. You
    A. Tell yourself to be more careful the next time
    B. Tell the nurse at once
    C. Do nothing
    D. Hope no one finds out
75. To protect a person's privacy, you should
    A. Keep all information about the person confidential
    B. Discuss the person's treatment with another nursing assistant in the lunch room
    C. Open the person's mail
    D. Keep the privacy curtain open when providing care to the person

PRACTICE EXAMINATION 2

This test contains 75 questions. For each question, circle the BEST answer.

1. You can refuse to do a delegated task when
   A. You are too busy
   B. You do not like the task
   C. The task is not in your job description
   D. It is the end of the shift

2. Mr. Smith does not want life-saving measures. You
   A. Explain to Mr. Smith why he should have life-saving measures
   B. Respect his decision
   C. Explain to Mr. Smith's family why life-saving measures are needed
   D. Tell your friend about Mr. Smith's decision

3. You are walking by a resident's room. You hear a nurse shouting at a person. This is
   A. Battery
   B. Malpractice
   C. Verbal abuse
   D. Neglect

4. When communicating with a foreign-speaking person, you
   A. Speak loudly or shout
   B. Use medical terms the person may not understand
   C. Use words the person seems to understand
   D. Speak quickly and mumble

5. To protect a person from getting burned, you
   A. Allow smoking in bed
   B. Turn hot water on first, then cold water
   C. Assist the person with drinking or eating hot food
   D. Let the person sleep with a heating pad

6. To prevent equipment accidents, you should
   A. Use two-pronged plugs on all electrical devices
   B. Follow the manufacturer instructions
   C. Wipe up spills when you have time
   D. Use unfamiliar equipment without training

7. To prevent a person from falling, you should
   A. Ignore call lights
   B. Use throw rugs on the floor
   C. Keep the bed in a high position
   D. Use grab bars in showers

8. You need to wash your hands
   A. Before you document a procedure
   B. After you remove gloves
   C. After you talk with a person
   D. After you talk with a co-worker

9. You need to turn a heavy person in bed. You
   A. Do the procedure alone
   B. Keep the privacy curtain open
   C. Ask the person to lie still
   D. Use good body mechanics

10. When transferring a person from a bed to a wheelchair, you never
   A. Ask a co-worker to help you
   B. Use a transfer or gait belt
   C. Have the person put his or her arms around your neck
   D. Lock the wheels on the wheelchair

11. When making a bed, you
   A. Keep the bed in the low position
   B. Wear gloves when removing linens
   C. Raise the head of the bed
   D. Raise the foot of the bed

12. To give perineal care to a male, you
   A. Use a circular motion and work toward the meatus
   B. Use a circular motion and start at the meatus and work outward
   C. Wear gloves only if there is drainage
   D. Use only water

13. A person with a weak left arm wants to put his or her sweater on. You
   A. Let the person do it without any assistance
   B. Help the person put the sweater on his or her right arm first
   C. Help the person put the sweater on his or her left arm first
   D. Tell the person to keep the sweater off

14. A person has an indwelling catheter. You
   A. Let the drainage bag touch the floor
   B. Keep the drainage bag higher than the bladder
   C. Hang the drainage bag on a bed rail
   D. Have the drainage bag hang from the bed frame or chair

15. A person needs to eat a diet that contains protein. Protein
   A. Is needed for tissue repair and growth
   B. Provides energy and fiber for bowel elimination
   C. Adds flavor to food and helps the body use certain vitamins
   D. Is needed for nerve and muscle function

16. Older persons
   A. Have an increased sense of thirst
   B. Need less water than younger persons
   C. May not feel thirsty
   D. Seldom need to have water offered to them

486

17. A person is NPO. You
    A. Post a sign in the bathroom
    B. Keep the water pitcher filled at the bedside
    C. Remove the water pitcher and glass from the room
    D. Provide oral hygiene every day
18. A person drank 3 oz of milk at lunch. He or she drank
    A. 30 mL
    B. 60 mL
    C. 90 mL
    D. 120 mL
19. When feeding a person, you
    A. Offer fluids at the end of the meal
    B. Use forks
    C. Do not talk to the person
    D. Allow time for chewing and swallowing
20. You need to do range-of-motion (ROM) exercises to a person's right shoulder. You
    A. Force the joint beyond its present ROM
    B. Move the joint quickly
    C. Force the joint to the point of pain
    D. Support the part being exercised
21. A person has a weak left leg. The person should
    A. Hold the cane in his or her left hand
    B. Hold the cane in his or her right hand
    C. Hold the cane in either hand
    D. Use a walker
22. To promote comfort and relieve pain, you
    A. Keep wrinkles in the bed linens
    B. Position the person in good alignment
    C. Talk loudly to the person
    D. Make sudden and jarring movements of the bed or chair
23. A person is receiving oxygen through a nasal cannula. You
    A. Turn the oxygen higher when he or she is short of breath
    B. Fill the humidifier when it is not bubbling
    C. Check behind the ears and under the nose for signs of irritation
    D. Remove the cannula when the person goes to the dining room
24. When taking an apical pulse, count the pulse for
    A. 1 minute
    B. 30 seconds
    C. 2 minutes
    D. 1 minute 30 seconds
25. When taking a person's pulse, you
    A. Use the brachial pulse
    B. Take the pulse for 30 seconds if it is irregular
    C. Tell the nurse if the pulse is less than 60
    D. Use your thumb to take a pulse

26. You are counting respirations on a person. You
    A. Tell the person you are counting his or her respirations
    B. Count for 1 minute if an abnormal breathing pattern is noted
    C. Report a rate of 16 to the nurse at once
    D. Count for 30 seconds if an abnormal breathing pattern is noted
27. You are taking blood pressures on people assigned to you. An older person has a blood pressure (BP) of 188/96 mm Hg. You
    A. Report the BP to the nurse at once
    B. Finish taking all the blood pressures before telling the nurse
    C. Retake the BP in 30 minutes before telling the nurse
    D. Ask the unit secretary to tell the nurse about the BP
28. When would you take a rectal temperature?
    A. The person has diarrhea.
    B. The person is confused.
    C. The person is unconscious.
    D. The person is agitated.
29. A person has been admitted to the nursing center recently. You
    A. Look through his or her belongings
    B. Ignore his or her questions
    C. Speak in a gentle, calm voice
    D. Enter the person's room without knocking
30. When taking a person's height and weight, you
    A. Let the person wear shoes
    B. Have the person void before being weighed
    C. Weigh the person at different times of the day
    D. Balance the scale every 6 months
31. A person is bedfast. To prevent pressure ulcers, you
    A. Re-position the person at least every 3 hours
    B. Massage reddened areas
    C. Let heels and ankles touch the bed
    D. Keep the skin free of moisture from urine, stools, or perspiration
32. A person has a hearing problem. When talking with the person, you
    A. Keep the TV or radio on
    B. Shout
    C. Face the person
    D. Speak quickly
33. When caring for a person who is blind or visually impaired, you
    A. Place furniture and equipment where the person walks
    B. Keep the lights off
    C. Explain the location of food and beverages
    D. Re-arrange furniture and equipment

34. You are caring for a person with dementia. You
    - A. Share information about the person's care
    - B. Share information about the person's condition
    - C. Protect confidential information
    - D. Expose the person's body when you provide care

35. When caring for a confused person, you
    - A. Call the person "Honey"
    - B. Do not need to explain what you are doing
    - C. Ask clear, simple questions
    - D. Remove the calendar from the person's room

36. A person with Alzheimer's disease likes to wander. You
    - A. Keep the person in his or her room
    - B. Restrain the person
    - C. Argue with the person who wants to leave
    - D. Exercise the person as ordered

37. Restorative nursing programs
    - A. Help maintain the lowest level of function
    - B. Promote self-care measures
    - C. Focus on the disability, not the person
    - D. Help the person lose strength and independence

38. When caring for a person with a disability, you
    - A. Focus on his or her limitations
    - B. Expect progress in a rehabilitation program to be fast
    - C. Remind the person of his or her progress in the rehabilitation program
    - D. Deny the disability

39. After a person dies, you
    - A. Can expose his or her body unnecessarily
    - B. Can discuss the person's diagnosis with your family
    - C. Can talk about the family's reactions to your friends
    - D. Respect the person's right to privacy

40. You enter a person's room and find a fire in the wastebasket. Your first action is to
    - A. Remove the person from the room
    - B. Close the door
    - C. Call for help
    - D. Activate the fire alarm

41. You leave a person lying in urine and he or she develops a bedsore. This is
    - A. Fraud
    - B. Neglect
    - C. Assault
    - D. Battery

42. A nurse asks you to place a medication and a sterile dressing on a small foot wound. You
    - A. Agree to do the task
    - B. Ask another nursing assistant to do the task
    - C. Politely tell the nurse you cannot do that task
    - D. Report the nurse to the director of nursing

43. You observe that a person's urine is foul-smelling and dark amber. Your first action is to
    - A. Tell the other nursing assistant
    - B. Tell the person
    - C. Tell the nurse
    - D. Record the observation

44. A daughter asks you for water for her mom. Your response is
    - A. "I am not caring for your mom. I will get her nursing assistant for you."
    - B. "I do not have time to do that."
    - C. "That's not my job."
    - D. "I will be happy to do that."

45. A person has a restraint on. You
    - A. Observe the person for breathing and circulation complications every 30 minutes
    - B. Know that unnecessary restraint is false imprisonment
    - C. Use the most restrictive type of restraint
    - D. Know that restraints decrease confusion and agitation

46. The nurse asks you to place a person in the supine position. You
    - A. Elevate the head of the bed 45 degrees
    - B. Elevate the foot of the bed 15 degrees
    - C. Place the person on his or her back with the bed flat
    - D. Place the person on his or her abdomen

47. The most important way to prevent or avoid spreading infection is to
    - A. Wash your hands
    - B. Cover your nose when coughing
    - C. Use disposable gloves
    - D. Wear a mask

48. You are eating lunch and a nursing assistant begins to gossip about another person. You
    - A. Join the conversation and talk about the person
    - B. Remove yourself from the group
    - C. Tell your roommate about the gossip you heard at lunch
    - D. Tell another nursing assistant about the gossip you heard

49. When moving a person up in bed, you should
    - A. Raise the head of the bed
    - B. Ask the person to keep his or her legs straight
    - C. Cause friction and shearing
    - D. Ask a co-worker to help you

50. A person is on a sodium-controlled diet. This means
    - A. Canned vegetables are omitted from his or her diet
    - B. Salt may be added to food at the table
    - C. Large amounts of salt are used in cooking
    - D. Ham is eaten regularly

51. Elastic stockings
    A. Are applied after a person gets out of bed
    B. Should not have wrinkles or creases after being applied
    C. Come in one size only
    D. Are forced on the person

52. While walking, the person begins to fall. You
    A. Call for help
    B. Reach for a chair
    C. Ease the person to the floor
    D. Ask a visitor to help

53. Before bathing a person, you should
    A. Offer the bedpan or urinal
    B. Partially undress the person
    C. Raise the head of the bed
    D. Open the privacy curtain

54. When taking a rectal temperature, you insert the thermometer
    A. ½ inch
    B. 1.5 inches
    C. 2 inches
    D. 2.5 inches

55. Touch
    A. Is a form of nonverbal communication
    B. Is a form of verbal communication
    C. Means the same thing to everyone
    D. Should be used for all persons

56. You may share information about a person's care and condition to
    A. The staff caring for the person
    B. The person's daughter
    C. Your family members
    D. The volunteer in the gift shop

57. A person tells you he or she has pain upon urination. You
    A. Tell the nurse
    B. Let the nurse document this information
    C. Ask the person to tell you if it happens again
    D. Tell the person's son

58. A person's culture and religion are different from yours. You
    A. Laugh about the person's customs
    B. Tell your family about the person's customs
    C. Ask the person to explain his or her beliefs and practices to you
    D. Tell the person his or her beliefs and customs are silly

59. You need to wear gloves when you
    A. Do range-of-motion exercises
    B. Feed a person
    C. Give perineal care
    D. Walk a person

60. An older person is normally alert. Today he or she is confused. What should you do?
    A. Ask the person why he or she is confused
    B. Ignore the confusion
    C. Check to see if the person is confused later in the day
    D. Tell the nurse

61. While walking with a person, he tells you he feels faint. What do you do first?
    A. Have the person sit down.
    B. Call for the nurse.
    C. Open the window.
    D. Ask the person to take a deep breath.

62. You are asked to encourage fluids for a person. You
    A. Increase the person's fluid intake
    B. Decrease the person's fluid intake
    C. Limit fluids to meal times
    D. Keep fluids where the person cannot reach them

63. Communication fails when you
    A. Use words the other person understands
    B. Talk too much
    C. Let others express their feelings and concerns
    D. Talk about a topic that is uncomfortable

64. During bathing, a person may
    A. Decide what products to use
    B. Be exposed in the shower room
    C. Have visitors present without his or her permission
    D. Have no personal choices

65. People in late adulthood need to
    A. Adjust to increased income
    B. Adjust to their health being better
    C. Develop new friends and relationships
    D. Adjust to increased strength

66. When measuring blood pressure, you should do the following except
    A. Apply the cuff to a bare upper arm
    B. Turn off the TV
    C. Locate the brachial artery
    D. Use the arm with an intravenous (IV) infusion

67. You find clean linens on the floor in a person's room. You
    A. Use the linens to make the bed
    B. Return the linens to the linen cart
    C. Put the linens in the laundry
    D. Tell the nurse

68. When doing mouth care on an unconscious person, you
    A. Use a large amount of fluid
    B. Position the person on his or her side
    C. Do the task without telling the person what you are doing
    D. Insert his or her dentures when done

69. When brushing or combing a person's hair, you
    A. Cut matted or tangled hair
    B. Encourage the person to do as much as possible
    C. Style the hair as you want
    D. Perform the task weekly
70. When providing nail and foot care, you
    A. Cut fingernails with scissors
    B. Trim toenails for a diabetic person
    C. Trim toenails for a person with poor circulation
    D. Check between the toes for cracks and sores
71. An indwelling catheter becomes disconnected from the drainage system. You
    A. Reconnect the tubing to the catheter quickly without gloves
    B. Tell the nurse at once
    C. Get a new drainage system
    D. Touch the ends of the catheter
72. Urinary drainage bags are
    A. Hung on the bed rail
    B. Emptied and measured at the end of each shift
    C. Kept on the floor
    D. Kept higher than the person's bladder

73. A person needs a condom catheter applied. You remember to
    A. Apply it to a penis that is red and irritated
    B. Use adhesive tape to secure the catheter
    C. Use elastic tape to secure the catheter
    D. Act in an unprofessional manner
74. For comfort during bowel elimination
    A. Have the person use the bedpan rather than the bathroom or commode if possible
    B. Permit visitors to stay
    C. Keep the door and privacy curtain open
    D. Leave the person alone if possible
75. You are transferring a person with a weak right side from the wheelchair to the bed. You
    A. Place the wheelchair on the left side of the bed
    B. Place the wheelchair on the right side of the bed
    C. Keep the person in the wheelchair
    D. Ask the person which side moves first

SKILLS EVALUATION REVIEW

Each state has its own policies and procedures for the skills test. The following information is an overview of what to expect:

- To pass the skills evaluation, you will need to perform all 5 skills correctly.
- A nurse evaluates your performance of certain skills. Having someone watch as you work is not a new experience. Your instructor evaluated your performance during your training program. While you are working, your supervisor evaluates your skills.
- Mannequins and people are used as "patients" or "residents," depending on the skills you are performing.
- If you make a mistake, tell the evaluator what you did wrong. Then perform the skill correctly. Do not panic.
- Take whatever equipment you normally take or use at work. Wear a watch with a second hand. You may need it to measure vital signs and check how much time you have left.

BEFORE AND DURING THE PROCEDURE

- Hand washing is evaluated at the beginning of the skills test. You are expected to know when to wash your hands. Therefore, you may not be told to do so. Follow the rules for hand hygiene during the test.
- Before entering a person's room, knock on the door. Greet the person by name and introduce yourself before beginning a procedure. Check the identification (ID) bracelet or the photo ID to make certain you are giving care to the right person.
- Explain what you are going to do before beginning the procedure and as needed throughout the procedure.
- Always follow the rules of medical asepsis. For example, remove gloves and dispose of them properly. Keep clean linens separated from dirty linens.
- Always protect the person's rights throughout the skills test.
- Communicate with the person as you give care. Focus on the person's needs and interests. Always treat the person with respect. Do not talk about yourself or your personal problems.

- Provide privacy. This involves pulling the privacy curtain around the bed, closing doors, and asking visitors to leave the room.
- Promote safety for the person. For example, lock the wheelchair when you transfer a person to and from it. Place the bed in the lowest horizontal position when the person must get out of bed or when you are done giving care.
- Make sure the call light is within the person's reach. Attaching it to the bed or bed rail does not mean the person can reach it.
- Use good body mechanics. Raise the bed and over-bed table to a good working height.
- Provide for comfort:
  - Make sure the person and linens are clean and dry. The person may have become incontinent during the procedure.
  - Change or straighten bed linens as needed.
  - Position the person for comfort and in good alignment.
  - Provide pillows as directed by the nurse and the care plan.
  - Raise the head of the bed as the person prefers and allowed by the nurse and the care plan.
  - Provide for warmth. The person may need an extra blanket, a lap blanket, a sweater, socks, and so on.
  - Adjust lighting to meet the person's needs.
  - Make sure eyeglasses, hearing aids, and other devices are in place as needed.
  - Ask the person if he or she is comfortable.
  - Ask the person if there is anything else you can do for him or her.
  - Make sure the person is covered for warmth and privacy.

SKILLS

Ask your instructor to tell you which of the following skills are tested in your state. Place a checkmark in the box in front of each tested skill so it will be easy for you to reference. The skills marked with an asterisk (*) are used with permission of National Council of State Boards of Nursing (NCSBN). These skills are offered as a study guide to you. The word "client" refers to the resident or person receiving care. You are responsible for following the most current standards, practices, and guidelines of your state.

The steps in boldface type are critical element steps. Critical element steps must be done correctly to pass the skill. If you miss a critical element step, you will not pass the skills evaluation. For example, you are to transfer a client from the bed to a wheelchair. You will fail if you do not lock the wheels on the wheelchair before transferring the person. An automatic failure is one that could potentially cause harm to a person. Your state may mark critical element steps in another way—underline or italics. If your state has one, review the candidate's handbook.

☐ *HAND HYGIENE (HAND WASHING) (CHAPTER 13)

1. Addresses client by name and introduces self to client by name
2. Turns on water at sink
3. Wets hands and wrists thoroughly
4. Applies soap to hands
5. **Lathers all surfaces of hands, wrists, and fingers, producing friction for at least 15 (fifteen) seconds keeping hands lower than elbows and the fingertips down**
6. Cleans fingernails by rubbing fingertips against palms of the opposite hand
7. After lathering for at least 15 seconds, rinses all surfaces of wrists, hands, and fingers, keeping hands lower than the elbows and the fingertips down
8. Uses clean, dry paper towel to dry all surfaces of hands, wrists, and fingers then disposes of paper towel into waste container
9. Uses clean, dry paper towel to turn off faucet then disposes of paper towel into waste container or uses knee/foot control to turn off faucet
10. Does not touch inside of sink at any time
11. Disposes of used paper towel(s) in wastebasket immediately after shutting off faucet

☐ *APPLIES ONE KNEE-HIGH ELASTIC STOCKING (CHAPTER 30)

1. Explains procedure, speaking clearly, slowly, and directly, maintaining face-to-face contact whenever possible
2. Privacy is provided with a curtain, screen, or door
3. Client is in supine position (lying down in bed) while stocking is applied
4. Turns stocking inside-out or at least to the heel
5. Places foot of stocking over toes, foot, and heel
6. Pulls top of stocking over foot, heel, and leg

7. Moves foot and leg gently and naturally, avoiding force and over-extension of limb and joints
8. **Finishes procedure with no twists or wrinkles and heel of stocking (if present) is over heel and opening in toe area (if present) is either over or under toe area**
9. Signaling device is within reach and bed is in low position
10. After completing skill, washes hands

☐ *ASSISTS CLIENT TO AMBULATE USING TRANSFER BELT (CHAPTER 14)

1. Explains procedure, speaking clearly, slowly, and directly, maintaining face-to-face contact whenever possible
2. **Before assisting to stand, candidate ensures client is wearing shoes**
3. Before assisting to stand, bed is at a safe level
4. Before assisting to stand, checks and/or locks bed wheels
5. **Before assisting to stand, client is assisted to sitting position with feet flat on the floor**
6. Before assisting to stand, applies transfer belt securely over clothing/gown
7. Before assisting to stand, provides instructions to enable client to assist in standing including prearranged signal to alert client to begin standing
8. Stands facing client positioning self to ensure safety of candidate and client during transfer. Counts to three (or says other prearranged signal) to alert client to begin standing
9. On signal, gradually assists client to stand by grasping transfer belt on both sides with an upward grasp (candidate's hands are in upward position), and maintaining stability of client's legs
10. Walks slightly behind and to one side of client for a distance of ten (10) feet, while holding onto the belt
11. After ambulation, assists client to bed and removes transfer belt
12. Signaling device is within reach and bed is in low position
13. After completing skill, washes hands

☐ ASSISTS WITH USE OF BEDPAN (CHAPTER 22)

1. Explains procedure speaking clearly, slowly, and directly, maintaining face-to-face contact whenever possible
2. Privacy is provided with a curtain, screen, or door
3. Before placing bedpan, lowers head of bed
4. Puts on clean gloves before handling bedpan

5. **Places bedpan correctly under client's buttocks**
6. Removes and disposes of gloves (without contaminating self) into waste container and washes hands
7. After positioning client on bedpan and removing gloves, raises head of bed
8. Toilet tissue is within reach
9. Hand wipe is within reach and client is instructed to clean hands with hand wipe when finished
10. Signaling device within reach and client is asked to signal when finished
11. Puts on clean gloves before removing bedpan
12. Head of bed is lowered before bedpan is removed
13. Avoids overexposure of client
14. Removes, empties, and rinses bedpan and pours rinse into toilet
15. After rinsing bedpan, places bedpan in designated dirty supply area
16. After placing bedpan in designated dirty supply area, removes and disposes of gloves (without contaminating self) into waste container and washes hands
17. Signaling device is within reach and bed is in low position

☐ *CLEANS UPPER OR LOWER DENTURE (CHAPTER 17)

1. Puts on clean gloves before handling dentures
2. Bottom of sink is lined and/or sink is partially filled with water before denture is held over sink
3. Rinses denture in tepid/moderate temperature running water before brushing them
4. Applies toothpaste to toothbrush
5. Brushes surfaces of denture
6. Rinses surfaces of denture under tepid/moderate temperature running water
7. Before placing denture into cup, rinses denture cup and lid
8. Places denture in denture cup with tepid/moderate temperature water and places lid on cup
9. Rinses toothbrush and places in designated toothbrush basin/container
10. Maintains clean technique with placement of toothbrush and denture
11. Sink liner is removed and disposed of appropriately and/or sink is drained
12. After rinsing equipment and disposing of sink liner, removes and disposes of gloves (without contaminating self) into waste container and washes hands

☐ *COUNTS AND RECORDS RADIAL PULSE (CHAPTER 26)**

1. Explains procedure, speaking clearly, slowly, and directly, maintaining face-to-face contact whenever possible
2. Places fingertips on thumb side of client's wrist to locate radial pulse
3. Count beats for one full minute
4. Signaling device is within reach
5. Before recording, washes hands
6. **After obtaining pulse by palpating in radial artery position, records pulse rate within plus or minus 4 beats of evaluator's reading**

☐ *COUNTS AND RECORDS RESPIRATIONS (CHAPTER 26)†

1. Explains procedure (for testing purposes), speaking clearly, slowly, and directly, maintaining face-to-face contact whenever possible
2. Counts respirations for one full minute
3. Signaling device is within reach
4. Washes hands
5. **Records respiration rate within plus or minus 2 breaths of evaluator's reading**

☐ *DRESSES CLIENT WITH AFFECTED (WEAK) RIGHT ARM (CHAPTER 18)

1. Explains procedure, speaking clearly, slowly, and directly, maintaining face-to-face contact whenever possible
2. Privacy is provided with a curtain, screen, or door
3. Asks which shirt he/she would like to wear and dresses him/her in top shirt of choice
4. While avoiding overexposure of client, removes gown from the unaffected side first, then removes gown from the affected side and disposes of gown into soiled linen container
5. **Assists to put the right (affected/weak) arm through the right sleeve of the top before placing garment on left (unaffected) arm**
6. While putting on shirt, moves body gently and naturally, avoiding force and over-extension of limbs and joints
7. Finishes with clothing in place
8. Signaling device is within reach and bed is in low position
9. After completing task, washes hands

*From the candidate handbook. Copyright © 2011 National Council of State Boards of Nursing, Inc. (NCSBN), Chicago, Ill.
**Count for one full minute.
†Count for one full minute. For testing purposes you may explain to the client that you will be counting the respirations.

☐ *FEEDS CLIENT WHO CANNOT FEED SELF (CHAPTER 19)

1. Explains procedure to client, speaking clearly, slowly, and directly, maintaining face-to-face contact whenever possible
2. Before feeding, candidate looks at name card on tray and asks client to state name
3. **Before feeding client, client is in an upright sitting position (75–90 degrees)**
4. Places tray where it can be easily seen by client
5. Candidate cleans client's hands with hand wipe before beginning feeding
6. Candidate sits facing client during feeding
7. Tells client what foods are on tray and asks what client would like to eat first
8. Using spoon, offers client one bite of each type of food on tray, telling client the content of each spoonful
9. Offers beverage at least once during meal
10. Candidate asks client if they are ready for next bite of food or sip of beverage
11. At end of meal, candidate client's mouth is wiped and hands are cleaned with hand wipe
12. Removes food tray and places tray in designated dirty supply area
13. Signaling device is within client's reach
14. After completing skill, washes hands

☐ *GIVES MODIFIED BED BATH (FACE AND ONE ARM, HAND, AND UNDERARM) (CHAPTER 17)

1. Explains procedure, speaking clearly, slowly, and directly, maintaining face-to-face contact whenever possible
2. Privacy is provided with a curtain, screen, or door
3. Removes gown and places in soiled linen container while avoiding overexposure of the client
4. Before washing, checks water temperature for safety and comfort and asks client to verify comfort of water
5. Puts on clean gloves before washing client
6. **Beginning with eyes, washes eyes with wet washcloth (no soap), using a different area of the washcloth for each eye, washing inner aspect to outer aspect then proceeds to wash face**
7. Dries face with towel
8. Exposes one arm and places towel underneath arm
9. Applies soap to wet washcloth
10. Washes arm, hand, and underarm, keeping rest of body covered

11. Rinses and dries arm, hand, and underarm
12. Moves body gently and naturally, avoiding force and over-extension of limbs and joints
13. Puts clean gown on client
14. Empties, rinses, and dries basin
15. After rinsing basin, places basin in designated dirty supply area
16. Disposes of used gown and linen into soiled linen container
17. Avoids contact between candidate clothing and used linens
18. After placing basin in designated dirty supply area, and disposing of used linen, removes and disposes of gloves (without contaminating self) into waste container and washes hands
19. Signaling device is within reach and bed is in low position

☐ *MAKES AN OCCUPIED BED (CHAPTER 16)

1. Explains procedure, speaking clearly, slowly, and directly, maintaining face-to-face contact whenever possible
2. Privacy is provided with a curtain, screen, or door. Locks bed brakes and raises bed to comfortable working height
3. Lowers head of bed before moving client. Directs RN observer to stand on opposite side of bed for safety
4. Client is covered while linens are changed
5. Loosens top linen from the end of the bed
6. Raises side rail on side to which client will move and client moves toward raised side rail
7. Loosens bottom used linen on working side and moves bottom used linen toward center of bed
8. Places and tucks in clean bottom linen or fitted bottom sheet on working side and tucks under client
9. Before going to other side, client moves back onto clean bottom linen
10. Raises side rail then goes to other side of bed
11. Removes used bottom linen. Client body never touches bare mattress
12. Pulls and tucks in clean bottom linen, finishing with bottom sheet free of wrinkles
13. Client is covered with clean top sheet and bath blanket/used top sheet has been removed
14. Changes pillowcase with zips and tags to inside
15. Linen is centered and tucked at foot of bed
16. Avoids contact between candidate's clothing and used linen
17. Disposes of used linen into soiled linen container and avoids putting linen on floor

*From the candidate handbook. Copyright © 2011 National Council of State Boards of Nursing, Inc. (NCSBN), Chicago, Ill.

18. Signaling device is within reach and bed is in low position and brakes locked
19. Washes hands

☐ *MEASURES AND RECORDS BLOOD PRESSURE (CHAPTER 26)‡

1. Explains procedure, speaking clearly, slowly, and directly, maintaining face-to-face contact whenever possible
2. Before using stethoscope, wipes bell/diaphragm and earpieces of stethoscope with alcohol
3. Assists client into a comfortable sitting or recumbent position with forearm relaxed and client's arm is positioned with palm up at level of the heart and upper arm is exposed
4. Feels for brachial artery on inner aspect of arm, at bend of elbow
5. Places blood pressure cuff snugly on client's upper arm, with sensor/arrow over brachial artery site
6. Earpieces of stethoscope are in ears and bell/diaphragm is over brachial artery site
7. Candidate does one of the following: a. Inflates cuff between 160 mm Hg to 180 mm Hg. (If beat heard immediately upon cuff deflation, completely deflate cuff.) Re-inflate cuff to no more than 200 mm Hg. OR b. Inflates cuff 30 mm Hg beyond where radial or brachial pulse was last heard or felt or RN test observer may provide loss of pulse number
8. Deflates cuff slowly and notes the first sound (systolic reading), and last sound (diastolic reading) (If rounding needed, measurements are rounded UP to the nearest 2 mm of mercury)
9. Removes cuff
10. Signaling device is within reach
11. Washes hands
12. **After obtaining reading using BP cuff and stethoscope, records both systolic and diastolic pressures each within plus or minus 8 mm of evaluator's reading**

☐ *MEASURES AND RECORDS URINARY OUTPUT (CHAPTER 21)

1. Puts on clean gloves before handling bedpan
2. Pours the contents of the bedpan into measuring container without spilling or splashing urine outside of container
3. Measures the amount of urine at eye level with container on flat surface

4. After measuring urine, empties contents of measuring container into toilet
5. Rinses measuring container and pours rinse into toilet
6. Rinses bedpan and pours rinse into toilet
7. After rinsing equipment, and before recording output, removes and disposes of gloves (without contaminating self) into waste container and washes hands
8. **Records contents of container within plus or minus 25 mL/cc of evaluator's reading**

☐ *MEASURES AND RECORDS WEIGHT OF AMBULATORY CLIENT (CHAPTER 27)

1. Explains procedure, speaking clearly, slowly, and directly, maintaining face-to-face contact whenever possible
2. Candidate ensures client has shoes on before walking to scale
3. Before client steps on scale, candidate sets scale to zero then obtains client's weight
4. While client steps onto scale, candidate stands next to scale and assists client, if needed, onto center of scale, then determines client's weight
5. While client steps off scale, candidate stands next to scale and assists client, if needed, off scale before recording weight
6. **Records weight based on indicator on scale. Weight is within plus or minus 2 lbs of evaluator's reading (If weight recorded in kg weight is within plus or minus 0.9 kg of evaluator's reading)**
7. Before recording, washes hands

☐ *POSITIONS ON SIDE (CHAPTER 14)

1. Explains procedure, speaking clearly, slowly, and directly, maintaining face-to-face contact whenever possible
2. Privacy is provided with a curtain, screen, or door. Locks bed brakes
3. Before turning, lowers head of bed, raises bed to appropriate working height
4. Raises side rail on side to which body will be turned
5. Slowly rolls onto side as one unit toward raised side rail
6. Places or adjusts pillow under head for support
7. Client is positioned so that client is not lying on arm. Maintains correct body alignment

*From the candidate handbook. Copyright © 2011 National Council of State Boards of Nursing, Inc. (NCSBN), Chicago, Ill.
‡This is a one-step blood pressure procedure. However, if a candidate correctly performs a two-step blood pressure procedure that includes step 7b, the candidate will not be penalized and will be given credit for step 7.

8. Supports top arm with supportive device
9. Places supportive device behind client's back
10. Places supportive device between legs with top knee flexed; knee and ankle supported
11. Signaling device is within reach and bed is in low position with bed brakes locked
12. Washes hands

☐ *PROVIDES CATHETER CARE FOR FEMALE (CHAPTER 21)

1. Explains procedure, speaking clearly, slowly, and directly, maintaining face-to-face contact whenever possible
2. Privacy is provided with a curtain, screen, or door
3. Before washing checks water temperature for safety and comfort and asks client to verify comfort of water
4. Puts on clean gloves before washing
5. Places linen protector under perineal area before washing
6. Exposes area surrounding catheter while avoiding overexposure of client
7. Applies soap to wet washcloth
8. **While holding catheter near meatus without tugging, cleans at least four inches of catheter nearest meatus, moving in only one direction, away from meatus, using a clean area of the cloth for each stroke**
9. **While holding catheter near meatus without tugging, rinses at least four inches of catheter nearest meatus, moving only in one direction, away from meatus, using a clean area of the cloth for each stroke**
10. While holding catheter near meatus without tugging, dries at least four inches of catheter moving away from meatus
11. Empties, rinses, and dries basin
12. After rinsing basin, places basin in designated dirty supply area
13. Disposes of used linen into soiled linen container and disposes of linen protector appropriately
14. Avoids contact between candidate clothing and used linen
15. After disposing of used linen and cleaning equipment, removes and disposes of gloves (without contaminating self) into waste container and washes hands
16. Signaling device is within reach and bed is in low position

☐ *PROVIDES FINGERNAIL CARE ON ONE HAND (CHAPTER 18)

1. Explains procedure, speaking clearly, slowly, and directly, maintaining face-to-face contact whenever possible
2. Before immersing fingernails, checks water temperature for safety and comfort and asks client to verify comfort of water
3. Basin is in a comfortable position for client
4. Puts on clean gloves before cleaning fingernails
5. Fingernails are immersed in basin of water
6. Cleans under each fingernail with orangewood stick
7. Wipes orangewood stick on towel after each nail
8. Dries fingernail area
9. Candidate feels each nail and files as needed
10. Disposes of orangewood stick and emery board into waste container (for testing purposes)
11. Empties, rinses, and dries basin
12. After rinsing basin, places basin in designated dirty supply area
13. Disposes of used linen into soiled linen container
14. After cleaning nails and equipment, and disposing of used linen, removes and disposes of gloves (without contaminating self) into waste container and washes hands
15. Signaling device is within reach

☐ *PROVIDES FOOT CARE ON ONE FOOT (CHAPTER 18)

1. Explains procedure, speaking clearly, slowly, and directly, maintaining face-to-face contact whenever possible
2. Privacy is provided with a curtain, screen, or door
3. Before washing, checks water temperature for safety and comfort and asks client to verify comfort of water
4. Basin is in a comfortable position for client and on protective barrier
5. Puts on clean gloves before washing foot
6. Client's bare foot is placed into the water
7. Applies soap to wet washcloth
8. Lifts foot from water and washes foot, including between the toes
9. Foot is rinsed, including between the toes
10. Dries foot, including between the toes
11. Applies lotion to top and bottom of foot, removing excess (if any) with a towel
12. Supports foot and ankle during procedure
13. Empties, rinses, and dries basin
14. After rinsing basin, places basin in designated dirty supply area

15. Disposes of used linen into soiled linen container
16. After cleaning foot and equipment, and disposing of used linen, removes and disposes of gloves (without contaminating self) into waste container and washes hands
17. Signaling device is within reach

☐ *PROVIDES MOUTH CARE (CHAPTER 17)

1. Explains procedure, speaking clearly, slowly, and directly, maintaining face-to-face contact whenever possible
2. Privacy is provided with a curtain, screen, or door
3. Before providing mouth care, client is in upright sitting position (75–90 degrees)
4. Puts on clean gloves before cleaning mouth
5. Places clothing protector across chest before providing mouth care
6. Secures cup of water and moistens toothbrush
7. Before cleaning mouth applies toothpaste to toothbrush
8. **Cleans mouth (including tongue and surfaces of teeth) using gentle motions**
9. Maintains clean technique with placement of toothbrush
10. Candidate holds emesis basin to chin while client rinses mouth
11. Candidate wipes mouth and removes clothing protector
12. After rinsing toothbrush, empty, rinse and dry the basin and place used toothbrush in designated basin/container
13. Place basin and toothbrush in designated dirty supply area
14. Disposes of used linen into soiled linen container
15. After placing basin and toothbrush in designated dirty supply area, and disposing of used linen, removes and disposes of gloves (without contaminating self) into waste container and washes hands
16. Signaling device is within reach and bed is in low position

☐ *PROVIDES PERINEAL CARE (PERI-CARE) FOR FEMALE (CHAPTER 17)

1. Explains procedure, speaking clearly, slowly, and directly, maintaining face-to-face contact whenever possible
2. Privacy is provided with a curtain, screen, or door
3. Before washing checks water temperature for safety and comfort and asks client to verify comfort of water
4. Puts on clean gloves before washing perineal area

5. Places pad/linen protector under perineal area before washing
6. Exposes perineal area while avoiding overexposure of client
7. Applies soap to wet washcloth
8. **Washes genital area, moving from front to back, while using a clean area of the washcloth for each stroke**
9. **Using clean washcloth, rinses soap from genital area, moving from front to back, while using a clean area of the washcloth for each stroke**
10. Dries genital area moving from front to back with towel
11. **After washing genital area, turns to side, then washes and rinses rectal area moving from front to back using a clean area of washcloth for each stroke. Dries with towel**
12. Repositions client
13. Empties, rinses, and dries basin
14. After rinsing basin, places basin in designated dirty supply area
15. Disposes of used linen into soiled linen container and disposes of linen protector appropriately
16. Avoids contact between candidate clothing and used linen
17. After disposing of used linen, and placing used equipment in designated dirty supply area, removes and disposes of gloves (without contaminating self) into waste container and washes hands
18. Signaling device is within reach and bed is in low position

☐ *TRANSFERS CLIENT FROM BED TO WHEELCHAIR USING TRANSFER BELT (CHAPTER 14)

1. Explains procedure, speaking clearly, slowly, and directly, maintaining face-to-face contact whenever possible
2. Privacy is provided with a curtain, screen, or door
3. Before assisting to stand, wheelchair is positioned along side of bed, at head of bed, and facing the foot of the bed
4. Before assisting to stand, footrests are folded up or removed
5. Before assisting to stand, bed is at a safe level
6. **Before assisting to stand, locks wheels on wheelchair**
7. Before assisting to stand, checks and/or locks bed wheels
8. **Before assisting to stand, client is assisted to a sitting position with feet flat on the floor**
9. Before assisting to stand, candidate ensures client is wearing shoes

10. Before assisting to stand, applies transfer belt securely over clothing/gown
11. Before assisting to stand, provides instructions to enable client to assist in transfer including prearranged signal to alert when to begin standing
12. Stands facing client, positioning self to ensure safety of candidate and client during transfer. Counts to three (or says other prearranged signal) to alert client to begin standing
13. On signal, gradually assists client to stand by grasping transfer belt on both sides with an upward grasp (candidates hands are in upward position) and maintaining stability of client's legs
14. Assists client to turn to stand in front of wheelchair with back of client's legs against wheelchair
15. Lowers client into wheelchair
16. Positions client with hips touching back of wheelchair and transfer belt is removed
17. Positions feet on footrests
18. Signaling device is within reach
19. After completing skill, washes hands

❏ *PERFORMS MODIFIED PASSIVE RANGE-OF-MOTION (PROM) FOR ONE KNEE AND ONE ANKLE (CHAPTER 41)

1. Explains procedure, speaking clearly, slowly, and directly, maintaining face-to-face contact whenever possible
2. Privacy is provided with a curtain, screen, or door
3. Instructs client to inform nurse aide if pain is experienced during exercise
4. Supports leg at knee and ankle while performing range of motion for knee
5. Bends the knee and then returns leg to client's normal position (extension/flexion) (AT LEAST 3 TIMES unless pain is verbalized)
6. Supports foot and ankle close to the bed while performing range of motion for ankle
7. Pushes/pulls foot toward head (dorsiflexion), and pushes/pulls foot down, toes point down (plantar flexion) (AT LEAST 3 TIMES unless pain is verbalized)
8. **While supporting the limb, moves joints gently, slowly, and smoothly through the range of motion, discontinuing exercise if client verbalizes pain**
9. Signaling device is within reach and bed is in low position
10. Washes hands

❏ *PERFORMS MODIFIED PASSIVE RANGE-OF-MOTION (ROM) FOR ONE SHOULDER (CHAPTER 41)

1. Explains procedure, speaking clearly, slowly, and directly, maintaining face-to-face contact whenever possible
2. Privacy is provided with a curtain, screen, or door
3. Instructs client to inform nurse aide if pain is experienced during exercise
4. Supports client's arm at elbow and wrist while performing range of motion for shoulder
5. Raises client's straightened arm from side position upward toward head to ear level and returns arm down to side of body (extension/flexion) (AT LEAST 3 TIMES unless pain is verbalized)
6. Moves client's straightened arm away from the side of body to shoulder level and returns to side of body (abduction/adduction) (AT LEAST 3 TIMES unless pain is verbalized)
7. **While supporting the limb, moves joint gently, slowly, and smoothly through the range of motion, discontinuing exercise if client verbalizes pain**
8. Signaling device is within reach and bed is in low position
9. After completing skill, washes hands

❏ PERFORMS PASSIVE RANGE-OF-MOTION (ROM) OF LOWER EXTREMITY (HIP, KNEE, ANKLE) (CHAPTER 41)

1. Washes hands before contact with client
2. Identifies self to client by name and addresses client by name
3. Explains procedure to client, speaking clearly, slowly, and directly, maintaining face-to-face contact whenever possible
4. Provides for client's privacy during procedure with curtain, screen, or door
5. Positions client supine and in good body alignment
6. Supports client's leg by placing one hand under knee and other hand under heel
7. Moves entire leg away from body (performs AT LEAST 3 TIMES unless pain occurs)
8. Moves entire leg toward body (performs AT LEAST 3 TIMES unless pain occurs)
9. Bends client's knee and hip toward client's trunk (performs AT LEAST 3 TIMES unless pain occurs)
10. Straightens knee and hip (performs AT LEAST 3 TIMES unless pain occurs)
11. Flexes and extends ankle through range-of-motion exercises (performs AT LEAST 3 TIMES unless pain occurs)

12. Rotates ankle through range-of-motion exercises (performs AT LEAST 3 TIMES unless pain occurs)
13. **While supporting limb, moves joints gently, slowly, and smoothly through range-of-motion to point of resistance, discontinuing exercise if pain occurs**
14. Provides for comfort
15. Signaling device within reach and bed is in low position
16. Washes hands

☐ PERFORMS PASSIVE RANGE-OF-MOTION (ROM) OF UPPER EXTREMITY (SHOULDER, ELBOW, WRIST, FINGER) (CHAPTER 41)

1. Washes hands before contact with client
2. Identifies self to client by name and addresses client by name
3. Explains procedure to client, speaking clearly, slowly, and directly, maintaining face-to-face contact whenever possible
4. Provides for client's privacy during procedure with curtain, screen, or door
5. Supports client's extremity above and below joints while performing range-of-motion
6. Raises client's straightened arm toward ceiling and back toward head of bed and returns to flat position (flexion/extension) (performs AT LEAST 3 TIMES unless pain occurs)
7. Moves client's straightened arm away from client's side of body toward head of bed, and returns client's straightened arm to mid-line of client's body (abduction/adduction) (performs AT LEAST 3 TIMES unless pain occurs)
8. Moves client's shoulder through rotation range-of-motion exercises (performs AT LEAST 3 TIMES unless pain occurs)
9. Flexes and extends elbow through range-of-motion exercises (performs AT LEAST 3 TIMES unless pain occurs)
10. Provides range-of-motion exercises to wrist (performs AT LEAST 3 TIMES unless pain occurs)
11. Moves finger and thumb joints through range-of-motion exercises (performs AT LEAST 3 TIMES unless pain occurs)
12. **While supporting body part, moves joint gently, slowly, and smoothly through range-of-motion to point of resistance, discontinuing exercise if pain occurs**
13. Signaling device is within reach and bed is in low position
14. After completing skill, washes hands

☐ MAKES AN UNOCCUPIED BED (CHAPTER 16)

1. Washes hands
2. Collects clean linens in order to be placed on bed
3. Places clean linens on a clean waterproof barrier/surface
4. Raises the bed for good body mechanics
5. Puts on gloves
6. Removes linens without contaminating uniform. Rolls each piece away from self
7. Discards linens into laundry bag
8. Moves the mattress to the head of the bed
9. Applies mattress pad
10. Applies bottom sheet, keeping it smooth and free of wrinkles
11. Places the top sheet and bedspread on the bed, keeping them smooth and free of wrinkles
12. Tucks in top linens at the foot of the bed. Makes mitered corners
13. Applies clean pillowcase with zippers and/or tags to inside of pillowcase
14. Lowers the bed to its lowest position. Locks the bed wheels
15. Washes hands

☐ *DONNING AND REMOVING PPE (GOWN AND GLOVES) (CHAPTER 13)

1. Picks up gown and unfolds
2. Facing the back opening of the gown, places arms through each sleeve
3. Fastens the neck opening
4. Secures gown at waist making sure that back of clothing is covered by gown (as much as possible)
5. Puts on gloves
6. Cuffs of gloves overlap cuffs of gown
7. **Before removing gown, with one gloved hand, grasps the other glove at the palm, removes glove**
8. **Slips fingers from ungloved hand underneath cuff of remaining glove at wrist, and removes glove turning it inside out as it is removed**
9. Disposes of gloves into designated waste container without contaminating self
10. After removing gloves, unfastens gown at neck and waist
11. Removes gown without touching outside of gown
12. While removing gown, holds gown away from body, turns gown inward and keeps it inside out
13. Disposes of gown in designated container without contaminating self
14. After completing skill, washes hands

*From the candidate handbook. Copyright © 2010 National Council of State Boards of Nursing, Inc. (NCSBN), Chicago, Ill.

☐ PERFORMS ABDOMINAL THRUSTS (CHAPTER 10)

1. Asks client if he or she is choking
2. Stands behind client
3. Wraps arms around client's waist
4. Makes a fist with one hand
5. Places thumb side of fist against client's abdomen
6. Positions fist in middle above navel and below sternum (breastbone)
7. Grasps fist with other hand
8. Presses fist and other hand into client's abdomen with quick upward thrusts
9. Repeats thrusts until object is expelled or client becomes unresponsive

☐ AMBULATION WITH CANE OR WALKER (CHAPTER 14)

1. Explains procedure to client, speaking clearly, slowly, and directly, maintaining face-to-face contact whenever possible
2. Locks bed wheels or wheelchair brakes
3. Assists client to a sitting position
4. **Before ambulating, puts on and properly fastens non-skid footwear**
5. Positions cane or walker correctly. Cane is on client's strong side
6. Assists client to stand, using correct body mechanics
7. Stabilizes cane or walker and ensures client stabilizes cane or walker
8. Stands behind and slightly to the side of client
9. Ambulates client
10. Assists client to pivot and sit, using correct body mechanics
11. Before leaving client, places signaling device within client's reach
12. Washes hands

☐ FLUID INTAKE (CHAPTER 19)

1. Observes dinner tray
2. Determines, in milliliters (mL), the amount of fluid consumed from each container
3. Determines total fluid consumed in mL
4. Records total fluid consumed on intake and output (I&O) sheet
5. Calculated total is within required range of evaluator's reading

☐ BRUSHES OR COMBS CLIENT'S HAIR (CHAPTER 18)

1. Explains procedure to client, speaking clearly, slowly, and directly, maintaining face-to-face contact whenever possible
2. Collects brush or comb and bath towel
3. Places towel across client's back and shoulders or across the pillow
4. Asks client how he or she wants his or her hair styled
5. Combs/brushes hair gently and completely
6. Leaves hair neatly brushed, combed, and/or styled
7. Removes towel
8. Removes hair from comb or brush
9. Before leaving client, places signaling device within client's reach
10. Washes hands

☐ TRANSFERS CLIENT USING A MECHANICAL LIFT (CHAPTER 14)

1. Assembles required equipment; performs safety check of slings, straps, hooks, and chains
2. Checks client's weight to ensure it does not exceed the lift's capacity
3. Asks a co-worker to help
4. Explains procedure to client, speaking clearly, slowly, and directly, maintaining face-to-face contact whenever possible
5. Provides for privacy during procedure with curtain, screen, or door
6. Locks the bed wheels
7. Raises the bed for proper body mechanics
8. Lowers the head of the bed to a level appropriate for client
9. Stands on one side of the bed; co-worker stands on the other side
10. Lowers the bed rails if up
11. Centers the sling under client following the manufacturer instructions
12. Ensures that the sling is smooth
13. Positions client in semi-Fowler's position
14. Positions a chair to lower client into it
15. Lowers the bed to its lowest position
16. Raises the lift to position it over client
17. Positions the lift over client
18. Attaches the sling to the swivel bar; checks fasteners for security
19. Crosses client's arms over the chest
20. Raises the lift high enough until client and sling are free of the bed
21. Instructs co-worker to support client's legs as candidate moves the lift and client away from the bed
22. Positions the lift so client's back is toward the chair
23. Slowly lowers client into the chair
24. Places client in comfortable position, in correct body alignment
25. Lowers the swivel bar and unhooks the sling
26. Removes the sling from under client unless otherwise indicated. Moves lift away from client
27. Puts footwear on client

28. Covers client's lap and legs with a lap blanket
29. Positions the chair as client prefers
30. Places signaling device within client's reach
31. Washes hands

☐ PROVIDES MOUTH CARE FOR AN UNCONSCIOUS CLIENT (CHAPTER 17)

1. Explains procedure to client, speaking clearly, slowly, and directly, maintaining face-to-face contact whenever possible
2. Provides for privacy during procedure with curtain, screen, or door
3. Washes hands
4. Positions client on side with head turned well to one side
5. Puts on gloves
6. Places the towel under client's face
7. Places the kidney basin under the chin
8. Uses swabs or toothbrush and toothpaste or other cleaning solution
9. Cleans inside of mouth including the gums, tongue, and teeth
10. Cleans and dries face
11. Removes the towel and kidney basin
12. Applies lubricant to the lips
13. Positions client for comfort and safety
14. Removes and discards the gloves
15. Places signaling device within client's reach
16. Washes hands

☐ PASSING FRESH WATER (CHAPTER 19)

1. Washes hands
2. Assembles equipment—ice, scoop, pitcher
3. Explains procedure to client, speaking clearly, slowly, and directly, maintaining face-to-face contact whenever possible
4. Uses the scoop to fill the pitcher with ice; does not let the scoop touch the rim or inside of the pitcher
5. Places scoop in appropriate receptacle after each use
6. Adds water to pitcher
7. Places the pitcher, disposable cup, and straw (if used) on the over-bed table, within client's reach
8. Before leaving, places signaling device within client's reach
9. Washes hands

☐ PROVIDES PERINEAL CARE FOR UNCIRCUMCISED MALE (CHAPTER 17)

1. Explains procedure to client, speaking clearly, slowly, and directly, maintaining face-to-face contact whenever possible
2. Provides for privacy during procedure with curtain, screen, or door

3. Washes hands
4. Fills basin with comfortably warm water
5. Puts on gloves
6. Elevates bed to working height
7. Places waterproof pad under buttocks
8. Gently grasps penis
9. Retracts the foreskin
10. Using a circular motion, cleans the tip by starting at the meatus of the urethra and working outward
11. Rinses the area with another washcloth, pats dry
12. Returns the foreskin to its natural position
13. Cleans the shaft of the penis with firm, downward strokes and rinses the area
14. Cleans the scrotum
15. Pats dry the penis and the scrotum
16. Cleans the rectal area
17. Removes the waterproof pad
18. Lowers the bed, locks bed brakes
19. Removes and discards the gloves
20. Washes hands
21. Before leaving, places signaling device within client's reach

☐ EMPTIES AND RECORDS CONTENT OF URINARY DRAINAGE BAG (CHAPTER 21)

1. Explains procedure to client, speaking clearly, slowly, and directly, maintaining face-to-face contact whenever possible
2. Washes hands
3. Puts on gloves
4. Places a paper towel on the floor
5. Places the graduate on the paper towel
6. Places the graduate under the collection bag
7. Ensures the bag is below the bladder and the drainage tube is not kinked
8. Opens the clamp on the drain, cleans drainage tube with alcohol wipe
9. Lets all urine drain into the graduate—does not let the drain touch the graduate, cleans drainage tube with alcohol wipe before replacing in pouch
10. Closes and positions the clamp
11. Measures urine
12. Removes and discards the paper towel
13. Empties the contents of the graduate into the toilet and flushes
14. Rinses the graduate
15. Returns the graduate to its proper place
16. Removes the gloves
17. Washes hands
18. Records the time and amount on the intake and output (I&O) record
19. Provides for client comfort
20. Places the signaling device within reach of client

❑ APPLYING A VEST RESTRAINT (CHAPTER 12)

1. Obtains the correct type and size of restraint
2. Checks straps for tears or frays
3. Washes hands
4. Explains procedure to client, speaking clearly, slowly, and directly, maintaining face-to-face contact whenever possible
5. Provides for privacy during procedure with curtain, screen, or door
6. Makes sure client is comfortable and in good alignment
7. Assists client to a sitting position
8. Applies the restraint following the manufacturer instructions—the "V" part of the vest crosses in front
9. Makes sure the vest is free of wrinkles in the front and back
10. Brings the straps through the slots
11. Makes sure client is comfortable and in good alignment
12. Secures the straps to the chair or to the movable part of the bed frame
13. Uses a secure knot that can be released with one pull
14. Makes sure the vest is snug—slide an open hand between the restraint and client
15. Places the signaling device within client's reach
16. Washes hands

❑ PERFORMS A BACK RUB (MASSAGE) (CHAPTER 17)

1. Washes hands
2. Explains procedure to client, speaking clearly, slowly, and directly, maintaining face-to-face contact whenever possible
3. Provides for privacy during procedure with curtain, screen, or door
4. Raises the bed for good body mechanics
5. Lowers the bed rail near the candidate, if up
6. Positions client in the prone or side-lying position
7. Exposes the back, shoulders, upper arms, and buttocks
8. Warms the lotion
9. Rubs entire back in upward, outward motion for approximately 2 to 3 minutes; does not massage reddened bony areas
10. Straightens and secures clothing or sleepwear
11. Returns client to comfortable and safe position
12. Places the signaling device within reach
13. Lowers the bed to its lowest position
14. Washes hands

❑ POSITIONS FOLEY CATHETER (CHAPTER 21)

1. Explains procedure to client, speaking clearly, slowly, and directly, maintaining face-to-face contact whenever possible
2. Washes hands
3. Puts on gloves
4. Secures catheter and drainage tubing according to facility procedure
5. Places tubing over leg
6. Positions drainage tubing so urine flows freely into drainage bag and has no kinks
7. Attaches bag to bed frame, below level of bladder, does not allow bag to touch floor
8. Washes hands

❑ APPLY COLD PACK OR WARM COMPRESS (CHAPTER 30)

1. Washes hands
2. Collects needed equipment
3. Explains procedure to client, speaking clearly, slowly, and directly, maintaining face-to-face contact whenever possible
4. Provides for privacy during procedure with curtain, screen, or door
5. Positions client for the procedure
6. Covers cold pack or warm compress with towel or other protective cover
7. Properly places cold pack or warm compress on site
8. Checks client for complications every 5 minutes
9. Checks the cold pack or warm compress every 5 minutes
10. Removes the application at the specified time— usually after 15 to 20 minutes
11. Provides for comfort
12. Places the signaling device within reach
13. Washes hands

❑ POSITIONS FOR AN ENEMA (CHAPTER 22)

1. Washes hands
2. Explains procedure to client, speaking clearly, slowly, and directly, maintaining face-to-face contact whenever possible
3. Provides for privacy
4. Positions client in Sims' position or in a left side-lying position
5. Covers client appropriately
6. Provides for comfort
7. Places the signaling device within reach
8. Washes hands

☐ POSITIONS CLIENT FOR MEALS (CHAPTER 19)

1. Washes hands
2. Explains procedure to client, speaking clearly, slowly, and directly, maintaining face-to-face contact whenever possible
3. If client will eat in bed:
   a. Raises the head of the bed to a comfortable position—usually Fowler's or high Fowler's position is preferred
   b. Removes items from the over-bed table and cleans the over-bed table
   c. Adjusts the over-bed table in front of client
   d. Places client in proper body alignment
4. If client will sit in a chair:
   a. Positions client in a chair or wheelchair
   b. Provides support for client's feet
   c. Removes items from the over-bed table and cleans the over-bed table
   d. Adjusts the over-bed table in front of client
   e. Places client in proper body alignment
5. Places the signaling device within reach
6. Washes hands

☐ TAKES AND RECORDS AXILLARY TEMPERATURE, PULSE, AND RESPIRATIONS (CHAPTER 26)

1. Washes hands before contact with client
2. Identifies self to client by name and addresses client by name
3. Explains procedure to client, speaking clearly, slowly, and directly, maintaining face-to-face contact whenever possible
4. Provides for client's privacy during procedure with curtain, screen, or door
5. Turns on digital oral thermometer
6. Dries axilla and places thermometer in the center of the axilla
7. Holds thermometer in place for appropriate length of time
8. Removes and reads thermometer
9. Records temperature on pad of paper
10. **Recorded temperature is within required range**
11. Discards sheath from thermometer
12. Places fingertips on thumb side of client's wrist to locate radial pulse
13. Counts beats for 1 full minute
14. Records pulse rate on pad of paper
15. **Recorded pulse is within required range**
16. Counts respirations for 1 full minute
17. Records respirations on pad of paper

18. **Recorded respirations are within required range**
19. Before leaving client, places signaling device within client's reach
20. Washes hands

☐ TRANSFERS CLIENT FROM WHEELCHAIR TO BED (CHAPTER 14)

1. Washes hands before contact with client
2. Identifies self to client by name and addresses client by name
3. Explains procedure to client, speaking clearly, slowly, and directly, maintaining face-to-face contact whenever possible
4. Provides for client's privacy during procedure with curtain, screen, or door
5. Positions wheelchair close to bed with arm of wheelchair almost touching bed
6. Before transferring client, ensures client is wearing non-skid footwear
7. Before transferring client, folds up footplates
8. Before transferring client, places bed at safe and appropriate level for client
9. **Before transferring client, locks wheels on wheelchair and locks bed brakes**
10. With transfer (gait) belt: Stands in front of client, positioning self to ensure safety of candidate and client during transfer (for example, knees bent, feet apart, back straight), places belt around client's waist, and grasps belt. Tightens belt so that fingers of candidate's hand can be slipped between transfer/gait belt and client

    Without transfer belt: Stands in front of client, positioning self to ensure safety of candidate and client during transfer (for example, knees bent, feet apart, back straight, arms around client's torso under arms)
11. Provides instructions to enable client to assist in transfer, including prearranged signal to alert client to begin standing
12. Braces client's lower extremities to prevent slipping
13. Counts to three (or says other prearranged signal) to alert client to begin transfer
14. On signal, gradually assists client to stand
15. Assists client to pivot and sit on bed in manner that ensures safety
16. Removes transfer belt, if used
17. Assists client to remove non-skid footwear
18. Assists client to move to center of bed
19. Provides for comfort and good body alignment
20. Before leaving client, places signaling device within client's reach
21. Washes hands

☐ WEIGHING AND MEASURING HEIGHT OF AN AMBULATORY CLIENT (CHAPTER 27)

1. Washes hands before contact with client
2. Identifies self to client by name and addresses client by name
3. Explains procedure to client, speaking clearly, slowly, and directly, maintaining face-to-face contact whenever possible
4. Starts with scale balanced at zero before weighing client
5. Assists client to step up onto center of scale
6. Determines client's weight and height
7. Assists client off scale before recording weight and height
8. Before leaving client, places signaling device within client's reach
9. Records weight and height within required range
10. Washes hands

AFTER A PROCEDURE

After you demonstrate a skill, complete a safety check of the room:

- The person is wearing eyeglasses, hearing aids, and other devices as needed.
- The call light is plugged in and within reach.
- Bed rails are up or down according to the care plan.
- The bed is in the lowest horizontal position.
- The bed position is locked if needed.
- Manual bed cranks are in the down position.
- Bed wheels are locked.
- Assist devices are within reach. Walker, cane, and wheelchair are examples.
- The over-bed table, filled water pitcher and cup, tissues, phone, TV controls, and other needed items are within reach.
- Un-needed equipment is unplugged or turned off.
- Harmful substances are stored properly. Lotion, mouthwash, shampoo, after-shave, and other personal care products are examples.

AFTER THE TEST

Celebrate—you have completed the competency evaluation! The length of time for you to get your test results varies with each state. In the meantime, try to relax. Continue your daily routine and be the best nursing assistant you can be.

ANSWERS TO REVIEW QUESTIONS IN TEXTBOOK CHAPTERS REVIEW

NOTE: Review questions included for selected chapters only based on competency evaluation requirements.

Chapter 1
1. c
2. b
3. a
4. a
5. a
6. b
7. d
8. a
9. b
10. b

Chapter 2
1. d
2. b
3. a
4. b
5. c
6. c
7. b
8. a
9. d
10. b
11. c
12. a

Chapter 3
1. c
2. c
3. a
4. d
5. d
6. b

Chapter 4
1. a
2. c
3. d

Chapter 5
1. d
2. a

Chapter 6
1. b
2. d
3. d
4. c
5. d
6. b
7. a
8. c
9. d
10. c
11. c
12. d
13. a
14. b

Chapter 8
1. b
2. d
3. c
4. c
5. d
6. c
7. d

Chapter 10
1. b
2. d
3. a
4. d
5. c
6. c
7. b
8. c
9. b
10. c
11. b

Chapter 11
1. a
2. d
3. b
4. c
5. c
6. c

Chapter 12
1. a
2. c
3. a
4. a
5. b
6. b

Chapter 13
1. b
2. d
3. d
4. a
5. a
6. c

Chapter 14
1. c
2. b
3. c
4. c
5. c
6. a
7. c
8. b
9. a
10. d

Chapter 15
1. a
2. a
3. a
4. c
5. b
6. c
7. d

Chapter 16
1. b
2. a
3. a
4. d
5. c

Chapter 17
1. c
2. d
3. b
4. d
5. c
6. b
7. a
8. c
9. d
10. a
11. a

Chapter 18
1. a
2. b
3. a
4. a
5. b
6. a
7. a
8. a
9. b
10. b
11. d

Chapter 19
1. d
2. a
3. b
4. a
5. d
6. d
7. a
8. c
9. c

Chapter 21
1. b
2. d
3. c
4. a
5. b
6. c
7. c

Chapter 22
1. b
2. d
3. d
4. a

Chapter 23
1. c
2. a
3. b
4. a

Chapter 24
1. d
2. c
3. a
4. d

Chapter 25
1. c
2. b
3. a
4. c
5. d

Chapter 26
1. c
2. b
3. a
4. c
5. d

Chapter 30
1. d
2. c
3. d
4. d
5. c

Chapter 31
1. c
2. c
3. a
4. a

Chapter 32
1. d
2. b
3. c
4. c

Chapter 33
1. b
2. c
3. a

Chapter 34
1. b
2. a
3. a
4. b
5. b

Chapter 35
1. d
2. c
3. a
4. c

Chapter 36
1. b
2. a
3. d

Chapter 37
1. c
2. a
3. b

Chapter 38
1. a
2. a
3. a
4. c
5. b
6. d

Chapter 39
1. c
2. d
3. a
4. d

Chapter 41
1. a
2. a
3. d
4. a
5. b